T0259273

RESEARCH METHODS IN HUMAN SKELETAL BIOLOGY

Dedicated to the memory of

Dr. Karen Ramey Burns

Friend, Colleague, and Anthropologist Extraordinaire

RESEARCH METHODS IN HUMAN SKELETAL BIOLOGY

Edited by

ELIZABETH A. DIGANGI
International Criminal Investigative Training Assistance Program (ICITAP)
Bogotá, Colombia

MEGAN K. MOORE
Department of Behavioral Sciences, University of Michigan-Dearborn
Dearborn, Michigan, USA

AMSTERDAM • BOSTON • HEIDELBERG • LONDON
NEW YORK • OXFORD • PARIS • SAN DIEGO
SAN FRANCISCO • SINGAPORE • SYDNEY • TOKYO
Academic Press is an Imprint of Elsevier

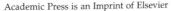

Academic Press is an imprint of Elsevier
The Boulevard, Langford Lane, Kidlington, Oxford, OX5 1GB, UK
225 Wyman Street, Waltham, MA 02451, USA

First published 2013

Notices

Knowledge and best practice in this field are constantly changing. As new research and experience
broaden our understanding, changes in research methods, professional practices, or medical treatment
may become necessary.

Practitioners and researchers must always rely on their own experience and knowledge in evaluating
and using any information, methods, compounds, or experiments described herein. In using such
information or methods they should be mindful of their own safety and the safety of others, including
parties for whom they have a professional responsibility.

To the fullest extent of the law, neither the Publisher nor the authors, contributors, or editors, assume
any liability for any injury and/or damage to persons or property as a matter of products liability,
negligence or otherwise, or from any use or operation of any methods, products, instructions, or ideas
contained in the material herein.

British Library Cataloguing in Publication Data
A catalogue record for this book is available from the British Library

Library of Congress Control Number: 2012940401

ISBN: 978-0-12-385189-5

Cover Art by Megan K. Moore

For information on all Academic Press publications
visit our website at **store.elsevier.com**

Working together to grow
libraries in developing countries

www.elsevier.com | www.bookaid.org | www.sabre.org

ELSEVIER   BOOK AID International   Sabre Foundation

Contents

III
TECHNOLOGICAL
ADVANCES

IV

COMPLETING AND CULTIVATING THE SCIENTIFIC PROCESS

Foreword

As anthropologists grounded in evolutionary theory, we know that vacant niches are soon filled. And so it is with this text, designed to fill a niche between the introductory text for undergraduates and the more advanced texts designed for graduate students. Its purpose is to provide guidance for identifying research projects, acquiring data, executing the analysis and presenting the results in published form.

A notable feature of the book is the use of case studies to provide concrete examples of the kinds of research projects that can be undertaken in the various areas covered. Case studies have long been used in forensic anthropology as a means to illustrate and teach. This book expands that approach to cover all the areas of skeletal biology, and the cases are not problematic individual skeletons but rather examples of how and why broader problems have been addressed.

The editors and many of the contributors are at the beginning of their professional careers. One might argue that the new generation lacks the experience and insight that comes with age, especially concerning historical matters, and they should wait until they are properly seasoned before embarking on such projects. On the contrary, the editors have provided historical context against which to view the modern discipline. Their treatment of our founders is insightful and fair, judging them by the standards of their time rather than the standards of the present. And the other side of that coin is that memories of their own graduate student experience are still fresh, allowing them to define what they would have found useful had it existed. Addressing the needs of those just embarking on a research career is the principal objective of the book and one in which the editors and contributors admirably succeed.

Just about any topic one could hope would be covered in a skeletal biology text is covered. The 18 chapters deal with topics from A to Z, from aging to Z-scores, from molecular methods to morphometry, from demography to distance and dentition, from histology to history, and many others. The chapters are thoughtfully and thoroughly developed. This is not a hastily assembled text. The editors and the authors have clearly invested a lot of effort and it shows. What has emerged is a book that will serve not only the interests of the target audience, students beginning the process of becoming researchers, but of their professors as well, who will find it easier to guide their students into meaningful research projects.

Richard L. Jantz
Professor Emeritus
University of Tennessee, Knoxville, USA

Preface

"Do not undertake a scientific career in quest of fame or money. There are easier and better ways to reach them. Undertake it only if nothing else will satisfy you; for nothing else is probably what you will receive. Your reward will be the widening of the horizon as you climb. And if you achieve that reward you will ask no other." — *Dr. Cecelia Payne-Gaposchkin (1996:227).*

The idea for this book occurred in a flash of inspiration. In April of 2009, we were teaching a research methods course we had developed for forensic anthropologists in Bogotá, Colombia. We first wrote a course manual and during the process of the one-week course, one of us looked at the other and asked, "Does a book exist for everything we are teaching right now?" Upon our realization that one did not, we agreed that we would set to the task and create a textbook geared towards an audience of students just starting out in research. The existing advanced texts in skeletal biology read primarily like a collection of research articles that assume the reader already understands the process, and we recognized the need for a text bridging the gap between introductory texts for undergraduates and advanced texts for graduates and postgraduates.

The participants in the research methods course were professional forensic anthropologists from all over Colombia. They represented diverse backgrounds and levels of experience in the field of forensic anthropology. Some had been working in the field for over 20 years; others had only a few months of experience. Some had been trained in cultural anthropology and others

in biological anthropology, most with only an undergraduate degree. All of them handle skeletal cases frequently, doing an average of about 50 cases individually each year. As casework is copious, it takes precedence over research, with very little research being done. The course we taught was designed to begin to address this deficit.

To accommodate the varying knowledge levels of the students in the course, we chose to introduce the basics of skeletal biological theory along with in-depth discussions of the scientific method and more recent applications of skeletal biology, such as the utility of isotopic analysis. We follow the same model for this textbook.

The practice of forensic anthropology in Colombia has greatly expanded in the past 20 years. In 1991, there was one forensic anthropologist working for a Colombian government agency and today there are over 50 practicing forensic anthropologists working for either the government or nongovernmental organizations. Due to the ongoing internal conflict between the Colombian government, illegally armed groups, and drug traffickers that has waged for the past 50 odd years, it is estimated that there may be as many as hundreds of thousands of disappeared individuals, a figure much larger than the 27,000 reported missing persons to the government as of 2009, although it is most likely in the tens of thousands (Gómez and Patiño, 2007; Equitas, 2010). The majority of the missing have in all likelihood been murdered and buried in clandestine graves or as John/Jane Does in cemeteries throughout the country.

Around the same time that we taught the first research course, one Colombian forensic anthropologist, Dr. César Sanabria, had begun efforts to assemble a modern skeletal collection of known individuals. One of the major obstacles facing Colombian forensic anthropologists is the paucity of Colombian standards for use in skeletal analyses. Like many forensic anthropologists around the world, Colombian forensic anthropologists use formulae and other standards developed decades ago in the United States, most notably Todd (1920), Trotter and Gleser (1952, 1958), Lovejoy et al. (1985), and İşcan et al. (1984a, 1984b, 1989). As with any other application of methods developed on one population and applied to another, the applicability of these methods to the Colombian population must be tested. As we learned about the development of this modern collection during the research course, we agreed that a data collection workshop utilizing the collection once ready would be the perfect hands-on complement to the theoretical research methods course.

The Colombian Modern Skeletal Collection is composed of individuals from cemeteries in Bogotá curated by the National Institute of Legal Medicine and Forensic Sciences (Colombia's national medical examiner office). This collection of known individuals has antemortem data available on age, sex, stature, place of birth, and cause/manner of death. The remains in the collection were unclaimed by next-of-kin after a four-year burial period and were collected before being cremated in accordance with Colombian law and custom (Sanabria and DiGangi, 2011). As of this writing, the collection has approximately 500 individuals and counting. This skeletal collection offers a unique opportunity to develop the first population-specific standards for modern Colombians.

As a result, in February 2011, four forensic anthropologists from the United States joined 30 forensic anthropologists, odontologists, and pathologists from Colombia in a collaborative effort to study this new skeletal collection. Data collected included standard measurements from the postcranial elements, three-dimensional coordinates from the skull, analysis of pathology, trauma, and nonmetric dental traits, subadult age estimation using epiphyseal fusion, and adult age estimation from the pubic symphyses and rib ends. The inspiration for this textbook came from the initial research course that later evolved into this massive collaborative effort to develop standards for Colombia.

From our completed years of graduate school tenure (18 years between us), we are familiar with the academic process of attaining intellectual maturity. Knowing how to do research is not a skill one necessarily acquires during undergraduate education, although the production of original research is a major expectation of graduate school. Conducting research can be a daunting task for many new professionals. Even seasoned investigators will hit roadblocks with details of research design. Many new investigators fall short of producing good quality work due to the lack of strong guidance. While this book should not take the place of an advisor, it can be viewed as a mentor in print form that will enable students to narrow down a topic of interest and work out initial research design that can then be discussed in detail with their advisors.

It is our hope that this book fills a gap within the literature of human skeletal biology and that students and professors alike will find its contents useful. Both of us wish we had had a resource such as this when we started graduate school, and perhaps the ideas presented herein will serve as their own flashes of inspiration for students of human skeletal biology.

Elizabeth A. DiGangi, PhD

Megan K. Moore, PhD

REFERENCES

Equitas, 2010. Propuestas Metodológicas para la Documentación y Búsqueda de Personas Desaparecidas en Colombia (Methodological Proposals for the Documentation and Search of Disappeared Persons in Colombia). Equitas, Bogotá.

Gómez, A.M., Patiño, A., 2007. Who is missing? Problems in the application of forensic archaeology and anthropology in Colombia's conflict. In: Ferllini, R. (Ed.), Forensic Archaeology and Human Rights Violations. Charles C. Thomas, Springfield, IL, pp. 170–204.

İşcan, M., Loth, S., Wright, R., 1984a. Age estimation from the rib by phase analysis: white males. Journal of Forensic Sciences 29 (4), 1094–1104.

İşcan, M., Loth, S., Wright, R., 1984b. Metamorphosis at the sternal rib end: a new method to estimate age at death in white males. American Journal of Physical Anthropology 65 (2), 147–156.

İşcan, M., Loth, S., Wright, R., 1985. Age estimation from the rib by phase analysis: white females. Journal of Forensic Sciences 30 (3), 853–863.

Lovejoy, C.O., Meindl, R., Pryzbeck, T., Mensforth, R., 1985. Chronological metamorphosis of the auricular surface of the ilium: a new method for the determination of adult skeletal age at death. American Journal of Physical Anthropology 68, 15–28.

Payne-Gaposchkin, C., 1996. The dyer's hand: an autobiography. In: Haramundanis, K. (Ed.), Cecelia Payne-Gaposchkin: An Autobiography and Other Recollections, 2nd ed. Cambridge University Press, Cambridge.

Sanabria, C., DiGangi, E., 2011. Development of the Colombian Skeletal Collection. Proceedings of the American Academy of Forensic Sciences 17, 338–339.

Todd, T., 1920. Age changes in the pubic bone: I. The male white pubis. American Journal of Physical Anthropology 3, 285–334.

Trotter, M., Gleser, G.C., 1952. Estimation of stature from long bones of American Whites and Negroes. American Journal of Physical Anthropology 10, 463–514.

Trotter, M., Gleser, G.C., 1958. A re-evaluation of estimation of stature based on measurements of stature taken during life and long bones after death. American Journal of Physical Anthropology 16, 79–124.

Acknowledgments

Any project such as this is the result of a large group effort. We would like to thank the individuals who attended the first research methods course we taught, as the idea for this project would not have surfaced without them. Francis Niño was a co-instructor during the course and helped design some of its contents. The National Institute of Legal Medicine and Forensic Sciences and Dr. César Sanabria granted permission for research on the Colombian Modern Skeletal Collection. Dr. Natalie Shirley and Dr. Jonathan Bethard led the data collection workshop (mentioned in the Preface) along with us.

We are grateful to EAD's employer for resources provided for forensic anthropology courses in Colombia that have informed this work. We have been privileged to work with forensic anthropologists and other forensic professionals in Colombia, whose professionalism and dedication under arduous conditions deserve recognition. We especially thank Dr. Dan Garner and Gary Sheridan for their support of this endeavor and others in Colombia.

Our editors at Academic Press, Kristi Anderson and Liz Brown, have our gratitude for their infinite patience and encouragement. Drs. Lynne Sullivan and Lydia Pulsipher gave us valuable advice on the publishing process. Brannon Hulsey and Frankie Pack helped with various editorial tasks, such as fact hunting; and Ruth Mendez assembled and alphabetized the glossary from each chapter. Dayna Anderegg, Emma Van Hoet, Amira Nasser, and Aaron Noles assisted with checking references and general chapter formatting. We are immensely grateful for each person's assistance.

We have assembled a diverse and accomplished group of contributors, and the quality of their contributions to this work is testament to their knowledge. We are thankful for their contribution, time, and effort spent. We are indebted to each of them for seeing our vision through to fulfillment. Any errors or omissions in the volume fall on us as editors.

EAD would like to thank her colleagues and friends for making Colombia feel more like home and for their moral support during this process, especially Adriana Otero and Ruth Mendez; and her furry family: Jake, Jeepers, and Simón, the best editorial assistants around.

MKM would like to thank her husband John and newborn son Jameson for the many sacrifices they endured during her emotional and physical absence. Their love and support provided the necessary stability for the completion of this volume. John Nipper also contributed several photographs to the volume. None of this would have been possible without the amazing childcare provided by Stephanie Soliz and her family. During the last few weeks of manuscript preparation, Stephanie and her mother Belinda were more than generous with their time. Their assistance provided the necessary peace of mind to endure the most grueling of workdays (and nights).

About the Contributors

Jonathan D. Bethard, PhD is a biological anthropologist currently working as an instructor of forensic anthropology at Boston University School of Medicine. He earned his doctorate in anthropology from the University of Tennessee, Knoxville in 2012 and his research interests include various topics in forensic anthropology and bioarchaeology. His first published research project was a coauthored project that investigated age-related change of the first rib.

Graciela S. Cabana, PhD is assistant professor of anthropology at the University of Tennessee, Knoxville, and director of the Molecular Anthropology Laboratories. She earned her doctorate degree in anthropology from the University of Michigan in Ann Arbor. Her first research project explored methods of inferring ancient demographic history — particularly ancient migrations - through the use of simulation modeling and ancient DNA analysis. Her current research agenda builds on her dissertation work to address both the biological consequences of migration (e.g., genetic admixture and genotype-phenotype interactions) and social consequences of migration (e.g., formation of identity/ies in relation to historical admixture events).

Elizabeth A. DiGangi, PhD is an anthropology advisor in Bogotá, Colombia where she consults and trains the country's forensic science professionals. She earned her doctorate in biological anthropology from the University of Tennessee, Knoxville in 2008. Her first research project explored the relationship between maxillary sinusitis and dental infection for a nineteenth century almshouse population in New York. While paleopathological questions still pique her interest, she is currently co-Principal Investigator on a multidisciplinary project to develop biological profile standards for the country of Colombia.

Susan R. Frankenberg, PhD coordinates the Museum Studies Program at the University of Illinois, Urbana-Champaign. She earned her doctorate in anthropology from Northwestern University in 1990, and has worked on demographic and collections issues in bioanthropology, archaeology, and museums in both academia and the private sector over the past 20+ years. Her research spans diverse populations, from the Eastern United States to Europe and the Mediterranean, and from the Middle Bronze Age/Early Woodland to the current day.

William D. Haglund, PhD is a death investigator and biological anthropologist with an interest in taphonomy. He earned his doctorate in physical anthropology from The University of Washington while serving as Chief Medical Investigator of the King County Medical Examiner's Office in Seattle. His dissertation was "Applications of Taphonomic Models to Forensic Investigations." Over the past 15 years he has been dedicated to international forensic investigations, including work as a senior forensic advisor with the United Nations and the international courts, and more recently with Physicians for Human Rights. His field investigations have included countries such as Rwanda, Bosnia, Nigeria, Sierra Leone, Cyprus, Afghanistan, and Iraq.

Emily Hammerl, PhD earned her PhD from the State University of New York at

Buffalo, and is a Research Assistant Professor for the Anthropology Department and for the Forensic Sciences Degree Program at the University of Nebraska-Lincoln. Her first research project examined the growth and development of the deciduous teeth in *Macaca nemestrina*. Her ongoing research examines growth of the mixed primary and permanent dentition of living primates as a proxy for establishing life history profiles of fossil hominins.

Joseph T. Hefner, PhD is a forensic anthropologist for the Joint POW/MIA Accounting Command Central Identification Laboratory at Joint Base Pearl Harbor-Hickam in Hawaii. He earned his doctorate in biological anthropology from the University of Florida, Gainesville, FL. His first research project explored the distribution of human remains at mass fatality scenes using geographic information systems. Currently, ancestry assessment and morphoscopic trait analysis is his primary research interest, within which he is exploring nonparametric classification statistics and other quantitative methods useful for categorical data analysis.

Brannon I. Hulsey, MA, is a PhD candidate at the Department of Anthropology at the University of Tennessee, Knoxville; she is also a key member of the Molecular Anthropology Laboratories' research team. She is broadly interested in the relationship between genotype and phenotype in humans, with a current focus on limb morphology in humans and other primates for her dissertation work.

Lyle W. Konigsberg, PhD is a Professor of Anthropology and of Surgery at the University of Illinois, Urbana-Champaign. He earned his doctorate in anthropology from Northwestern University in 1987. His first published research project was a paleodemographic study of the cremated remains from a classic Ohio Hopewell site. Nearly 30 years later, he continues to work on paleodemographic analyses as well as on statistical problems in forensic anthropology.

Anne M. Kroman, DO, PhD is a resident physician at Northside Hospital and Heart Institute in St. Petersburg, Florida. She earned her doctorate in biological anthropology from the University of Tennessee, Knoxville in 2007. After graduate school, she continued on to medical school at DeBusk College of Osteopathic Medicine completing her degree in 2012. Her research interests include skeletal trauma, cardiovascular physiology, and interventional medicine. Her first research project was on the analysis of knife wounds to the rib cage.

Kerriann Marden, PhD is an Assistant Professor and Director of the Biological and Forensic Anthropology Laboratory at the University of West Georgia. Her first research project was a Program Ethnography of the Police Corps Pilot Project in the Western Police District of Baltimore, MD. Upon entering the doctoral program at Tulane University, her interests shifted to biological anthropology. She volunteered in local morgues and eventually became a registered Medicolegal Death Investigator. Her dissertation applied forensic methods to an archaeological context, focusing on taphonomic and pathological changes in the human remains from the pre-Columbian Southwestern site of Pueblo Bonito in Chaco Canyon, New Mexico.

Ashley H. McKeown, PhD is an Associate Professor in the Department of Anthropology at the University of Montana and specializes in morphometric analyses, bioarchaeology, and forensic anthropology. She earned her doctorate in biological anthropology from the University of Tennessee, Knoxville where her dissertation research employed geometric morphometrics to conduct a large-scale biological distance analysis. Her first research project investigated the relationship between time since death and the separation of single rooted teeth from the alveolar bone for the purposes of estimating the postmortem interval.

Megan K. Moore, PhD works as an Assistant Professor of Anthropology at the University of Michigan-Dearborn where she teaches diverse courses in biological anthropology and human biology. She earned her doctorate from the University of Tennessee, Knoxville in 2008. Her undergraduate honors thesis research investigated dental anthropology and biodistance of a fifteenth century cemetery in Cyprus in 1996. More recently, she has taught forensic anthropology and research methods courses in Bogotá, Colombia, collaborating on several research projects to develop Colombian population standards for sex and stature estimation. Her research passion, however, stems from her dissertation on functional morphology and the effects of body mass (especially obesity) on the skeleton.

Frankie L. Pack is an MA/PhD candidate in the Department of Anthropology and research team member of the Molecular Anthropology Laboratories at the University of Tennessee, Knoxville. Her current research explores genotype-phenotype relationships in humans using matched DNA-dermatoglyphic and DNA-craniodental samples.

Ann H. Ross, PhD is a Professor, Director of Graduate Programs in Anthropology, and Co-Director of the Forensic Sciences Institute at North Carolina State University. She earned her doctorate in biological anthropology from the University of Tennessee, Knoxville. Her areas of research include developing new population-specific standards for various aspects of the biological profile and human rights. Her first project, a thesis project, was a gunshot wound study on estimating caliber from entrance wound defects.

Ryan W. Schmidt, PhD earned his doctorate at the Department of Anthropology, University of Montana. His main interests include quantitative genetics and the population history of ancient nomadic groups in Mongolia and China. His first research project dealt with exploring the history of Chinese-Americans from Nevada using craniometrics as part of his thesis research at the University of Nevada, Las Vegas.

Maria Ostendorf Smith, PhD is an Associate Professor of Anthropology in the Sociology and Anthropology Department of Illinois State University. She received her doctorate in biological anthropology from the University of Tennessee, Knoxville. Her research interest is the bioarchaeology of pre-Columbian cultures of the upper and lower Tennessee River Valley in Tennessee as well as the Upper Mississippi River Valley of Illinois. Topics include temporal and spatial patterns of intergroup violence, community health (sex and social roles), treponemal disease, and the social and economic correlates of oral health.

Marcella H. Sorg, PhD, D-ABFA is Research Associate Professor of Anthropology, Public Policy, and Climate Change at the University of Maine. She is the consulting forensic anthropologist for the Offices of Chief Medical Examiner of Maine, New Hampshire, and Delaware. She earned her doctorate in physical anthropology from The Ohio State University in 1979 and was certified by the American Board of Forensic Anthropology in 1983. Her first research project in forensic anthropology explored the taphonomic role of scavenger modification in forensic cases. She is currently Principal Investigator on a National Institute of Justice funded project to develop and validate regional taphonomic standards for northern New England forensic death investigations.

Steven A. Symes, PhD, D-ABFA is a forensic anthropologist best known for his expertise in interpreting trauma to bone and a leading authority on saw and knife mark analysis. He has been involved with hands-on forensic anthropology since 1979, when he became the graduate assistant to Dr. William M. Bass, founder of the Forensic Anthropology Center at the University of Tennessee, Knoxville. Both Dr. Symes' Master's and doctoral degrees in physical anthropology were earned at UT, Knoxville. Dr. Symes' current research, supported by the National Institute of Justice, involves establishing a gold standard methodology for analyzing saw and knife marks in bone.

Lindsay H. Trammell, PhD is a Medicolegal Death Investigator for the Pima County Office of the Medical Examiner in Tucson, Arizona. She earned her doctorate in biological anthropology from the University of Tennessee, Knoxville. Her first research project was a comparative study of the histological features of faunal species endemic to South Carolina.

Natalie M. Uhl, MS is a graduate student at the University of Illinois at Urbana-Champaign. She earned her Master's in human biology from the University of Indianapolis. While her research interests include forensic anthropology and age-at-death estimation, her dissertation uses multivariate calibration to explore the relationship between brain and body size in fossil hominins.

INTRODUCTION TO RESEARCH
IN SKELETAL BIOLOGY

Introduction to Skeletal Biology

Elizabeth A. DiGangi, Megan K. Moore

GOALS OF THIS TEXTBOOK

This book is designed as an intermediary text to fit between introductory textbooks for new undergraduates and advanced texts for graduate students and professors. Advanced undergraduates or first-year graduate students are often expected to generate their own original research project. However, no comprehensive texts geared towards this specific student demographic previously existed for skeletal biology that unified the following six themes: (1) the specifics of the scientific method; (2) overviews and theory behind each subfield within skeletal biology; (3) the types of scientific questions that each subfield seeks to answer; (4) the specific methods used in each subfield for research; (5) how to narrow down an area of interest and steps to take once that has occurred; and (6) how to present and publish results. This book addresses all of these aforementioned topics and therefore aims to act as a "pocket" advisor.

Some of the readers of this volume will have outstanding advisors who provide sage and timely advice throughout the entire academic process, others will have advisors who take less of a hands-on approach. This book has been written for students in both of the above situations, as well as for those who fall somewhere in the middle. We hope to shed light on how research projects are developed by walking students through the process of choosing a research direction, highlighting not only background but exciting new developments in each area of skeletal biology. Each chapter presents one or more case studies that break down a research project in different ways for the reader. Finally, the ultimate responsibility of scientists is to share their results, so at the end of the volume we offer suggestions about how to present papers and submit manuscripts for publication. Reading these pages will hopefully reduce the mystery of the research process and set the student reader on the path towards becoming a successful skeletal biologist. This chapter will therefore begin the journey by providing a brief introduction and history of biological anthropology and the specialization of skeletal biology.

There are several authoritative books that should be used as complements to this one. We recommend *Standards for Data Collection from Human Skeletal Remains* by Buikstra and Ubelaker (1994) for a detailed treatment on how to record the cranial and postcranial skeleton. In addition, there are other excellent resources covering many of the topics herein;

however, these works assume that the reader already understands how to develop a problem-oriented question (e.g., Katzenberg and Saunders, 2008; Blau and Ubelaker, 2011). The text here is rather directed to the new researcher early in their academic career to guide them in developing a research focus that will later develop into a research program. Each chapter either specifically recommends further reading, or the bibliographies can be used as starting points for further exploration.

This text is not exclusively geared towards either bioarchaeology or forensic anthropology. We chose to focus on skeletal biology because the inherent themes are relevant for practitioners of both fields within biological anthropology, with potential relevance for other areas as well. This book assumes that the reader's knowledge of biological anthropology is at or above the level of an undergraduate major or minor in anthropology. Specific anthropological terms and concepts are therefore used with the presupposition that the reader understands the context. We do not cover anatomical orientations, names of bones and features, or how to measure bones. For bone features, several authoritative textbooks are available, including *Human Osteology* (White et al., 2012), and *Developmental Juvenile Osteology* (Scheuer and Black, 2000), which you should have on your bookshelf. A glossary containing bolded terms throughout the volume is found at the end of the book to serve as a reference for terminology.

One of the key figures in the development of our discipline, Aleš Hrdlička, famously asked a colleague to make an announcement following a paper at the *American Association of Physical Anthropologists'* meeting in 1940: "Statistics will be the ruination of the science" (quoted in Brace, 2005:226). Despite this proclamation, much has changed over the decades. Today, to be a successful researcher in skeletal biology, comfort with statistical analysis is a requirement. However, comprehensive coverage of statistical methods applicable for skeletal biology projects is beyond this book's scope. Therefore, while quantitative statistical analysis is essential to research methods in biological anthropology, only the chapters for which statistics is inextricably linked with method go into the details for conducting specific analyses (e.g., Konigsberg and Frankenberg [Chapter 11]).

For a detailed introduction to statistics, the following texts are written for the novice: *Introduction to the Practice of Statistics* (Moore et al., 2010) and *Discovering Statistics Using SPSS* (Field, 2009). For more advanced **multivariate analyses,**[1] *Using Multivariate Statistics* (Tabachnick and Fidell, 2012) and *Principles of Multivariate Analysis* (Krzanowski, 2000) are recommended. We additionally suggest that college statistics courses be taken to increase competency in this area.

WHY STUDY THE HUMAN SKELETON?

Skeletal biology is, quite simply, the study of the biology of the human skeleton. The study of the skeleton therefore includes its evolution, its structure, its function, its growth and development, and how it is affected by the environment. Biology itself is the study of life, and as such, remember that the skeleton is (or once was) a living thing. Muscles attach to it via tendons, bones articulate with other bones, and it receives nutrients from the bloodstream. Due to the durability of skeletal tissues, bones and teeth are often all that remains

---

[1]All bolded terms are defined in the glossary at the end of this volume.

of a once living person. When faced with dry bones, it can be easy to forget that the skeleton once was not only a dynamic living thing, but it had a very specific purpose, reflected in its morphology. This was not just on the level of the individual, but reflecting long-term evolution, on the level of the population (defined below) as well. We therefore study the skeleton to learn about the individual and the population overall.

In biological anthropology, we are interested in studying human populations, as stated. A human **population** can be defined as a group of individuals who are contemporaneous, occupy relatively the same area geographically, have a shared culture (language, traditions, belief systems, etc.), and who tend to find mates from within the same group. For example, a population in prehistory can consist of all of the people under Inca rule in South America between 1400 and 1532 A.D., or it can be the people who lived in the city of Cuzco (the Inca capital) during the same time. We also make a distinction between the population and the *sample* that we have access to as a result of what was recovered archaeologically. Recovery and preservation bias will affect which individuals of the population are recovered,[2] and therefore this will affect the types of questions we are able to pose. We try to comprise our samples so that they are representative of the population overall, but as stated, sometimes this is not possible. We may also choose specific demographics of individuals from within the sample to study. Therefore, a sample can be individuals falling into each **age cohort** from an Incan cemetery in Cuzco, or all the females of child-bearing age from that same cemetery in Cuzco, or only the high-status individuals who were ethnically Inca (as opposed to high-status people of other ethnicities ruled by the Inca), and so forth.

Because each population of people experiences life in a particular way given environmental (e.g., nutrition, climate, presence of disease), cultural[3] (e.g., differential access to resources, psychosocial stress, activity level), and evolutionary forces (e.g., **gene flow** resulting from people from different populations mating with each other[4]), populations differ from one another and this is often recorded in many ways in the bones of individuals in the archaeologically recovered skeletal sample. We refer to the experience of each population as **population history**.

Bones record basic biological characteristics of an individual (age, sex, ancestry, and stature);[5] how that individual may have fit into their society or experienced life (via social status, occupation, diet, disease, etc.);[6] and other aspects such as a person's geographical place of origin;[7] the demographic profile of populations and relationships between different

[2]See DiGangi and Moore (Chapter 2) and Smith (Chapter 7), this volume.

[3]Cultural and environmental factors are inextricably linked. For example, while diet (foods eaten) may be dictated by the environment (what can grow and what types of animals are present), the culture (society) decides what is edible, what will be grown (for horticultural or agricultural societies), and who will have access to the most preferential food items.

[4]See Cabana et al. (Chapter 16), this volume, for a discussion of evolutionary forces and how they affect populations.

[5]See Uhl (Chapter 3); Moore (Chapter 4); DiGangi and Hefner (Chapter 5); Moore and Ross (Chapter 6); Hammerl (Chapter 10); Trammell and Kroman (Chapter 13), this volume.

[6]See Smith (Chapter 7); Hammerl (Chapter 10); Bethard (Chapter 15), this volume.

[7]See DiGangi and Hefner (Chapter 5); Bethard (Chapter 15); Cabana et al. (Chapter 16), this volume.

populations (**biological distance**);[8] and adaptations to behavior and activity in addition to insults that may have occurred to the individual during or after life.[9] Thus, skeletal biology overall is a major focus in many aspects of biological anthropology: bioarchaeology, forensic anthropology, paleoanthropology, and comparative primate anatomy. This volume, however, has as its focus skeletal biology as it relates to modern humans.

The Biocultural Perspective

The **biocultural** perspective, as defined by Armelagos and Van Gerven (2003), is that culture is an environmental force affecting and interacting with biological adaptation. Humans therefore have a unique biocultural evolutionary history as a result of the mutual interaction of biology and culture. While early physical anthropology (with the notable exception of Franz Boas, discussed below) largely ignored the influence of culture on biology,[10] biological anthropology today is increasingly cognizant of the interrelationship between (1) environment, (2) culture, and (3) biology. Cartmill (1999:658) states (emphasis added), "… culture *always* affects the interaction between genes and environment in our species." This is because human experience is constrained by the three major factors mentioned above.

You are able to read this text because (1) reading exists in your culture and (2) your culture has decided that literacy is important; and therefore you were taught how to read as a child. However, your environment, including the social environment of where you were raised played a role as well: your parents or caretakers made the decision for you that you would learn to read, and they provided the necessary resources for you to be able to do so (transportation to school, school supplies, shelter at night, proper nutrition, preventive and curative medical care, etc.). Further, the fact that you *were* provided with proper nutrition and medical care affected your biology so that your brain and body could focus on more than just staying alive. Had you been born into a different culture where written language did not exist, you would not have learned how to read, even given your biological potential to be able to do so (a functioning human brain and sensory organs). If you had experienced different sociocultural circumstances as a child, perhaps the same would be true. Therefore, all three variables are inextricably linked: your sociocultural surroundings are just as much a part of your environment as climate, nutrition, diet, and exposure to pathogens are due to their mutual interaction. Therefore, biology is affected by both culture and physical environment.

As a result, in biological anthropology our analyses are focused on this dynamic interaction. We cannot understand the individual, never mind the population to which the individual belonged if we do not attempt to uncover the cultural and environmental factors that have affected the biology of the skeletons we analyze. This biocultural interaction is not only preserved in the composition of the bones themselves, but recorded in the context of the remains' deposition. The study of the human skeleton can therefore

---

[8]See Konigsberg and Frankenberg (Chapter 11); McKeown and Schmidt (Chapter 12); and Cabana et al. (Chapter 16), this volume.

[9]See Moore (Chapter 14); Kroman and Symes (Chapter 8); and Marden et al. (Chapter 9), this volume.

[10]See discussion in DiGangi and Hefner (Chapter 5), this volume.

contribute a unique perspective of the life and health of a person who was a member of a larger society.

A CONCISE (AND ABRIDGED) OVERVIEW AND HISTORY OF THEMES IN PHYSICAL/BIOLOGICAL ANTHROPOLOGY RELEVANT TO HUMAN SKELETAL BIOLOGY[11]

At the end of the nineteenth century, physical anthropology emerged as a subdiscipline of anthropology that focused on the physical anatomy of *Homo sapiens* (e.g., Hrdlička, 1914; Spencer, 1986, 1997; Cook, 2006). However, in recent years, the use of the designator "biological" has begun to replace "physical" to describe this subdiscipline of anthropology. This shift is meant to demonstrate the discipline's emphasis on the population and its biocultural aspects in addition to the evolutionary history of the entire species as the object of study rather than on physical types of human beings. The two terms are used interchangeably throughout the text; however, "physical anthropology" is used in reference to the discipline's past while "biological anthropology" is used in reference to the present and the future. We have made this decision because the term "biological" is more general and inclusive than "physical," hinting at not just the physical form but the underlying evolutionary processes as well. As an aside, the National Science Foundation in the United States recently changed the Physical Anthropology program name to "Biological Anthropology," citing as the reason the diversity of the field.[12]

Typology and its Consequences

The following discussion is a brief historical review of the evolution of physical anthropology as a field focused on types of human beings and their hierarchical arrangement to one that has instead become focused on populations and **human variation**. Brace (1982) asserts that delving into historical background is valuable, but that we must consider what to do about the facts we uncover rather than be ashamed of them. Therefore, biological anthropologists must be both aware of the beginnings of our subdiscipline and self-aware that each scientist is a product of their own culture, which includes contemporary sociopolitical convention.

Research in physical anthropology initially was focused on early scientists using a **typological approach** borrowed from biologists and naturalists. Typology is the use of characteristics of one individual or a few individuals to characterize an entire population. As Western scientists had been dividing humans into races or categories for centuries (e.g., see Linnaeus, 1758; Blumenbach, 1806), it was therefore assumed that races did exist, that there were features that were typical of each race (physical <u>and</u> sociocultural), and that the races could be organized hierarchically. Stemming out of this was the idea that physical characteristics

---

[11]Much of the information presented in this section up to "Processualism" (especially related to the race concept) is covered in more detail in DiGangi and Hefner (Chapter 5), this volume. Please read that chapter for more information and consult the references cited therein.

[12]See http://www.nsf.gov

(skin color, head shape) and cultural characteristics (language, social status, "level" of civilization) were **biologically determined** (Caspari, 2003), meaning that sociocultural traits in addition to physical traits were inherited.

Physical anthropologists practicing in the late nineteenth century such as Samuel Morton (in the United States) and Paul Broca (in France) measured physical attributes (e.g., cranial shape and cranial capacity) for scientific justification of the existing hierarchical race rankings (Haller, 1995; Gould, 1996). They assumed races existed and therefore attempted to describe and measure the characteristics that could clearly define or type each racial group.

This use of science to justify differences (physical and cultural) between different groups of people continues and is known as **scientific racism**. Scientific racism has had tragic consequences, perhaps most notably with the *eugenics movement* of the late nineteenth century and early twentieth century. The goal of eugenics was to prevent undesirable traits from accumulating in the population by preventing people with such traits from reproducing (Shipman, 1994; Gould, 1996). In this sense, "undesirable" included poverty, alcoholism, homosexuality, and/or being physically disabled in addition to membership in certain races—so the definition includes traits that we now know are not necessarily heritable or those that are heavily influenced by sociocultural factors. The eugenics movement was actualized most brutally and tragically through the Holocaust perpetrated by Nazi Germany. But there were tragic consequences felt in the United States as well. Forced sterilizations and strict immigration policies were two such results (Gould, 1996).

The Roles of Hooton, Hrdlička, and Boas in Early Physical Anthropology

The fledgling discipline of physical anthropology in the United States during the first half of the twentieth century owes its development and solidification as a discipline in large part to the major contributions of three anthropologists: Earnest Hooton, Aleš Hrdlička, and Franz Boas.[13] Hooton and Hrdlička had similar ideas regarding the race concept, while Boas was on the opposite end of the spectrum. Hooton and Hrdlička both used typological approaches to human variation, believing that races could be hierarchically arranged and that types existed. Conversely, Boas was the first to argue against types and for the critical role that culture had to play with influencing human differences. As a result, two separate schemata of physical anthropology developed: "Washingtonian" and "Boasian." Given that Hrdlička was on staff at the Smithsonian Institution in Washington, D.C., his ideas typified the Washingtonian camp, with Boas' contrary ideas making up the Boasian camp.

As mentioned, Hrdlička and Hooton both considered the history of races as central to anthropology (Armelagos and Van Gerven, 2003) with Hrdlička defining "physical anthropology" as the study of comparative human racial anatomy (Blakey, 1987). However, while Hrdlička did not produce students in his position at the museum, his legacy in addition to his scholarship is in the founding of the *American Journal of Physical Anthropology* (AJPA) in 1918 and the *American Association of Physical Anthropologists* (AAPA) in 1929 (Brace, 2005).

---

[13]There is much, much more to learn about the contributions and philosophies of each of these scholars and how they have shaped biological anthropology that cannot be summed up in a few paragraphs here. Some authoritative sources are Krogman (1976), Spencer (1979), and Birdsell (1987). Further, do not neglect to read the contributions of each scholar.

Hooton, professor at Harvard, was interested in the use of cranial nonmetric traits to typify groups and to answer his research questions about body form. He used the prevalence of such traits and other cranial features in his descriptions of different groups for comparative purposes (e.g., Hooton, 1918). Arguably, however, his most important contribution to the development of the field was that he produced a large number of PhD physical anthropologists in a relatively short time, being the major professor of 28 students, the first of whom graduated in 1925 (Giles, 1997; Caspari, 2003).[14] Many of his students went on to found or lead physical anthropology departments at colleges and universities around the United States (Spencer, 1981).

When Franz Boas started at Columbia University in 1896, he had already developed ideas of **cultural relativism**. He strongly believed in a four-field anthropological approach, was the first to question the race concept, and vehemently rejected biological determinism, preferring emphasis on the culture concept as an explanation for human social differences (Caspari, 2003). While many of his contemporaries including Hooton and Hrdlička accepted *a priori* that races existed and therefore humans could be thusly classified, Boas questioned this assumption and proposed that critical questions should be asked regarding these assumptions, especially those related to the types of measurements that were taken and their significance (Montagu, 1964). His influence on the field therefore still resonates today, as we use a biocultural approach as the basis for the scientific questions we pose.

Resolutions against the Race Concept: UNESCO and AAPA, AAA Statements

While typology defined a large part of the early years of physical anthropology, it was not always to be so. In 1949, a new organization, the United Nations, asked one of its committees, the United Nations Educational, Scientific, and Cultural Organization (UNESCO), to consider a public statement that would use scientific facts to combat racism (Shipman, 1994). The recent end of World War II and the horrors of the Holocaust—racism's ultimate consequence—were the likely provocation. Panel members consisted mainly of anthropologists and sociologists, notably including Ashley Montagu (a former Boas student), a professor of anthropology at Rutgers University and race critic (Brace, 2005). This collaboration resulted in the 1950 Statement on Race, which (among other points) declared (1) that all humans belonged to one species, (2) that the differences between them were due to evolutionary forces, (3) that the species was therefore divided into populations, and (4) that races defined populations that shared a number of physical characteristics but did not define those groups sharing cultural characteristics (Montagu, 1964). However, it also stated that human variation is inherent and changing, and that culture explains social differences between groups of people, and therefore the term "ethnic group" should be used in lieu of "race." Further, the statement went on to reject biological determinism and asserted that mental capabilities were not connected with race (Montagu, 1964).

---

[14]There were only six PhD degrees awarded in physical anthropology in the U.S. prior to 1925 (Caspari, 2003).

Several scholars at the time protested the conclusions in the 1950 statement, especially the assertion that intelligence did not differentially characterize some races over others and that the term "ethnic group" would work as a substitute for the term "race" (Shipman, 1994). This led to a revision of the 1950 statement, which was released in 1952, this time under a committee of mostly physical anthropologists and geneticists (although Montagu was still involved). This revised statement backtracked somewhat on the earlier one, implying science had not yet agreed on the invalidity of the use of "race" to describe human differences (Graves, 2001). Based on a review of popular introductory textbooks at the time, physical anthropologists still disagreed whether or not race was a legitimate way to characterize human differences even given these statements (Littlefield et al., 1982). However, after 1970, more textbooks than not began including arguments for the rejection of the race concept (Littlefield et al., 1982), probably as a reaction to the sociopolitical climate and the subsequent UNESCO statements, outlined below.

The Civil Rights Movement in the United States in the 1950s and 1960s contributed further pressure on physical anthropology to take a public stance against the race concept, illustrating how contemporary sociocultural and political views can influence science and its practitioners. In addition, the publication of the book *The Origin of Races* (Coon, 1962) prompted intense dialogue within anthropology about the race concept (Jackson, 2001; Caspari, 2003). The main thesis by Carleton Coon (a Hooton student) was that five major races of *H. sapiens* evolved separately from *Homo erectus*, with Caucasoids (the term he used) evolving first, and this antiquity of Caucasoids compared to other races was therefore correlated with their cultural achievement (Coon, 1962; Jackson, 2001; Caspari, 2003). Debate was thus sparked about Coon's conclusions, their social implications, and the need to reevaluate the race concept in anthropology (Shipman, 1994; Jackson, 2001; Caspari, 2003).

Soon thereafter, UNESCO released two new statements in 1964 and 1967, which rejected typology, races, and biological determinism, while emphasizing the importance of cultural relativism for understanding the differences between cultures and stating that racist doctrines have no basis in science. The 1967 statement further maintained that scientists have a responsibility to ensure that their research is not misused towards racist ends, perhaps a particularly important point for biological anthropology given that we are fundamentally interested in human variation as it informs us about human populations and the human experience.

Several decades later, the AAPA and *American Anthropological Association* (AAA) passed resolutions rejecting the race concept in 1996 and 1999, respectively. The AAA statement focuses on the social meaning of race and its socioeconomic consequences, while the AAPA statement maintains that (1) it is time to discard antiquated nineteenth century ideas, (2) that biological differences between groups are due to the interaction of heredity and environment, (3) that humans cannot be neatly classified into distinct bounded geographic groups, and (4) that one group is not superior to another (AAPA, 1996; AAA, 1999). It is clear that as our understanding of human variation and its causes continues to be enhanced, so will our thinking on how to best communicate this with the public and with our colleagues. However, typology, biological determinism, and the biological concept of race have definitively been rejected as viable explanations for human differences. Current and future research in this area will focus on the patterns behind human variation, with the goal of answering anthropology's central question: "What makes us human?"

The Evolutionary Perspective

The Modern Synthesis and the New Physical Anthropology

The **modern synthesis** of evolution merged the theories of **genetics** with Darwinian natural selection between 1936 and 1947 (Mayr, 1998). Notable figures in the modern evolutionary synthesis were Julian Huxley (who coined the term), and Theodosius Dobzhansky. This synthesis emerged when Mendelian genetics was found to be consistent with natural selection and a seemingly gradual tempo for **evolution**. Ernst Mayr, who helped conceptualize the modern synthesis, hoped that the new perspective on population genetics could serve as a weapon against public racism (Caspari, 2003; Mayr, 1998; Gould, 2002; Pigliucci and Müller, 2010).

Given the winds of change socially and politically within the United States and in the biological sciences in general as discussed above, one of Hooton's students, Sherwood Washburn (1951), published a famous call to action for physical anthropology to discard its use of the typological approach. Washburn suggested that the "new physical anthropology" should change its focus from typology to the study of populations, with the goal of research being to understand human variation and the process of evolution rather than continued focus on types. Washburn, among others, wanted to see a change in emphasis from the simple recording of a trait to asking the question of *why* the trait exists and what function it serves. Washburn observed that the old physical anthropology was 80% measurement and 20% heredity and he advised that the "new physical anthropology" should reverse this proportion (Washburn, 1951).

In addition, many anthropologists replaced the race concept with the concept of geographical **clines** (a gradual change of a character or feature in a species over a geographical area, e.g., skin color being darker near the equator and lighter in more northern latitudes). Frank Livingstone's declaration, "There are no races, only clines" began this trend (1962:279). Many other workers focused research efforts towards discovering the patterning of human variation. For example, Richard Lewontin, evolutionary biologist and population geneticist, famously demonstrated in 1972 that there is more genetic variation *within* human populations than *between* them, meaning that human populations are more similar to each other than they are different. While some contemporary scholars disagree with Lewontin's conclusions and the cline concept as they relate to the geographic patterning of human variation, all agree that race is neither a useful, accurate, nor scientific way to characterize human variation (Edgar and Hunley, 2009; and see discussions in DiGangi and Hefner [Chapter 5]; and Cabana et al. [Chapter 16], this volume).

Processualism and Post-processualism

By the 1950s, due to the restricted primary role of skeletal analysis to the typological classification of skulls, the specific application of skeletal analysis to archaeological questions had decidedly stagnated when Washburn recommended a "new physical anthropology." (Jarcho, 1966; and see Smith [Chapter 7], this volume). In the late 1960s, the archaeologist Louis Binford helped propel the discipline in a new direction (known as the "New Archaeology" or "processualism") by arguing that cultural systems adapt to the environment. This new theoretical perspective for archaeology premised a biocultural approach in skeletal analysis (i.e., the ideas that mortuary context and skeletal biology also reflect culture and environment) (Buikstra and Cook, 1980; Armelagos et al., 1982, and Van Gerven, 2003; Cook and Powell, 2006).

In the decades following Washburn's call to change, there was an explosive increase in the number of studies using a more functional or analytic approach addressing issues of trauma, growth patterns, and differential mortality (see Smith [Chapter 7], this volume). Further paradigm shifts in archaeology (i.e., post-processualism, agency theory, gender studies) have introduced broader interpretive frameworks for data from skeletal analysis, which has resulted in a more robust discipline. Although there are certainly investigative limitations imposed by skeletonized and mummified human remains, there is much that remains to be addressed, quantified, and hypothesized.

The Osteological Paradox

Wood and colleagues (1992) proposed "the **osteological paradox**," perhaps one of the most important interpretive issues in *bioarchaeology* (defined below). The paradox addresses fundamental problems relative to interpreting health and disease prevalence in the past. Wood and colleagues (1992) discussed three major issues that influence conclusions when analyzing historic and prehistoric skeletal series: (1) demographic nonstationarity, (2) selective mortality, and (3) differential frailty (see also Smith [Chapter 7], this volume).

The first issue addressed by the paradox, *demographic nonstationarity*, means that populations cannot be argued to maintain a constant size over time, therefore the age-at-death distribution in a cemetery sample is more indicative of fertility, rather than mortality. That is, the differential representation of individuals by age has more to do with the number of people entering the population (intrapopulation growth) than the factors that cause their deaths (disease, malnutrition, accidents, etc.).

The second point is of *selective mortality*, meaning that the presence of lesions on bone does not necessarily tell us about the prevalence of a given disease (because not all individuals will develop lesions) and individuals differ in their own **life history** in terms of other pathogens to which they have been exposed or other environmental or sociocultural factors that influence when they actually do die. The quandary then is whether skeletons without lesions represent (1) healthy individuals, or (2) those who were weak and died of a pathogen that could have affected the skeleton but they died before reaching that point (Wright and Yoder, 2003). In essence, the skeleton with the *least* pathology may actually represent the person who was the *least* healthy, and therefore died quickly before lesions could affect the skeleton. In contrast, those skeletons demonstrating the greatest pathology may reflect individuals who were able to survive longer, as the skeleton is typically the last tissue in the body to remodel as a response to disease.

The final point is of *differential frailty*. This means that individuals differ in their response to disease, so some will die from a given disease while others with the same disease will not die. This is perhaps the most difficult part of the paradox to handle when analyzing skeletal series, as the factors that led one person to be more susceptible to disease versus another (i.e., nutrition, access to resources, etc.) are multiple and intertwined. Wood and colleagues (1992) suggested that research on the causes of differential frailty in modern populations and research on how frailty contributes to death risk might lead towards a solution for this part of the paradox.

While several scholars have countered the arguments in the paradox (e.g., Goodman, 1993; Cohen, 1994), Wood and Milner (1994) conceded that while the model presented in the 1992 publication has pitfalls, the important point remains that models for making interpretations about the living population based on the dead (skeletal) population are lacking. They also stated (1994:635), "If a skeletal lesion has any relationship whatsoever to the risk of death … the skeletal population *must* be a biased sample for the living population" (emphasis in original). Essentially, people die for a reason—even accidental deaths can differentially affect certain individuals over others—and therefore the skeletal sample of those who have died (assuming the sample accumulated over time) tells us little about those who <u>did not</u> die (Wood and Milner, 1994).

While this is true, skeletal biologists who study the past are obviously limited in terms of the sample at their disposal. While a given skeletal series may be a snapshot in time of the deceased population, one of the facts of life is that everyone dies, sooner or later. While unfortunate for each individual, this gives us an opportunity to study health in the past—to observe populations across time and space. Via improved demographic methods (see Konigsberg and Frankenberg [Chapter 11], this volume) we can identify trends and patterns seen between and even within populations. Several publications have examined the osteological paradox in depth. For a review, see Wright and Yoder (2003) and refer to Smith (Chapter 7), this volume.

Bioarchaeology

Jane Buikstra was the first to use the term "bioarchaeology" in reference to the merging of physical anthropological methods with archaeology (Buikstra, 1977). While the term was first used in the 1970s, the methods nevertheless have a deep historical root (Buikstra et al., 2003). For example, researchers such as Hrdlička and Hooton were interested in the application of physical anthropology to the interpretation of archaeological sites. For instance, Hrdlička collected a large number of Native American skeletons to refute hypotheses regarding pre-Pleistocene occupation of the Americas (Armelagos and Van Gerven, 2003). Further, Hooton's analysis of skeletal remains from Pecos Pueblo, an archaeological site in New Mexico, was one of the first, if not the first, to approach skeletal analysis using an epidemiological and biocultural approach (Armelagos and Van Gerven, 2003; Beck, 2006). The subsequent publication, *The Indians of Pecos Pueblo* (Hooton, 1930) demonstrates that he critically examined the archaeological context to ask temporal questions about population change (Beck, 2006), part of the focus of bioarchaeology today.

Bioarchaeology helps to contextualize past populations and their individuals, by answering questions about behavior, quality of life, lifestyle, gender, and politics, among others (Larsen, 1997, Buikstra, 2006a,b). It also examines population history and biological distance, two themes important for elucidating the human experience. It does this via several main approaches, what Buikstra (2006b) calls the "bioarchaeologies." These "bioarchaeologies" were preceded historically by publications from scholars such as Wilton Krogman and J. Lawrence Angel. Krogman's contribution illustrated the use of skeletal analysis to show that bones record life's data and Angel's contributions included contextualizing questions about culture from biology (Buikstra, 2006b).

One of the "bioarchaeologies" is the biocultural approach, discussed earlier and championed by Buikstra, among others. In bioarchaeology, this approach is problem-oriented, has a holistic viewpoint as its centerpiece, and encourages interdisciplinary collaborations to examine the interrelationships between culture, environment, and biology in the past (Buikstra, 2006b). Recent volumes taking a biocultural approach include Gowland and Knüsel (2009), Knudson and Stojanowski (2010), Agarwal and Glencross (2011), Tung (2012), and Baadsgaard et al. (2012).

Another one of the "bioarchaeologies" is the osteobiography, as coined by Saul in 1961 (Saul and Saul, 1989; Buikstra, 2006b). The term seeks to encapsulate the fact that bones record several aspects of an individual's life, and that analysis should be focused on interpreting the combination of these features rather than age, sex, etc., separately (Buikstra, 2006b). Larsen (1997, 2006) further emphasizes the reconstruction of human behavior in his definition and approach to bioarchaeology. For more information on these approaches, see Smith (Chapter 7), this volume.

Regardless of the approach taken towards bioarchaeological inquiry, the questions being asked are the same, as outlined above. Further, research that utilizes paleodemography to accurately reconstruct the age and sex distributions of past populations as well as mortuary behavior is being explored (Buikstra, 2006a). Goldstein (2006), however, critiques current bioarchaeological practice, maintaining that workers should contextualize bioarchaeology itself by incorporating existing archaeological theory with skeletal interpretation. If the reader is an aspiring bioarchaeologist, this advice should be heeded.

The Native American Graves Protection and Repatriation Act of 1990[15]

We have gained valuable insight into past populations via the merging of skeletal analysis with archaeological site interpretation since Hooton's *Pecos Pueblo* in 1930, but political decisions have impacted the practice of bioarchaeology, especially in the United States. The most important major development that forced a reorganization of prehistoric skeletal analysis was the passage of the Native American Graves Protection and Repatriation Act (NAGPRA) in 1990. This federal law was in response to increased political activism by Native American tribes that had both religious and practical arguments against the excavation, museum curation, and study of their ancestral funerary objects and human remains (Buikstra, 2006c). The law was crafted to redress injustices to Native Americans by formalizing their access to information about ancestral remains and materials in addition to granting them decision-making ability with regard to those materials (White et al., 2012).

NAGPRA requires museums and laboratories that receive federal funding (1) to inventory all Native American remains and funerary objects, (2) to determine which of those can be culturally affiliated (via a preponderance of evidence that the remains or materials are or belong to the ancestors of a federally recognized tribe), (3) to then communicate with the tribe about the remains, and (4) to allow the tribe to decide what to do with them (NAGPRA, 1990; Buikstra, 2006c; White et al., 2012). That decision may include repatriation, whereby the tribe takes possession of the materials and no further scientific study is done, or it may include agreements with the museum or laboratory to allow continued curation and/or study of the materials.

---

[15]Public Law 101-601; 25 U.S.C. § 3001 et seq.

NAGPRA created sweeping changes for how Native American remains are studied in the United States.[16] However, it has had some beneficial and negative consequences for both Native American tribes and anthropologists. Benefits included the inventory of collections that had never previously been studied. The law also helped to forge new relationships between some anthropologists and Native American tribes (Buikstra, 2006c). However, a major disadvantage has been the nonregulation of the regulators, those individuals charged with enforcing the law. In many cases, osteologists or former collections curators have been discouraged from carrying out their duties, and for some museums and universities, this has resulted in an end to skeletal biology programs (White et al., 2012).

Previously, only recognized tribes that could demonstrate an affiliation to remains or mortuary goods were authorized to claim them. In 2010 new regulations were added (by the Department of the Interior) regarding culturally unidentified remains, stating that any tribe could claim unidentified remains. Museums, scientists, and professional organizations have protested *en masse*, stating (1) that these new regulations allow any tribe to claim materials, even those materials that are not from the geographic ancestral lands of the tribe; (2) that conceivably one tribe could claim *all* unidentified materials; (3) that tribes not federally recognized are preempted, meaning that their rightful materials may be claimed by another tribe; (4) that the ambiguity of the new regulations will result in vast expense; (5) that it is possible that some unidentified materials would be identified in the future given new technologies; (6) that there are constitutionality issues; and (7) that the loss to humanity and future posterity of the information we could gain from such materials (i.e., via stable isotope analysis) is immeasurable (see Bell, 2010; Gover and Samper, 2010; Smith et al., 2010).

Prior to these new regulations, the discovery of a skeleton in Washington State in 1996 (later dubbed "Kennewick Man") that was dated to be older than 9000 years caused controversy when several tribes made a claim to the remains under NAGPRA but anthropologists raised doubts about Kennewick Man's cultural affiliation due to his great antiquity (Owsley and Jantz, in press). Both anthropologists and tribes filed subsequent lawsuits, with the court deciding that there would be no repatriation since the remains were not Native American as defined by NAGPRA (White et al., 2012). However, access to the remains is controlled by the Army Corps of Engineers (ACE) (the landowner of the property where Kennewick Man was found) and the ACE has not yet been released from the lawsuit, so the remains cannot currently be studied; and future prospects are uncertain even once litigation has ended (R. Jantz, personal communication, 2012). The great importance of a skeleton such as Kennewick Man is in the ability to answer questions about lifestyle, behavior, quality of life, diet, health, geolocation, and so on from an individual who lived at the dawn of the peopling of the Americas. A rare skeleton such as this should be available for study by qualified scientists to reveal unique information about our past.

Overall, NAGPRA has exerted a great deal of pressure on biological anthropology and it was feared by many researchers that it would be the end of bioarchaeology in the United States. However, a massive effort ensued to collect as much data as possible from Native American skeletal series, which was facilitated by the standardized data collection procedures

[16]While this discussion focuses on a specific law in the U.S., the lessons learned (i.e., communication with descendant communities/the public, improved skeletal study/interpretation, and the irreplaceable nature of human skeletal remains) are germane for prehistoric skeletal study in all countries (see Buikstra, 2006c).

put forth by Buikstra and Ubelaker (1994). As a result, bioarchaeology has benefitted from NAGPRA in two important ways: (1) many collections have now been systematically studied,[17] and (2) importantly, there are now more collaborations between Native American groups and bioarchaeologists encouraging mutual understanding and respect (Buikstra, 2006c). It remains to be seen what the effects of the 2010 regulations on culturally unidentifiable remains will have on the practice of bioarchaeology in the United States.

One consequence of NAGPRA may be that more U.S. trained scholars will seek research opportunities abroad in countries without similar regulations, although a number of countries do have comparable policies in place (Larsen and Walker, 2005). However, this does not mean that international bioarchaeological work is free from other obstacles. Navigating the complexities and logistics of living abroad temporarily and local regulations for excavation, analysis, and/or transport permits must be considered. Further, Turner and Andrushko (2011) discuss particular issues related to international work and collaboration. Questions arise concerning how to properly communicate results with local communities and what politics are involved with local collaborations. Differences in expectations between collaborating scientists from different cultures must be contemplated, in addition to language barriers or other cultural barriers that add complications towards full participation of international scholars in the scientific process, including publication in American journals (Turner and Andrushko, 2011). Further, outsiders doing work in other countries must be respectful and grateful that they have been made welcome to investigate the past in a country other than their own.

Forensic Anthropology

Forensic anthropology is a relatively new field, having been practiced in earnest for about 40 years. Early definitions emphasized the applied nature of the field, of using concepts and techniques from physical anthropology to individuate human skeletal remains in medicolegal contexts (e.g., Stewart, 1979; and see Komar and Buikstra, 2008 for a discussion of the historical development of the field). However, given the evolution of the field over the past two decades, Dirkmaat and colleagues (2008:47) recently proposed an updated definition that encompasses the many different aspects of forensic anthropological work, stating that "[forensic anthropology is] the scientific discipline that focuses on the life, the death, and the postlife history of a specific individual, as reflected primarily in their skeletal remains and the physical and forensic context in which they are emplaced."

This definition reflects several themes as outlined by Komar and Buikstra (2008): (1) the actual identification of remains is no longer the main theme of forensic anthropology as analyses such as trauma analysis have become important as well; and (2) the archaeological context of where the remains are found is also an object of study. Further, Komar and Buikstra (2008) state that there are two additional departures from the original definitions of the field. The first is the humanitarian function that many forensic anthropological investigations have undertaken, as seen with the Argentine Forensic Anthropology Team founded by Dr. Clyde Snow (www.eaaf.org), other similar teams in Latin America, and nongovernmental organizations such as the International Committee of the Red Cross (www.icrc.org).

---

[17]One drawback to this, however, has been the urgency with which this has been done, in many cases with disregard for the archaeological contextual information (Buikstra, 2006c).

The second is that forensic anthropological investigations no longer focus on remains that are exclusively skeletal. Forensic anthropologists are used in cases where soft tissues are still present but have been altered, e.g., decomposed and burned remains (Komar and Buikstra, 2008).

Given the varied tasks involved in today's forensic anthropology, the field seems to be moving out from being relegated as an applied subfield of biological anthropology and perhaps into a fully fledged subdiscipline of anthropology in its own right (Dirkmaat et al., 2008). Dirkmaat and colleagues (2008) state that this evolution is a result of several developments that have occurred both inside and outside the field over the past several years. These developments include the advent of **DNA** analysis that has removed identification as being the primary task of forensic anthropologists. Other developments have included legal requirements[18] for increased accuracy and rigor with analyses and this has in part led to improved quantitative statistical methods (Komar and Buikstra, 2008; Dirkmaat et al., 2008). In addition, stress on the importance of the archaeological context has emerged and this has had an impact on the development of other areas of analysis, such as taphonomy.[19] Finally, trauma analysis has become a specialty in its own right, with forensic anthropologists being trained in bone biomechanics in order to assess the effect that a variety of traumatic forces have on bone (Dirkmaat et al., 2008).[20]

In addition, the recent publication by the National Research Council of the National Academies (2009) regarding the (poor) state of the forensic sciences in the United States has begun to spur changes. Specifically, recommendations include that all forensic laboratories be certified by some qualified agency, and research to improve methods should be a major focus. For forensic anthropology, this would include increasing our ability with determining how unique any given skeletal trait is that we use for identification, as well as with ascertaining the probability of identifications given the particular biological profile and other skeletal features in an individual case. Evidence of how this report has influenced the field can be seen with the recent creation of the Scientific Working Group for Forensic Anthropology (SWGANTH - www.swganth.org), charged with creating minimum standards and best practices for forensic anthropology.

Most recently, Boyd and Boyd (2011) united several theoretical perspectives for forensic anthropology, essential for any scientific discipline. They divided these into three hierarchical levels of theory. The first level of theory is that evolutionary forces affect human variation[21] and therefore affect **secular change,**[22] as well as skeletal growth, development, and

---

[18]In the United States, this includes the *Daubert* criteria, which essentially state that expert witnesses must demonstrate that scientific methods used to analyze evidence are reliable and accepted by the scientific community (Christensen, 2004). See Moore (Chapter 4), this volume for more information. Further, the Scientific Working Group for Forensic Anthropology (SWGANTH) was recently created to set best practices and minimum standards for forensic anthropology. www.swganth.org

[19]See Marden et al. (Chapter 9), this volume.

[20]See Kroman and Symes (Chapter 8), this volume.

[21]See Cabana et al. (Chapter 16), this volume.

[22]See Moore and Ross (Chapter 6) and McKeown and Schmidt (Chapter 12) for discussions of secular change.

degeneration (Boyd and Boyd, 2011). This is the same level of theory used for biological anthropology in general. It is also essential for forensic anthropology, as biological profiles (age-at-death, sex, ancestry, stature, etc.) are estimated for individuals. Generating such a profile requires a prior understanding of the processes that have affected human variation and therefore skeletal features.

The second level of theory has as its goal the interpretation of the archaeological (forensic) record (context) to determine what created it and therefore asks "who, what, where, when, how" to connect human behavior and explanations for that behavior with the material and organic remains (Boyd and Boyd, 2011). As such, several manifestations of theory can be applied to this goal: (1) *taphonomy* (what happens to remains after death), (2) *agency* (each individual's actions taken into account), (3) *behavior* (different agents and their activities and interactions with each other and with materials [i.e., tools]), and (4) *nonlinear systems* (the consequences arising from the interaction of multiple variables) (Boyd and Boyd, 2011:1408–1409). Applying these four theories in combination leads to a robust interpretation and understanding of the archaeological context.

Forensic anthropologists are involved with interpreting each of the above theoretical areas even if they may be unaware of it (Boyd and Boyd, 2011). While taphonomic interpretations seem obvious in terms of being part of the forensic anthropology toolkit, nonlinear systems and therefore agency and behavior are also considered when interpreting traumatic injuries from a mass graves site (for example). Multiple variables caused the site to be created, taphonomy is involved with the preservation of the remains, and perpetrators were ostensibly involved with the creation of the grave and the injury patterns on the remains.

Finally, the lowest level of theory as it relates to forensic anthropology involves forensic archaeological recovery and statistical induction (Boyd and Boyd, 2011). Regardless of what popular forensic science television shows depict, you probably already know that digging up a clandestine grave without using archaeological methods is taboo. There exists a standardized methodology for assessing and processing sites, from the scene confirmation to the scene excavation stage. Several texts have been published in this area (e.g., Cox et al., 2007; Hester et al., 2008). As a myriad number of techniques exist, justifying one excavation technique over another given a certain set of circumstances is known as *recovery theory* (Boyd and Boyd, 2011).

Statistical induction is the final theory that can be applied to forensic anthropology (Boyd and Boyd, 2011). As mentioned above, the increase in quantitative analyses is one of the aspects defining current forensic anthropology. We use standards for age-at-death, sex, ancestry, and stature based on our analyses of modern skeletal collections. These standards are then applied statistically to unknown remains in order to establish a biological profile. However, as will be discussed throughout this volume, it is essential that the standards are **population specific**, i.e., standards developed on one population should not be applied to another due to human variation and biological distance between populations, as errors may result in the accuracy of the results. When standards are properly applied, the results of the statistical analysis have a scientifically defensible theoretical foundation (Boyd and Boyd, 2011).

It is important to note that the goals of bioarchaeology and forensic anthropology are different within the framework of skeletal biology. The bioarchaeologist is concerned with reconstructing population history from a skeleton or group of skeletons, whereas the forensic anthropologist is attempting to individuate the skeleton, and to make statements about manner of death via analysis of trauma and archaeological context. The new conceptual framework discussed above also applies a strong biocultural emphasis to not only the biological profile, but also the environmental context, emphasizing individual agency and the interaction of the two. Future research in forensic anthropology, forensic taphonomy, trauma, and forensic archaeology will incorporate the aspects of theory discussed above while improving upon current methods and creating population-specific standards.

Ethical Considerations

The ethics of working with human remains must not be overlooked. Moral principles are culturally bound, i.e., what you consider ethical may not be considered ethical by someone else, and therefore making informed and proper decisions about research with human skeletal remains when different parties have an interest (i.e., descendant communities, scientists, local communities, the media, etc.) is complicated but crucial (White et al., 2012).

Research that uses human skeletal remains is not under the purview of most human subjects institutional review boards (IRB), as the subjects are no longer living. However, that does not mean that analyzing human skeletal material is free from ethical concerns. For example, the interests of all parties must be carefully considered. While biological anthropologists feel a responsibility to record for posterity the history of the human condition via analysis of skeletal remains, descendant communities may have certain beliefs about the dead, including prohibitions against outsiders touching the remains of the ancestors. A respectful balance needs to be reached between descendants and scientists, as in addition to the sacred and emotional significance of remains, there is also educational and scientific benefit (Larsen and Walker, 2005).

For forensic anthropologists, Walsh-Haney and Lieberman (2005) recommend that three tenets should always be strived for: (1) do no harm (i.e., handle the remains with care and respect); (2) avoid deception and misrepresentation in data collection, presentation, and publication; and (3) act impartially so that all parties are treated equally. For bioarchaeologists, fostering collaborations with indigenous groups can serve to avoid the political fallout that has occurred in the U.S. in the form of NAGPRA and other countries as well (e.g., Canada, Australia, New Zealand, Israel, Peru, and elsewhere) (Larsen and Walker, 2005). Giving the descendants/survivors respect and a voice has even resulted in the donation of human remains to bioarchaeological or modern skeletal collections (Larsen and Walker, 2005; Walsh-Haney and Lieberman, 2005). White and colleagues (2012:357–378) include a detailed discussion of ethics in human osteology with suggested readings to which you should refer for more information. Also refer to the discussion in DiGangi and Moore (Chapter 2), this volume.

FORMAT OF THIS BOOK

This book is divided into four sections. Each chapter within the four sections is geared towards an audience of advanced undergraduates or new graduate students in biological anthropology whose knowledge level of the discipline is at or above that of an undergraduate anthropology minor or major. Each chapter includes a literature review of its particular topic that, while not meant to be comprehensive, serves as an excellent point of departure for further exploration by the student. A sampling of the major references students should be familiar with to do a project in each area is included, enabling the interested reader to begin their own search of the literature. Overviews are given of each topic while tying the presented information into the details of research projects utilizing a "how-to" approach. For instance, each chapter addresses what the types of questions are for each subject (i.e. what we seek to ask via scientific methods), what the existent challenges are, the different types of research modalities that exist, and key points to consider when initiating and executing projects in each area.

Further, each chapter includes one or more case studies that vary in their design. Some focus on the logistics behind developing a question (e.g., Hammerl, Chapter 10; DiGangi and Moore, Chapter 2); others on method and critical analysis of results (e.g., Smith, Chapter 7); and yet others on strict application of methods to solve a specific problem (e.g., Cabana et al., Chapter 16; Trammell and Kroman, Chapter 8). We intentionally asked each contributor to create the case studies as they saw fit, as when taken together the entire volume then gives the reader a broad overview and understanding of each step of the scientific process from logistical considerations to technical aspects.

Part I: Introduction to Research in Skeletal Biology

Part I: Introduction to Research in Skeletal Biology includes two chapters that define the topic and purpose of the book. Following the current chapter, Chapter 2 introduces the scientific method and presents the theory and practice behind how it applies to skeletal biology. It provides an overview of the philosophy behind science and the scientific method, exploring how each step of the scientific method occurs in skeletal biology research. It additionally includes a section outlining the goals of science and its limitations. The second portion of the chapter is dedicated to specifically examining how research ideas are generated and the logistics that must be considered (including ethical considerations), which are vital topics for students embarking on their first project.

Part II: Research on Aspects of the Biological Profile

Part II: Research on Aspects of the Biological Profile includes nine chapters, all of which cover some aspect of what is known as the "biological profile"—specific characteristics of an individual that we can identify or estimate from bone. This section begins with four chapters on the traditional four components of the biological profile: age-at-death, sex, ancestry, and stature estimation.[23] However, there are multiple additional areas of analysis that can contribute information about the individual and/or their population. Demography, for example, fits into this section because it addresses population-wide questions and advanced demographic analyses can more accurately estimate aspects of the traditional biological profile. In addition, while taphonomy is relegated to what happened to an individual after death, taphonomic processes can confound or destroy indicators used in biological profile

---

[23]While some skeletal biologists may order the biological profile differently, we have chosen this arrangement because you must know if the individual is a juvenile or adult before proceeding with the subsequent analyses.

construction. Therefore this section continues with several chapters that cover other areas informing the reconstruction of an individual's biological profile: paleopathology, trauma, taphonomy, dental anthropology, and demography.

Chapter 3 examines adult and subadult skeletal age-at-death estimation. It concisely reviews growth so as to discuss the differences behind the theory of aging methods for juveniles and adults. Dental development and long bone growth are therefore reviewed and subadult aging methods discussed. Likewise, the chapter examines the major methods developed for adult age-at-death estimation. It further presents how anthropologists quantify developmental and degenerative changes, given the inherent difficulties involved to create more robust age estimates. It includes a discussion of multifactorial methods and the use of Bayesian statistics in age estimation.

Chapter 4 discusses the causes and consequences of sexual dimorphism in the human skeleton. This chapter elucidates the distinction between metric sex estimation and visual sex assessment from the adult skeleton, with an overview of the historical development for each. The accuracy of existing sexing methods for each bone is discussed, calling into question the preference for the skull when postcranial elements perform at least as well in discriminant function analyses. Sex estimation (metric analysis) offers the benefit of error estimates and reduced interobserver error. Other sex estimation research that has had varying degrees of success is discussed, including research on sexing subadults, sex estimation from skeletal pathology, and molecular methods for sex estimation.

Chapter 5 covers ancestry estimation and begins with a historical review of the race concept in physical anthropology and its social impact, especially in terms of the effect scientific racism has had on both society and the development of the discipline of biological anthropology into what it is today. Key historical figures who influenced the development of the concept in some way are discussed and the modern view of human variation is introduced. The chapter then outlines the practice of ancestry estimation by discussing metric and nonmetric trait analysis through the use of robust multivariate statistical methods.

Chapter 6 focuses on stature estimation and therefore presents the various anatomical and mathematical methods developed for its approximation. It explores the history of stature estimation including early femur/stature ratios, the development of regression formulae for various bones, and anatomical methods along with recent revisions. Secular trends are also discussed as their influence has resulted in a relative increase in stature over the last few centuries. Further, problems in methodology are presented in terms of incongruence between antemortem and postmortem data and the accuracy of various statistical approaches.

Chapter 7 addresses the skeletal analysis of paleopathology. Bioarchaeology and analytical paleopathology are defined and discussed in depth as to their importance with elucidating factors for past populations such as subsistence and community health. Differential diagnosis and specific and nonspecific stress indicators are explored. Further, discussion centers around selection of pathological parameters, accurate documentation of bony reactive changes, careful quantification of these continuous processes, and designing an appropriate analytical framework for paleopathological projects.

Chapter 8 investigates the analysis of skeletal trauma. It begins by reviewing basic bone biomechanics and proceeds to define major principles of trauma as seen with the categories of blunt force, sharp force, ballistic, and thermal trauma. A new viewpoint for the conceptualization of trauma as a continuum is presented. Case-based and experimental research is evaluated and discussed as two major avenues in which trauma research is conducted. Further, logistics particular to trauma research is reviewed.

Chapter 9 explores the field of taphonomy and its relevance to biological anthropology. It provides an overview of the postmortem perspective, presents the different types of research modalities used to explore taphonomic questions (e.g., actualistic research), and reviews how to recognize and interpret marks on bone. It further provides a discussion of outdoor research facilities that have greatly expanded our knowledge in this area. Two case studies are presented—one demonstrating how taphonomy can be used in a medicolegal context, and one that illustrates how taphonomic analyses can be applied to historical questions.

Chapter 10 tackles dental anthropology. It presents a basic overview of dental anatomy and tooth growth and development. The importance of such aspects as emergence patterns and conditions that may affect the teeth during their development is briefly discussed. It further includes treatment of how dental metrics and nonmetrics are used to generate valuable information, such as sex, age, and ancestry estimations from the teeth alone. It additionally demonstrates how analyses of dental disease, stable isotopes, and microwear from teeth have provided important data for a variety of anthropological studies.

Chapter 11 is dedicated to demography, crucial for skeletal biologists to consider when reconstructing population structure, morbidity, and mortality. The chapter takes the standpoint that demographic analysis should *precede* the estimation of individual ages-at-death or sex. The method of maximum likelihood is introduced as being able to estimate basic demographic parameters from skeletal data. These parameters can then be used to estimate age-at-death and sex. This chapter is the only one in the book that dives very specifically and purposefully into statistical analysis, necessary given the nature of generating demographic profiles. Case studies throughout the chapter therefore make use of Bayes' Theorem, hazard models, and maximum likelihood, all of which can be explored further by the reader through the website provided in the text.

Part III: Technological Advances

In recent years, the study of biological anthropology has been enhanced by the advent of advanced analytical methods. *Part III: Technological Advances* has five chapters, each of which covers a different area highlighting advanced applications of technology to the practice of biological anthropology. All of these subjects have been studied for some time in other fields, and anthropologists have been realizing and adapting their utility for skeletal biology. These chapters include geometric morphometrics, histology, functional morphology and medical imaging, isotopic analysis, and DNA.

Chapter 12 introduces geometric morphometrics—the analysis of geometry of form (most notably for the skull) via multidimensional data. The history of traditional morphometrics is presented and multivariate statistical methods for analysis of morphometric data are discussed. Further, the different types of landmarks and the utility of three-dimensional data (and how it is collected) are outlined. The chapter additionally provides specific discussion of methods particular to geometric morphometric analysis, such as Procrustes analysis, and a listing of statistical programs capable of analyzing such data. Further, the relevance and importance of such methods to biodistance analyses and uncovering population history is discussed.

Chapter 13 investigates bone and dental histology. It therefore first provides a review of histological structures and a discussion of the utility of histological methods to assist with development of the biological profile and human versus nonhuman animal determinations. The methods involved in this research area include embedding the material in resin and cutting thin sections of the tooth or bone, and this chapter provides useful step-by-step instructions for the aspiring histologist, which can be supplemented with information from the literature. Discussion includes how histological analyses can also inform investigations of taphonomy, biomechanics, and pathology.

Chapter 14 covers the theory of functional adaptation of human bone, often referred to as Wolff's Law (whether correctly or incorrectly), and in so doing, introduces the basics of bone biomechanics and functional morphology. Medical imaging technologies provide noninvasive and highly sophisticated methods to analyze bone strength properties via analysis of bone shape or density. Biplanar radiographs can provide rough approximations of three-dimensional shape. The preferred method, computed tomography (CT), provides essentially a three-dimensional digital radiograph and is the preferred noninvasive method in research on cross-sectional geometry. The material properties of bone density are investigated using dual energy X-ray absorptiometry (DEXA) or CT. Other methods reviewed, but less common for research in skeletal biology include peripheral quantitative CT, magnetic resonance imaging (MRI), and ultrasonography.

Chapter 15 evaluates the contribution that stable isotope analysis has made to skeletal biology over about the past 30 years. As the value of isotopes has been increasingly realized, they are more frequently being used for bioarchaeological applications. A number of questions are addressable via isotope analysis, in particular those pertaining to paleodiet, residential mobility, and migration patterns. This chapter discusses the types of questions answerable via isotope analysis in addition to presenting the anthropological significance of several isotopes. Standard methods for data collection (i.e., extraction of bone biological apatite and collagen) are presented in addition to an overview of the sophisticated analysis equipment involved. Further, the potential forensic applications of isotopes are briefly outlined.

Chapter 16 focuses on DNA analysis, beginning with a review of basic concepts in genetics. It provides a history of genetics in anthropology and evolutionary theory (in terms of population genetics), and therefore outlines the four forces of evolution with examples. Theory, methods used, and interpretation of molecular data are fully explored, including a discussion of the special case that degraded DNA presents to the researcher. It further tackles how the application of DNA analysis to the question of human variation has informed that debate.

Part IV: Completing and Cultivating the Scientific Process

Finally, *Part IV: Completing and Cultivating the Scientific Process* concludes the volume with two chapters. The end stage of the scientific process involves disseminating information to a wider audience. As such, the book would not be complete without a chapter covering in detail how to do library research, present original work, and publish journal articles. The subsequent and last chapter focuses on the concept that science advances and is cultivated not only via presentation and publication of results, but through conversations about themes and trends in the discipline, with a vision for the direction of the discipline towards the future.

Chapter 17 takes the reader through additional steps necessary to bring a project from its early stages through to presentation and/or publication. The art of doing library and database research is discussed in detail, and new database search engines and bibliographic software of use are listed. Following this discussion, the chapter outlines how to present posters and papers at scientific conferences and how to publish original research in peer-reviewed journals. It provides tables listing conferences and journals accepting work in skeletal biology as a starting point for the industrious researcher.

To conclude the volume, Chapter 18 presents an overview of recommendations for beginning researchers in addition to current trends and important considerations for research in skeletal biology. The conclusion ties everything together by emphasizing the direction in which research in skeletal biology is traveling—increased collaboration with other disciplines, standardization and validation of method application, and development of population-specific standards, all from a biocultural standpoint.

HOW TO USE THIS BOOK

We recommend that this book be incorporated into the curricula of first semester graduate level biological anthropology theory and methods courses, research methods courses, or advanced undergraduate seminars covering the above topics, including independent study. It can be used as a complement or precursor to other texts such as Katzenberg and Saunders (2008) and Stinson et al. (2012).

Beginning students who are trying to identify which specific area of skeletal biology piques their interest most should read the book in its entirety. Students who have already narrowed down their area of interest somewhat should read the chapters in Parts I and IV. Given that each chapter in Parts II and III is designed to stand on its own as an introduction, literature review, and "how-to" for methods in that specific area, they should also read the chapter(s) that correspond to the area(s) they have chosen for their research effort in these two middle sections.

FINAL THOUGHTS

As researchers who once wore the shoes of neophyte graduate students, we want you to learn from the information and case studies presented in this volume as they illustrate the diversity of the shared knowledge and experience of the contributors and within skeletal biology in general. There can be a great deal of uncertainty when choosing to pursue an advanced degree. You are probably already aware that a lucrative job is unlikely, and that this is the reality for a research-based career in anthropology. However, you are studying human skeletal biology because in all likelihood, you are amazed by the elegant complexity of the human skeletal system and what it can tell us about our shared past. Each of the contributors to this volume is living proof that following one's passion is possible. We therefore invite you to begin your own journey via exploration of the topics in this volume.

ACKNOWLEDGMENTS

We are grateful to Drs. Maria Smith and Jonathan Bethard, whose helpful comments and suggestions improved this chapter.

REFERENCES

Agarwal, S.C., Glencross, B.A. (Eds.), 2011. Social Bioarchaeology. Wiley-Blackwell, Malden, MA.

American Anthropological Association, 1999. AAA statement on race. American Anthropologist 100 (3), 712–713.

American Association of Physical Anthropologists, 1996. AAPA statement on biological aspects of race. American Journal of Physical Anthropology 101, 569–570.

Armelagos, G.J., Van Gerven, D.P., 2003. A century of skeletal biology and paleopathology: contrasts, contradictions, and conflicts. American Anthropologist 105 (1), 53–64.

Armelagos, G.J., Carlson, D.S., Van Gerven, D.P., 1982. The theoretical foundations and development of skeletal biology. In: Spencer, F. (Ed.), A History of American Physical Anthropology, 1930–1980. Academic Press, New York, pp. 305–328.

Baadsgaard, A., Boutin, A.T., Buikstra, J.E. (Eds.), 2012. Breathing New Life into the Evidence of Death: Contemporary Approaches to Bioarchaeology. SAR Press, Santa Fe, NM.

Beck, L.A., 2006. Kidder, Hooton, Pecos, and the birth of bioarchaeology. In: Buikstra, J.E., Beck, L.A. (Eds.), Bioarchaeology: The Contextual Analysis of Human Remains. Academic Press, San Diego.

Bell, F.W., 2010. Letter to Dr. Sherry Hutt, Manager, National NAGPRA Program, National Park Service, on behalf of the American Association of Museums. 13 May 2010. http://www.friendsofpast.org/nagpra/2010NAGPRA/AAM.pdf. Retrieval date 29 March 2012.

Bethard, J.D., 2013. Isotopes. In: DiGangi, E.A., Moore, M.K. (Eds.), Research Methods in Human Skeletal Biology. Academic Press, San Diego.

Birdsell, J., 1987. Some reflections on fifty years in biological anthropology. Annual Reviews of Anthropology 16 (1), 1–12.

Blakey, M.L., 1987. Skull doctors: intrinsic social and political bias in the history of American physical anthropology with special reference to the work of Ales Hrdlicka. Critique of Anthropology 7 (2), 7–35.

Blau, S., Ubelaker, D.H., 2011. Handbook of Forensic Anthropology and Archaeology. Left Coast Press, Walnut Creek, CA.

Blumenbach, J., 1806. Contributions to Natural History Part I. Heinrich Dieterich, Gottingen.

Boyd, C., Boyd, D.C., 2011. Theory and the scientific basis for forensic anthropology. Journal of Forensic Sciences 56 (6), 1407–1415.

Brace, C.L., 1982. The roots of the race concept in American physical anthropology. In: Spencer, F. (Ed.), A History of American Physical Anthropology, 1930–1980. Academic Press, New York.

Brace, C.L., 2005. "Race" Is a Four Letter Word: The Genesis of the Concept. Oxford University Press, Oxford.

Buikstra, J.E., 1977. Biocultural dimensions of archaeological study: a regional perspective. In: Blakely, R.L. (Ed.), Biocultural Adaptation in Prehistoric America, Southern Anthropological Society Proceedings, 11 (6), pp. 67–84.

Buikstra, J.E., 2006a. Emerging specialties: Introduction. In: Buikstra, J.E., Beck, L.A. (Eds.), Bioarchaeology: The Contextual Analysis of Human Remains. Academic Press, San Diego, pp. 195–205.

Buikstra, J.E., 2006b. On to the 21st century: Introduction. In: Buikstra, J.E., Beck, L.A. (Eds.), Bioarchaeology: The Contextual Analysis of Human Remains. Academic Press, San Diego, pp. 347–357.

Buikstra, J.E., 2006c. Repatriation and bioarchaeology: challenges and opportunities. In: Buikstra, J.E., Beck, L.A. (Eds.), Bioarchaeology: The Contextual Analysis of Human Remains. Academic Press, San Diego, pp. 389–415.

Buikstra, J.E., Cook, D.C., 1980. Paleopathology: an American account. Annual Review of Anthropology 9, 433–470.

Buikstra, J.E., Ubelaker, D.H., 1994. Standards for Data Collection from Human Skeletal Remains. Arkansas Archaeological Survey, Fayetteville, Arkansas, AR.

Buikstra, J.E., King, J.L., Nystrom, K.C., 2003. Forensic anthropology and bioarchaeology in the American Anthropologist: rare but exquisite gems. American Anthropologist 105 (1), 38–52.

Cabana, G.S., Hulsey, B.I., Pack, F.L., 2013. Molecular methods. In: DiGangi, E.A., Moore, M.K. (Eds.), Research Methods in Human Skeletal Biology. Academic Press, San Diego.

Cartmill, M., 1999. The status of the race concept in physical anthropology. American Anthropologist 100 (3), 651—660.

Caspari, R., 2003. From types to populations: a century of race, physical anthropology, and the American Anthropological Association. American Anthropologist 105 (1), 65—76.

Christensen, A.M., 2004. The impact of Daubert: implications for testimony and research in forensic anthropology (and the use of frontal sinuses in personal identification). Journal of Forensic Sciences 49, 427—430.

Cohen, M.N., 1994. The osteological paradox reconsidered. Current Anthropology 35 (5), 629—637.

Cook, D.C., 2006. The old physical anthropology and the New World: a look at the accomplishments of an antiquated paradigm. In: Buikstra, J.E., Beck, L.A. (Eds.), Bioarchaeology: The Contextual Analysis of Human Remains. Academic Press, San Diego, pp. 27—71.

Cook, D.C., Powell, M.L., 2006. The evolution of American paleopathology. In: Buikstra, J.E., Beck, L.A. (Eds.), Bioarchaeology: The Contextual Analysis of Human Remains. Academic Press, San Diego, pp. 281—322.

Coon, C.S., 1962. The Origin of Races. Knopf, New York.

Cox, M., Flavel, A., Hanson, I., Laver, J., 2007. The Scientific Investigation of Mass Graves: Towards Protocols and Standard Operating Procedures. Cambridge University Press, Cambridge.

DiGangi, E.A., Hefner, J.T., 2013. Ancestry estimation. In: DiGangi, E.A., Moore, M.K. (Eds.), Research Methods in Human Skeletal Biology. Academic Press, San Diego.

DiGangi, E.A., Moore, M.K., 2013. Application of the scientific method to skeletal biology. In: DiGangi, E.A., Moore, M.K. (Eds.), Research Methods in Human Skeletal Biology. Academic Press, San Diego.

Dirkmaat, D.C., Cabo, L.L., Ousley, S.D., Symes, S.A., 2008. New perspectives in forensic anthropology. Yearbook of Physical Anthropology 51, 33—52.

Edgar, J.H., Hunley, K.L., 2009. Race reconciled? How biological anthropologists view human variation. American Journal of Physical Anthropology 139, 1—4.

Field, A.P., 2009. Discovering Statistics Using SPSS. Sage Publications, Thousand Oaks, California.

Giles, E., 1997. Earnest Albert Hooton (1887—1954). In: Spencer, F. (Ed.), History of Physical Anthropology. Garland Publishing. New York.

Goldstein, L., 2006. Mortuary analysis and bioarchaeology. In: Buikstra, J.E., Beck, L.A. (Eds.), Bioarchaeology: The Contextual Analysis of Human Remains. Academic Press, San Diego.

Goodman, A.H., 1993. On the interpretation of health from skeletal remains. Current Anthropology 34 (3), 281—288.

Gould, S.J., 1996. The Mismeasure of Man, Revised Edition. W.W. Norton & Company, New York.

Gould, S.J., 2002. The Structure of Evolutionary Theory. Belknap Press of Harvard University Press, Cambridge.

Gover, K., Samper, C., 2010. Letter to Dr. Sherry Hutt, Manager, National NAGPRA Program, National Park Service on behalf of the Smithsonian Institution. 14 May 2010. http://www.friendsofpast.org/nagpra/2010NAGPRA/NMAI_NMNH.pdf. Retrieval date March 29 2012.

Gowland, R., Knusel, C., 2009. The Social Archaeology of Human Remains. Oxbow Books, Oxford.

Graves, J.L., 2001. The Emperor's New Clothes: Biological Theories of Race at the Millennium. Rutgers University Press, New Brunswick, New Jersey.

Haller, J.S., Jr., 1995. Outcasts from Evolution: Scientific Attitudes of Racial Inferiority, 1859—1900. Southern Illinois University Press, Carbondale.

Hammerl, E., 2013. Dental anthropology. In: DiGangi, E.A., Moore, M.K. (Eds.), Research Methods in Human Skeletal Biology. Academic Press, San Diego.

Hester, T.R., Shafer, H.J., Feder, K.L., 2008. Field Methods in Archaeology, 7th ed. Left Coast Press, Walnut Creek, CA.

Hooton, E.A., 1918. On certain Eskimoid characters in Icelandic skulls. American Journal of Physical Anthropology 1, 53—76.

Hooton, E.A., 1930. The Indians of Pecos Pueblo, A Study of Their Skeletal Remains, Vol. 4. Papers of the Southwestern Expedition. Yale University Press, New Haven.

Hrdlicka, A., 1914. Physical anthropology in America: an historical sketch. American Anthropologist 16 (4), 508—554.

Jackson, J.P., Jr., 2001. "In ways unacademical": the reception of Carleton S. Coon's The Origin of Races. Journal of the History of Biology 34, 247—285.

Jarcho, S., 1966. Human Palaeopathology. Yale University Press, New Haven.

Katzenberg, M.A., Saunders, S.R., 2008. Biological Anthropology of the Human Skeleton, 2nd ed. John Wiley & Sons. Hoboken, NJ.

Knudson, K.J., Stojanowski, C.M., 2010. Bioarchaeology and Identity in the Americas. University Press of Florida, Gainesville.

Komar, D.A., Buikstra, J.E., 2008. Forensic Anthropology: Contemporary Theory and Practice. Oxford University Press, New York.

Konigsberg, L.W., Frankenberg, S.R., 2013. Demography. In: DiGangi, E.A., Moore, M.K. (Eds.), Research Methods in Human Skeletal Biology. Academic Press, San Diego.

Krogman, W., 1976. Fifty years of physical anthropology: the men, the materials, the concepts, and the methods. Annual Reviews of Anthropology 5, 1—14.

Kroman, A.M., Symes, S.A., 2013. Investigation of Skeletal trauma. In: DiGangi, E.A., Moore, M.K. (Eds.), Research Methods in Human Skeletal Biology. Academic Press, San Diego.

Krzanowski, W.J., 2000. Principles of Multivariate Analysis. Oxford University Press, New York.

Larsen, C.S., 1997. Bioarchaeology: Interpreting Behavior from the Human Skeleton. Cambridge University Press, Cambridge.

Larsen, C.S., 2006. The changing face of bioarchaeology: an interdisciplinary science. In: Buikstra, J.E., Beck, L.A. (Eds.), Bioarchaeology: The Contextual Analysis of Human Remains. Academic Press, San Diego, pp. 359—374.

Larsen, C.S., Walker, P.L., 2005. The ethics of bioarchaeology. In: Turner, T.R. (Ed.), Biological Anthropology and Ethics: From Repatriation to Genetic Identity. State University of New York Press, Albany, New York, pp. 111—119.

Lewontin, R.C., 1972. The apportionment of human diversity. Evolutionary Biology 6, 381—398.

Linnaeus, C., 1758. Systema Naturae. 10th revised edition of 1758 [1956]. Laurentii Salvii, Stockholm.

Littlefield, A., Lieberman, L., Reynolds, L.T., 1982. Redefining race: the potential demise of a concept in physical anthropology. Current Anthropology 23 (6), 641—655.

Livingstone, F.B., 1962. On the non-existence of human races. Current Anthropology 3 (3), 279—281.

Marden, K., Sorg, M.H., Haglund, W.D., 2013. Taphonomy. In: DiGangi, E.A., Moore, M.K. (Eds.), Research Methods in Human Skeletal Biology. Academic Press, San Diego.

Mayr, E., 1998. The Evolutionary Synthesis: Perspectives on the Unification of Biology (with a new preface). Harvard University Press, Cambridge.

McKeown, A.H., Schmidt, R.W., 2013. Geometric morphometrics. In: DiGangi, E.A., Moore, M.K. (Eds.), Research Methods in Human Skeletal Biology. Academic Press, San Diego.

Montagu, A., 1964. Man's Most Dangerous Myth: The Fallacy of Race, 4th ed. The World Publishing Company, Cleveland and New York.

Moore, D.S., McCabe, G.P., Craig, B., 2010. Introduction to the Practice of Statistics. W.H. Freeman, New York.

Moore, M.K., 2013. Sex estimation and assessment. In: DiGangi, E.A., Moore, M.K. (Eds.), Research Methods in Human Skeletal Biology. Academic Press, San Diego.

Moore, M.K., 2013. Functional morphology and medical imaging. In: DiGangi, E.A., Moore, M.K. (Eds.), Research Methods in Human Skeletal Biology. Academic Press, San Diego.

Moore, M.K., Ross, A.H., 2013. Stature estimation. In: DiGangi, E.A., Moore, M.K. (Eds.), Research Methods in Human Skeletal Biology. Academic Press, San Diego.

National Research Council of the National Academies, 2009. Strengthening Forensic Science in the United States: A Path Forward. The National Academies Press, Washington, D.C.

Native American Graves Protection and Repatriation Act (NAGPRA), 1990. (Public Law 101—601; 25 U.S.C. 3001—3013; 104 Stat. 3048—3058).

Owsley, D., Jantz, R.L., in press. Kennewick Man. A&M Press, College Station, Texas.

Pigliucci, M., Muller, G.B., 2010. Evolution—The Extended Synthesis. MIT Press, Cambridge, MA.

Saul, F.P., Saul, J.M., 1989. Osteobiography: a Maya example. In: Iscan, M.Y., Kennedy, K.A.R. (Eds.), Reconstruction of Life from the Skeleton. Alan R. Liss, New York, pp. 287—302.

Scheuer, L., Black, S., 2000. Developmental Juvenile Osteology. Academic Press, San Diego.

Shipman, P., 1994. The Evolution of Racism: Human Differences and the Use and Abuse of Science. Harvard University Press, Cambridge.

Smith, B.D., Adams, R.M., Altmann, J., Asfaw, B., Bar-Yosef, O., Beall, C., Buikstra, J.E., Carneiro, R., Coe, M.D., Drennan, R.D., Flannery, K.V., Garruto, R.M., Goldstein, M.C., Hammel, E.A., Harpending, H., Hawkes, K., Hole, F., Hrdy, S.B., Kay, P., Kirch, P.V., Klein, R.G., Kottak, C.P., Marcus, J., Medin, D.L., Meltzer, D.J., Moseley, M., O'Connell, J.F., Partee, B.H., Piperno, D.R., Plog, S., Romney, A.K., Sabloff, J.A., Sahlins, M., Schild, R., Spencer, C.S., Spiro, M.E., Thomas, D.H., Watson, P.J., Wendorf, F., White, T., Yen, D., 2010. Letter to the Honorable Ken Salazar,

Secretary of the Interior, Department of the Interior, on behalf of 41 members of the National Academy of Sciences. 17 May 2010. http://www.friendsofpast.org/nagpra/2010NAGPRA/Smith517.pdf. Retrieval date 29 March 2012.

Smith, M.O., 2013. Paleopathology. In: DiGangi, E.A., Moore, M.K. (Eds.), Research Methods in Human Skeletal Biology. Academic Press, San Diego.

Spencer, F., 1979. Ales Hrdlicka M.D., 1869—1943: A Chronicle of the Life and Work of an American Physical Anthropologist. Unpublished PhD dissertation. University of Michigan, Ann Arbor.

Spencer, F., 1981. The rise of academic physical anthropology in the United States (1880—1980): A historical overview. American Journal of Physical Anthropology 56, 353—364.

Spencer, F., 1986. Ecce Homo: An Annotated Bibliographic History of Physical Anthropology. Greenwood Press.

Spencer, F., 1997. History of Physical Anthropology: An Encyclopedia. Garland, New York.

Stewart, T.D., 1979. Essentials of Forensic Anthropology, Especially as Developed in the United States. Charles C. Thomas, Springfield, IL.

Stinson, S., Bogin, B., O'Rourke, D., 2012. Human Biology: An Evolutionary and Biocultural Perspective. Wiley-Blackwell, Hoboken, NJ.

Tabachnick, B.G., Fidell, L.S., 2012. Using Multivariate Statistics. Prentice Hall, Upper Saddle River, NJ.

Trammell, L.H., Kroman, A.M., 2013. Bone and Dental Histology. In: DiGangi, E.A., Moore, M.K. (Eds.), Research Methods in Human Skeletal Biology. Academic Press, San Diego.

Tung, T.A., 2012. Violence, Ritual, and the Wari Empire: A Social Bioarchaeology of Imperialism in the Ancient Andes. University Press of Florida, Gainesville.

Turner, B.L., Andrushko, V.A., 2011. Partnerships, pitfalls, and ethical concerns in international bioarchaeology. In: Agarwal, S.C., Glencross, B.A. (Eds.), Social Bioarchaeology. John Wiley & Sons, Malden, MA, pp. 44—67.

Uhl, N.M., 2013. Age-at-death estimation. In: DiGangi, E.A., Moore, M.K. (Eds.), Research Methods in Human Skeletal Biology. Academic Press, San Diego.

United Nations Educational, Scientific, and Cultural Organization (UNESCO), 1969. Four Statements on the Race Question. Oberthur-Rennes, Paris.

Walsh-Haney, H., Lieberman, L., 2005. Ethical concerns in forensic anthropology. In: Turner, T.R. (Ed.), Biological Anthropology and Ethics: From Repatriation to Genetic Identity. State University of New York Press, New York, pp. 121—131.

Washburn, S.L., 1951. The new physical anthropology. Transactions of the New York Academy of Sciences, Series II 13 (7), 298—304.

White, T.D., Black, M.T., Folkens, P.A., 2012. Human Osteology. Academic Press, San Diego.

Wood, J.W., Milner, G.R., 1994. Reply (to M.N. Cohen: The osteological paradox reconsidered). Current Anthropology 35 (5), 629—637.

Wood, J.W., Milner, G.R., Harpending, H.C., Weiss, K.M., 1992. The osteological paradox: problems of inferring prehistoric health from skeletal samples. Current Anthropology 33, 343—358.

Wright, L.E., Yoder, C.J., 2003. Recent progress in bioarchaeology: approaches to the osteological paradox. Journal of Archaeological Research 11 (1), 43—70.

2

Application of the Scientific Method to Skeletal Biology

Elizabeth A. DiGangi, Megan K. Moore

It may seem obvious, but having an understanding of the scientific method before undertaking a research project is the most important preliminary step. Many new graduate students have a vague idea of where their interests lie and an even vaguer understanding of the steps of the scientific method. This chapter is therefore designed as a review, as discussing every aspect is beyond the scope of treatment here. The reader searching for additional information should refer to the many different volumes that cover the subject in detail, several of which are referenced herein. This chapter therefore will first outline what science is and is not and in the process, demonstrate how different areas of science (e.g., anthropology, medicine, chemistry, and so on) are connected to each other. Following this will be an introduction to the scientific method with a subsequent section exploring how researchers develop ideas. The chapter concludes with a case study to illustrate some of the points made.

INTRODUCTION TO SCIENCE

Science is the overall discipline that explores the *natural world*. It is divided into several major divisions: the natural or physical sciences (e.g., chemistry, computer science), the life sciences (e.g., biology, microbiology), the health sciences (e.g., medicine, pharmacology), and the social sciences (e.g., anthropology, psychology). The natural world includes the Earth, plants, animals, planets, atoms, elements, fossils, mountains, bacteria, DNA, human bones, things we have created using naturally occurring components (e.g., plastic, glass), and so on. In other words, the natural world consists of *physical* things—things that are tangible or that can be physically measured or observed in some way. Science investigates the natural world through *inquiry*, which is the search for unknown information. Scientists pose *questions* about the natural world when they come across phenomena that seem to pose a problem in some way. For example, "Can we see the effects of chronic obesity and anorexia on the skeleton?" is a question resulting from the problem of expanding the biological profile to include body mass estimation; and "Can we differentiate the effects of perimortem trauma from postmortem trauma when bones are subjected to fire?" is a question that results from the problem of how a phenomenon such as fire can affect bone postmortem (Moore, 2008; Schmidt and Symes, 2008).

Scientific inquiry is designed based on certain assumptions scientists have about nature itself. These assumptions are: a physical universe exists, the principles that govern it can be discovered through science, and our knowledge of the universe is constantly growing and changing when new knowledge is discovered (Graziano and Raulin, 2000). What we know about the natural world grows exponentially as our level of knowledge expands and new questions arise. To use an example from modern technology, the first computer capable of performing rapid calculations was functional in 1945 and took up the space of a small house (Rojas, 2001). Today, due to the fact that discoveries in computer science and engineering have continually built upon each other, many of us carry around very powerful computers that fit in our pockets in the form of our smart phones. An example that further illustrates this rapid growth of technology in an almost astonishing way is the fact that in terms of processing speed and memory, the laptops we are writing this chapter on are *millions of times* more powerful[1] than the computer on the first shuttle that went to the moon! All of the advances in just this one area of science have occurred in the span of only seven decades.

Furthermore, one new discovery, while answering one question, often poses several more unanswered questions, and can lead to several different lines of new inquiry. For example, when Todd (1920) showed that the human pubic bone is useful in age estimation of the skeleton, this served to pose the question, "Which other bones reflect chronological age?" Today, over 90 years later, skeletal biologists continue exploring this question for a number of different bones and features (refer to Uhl [Chapter 3], this volume).

Natural versus Supernatural

"A set of ideas that cannot ... be falsified is not science." (Gould, 1981a:35)

Note that a key part of the definition of science is the phrase "natural world"—this phrase is the cornerstone of what science is. Science has the capacity to inform us about this natural world. However, there is a limitation to what science can do: it cannot inform us about the *supernatural* world. The very definition of "supernatural" is "of or relating to an order of existence *beyond the visible observable* universe; departing from what is usual or normal especially so as to appear to *transcend the laws of nature*" (Merriam-Webster definition, 2003; emphasis added). As science is defined as dealing with the natural world, it cannot by definition make inquiries into the supernatural world.

Therefore, while we can use science to learn about things such as evolution, fossils, the age of the universe, etc. (all natural things), we cannot use it to learn about the existence of supernatural beings or phenomena. The reason for this is that science can only test things in the observable world. By "test" we are referring to the methods we use to seek scientific information (refer to hypothesis testing section, later in this chapter). There is no way to scientifically

---

[1]Hall (1963) lists the Apollo Guidance Computer characteristics, which when compared to modern computers, had five million times *less* memory and 250 million times *less* processing capability! (G. Westerwick, personal communication, 2012).

test something like faith or the existence of any given supernatural being, because the existence of either of these phenomena cannot be <u>disproved</u>. Science works by testing and disproving questions: there is no conceivable test that can show a supernatural being <u>does not</u> exist. You might *feel* faith, you might *know* a higher being exists, but you simply cannot test either through scientific means. For these reasons, scientific methods can only be applied to the natural world, which by definition is separate from the supernatural world.

The Law of Parsimony

This concept states that the simplest explanation is the likeliest one. By "simple" we mean the most logical and least complicated explanation for a given phenomenon or observation. If you find a skeleton in the woods of Tennessee and infer that the puncture marks you see all over the bones were caused by the individual's pet alligator when there is no evidence to suggest (1) the person's identity and (2) they had a pet alligator and (3) the pet alligator caused the person's demise, then the likelihood of this inference being correct is <u>very</u> low. In addition, this being the state of Tennessee where there are no alligators in the wild (and probably very few being kept as pets), the most likely and simplest explanation is that the puncture marks were caused by a dog that scavenged the remains. Parsimony is important for many steps of science, including hypothesis construction and critical analysis of the results. Remember the forensic pathologist's old adage, "If you see hoof prints in Texas, think horses, not zebras."

The Hypothesis

In science, a **hypothesis**[2] is a scientific statement that proposes an explanation about something in the natural world. The most important part about hypotheses is that they are designed in such a way that they can be *tested* and *falsified*. Statements that cannot be tested do not meet the criteria for a hypothesis. For example, a statement such as, "the first person to travel over the Bering Land Bridge to settle in North America did so on June 12, 8023 BCE" cannot be tested. This statement is way too narrow and there is no test that could show the exact date that the peopling of the New World commenced. However, a statement such as, "the peopling of the New World began around 10,000 years ago" can be tested. This statement is more general and radiometric dating methods (which give date ranges) applied to prehistoric archaeological sites can be used to test this latter hypothesis.

The second criterion for hypotheses, falsification, is important because as scientific knowledge grows, it should be possible to find that previous explanatory statements were not correct via new discoveries or evidence. If it were not for the falsifying principle, then valid hypotheses would not be able to replace invalid ones. As Gould sums up, "science advances primarily by *replacement*, not by addition" (1981b:322; emphasis added). In science we are trying to obtain valid explanations for different phenomena, and it must be the case that explanations found to be invalid are not competing with newer explanations in the testing stage or explanations already shown by the latest evidence to be the most valid. Whether

---

[2]All bolded terms are defined in the glossary at the end of this volume.

or not a hypothesis is falsified depends on the level of surety that you set with the test (often with the statistics chosen) and the critical analysis of the results. It is important to note that your results and thus your determination of falsifiability will not always be cut and dry. There are often gray areas where the results are inconclusive—which may indicate that you need to refine your hypothesis and/or your testing mechanism.

For example, a prevailing hypothesis that stood for centuries in the Western world was that the Earth was flat. This hypothesis was of course falsified when sea journeys began in earnest by European nations in the fifteenth and sixteenth centuries and the ships did not fall off the edge of the Earth. The new evidence of ships continuing to sail past the horizon without falling in part resulted in the replacement of the earlier hypothesis of the Earth being flat.

In addition, the very nature of science is that while we <u>can</u> show that a hypothesis is *not* always true, we <u>cannot</u> show that one is *always* true, because there might be some future test or evidence that could refute current knowledge and results. This is reflected in the language we use when analyzing the results—we either *reject* or *fail to reject* the hypothesis. A simpler way to think about this is that we can either state the hypothesis has been *supported* by the results, or that it has not been supported by the results. Refer to the hypothesis testing section later in this chapter for more detailed information about hypotheses.

Fact and Theory

Facts are essentially the world's data (Gould, 1981a): vertebrates have skeletal systems, most mammals give birth to live young, and humans need to breathe oxygen to survive are all examples. A *theory* results from a number of related hypotheses that have been tested and retested and not shown to be untrue (Gould, 1981a). Facts and theories differ because while facts are *always* true (all vertebrate animals have skeletal systems), theories have been shown to <u>not be false</u>, based on the preponderance of the existing evidence. Theories are therefore explanations, verified over time, that are based on many consistent observations from different and various experiments.

Note that this definition of "theory" is very different from the way we use the word in everyday language. The general public would define "theory" as meaning "guess." In science, a theory is not a guess. The Germ Theory of Disease is a valid *explanation* for what causes disease, not mere conjecture. Similarly, the Theory of Evolution is also a sound *explanation* for species change, not speculation. These theories came into existence after the testing and retesting of a variety of different hypotheses showing (1) the explanations were the simplest ones for the phenomenon, (2) the explanations made predictions that could be tested, and (3) the explanations had not been shown to be untrue (Graziano and Raulin, 2000). These two theories have stood the test of time because the vast accumulation of evidence has continued to support them and because they still meet the three criteria for a theory listed above.

We have entered into the preceding discussion about science versus religious belief and hypothesis versus theory because as an anthropologist, it is quite likely that you will be tasked with teaching the basics of science at some point in your career—and it is absolutely essential that you first, fully understand the principles, and second, are able to talk about it in a convincing and understandable way. There is no greater misunderstanding with regard to scientific principles among the general public than the points of what a scientific theory is and what science can and cannot do.

The Interconnected Nature of Science

It is important to demonstrate that each discovery in science builds upon a previous discovery, and skeletal biology is no exception. Biological anthropology, like many disciplines, is a field that taps into discoveries and advances in several other areas of science. For example, knowledge from anatomy, biology, and medicine is essential for understanding the human skeleton and the evolutionary processes that affect it. Paleoanthropologists rely heavily on knowledge from geology and paleontology. Forensic anthropologists who study taphonomy learn about some taphonomic processes from paleontological research. Chemistry is a key discipline with discoveries that have led to isotope analysis and radiometric dating, applicable for anthropologists working in past or prehistoric time periods. Advances in physics and engineering have led to the invention of advanced technologies we utilize, such as ground penetrating radar. It is essential to appreciate the importance of this multidisciplinary nature of science, how it relates to skeletal biology, and your particular interests. Do not neglect searching for information within related disciplines (or collaborating with scientists in other fields), as a method or discovery in a related field may positively contribute to your own inquiry. For an example, refer to the case study at the end of this chapter.

THE SCIENTIFIC METHOD

The development of the scientific method is often credited to Galileo due in part to his experiments with the physics of motion. While scholars debate this attribution, the fact remains that his experiments did follow the sequence of the method as we use it today (Shapere, 1974; Sharratt, 1994). The sequence is as follows: (1) make an *observation* about something; (2) state the *problem/question*; (3) formulate a *hypothesis*; (4) design and carry out the *methods*; (5) analyze the data to arrive at *results*; (6) come to a *conclusion*; and finally, (7) *communicate* with others. Steps 1–6 are covered below and Step 7 is covered by DiGangi (Chapter 17), this volume. See Table 2.1.

From a philosophical standpoint, there are several approaches we can take to any given scientific inquiry. The approach you take with your project will depend on the type of observation made and/or question that you have (see upcoming sections). The two major ways that we can approach scientific inquiry are through **induction** and **deduction**. Inductive approaches follow closely the organization of the scientific method as discussed throughout this chapter: an observation that leads to hypothesis formation, and later, theory (Snieder and Larner, 2009). For example, Charles Darwin's theory of natural selection followed an

TABLE 2.1 Steps of the Scientific Method

1. Observation
2. Problem/Question
3. Hypothesis
4. Methods
5. Results
6. Conclusion
7. Communication

inductive approach. Based on observations made of specialized adaptations in different animals, he developed a hypothesis that adaptations leading to the survival of an organism so that it could reproduce would be beneficial and therefore would be selected for (Darwin, 1859).

Deductive approaches work in an opposite manner, from theory to hypothesis to observations (Snieder and Larner, 2009). Scientific theory sometimes is based on inferences that may not have yet been directly observed. For example, the discovery of the structure of **DNA** to be a double helix in the 1950s took a deductive approach. Based on other evidence and inferences, scientific theory stated that a molecule of life existed. Several researchers therefore devised hypotheses as to what that molecule would look like and set out to make observations that ultimately revealed the double helix structure (Watson and Crick, 1953).

Each study in skeletal biology can fit into one of several broad categories of inquiry: (1) testing a hypothesis; (2) measuring a relationship or relationships; (3) constructing a model or models; or (4) generating a descriptive analysis or analyses. The first category is explained in detail in the upcoming section on hypotheses. Examples of studies that measure relationships are stature and craniometric studies. For instance, the study of craniometrics looks for relationships between measurements of the skull and certain aspects about either the individual or their population, such as ancestry or **biological distance** (see DiGangi and Hefner [Chapter 5]; and McKeown and Schmidt [Chapter 12], this volume). If a relationship exists, the study results will be used to construct a model (in the form of stature formulae, discriminant functions, biological distance, etc.). Model constructing can include experimental research, as seen in studies in taphonomy or trauma for example (refer to Marden et al. [Chapter 9]; and Kroman and Symes [Chapter 8], this volume) or when theory building, as seen in the **osteological paradox** for instance (Wood et al., 1992) (see DiGangi and Moore [Chapter 1]; Smith [Chapter 7], this volume). Descriptive analysis has been used most often in **paleopathology**, although there is a movement towards model building and hypothesis testing in this area (see Smith [Chapter 7], this volume).

Step 1: Observation and Inference

The first step of the scientific method is **observation**. Observations can be *qualitative* or *quantitative*. In general, qualitative observations focus on description, while quantitative observations focus on numbered amounts. We can further break down qualitative observations into the categories of *nominal* and *ordinal-categorical* variables. A *variable* is some characteristic that can be observed or measured in some way (Walsh and Ollenburger, 2001). Nominal variables have no logical ordering, at least not in the sense that numbered amounts do (L. Konigsberg, personal communication 2012). Presence/absence traits fall into this category, such as presence/absence of the metopic suture or presence/absence of parietal foramen. Ordinal-categorical variables have a relative ranking scale not associated with quantitative differences (Zar, 2010). An example would be the scoring system for sexually dimorphic cranial features from *Standards for Data Collection from Human Skeletal Remains* (Buikstra and Ubelaker, 1994): features such as the nuchal crest and mental eminence are scored on a scale from 1 to 5, with "1" being minimal expression and "5" being maximum expression.

Another way to think of quantitative variables is as *metric* variables (L. Konigsberg, personal communication 2012). Examples could be that the measurement of maximum cranial breadth is 136 millimeters or the mean value of maximum length of the radius from Colombian males is 232 millimeters. Any studies that measure something numerically use metric variables: studies of stature and of craniometrics are examples (see Moore and Ross [Chapter 6]; and McKeown and Schmidt [Chapter 12], this volume).

For all the examples listed above, the observation is clear and easy to make. However, what do we do when we cannot directly see or measure something? One principle we rely on is the **principle of uniformitarianism**, which states that the natural mechanisms by which processes occurred in the past are the same mechanisms by which processes occur today (i.e., wind erosion, mutation rates of genes, natural selection, and so on). Using this principle we are able to come to conclusions about things we cannot see or measure *directly* today. While initially posited by Hutton (1788) and Lyell (1830) for geological processes, scientists have adapted the concept for application to other sciences, such as biology. For example, how do we know that four and a half million years ago, the geographic locality of Aramis in East Africa consisted of a woodland environment as opposed to the arid environment it is today? How do we know *how* fractures on a bone were caused? How do we know that a particular prehistoric culture had a specific religious reason for burying bodies with heads facing a certain direction? Did anyone at the time make observations that they wrote down for us today? Obviously not—but that still begs the question of how we know the answers to any of these questions or ones similar. The answer lies in inference. An **inference** is an interpretation of an observation. For example, one can infer that bones feel lighter than usual because some of the mineral that gives them weight has been resorbed due to a disease the individual developed during life.[3]

Based on observations of things we can directly see and measure today, we are able to infer certain things about the natural world. Aramis contains an abundance of fossils of mammals that inhabit woodland areas. Based on this and other geological evidence, we can infer it was not always the arid environment it is now (White et al., 2009). We can look at fractures and infer the biomechanics behind how they were caused based on results from experiments designed to look at fracture mechanics (see Kroman and Symes [Chapter 8], this volume). Prehistoric archaeologists and bioarchaeologists can infer information about a culture's religious beliefs from comparative knowledge of other extant and extinct cultures, and from a variety of other lines of evidence, including artifacts.

Inference is something we use frequently in skeletal biology. Often we make inferences based on results from other studies and then test them, such as inferring that if one bone contains age-related information, then other bones must as well. Another important example that has resulted in some groundbreaking new research for forensic anthropology involves inferences that change in stature or cranial dimensions over several decades (known as **secular change**[4]) would affect our use of standards created from skeletal collections of individuals who died 50 or more years ago (Langley-Shirley and Jantz, 2010).

---

[3]The mineral is hydroxyapatite and the disease would be **osteoporosis**.

[4]Due to an improvement or deterioration over time in factors such as nutrition, access to medical care, infectious disease, etc. See discussion in Moore and Ross (Chapter 6) and McKeown and Schmidt (Chapter 12), this volume.

Step 2: The Problem and the Question

In science, we often talk about "the problem" or "the question." It is important to explain the distinction between these two terms, even though we often use them interchangeably. **The problem** refers to the larger, overall picture, while **the question** is more specific and contributes to resolving part of the problem. For example, Dr. William Bass founded the famous forensic anthropological research facility at the University of Tennessee in Knoxville because he had been approached by law enforcement with a time-since-death question for a body found after a cemetery flood that he underestimated by over a century (Bass and Jefferson, 2003). Therefore, the problem he was tackling with the creation of a specialized outdoor decomposition facility was that human decomposition is a phenomenon science knows nothing about. There are numerous questions that are specific to this particular problem. Examples include the following: How long does it take a human body to decompose in different temperatures? What are the stages of human decomposition? What are the different variables that affect decomposition?

There are two types of questions—*open-ended* or *closed-ended* ones (Marder, 2011). See Table 2.2. Closed questions typically already have answers that are known or can be found out. Examples include the following: How many bones does an adult human have? What is the range of maximum cranial breadth for nonpathological adult skulls? How many bony muscle attachments are there on the femur and what are they? Open questions on the other hand are more challenging and complex because multiple answers may exist (Marder, 2011). Examples include the following: Which bony features contain reliable information about age-related change? Can shape analysis of the skull reveal information about biological distance between populations? Can we determine what prehistoric health was like from examining skeletons?

Your research will most likely include some combination of closed and open questions. Even if you are only focusing on answering a closed question, consider that each closed question essentially ties into an open question (Marder, 2011) and therefore will in some way contribute to answering an open question. For example, a closed question in skeletal biology may be as follows: Within what age range does the distal femoral epiphysis close in modern Mexican males? This question has a simple answer that can be easily discovered. An open question that this would tie into would be the following: What are the driving

TABLE 2.2   Examples of Open and Closed Questions

Open-Ended Questions	Closed-Ended Questions
Which bones can be used to estimate stature?	How many bones does a 1-year-old have?
Are there features on the skeleton that can be used to estimate body mass?	How many muscle attachment sites are there on the os coxae?
Can analysis of cranial landmarks be used to estimate ancestry?	What are the cranial landmarks?
Can we tell what caused a particular lesion on a bone?	What are the diseases we already know that do affect bone?

factor(s) behind secular change affecting the timing of epiphyseal fusion in humans? This question is much more complex and would require a number of tests to answer it properly.

At this stage, you want to state your question in specific terms and you will further refine this into your hypothesis later. For example, don't ask, "What can lumbar vertebrae reveal about an individual?" Rather, ask, "Can the fifth lumbar vertebra (L5) be used to estimate stature?" You will base your question on the observation(s) you have already made and ask if it is testable given current knowledge and technology. If your question is whether or not the fifth lumbar vertebra can be used to estimate stature, then yes, that is a testable question. You could measure the height of several L5 bodies from a sample of individuals for whom you have living stature information. You could then perform a regression analysis to determine if the height of the vertebra correlates with living stature (refer to Moore and Ross [Chapter 6], this volume for more information on stature research).

If your question is technically testable but the test would require logistic planning and resources that would be prohibitive, then you will want to pose a different question. For example, if you wish to develop a stature equation based on the femur for a sample of 6000 skeletons but you will be working by yourself and you only have one week to do it, you will have to accept a smaller sample size or come up with a different project. Once you have determined whether or not your question is testable, begin thinking about *how* you will go about designing the test.

At this early stage, most likely all you have actually done is *think* about your observation and problem. What you must also do is background research on your problem and question (refer to section on library research in DiGangi [Chapter 17], this volume; and the upcoming section on developing ideas, this chapter). There is no point in reinventing the wheel if research has already been done on the exact same question. However, reasons to repeat a study might include testing different statistical techniques, to verify the results, to improve upon a method, or perhaps to validate a particular method for another population. Even if the same exact question has not been studied before, it is likely that similar questions have been, and you can use these studies to help you formulate your own research design. Science builds on what has been already done—there is no reason to come up with an entirely novel research design unless it is your goal to do so. Do not skip over this background research step. We attended a presentation once in which the researcher presented their hypothesis for unusual features found on some skulls. Unfortunately, it turned out that these unusual features were simply a normal anatomical variant, a fact that was pointed out to the person at the conclusion of their presentation. Doing library research initially after having first made the observation of the features would have saved them a lot of time and embarrassment.

Step 3: Hypothesis Testing

As outlined earlier, a hypothesis is a scientific statement based on an observation(s) that is both testable and falsifiable. Hypotheses that are valid meet these two criteria. This is important because as mentioned previously, science works by testing and disproving questions. For example, a statement such as, "osteophyte formation on the lumbar vertebrae is age-related" is both testable and falsifiable. You could use a sample of skeletons that have real-age information and look at presence/absence or even degree of osteophyte formation to see if there is a correlation with age. You might find out that there is a relationship, or you might falsify your statement by finding out there is not a relationship. On the other hand, a statement such as, "osteophytes on the lumbar vertebrae of males form more interesting patterns than those on females" is not testable or falsifiable. The determination of how aesthetically pleasing the formation of the osteophytes is subjective and therefore not scientifically testable.

Hypotheses should also be the simplest explanation for the observation. Making statements such as "osteophyte formation on lumbar vertebrae is due to the overconsumption of broccoli during life or the type of mattress slept on" are overly complicated explanations and additionally, these statements would be difficult if not impossible to test, depending on the type of antemortem information available. The simplest explanation is also the likeliest one because it is the least likely explanation to be a coincidence. Even if you were able to show that people who ate a lot of broccoli have osteophytes (as compared to people who did not eat a lot of broccoli), it remains a dubious relationship and it does not necessarily mean that the broccoli is *causing* the osteophytes. On the other hand, it is much more likely that based on what we know about skeletal degeneration, osteophytes would result from increasing age.

When undergoing hypothesis testing, we must define the **independent** and **dependent variables**. As stated previously, a variable is some characteristic that can be observed or measured (Walsh and Ollenburger, 2001). The dependent variable is the variable you will be measuring and the independent variable is what will change throughout the study. An exception would be in regression settings, where you have to measure bone length (the dependent variable) *and* real stature (the independent variable), for example. You can also view the relationship as one of cause and effect: the independent variable as causing a change in the dependent variable (Marder, 2011; but see Konigsberg et al., 1997 and Konigsberg and Frankenberg [Chapter 11], this volume). In our example of osteophyte formation, age is the independent variable and the formation of osteophytes is the dependent variable. The sample will be selected so that there is variation in the age-at-death structure (each skeleton you look at will have a different real age, ideally distributed from young adults to older adults); and you will be recording osteophyte formation. You also believe that age (the independent variable) will cause a change to the osteophyte formation (the dependent variable).

Co-variates

In skeletal biology, we often run into situations where the dependent variable (the one you are measuring) is correlated with other variables. These are known as **co-variates** (Huitema, 2011). Typical co-variates with the human skeleton include age, sex, ancestry, activity, diet, disease expression, traumatic injuries, musculoskeletal markers of stress, etc. Each of these variables could be tied to another variable inextricably. For example, males in one population may exhibit more trauma of a certain type (due to interpersonal violence) than females of the same age in the same population (e.g., see Smith, 2003). Biological research with humans (or any organism) will never eliminate every co-variate, but you need to try your best to limit (or control for) as many as possible. For example, if you want to just look at age, how do you eliminate sex from having a confounding effect on the results? The simplest way is to analyze individuals of each sex separately or use samples that are age and sex-matched.

With our example of osteophyte formation, possible co-variates could include sex, activity patterns, and diet (and possibly others). While we probably cannot control for the effect activity and diet may have had on the osteophyte formation (since that type of antemortem information may not be available), we can control for sex by analyzing males and females separately. Your construction of your hypothesis test needs to be done carefully so that co-variates and how to handle them are considered. Later the critical analysis of the results should examine whether any co-variates had an effect.

Null and Alternative Hypotheses

After you have the variables figured out, you will further divide your hypothesis into **null** and **alternative** hypotheses. The null hypothesis is stated in negative, or rather, conservative terms and will be that any changes in the independent variable will *not* lead to changes in the dependent variable (Marder, 2011). Essentially with the hypothesis test we are challenging the conservative viewpoint, namely, that one variable has no effect on the other. The alternative hypothesis will be the opposite: that changes in the independent variable *will* lead to changes in the dependent variable. With our example, the null hypothesis is that osteophyte formation on the lumbar vertebrae is not age-related. The alternative hypothesis is that osteophyte formation on the lumbar vertebrae is age-related.

You will either *reject* or *fail to reject* the null hypothesis. The term "fail to reject" in this sense is another way of saying "accept"; however, we usually do not use the term "accept" because that indicates some measure of complete truth, which may not necessarily be the case as other unknown factors may be at play—or the hypothesis may be accepted in one situation given certain variables but a slight variable change may change the outcome, even though the hypothesis itself has not changed. In addition, keep in mind that failure to reject the null hypothesis does not necessarily mean that the alternative hypothesis is the correct explanation. Another alternative hypothesis may exist. Remember that you cannot show that something is *always* true, but you *can* show that it is *not* always true. The logic here is that there may be some evidence yet undiscovered or a test yet undeveloped that would negate previous results. For example, skeletal biologists used to infer that pits on the dorsal side of the pubic symphysis, commonly seen in female adults, meant that a female had given birth. Even though not everyone was in agreement about this in the past, today the consensus is that further research is necessary given the fact that pitting can occur in males and there may be other causal factors at play (Ubelaker and De La Paz, 2012). Refer to Figure 2.1 for a flowchart diagram of hypothesis testing.

Step 4: Methods Development/Research Design

Once you have formulated your hypothesis and question (or determined what type of descriptive analysis you will undertake), it is time to set up your methods and research design. This is a critical step. Descriptive analysis is primarily used for paleopathology, trauma, or taphonomy case studies (see Smith [Chapter 7]; Kroman and Symes [Chapter 8]; and Marden et al. [Chapter 9], this volume). However, while case studies are valuable for describing novel findings, you should focus on a project that involves hypothesis testing for your thesis or dissertation so that you hone all of the associated research skills. Based on your library research and conversations with your advisor, you have probably already

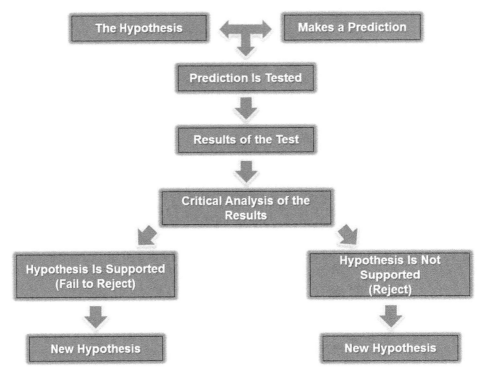

FIGURE 2.1 Hypothesis testing flowchart. Note that no matter the outcome of a test, new hypotheses are generated based on the critical analysis of the results.

identified the skeletal collection you wish to use for your project. Logistics with regards to access, permissions, travel, etc., all become important here. (Refer to the upcoming section on developing a research idea for more information.) Assuming that you have already worked all these issues out, you will need to sit down and figure out several things: (1) data collection method; (2) appropriate sample size; (3) possible sources of bias inherent to the sample; (4) how to contend with intra- or interobserver error; and (5) how to analyze the data. Each of these deserves further mention.

A good discussion of sample size and intra- and interobserver error as it relates to skeletal biology can be found in Buikstra and Ubelaker (1994). Consult this reference for a complete discussion; however, to summarize you need to conduct a statistical analysis of **intraobserver error** (if doing all the scoring/measuring by yourself) and/or a statistical analysis of **interobserver error** (if two or more individuals are scoring/measuring). This is to demonstrate the replicability of your study. If either you or between two or more observers are not measuring or scoring consistently, then this will negatively affect the results and introduce a lot of error. Ideally, your study will have a very low level of this type of error. See Smith (Chapter 7), this volume for more information on intra- and interobserver error.

Further, you need to consider the introduction of unintentional bias on the part of each observer. For example, if you are conducting an aging study but the real age of the individual is visible on the storage box before you open it, you *will* be affected by that whether or not you intend to. Ideally, you should cover up the age/sex/ancestry information on the boxes of those skeletons you will use for your study ahead of time (a day or so in advance so you will not remember information about specific cases). If time is a factor, then have a helper do this for you. Additionally, other bones in the box that you are not analyzing will also cause bias as you see them while unpacking the box to pull out the bone(s) you need. If you can, have a helper pull out the bones you will be analyzing. This will ensure that each observer is "blind" to other information that may lead to bias.

Each study will be different with regard to sample size. For some, such as certain paleo-pathological case studies, the sample size is obviously one. For other studies, a sample size of one is unacceptable. In order to have statistical significance, you must choose a sample size that will be appropriate based on the population variance of the measurements or traits being studied (Buikstra and Ubelaker, 1994). Choosing an appropriate sample size can be tricky and confusing, especially since many introductory statistics courses teach that a sample of 30 is large enough for statistical significance, which is unwise (L. Konigsberg, personal communication 2012). Referring to statistical texts and previously published articles in your topic will help you choose the most appropriate sample size for your study. For information on important factors to consider when choosing a collection and sample, especially with regard to inherent bias, see Box 2.1.

The data collection method will rarely be something novel. If you are validating a stature equation for example, then you will follow the same method for measuring

---

BOX 2.1

BIAS

Types of Bias

In addition to the **osteological paradox** (see DiGangi and Moore [Chapter 1] and Smith [Chapter 7], this volume for detailed discussion), there are several types of bias with skeletal collections: (1) interment, (2) archaeological, (3) recovery, and (4) taphonomic.

Interment bias refers to the fact that not all individuals have an equal chance of being buried at a certain location due to the particular mortuary program in place. For example, infants may not be buried at all and social status or other cultural reasons may determine who is buried where. See Smith (Chapter 7), this volume for details.

For archaeological bias, only those sites discovered and excavated will contribute to the sample. If the archaeological recovery was focused on houses for example, burials located elsewhere may have been overlooked. See Smith (Chapter 7), this volume for more information.

In terms of recovery bias, only so many sites are discovered and excavated for a variety of reasons, resulting in collections that are mere fractions of once living populations (White et al., 2012). We then use the individuals in these collections as

(Continued)

BOX 2.1 (cont'd)

representative of the entire population, bias notwithstanding, because that is all that exists.

Taphonomic bias results from everything that happens to remains after the moment of death. A variety of factors influence remains preservation—some will not be preserved at all, some will be deteriorated, and others will have excellent preservation. In some cases, this may affect the preservation of remains from a single site (i.e., infant remains not being preserved as well as adult remains—see Walker et al., 1988). Refer to Marden et al. (Chapter 9), this volume for more information on taphonomy.

There are other sources of bias. Modern collections may be disproportionately composed of individuals falling into one demographic versus another because there are cultural reasons for individuals being in the collection (e.g., who decides to donate themselves and why; whose decision has been made for them by someone else and why).

The Sample and Bias

We use samples to make statements about populations. A "**population**" is a group of individuals who are contemporaneous, occupy relatively the same area geographically, have a shared culture (language, traditions, belief systems, etc.), and who tend to find mates from within the same group. An ideal sample is both (1) smaller than the population and (2) representative of the population; and is used to derive conclusions about the entire population. This is a necessary strategy in skeletal biology and biology in general, because we could never analyze every individual in the population.

It is therefore first necessary to identify the population (which group of people you are interested in studying) and then draw the sample. Ideally the sample should be drawn in such a way that the entire population is characterized, e.g., having an equal number of males and females and all **age cohorts** represented. However, the sample you analyze is obviously limited by the skeletons available in the collection. Further, if the sample originated from a cemetery, remember that the age-at-death profile does not mirror the proportions from the living population (because the cemetery represents those who *died*). See DiGangi and Moore (Chapter 1) and Smith (Chapter 7) for more information on this part of the osteological paradox.

Each collection is the result of a mixture of the sources of bias discussed above, in addition to the respective social and political climate present during its initial curation. For example, some modern collections are composed of individuals who were impoverished during life. This makes extrapolating conclusions about the population in general from such a specific group problematic given the particular environmental conditions they may have been overly exposed to as a result of their impoverishment, disproportionately altering their skeletal features. As another example, the prehistoric skeletal collection curated by the Archaeological Museum in La Serena, Chile has one archaeological site represented by only skulls, as the archaeologists who did the excavations in the 1940s did not think recovering the rest of the bones was important (not an uncommon practice in the early twentieth century given the emphasis on **typology**—see DiGangi and Moore [Chapter 1]; DiGangi and Hefner [Chapter 5]; and Smith [Chapter 7], this volume).

the bones that the authors of the study you are validating did. If measuring or scoring bone features, you should refer to Buikstra and Ubelaker (1994) for the appropriate method to use. *You will want to ensure that you understand the scoring or measurement definitions of whatever feature you will be analyzing.* Ideally, you should do a trial run-through with about 10–30 skeletons to practice the scoring/measuring method prior to actual data collection. This becomes especially important if you are using a piece of equipment that requires practice and expertise such as a 3-D digitizer for the first time (refer to McKeown and Schmidt [Chapter 12], this volume). If you collect data differently from the way everyone else has done it, then your results will not be comparable to anything already done (or that will be done). If you will be using any kind of equipment (from calipers to a mass spectrometer) then ensure that the equipment has been calibrated properly and is in working order. Further, if you are using calipers for example, do not switch tools in the middle of data collection for consistency—i.e., use the same calipers for all the observations. If you forgot to calibrate your calipers and they are off by 1 mm for example, then all the measurements will be off by 1 mm and you might be able to detect the error and correct it later.

You will need to begin considering how you will analyze the data at this stage. This is important because your analysis method may be impacted by your data collection method. For example, certain statistics packages may only accept a certain number format (i.e., periods or commas for decimal points, a certain number of digits, or empty fields may not be allowed). You may not be able to import your data into certain packages directly from Microsoft Excel or other file formats. You want to know these things at the outset, before you have collected your data. Again, keep your analysis plan simple. Choose the statistical tests that are most appropriate for your hypothesis and data. If you are new to statistics, then now is the time to take one or two courses to catch up. Introductory statistical texts, especially those geared towards students in the social sciences, will also help in this regard. For example, Agresti and Finlay (2009) and Walsh and Ollenburger (2001) are good starting points.

In addition, you should set up your data collection sheet now. If possible, do a test run-through with the data sheet and a small sample of ten skeletons or so to make sure that the sheet is set up logically for what you will be doing. If you have enough time and resources, it is also a good idea to do a miniature pilot project using a smaller sample size so that you can work out all the logistical and analysis issues before beginning your larger project.

When you have worked through these steps and are finally ready to begin data collection, remember to stay organized. Document everything you do. Each day, keep a record of which skeletons you look at or samples you take. Your data collection sheet can include this information. This will help if later on you realize you have to go back for some reason and look at a particular skeleton again. If you take photographs, keep a detailed photo log that includes the date, photograph exposure number, individual skeleton number, the bone and side, the part of the bone (distal, proximal, etc.), and the anatomical position of the bone or feature being depicted (i.e., view of anterior side, etc.). You will not remember later and you may not be able to tell from the photograph. Refer to Smith (Chapter 7), this volume, for further recommendations regarding photographs. Being organized and keeping excellent records will also assist you later when it is time to write up your study. See Table 2.3.

TABLE 2.3   Documentation Checklist for Data Collection

For datasheet:	For photo log:
✔ Date and your name	✔ Date
✔ Individual number	✔ Individual number
✔ Site name/location if applicable	✔ Bone name and side
✔ Samples taken if applicable	✔ Anatomical part of bone
✔ Photos taken? If so, photo numbers	✔ Detailed photo description
✔ The data itself	✔ View photo taken from

Steps 5 and 6: Analysis, Results, and Conclusion

Now comes one of the best parts—analyze your data! You already decided what tests you would undertake when you were in the research design stage. As mentioned earlier, if you are not strong in statistics, now is the time to review. Refer to statistics books and take a statistics course so that you understand the output and interpret it correctly. You will need to *critically analyze* your results. This means that you will thoughtfully scrutinize the output and decide whether your hypothesis was supported or not. Statistics packages will generate a series of numbers and tables or graphs that you need to be able to interpret and put the significance of these numbers into words. It is always a good idea to show your results to someone else before you write them up—your advisor, for example—so that you can make sure there were no problems with the data collection stage or with analysis. Someone with more experience with your topic should be able to pick up on any subtle inconsistencies with the results.

Based on your results, determine if there were any sources of error (contamination, inaccurate measurements, interobserver/intraobserver error, etc.). If so, how might you avoid this error in the future? Depending on the study undertaken, you may want to repeat your study later, on a subset of the original sample. You may do this to check intraobserver error for example. If you developed or tested a method, you may want to repeat the study on a completely different sample in order to validate your original results. Perhaps there will be different results when a different sample or population is used, or maybe there will be different (unknown) variables that create a different outcome. There may also be legal reasons to repeat or validate a study. For example, consider the precedent set by the war crimes trials for the former Yugoslavia where the use of standards created on North American populations was questioned as to their validity when being used to identify Eastern Europeans (Kimmerle and Jantz, 2008).

Consider that your results will not be valid if they are based on opinions and not data; if you draw conclusions that do not logically follow from the evidence; if you overgeneralize; or if your sample size is too small or overly biased in some way. When you do draw your conclusions, make sure they follow logically from the results. Decide whether or not your hypothesis is supported and what the further questions are which arose based on your results (there always are some). In addition, state what your suggestions are for future studies based on what you found and the new questions that surfaced.

Scientific Integrity

You are already familiar with the concept of integrity in general. Academic honesty consists of not fabricating data or results and not stealing or copying someone else's original ideas, data, or results. Your data that include photographs, actual data collected, results, write-ups, and so on all fall into the category of intellectual property. If someone else wants to use your intellectual property they must receive permission from either you or the copyright holder and cite it properly. The consequences for violating academic honesty range from a guilty conscience to a potentially life-destroying event. The scientist who fabricated his data and results with cloning research and narrowly avoided prison for it comes to mind (Sang-Hun, 2009). Be particularly careful when referencing. When taking notes from articles or books, use bullet points in your own words. When you do your write-up, you will have to formulate your own original sentences. Learn how to paraphrase, use quotes when necessary, and always cite the sources of your information.[5]

Data Curation

While your data are part of your intellectual property, that doesn't mean that they exclusively belong to only you. You generated data as part of an inquiry for new scientific information (which technically belongs to everyone), and therefore, you must care for them so they remain accessible to you and others later on. Today we save most of our data (measurements, observations, photographs, write-ups, etc.) digitally. However, as technology grows and programs or file formats change, at some point your files will no longer be able to be opened—making all your hard work disappear. Make sure that you update your digital files to newer versions as applicable and/or save hard paper copies of everything (preferably on acid-free paper) for long-term curation. Saving files to a program in the Internet cloud is also advised, especially while the project is in progress, so that you do not lose any work as a result of hard drive failure or other disasters.

DEVELOPING A RESEARCH QUESTION: HOW TO THINK OF AND DEVELOP IDEAS

As an advanced undergraduate or new graduate student, this is probably the main question on your mind when it comes to doing your research project. During your first year in graduate school you learn very quickly that the production of original research is a major expectation and that you have to develop your own project that you will primarily work on by yourself, with guidance from your professors. However, most likely you have little

---

[5]For more information, refer to the National Academy of Sciences' volume on Responsible Science (1992).

to no experience with conducting your own project. In rare cases, your advisor will hold your hand through the entire process. In all likelihood however, your advisor will take the stance that as a graduate student, you must begin taking responsibility for your own education and intellectual development and therefore you must do the major critical thinking and analysis work yourself. You are not alone, however. Ask questions in class. Talk to your classmates, particularly those further along in the program. Take advantage of your professors' office hours. Read this book.

It is the rare student who enters graduate school after four (or five) years of undergraduate work where the emphasis was first on rote memorization and later, critical thinking, who has developed their intellectual maturity to the point where they already know exactly what they want to do their thesis or dissertation on and how to go about it. Most first-year graduate students in anthropology basically know that they are interested in anthropology and probably which subfield they are leaning towards. While you probably had to identify where your interests lay when you applied to graduate school, this was probably a generalization. You might even find that after your first semester of graduate school you are no longer interested in what you stated in your letter of intent. Moving the several steps from what you are generally interested in to narrowing down a specific research project is challenging and takes some work. Do not despair if you have no idea yet where to focus your research efforts. This chapter and book are designed to help you work out the steps you need to take in order to answer that ever-elusive question, "Just how do I think of an idea?"

Observation

As with the first step of the scientific method, the first step towards thinking of an idea is observation. This can be done in a variety of ways. Pay attention to interesting or seemingly unusual features on the skeleton, to comments your peers make, to things you've read, to what your professors say in class. You never know when a simple observation will spark an idea. As you take your upper division biological anthropology courses, we recommend that you write down any questions or thoughts you have in your notebook. At least once per class there should be something that really sparks your interest. At the end of the semester, collect all of these thoughts into a single journal. This will be your "thesis/research development journal." Perhaps some of your questions were answered later on in the semester, but maybe not to your satisfaction, and you would be interested in exploring one of these questions for yourself. Further, be aware of what resources your college or university or any other nearby institutions have for research. Are there skeletal collections available? What kinds of laboratories exist? Knowing this at the outset and perhaps taking a tour when possible might help you focus your thinking at this point—whether or not you will use these resources for your project.

Ask Questions

Further, you have probably been exposed to dozens or maybe even hundreds of skeletons by now. You already know that you find the skeleton very interesting; otherwise you would not have opted to embark on its advanced study. Ask yourself a series of questions regarding your interests about the skeleton. What are a few things that you find <u>most</u> interesting about it? How it ages? Morphological differences that can hint at ancestry or the distance between populations (biological distance)? Sex differences? Trauma? Its DNA? Do you prefer juvenile skeletons to adult ones? Is there a particular bone that is your favorite?[6] What about the teeth? Think about and write down your top three interests with regard to the skeleton. See Table 2.4 for example questions. Next take this exercise a step further and ask yourself if there is a particular time period or area of the world to which you are drawn. Are you interested in the lifeways of prehistoric or historic people? If so, do you find the prehistory of Peru particularly attractive? Have you always been enthralled by historic European cultures or perhaps ancient Egypt? Or maybe you prefer prehistoric North America? Perhaps you are less drawn by prehistoric or historic questions and instead find yourself more attracted to applied biomedical or forensic queries. Rank your answers in a hierarchy according to your preference or curiosity.

Read Articles and Narrow it Down

Once you have made your two lists of interests, you need to start reading some articles that cover your top three areas of interest on each list. Previous findings essentially provide a road map for researchers, outlining what is already known and what is still needed to fill in the blanks—this will help you with learning about possible research questions you could ask. Three or four articles/chapters in each area should be sufficient for this part of the process. As you're reading, keep track of your response to each article (did you find it engaging/not as engaging as something else, did it create more questions for you?). In addition to reading, think about which areas you found most interesting in the classes you've had and are taking now. What were the specific topics that kept your attention the most and sparked the most questions for you? This will help you determine which of the areas on each of your lists you find the *most* engaging. At this point—congratulations! You have at least narrowed down the broad area in which you wish to focus your research. It is **absolutely imperative** that you find whatever topic you decide on to be exciting—so choose carefully. You will be spending a lot of time working on each aspect of the project and if you are not passionate

TABLE 2.4   *What Do You Find Most Interesting About the Skeleton?*

- Bones on a cellular level?
- Trauma?
- Its growth and development?
- Chemical signatures locked inside?
- Evidence of health/disease?
- Cranial/postcranial morphology?
- Agents of postmortem change?
- Juvenile or adult remains?
- Its DNA?
- The biological profile?

[6]The first author's is the sphenoid, in case anyone wants to know.

about your topic and feel invested in it, not only will the process be agonizing for you, but it will be less likely that you will see it through to completion.

Let's say you have decided that you want to focus on interpersonal violence in prehistory, and you are most interested in specifically exploring this topic for a Latin American population. You will need to ensure that (1) there are skeletal collections that will be accessible (with a sufficient number of individuals exhibiting trauma); (2) local authorities (i.e., at the museum) would be interested in your research topic for their collection; (3) you can obtain an invitation/permission to do research; and (4) you can obtain the resources needed for travel (if applicable). Speak to your advisor at this point—they will be able to help guide you in terms of key references you should read and perhaps with a certain direction you should explore or with setting up contacts in the country, museum, and/or university where you wish to work. Make sure you stay in touch with your advisor through the different steps of the process. Not only will you need their support while you are working on your project, but they will be one of the people who signs your completed thesis or dissertation and therefore you have to make sure they approve of what you decide to work on.

Travel Possibilities

As a side note, we strongly recommend that you seriously consider traveling to do your research. You became (or are considering becoming) an anthropologist for a reason, part of which probably involved reading about anthropologists who travel to all corners of the world and the adventures that ensue. Even if you are fortunate enough to be at a university with a skeletal collection, do not disregard the fact that there are other skeletal collections, of prehistoric, historic, and modern individuals, available for research literally all over the world.[7] Your research project should be about more than your education—it should be about your own personal development as well. Travel contributes to personal development almost like nothing else. If you travel to do your data collection, not only will you develop a passion for the area of the world to which you travel and the collection you are studying, but you will create contacts in that country for your future career. Further, part of the nature of anthropology is its cross-cultural perspective. Take advantage of travel to foster this in your own work if possible.

Full Literature Review

You will need to do a full literature review on whichever area you have decided to direct your focus. This sounds like a lot of work—and it is—but being prepared will pay off later. First, you will have to do an exhaustive literature review for your thesis or dissertation anyway, so you might as well get started reading the literature now. Second, reading the literature will spark a lot of specific ideas. Many studies will state in the conclusion something similar to, "we recommend that future studies examine ..." or "further work is needed

---

[7]Refer to the online Skeletal Collections Database: http://skeletal.highfantastical.com/. This lists several, but not all, skeletal collections available (link current as of publication). In addition, see Usher (2002); White et al. (2012:382–383); and Ubelaker (in press) for listings of skeletal collections.

to ...." This exercise will educate you about the state of the area you are interested in and will direct you toward the things that are still unknown about it. Creating an annotated bibliography of everything you read is a useful way to keep all of the information together and easily accessible (refer to DiGangi [Chapter 17], this volume).

Brainstorming

Another way to think of ideas is brainstorming. This can be an effective tool for coming up with projects, especially when conducted with peers or colleagues (at happy hour perhaps). Write down everything you like about the skeleton and things you wish you knew about it. Allow your brainstorming to branch out from the previous exercises you have completed: the observation, research journal, and literature review steps. The crazier and more outrageous you get in your brainstorming, the better. You never know when a crazy idea will spark a viable one. Taking this three-tiered approach (observation, library research, and brainstorming) to thinking about developing your research project will help you narrow down a specific problem to focus on. See Table 2.5.

Simplicity is Key

Once you have gotten to this point, there are a few things you will need to do to further refine your idea. Particularly for your first project, you want it to be manageable, feasible, and simple. Choosing a project that you know at the outset will take five years for data collection alone for your Master's thesis is not a good idea because there is a low likelihood that

TABLE 2.5   How to Think of Ideas

Step	Exercise
1	Observation based on:
	Reading articles
	Things said in class
	Things you notice about the skeleton
2	Focus your thinking:
	Create a research journal
	Make a list of most interesting things about the skeleton
	Make a list of time periods/locations you find interesting
	Read articles in the above areas
	Narrow down your interest based on readings
3	Use brainstorming to supplement the above
4	Logistics:
	Talk to your advisor
	Consider traveling
	Can you obtain permission/access to collection?
	Can you obtain resources for travel/analysis?
5	Full literature review on your topic

you will follow it through to the end. You want to succeed with your first project, particularly because it is going to lead toward a Master's or doctorate. Coming up with a complicated project to start out with makes completion less likely and it will discourage you from continuing on in the field. Your advisor will be able to make suggestions with regard to how to make your particular project as feasible and manageable as possible.

PROJECT LOGISTICS

Thinking about the logistics that will be involved will help you determine how manageable your project will be. See Table 2.6. Do you have access to the proper equipment you will need? For example, if you want to do a stable isotope or DNA analysis, you will need access to very specialized equipment. Will you need special permission to access the sample? How will you go about obtaining that permission? How much time will data collection take? Will you have that time available based on your schedule? Will the study involve destructive analysis, and if so, is it absolutely necessary and can you receive permission for this? (Refer to the section on ethical considerations, later in this chapter.) Can you receive permission for transport of samples (teeth, etc.) to the laboratory for stable isotope or other specialized analysis? (See, for example, Bethard [Chapter 15], this volume.) Will you need any technical or specialized help (with data collection, with sample preparation, with analysis, etc.)? Will you be allowed to publish the data? Will you need money for analysis, travel, etc., and if so, where will you get it from? Answering these questions will help you refine your idea even further depending upon the answers. Sometimes your idea may come to a standstill if for example you do not receive permission to carry it out. Other times it might be delayed if you need to apply for funding. Again, your advisor can help you during this process with suggestions and guidance if you do hit any roadblocks.

Locating a Sample

Finding a sample can be one of the simplest parts of your logistics if you intend to study skeletal collections. As mentioned earlier, by this point you should have an idea of which part of the world you wish to focus on. During your review of the literature, many papers will list the name of the collection used—let that serve as your starting point. However, if you plan on

TABLE 2.6 Refining Your Idea: Logistics Involved

- Is your project manageable and feasible?
- Do you have/can you obtain access to necessary equipment?
- Do you need special permission? How do you obtain permission?
- Is destructive analysis involved? Do you need permission for this?
- How much time will it take—do you have the time available?
- How will you transport the samples if applicable?
- Will you need special technical assistance?
- Will you need permission to publish the data/results?
- Do you have/can you obtain the resources to carry out the study?
- Does the project meet accepted ethical standards?

some sort of destructive analysis, your search for a suitable collection will be more difficult. Keep in mind that destructive analysis requests will be strongly scrutinized by the curator of the collection, and therefore you must ensure it is absolutely necessary for data collection and moreover, necessary to answer a question of importance. Whether or not your plans include destructive analysis, contact the curator of the collection first to ascertain their interest in having you conduct your project on their collection and follow their protocol for writing a research proposal carefully. This will require that you organize your methodology before collecting any data. You may need to provide a letter of recommendation from your advisor or other committee member as well.

Funding

Although you may not need funding, it may behoove you to apply for funding from a notable institution, such as the National Science Foundation or National Institutes of Health (in the United States). Any grant on your curriculum vitae (CV) demonstrates a productive research portfolio. Having a grant from a renowned institution, however small, is a bright feather for your cap (and CV). This will be important as you apply for jobs in the future. If your project is costly (e.g., DNA or stable isotopes analysis), applying for and receiving funding will be essential. Refer to DiGangi (Chapter 17), this volume, for information on funding organizations.

The Importance of Remaining Flexible

Every research endeavor requires a high degree of creativity and flexibility so unavoidable setbacks can be dealt with successfully. These can be among the most useful skills you will learn for your research career. Research can be derailed for a variety of reasons: conflicts break out in regions of interest, access to collections can be tenable, having multiple advisors can become tumultuous, and money can dry up. Just remember that a good research project is a COMPLETED research project that includes the signatures of your committee members. Be flexible with your research question and be ready to switch directions or collections as need be.

Creativity with your logistics can ultimately save you a lot of time. For example, if you had planned to travel for your project and the collection will no longer be available (or you no longer have funding), perhaps there is a collection containing individuals from the same population located closer to home, or perhaps you can ask the same research question of a different population in a local collection, negating the need to rework the entire project from scratch. See Hammerl (Chapter 10), this volume, for a case study example of the importance of flexibility with research questions.

Being a Professional Student—When does it End?

Another thing to think about will be your timeline for completion. Many Master's degree programs have a set timeline within which students must finish, usually ranging from one to three years; but PhD programs in many cases seem to be endless. It will be up to you to decide how long you want to be a student beyond the period of mandatory residency set by your college or university. Several factors will go into your decision, including your goals for your project and the future, family responsibilities, finances, and so on. However, it has been our observation that those students who do not set a timeline or goal for completion either never finish or finish several years beyond when they should have (paying several thousand dollars more of tuition along the way).

Create a research outline and then continue to elaborate on that outline until you have a detailed schedule. Set up a timeline for how long it will take you to complete each task. Be realistic about your own productivity. How long does it take you to measure a femur or read an article? Keep in mind that some tasks will require more time investment and concentration than others. Become familiar with your own productivity; some days and timeslots are more fruitful than others depending on your mood, your stress level, other commitments, and so on. Make sure you build in "off" days and timeslots to give your brain a break. With this timeline established, stick to it. Each time you complete reading a large amount of references, a major aspect of data collection, analysis, writing a chapter, or even a paragraph that was particularly challenging, put a checkmark on your timeline and treat yourself in some way. Take a break and do something to relax before diving back in. Breaking down your timeline in this manner will help divide the massive endeavor into manageable parcels.

Last but not least, know when to say enough. There will always be another paper to read and cite or a few more skeletons to analyze. However, your advisor and committee will have the ultimate say in whether you have collected enough data or included enough citations. You and your advisor should maintain open lines of communication as you progress through the program. Make sure you run your ideas by your committee regularly so there will be no unpleasant surprises from them at the end and do not be afraid to ask for help when you need it. At least one of your committee members should give you some sort of feedback along the way to let you know if you are going in the right (or wrong) direction. If your committee is not very communicative, develop a group of peers as an alternative sounding board.

You will come to the realization that your thesis or dissertation does not have to be the most brilliant one ever completed, but it does have to demonstrate your mastery of research skills and the subject matter. You will have plenty of time to do brilliant work after you've hung your diploma on the wall. Accept this when you are ready. As a graduate student, having that M.A., M.S., or PhD diploma should be your ultimate goal—because it will lead you onwards to your career in skeletal biology.

Ethical Considerations

Do not just ask if you *can* do the project, but ask if you *should* do the project. There are **always** ethical considerations when studying living humans[8] and animals, and many of these considerations spill over to studying the remains of human beings.

---

[8]While unusual for skeletal biology projects, you may have a project that involves living human subjects. In that case, you will have to complete an institutional review board (IRB) proposal through your college or university to receive permission for your study. The IRB process will improve the quality of your proposal and help simplify your methods while preventing potential ethical problems.

We often have access to skeletal samples of indigenous groups. This is becoming less common in the United States due to laws such as the Native American Graves Protection and Repatriation Act of 1990[9] and recent additions regarding culturally unaffiliated human remains, but for some countries in Latin America for example cultural heritage laws either do not exist, are not enforced, or do not protect skeletal remains. In these instances, it is up to us to protect the remains. Many cultures have or had very specific beliefs about the dead and you **must** respect that. You cannot dig up every cemetery to look at skeletons "just because." You must have a compelling reason to do so, such as the site being in danger or the overwhelming scientific impact the information we could glean would have.

Even when there is no evidence suggesting that the culture a particular set of skeletons belonged to attached specific meaning to the remains themselves, you must always treat all remains with respect. That is, you should view the fact that you are able to touch the bones of a fellow human being as a privilege.

Different cultures will have different standards for treatment and respect of human remains. Some descendant communities may not want non-group members touching their ancestors' remains and others will not want the remains handled by anyone, regardless of group membership. In other cases, the descendants may want trained investigators to do research so that they can learn more about their ancestors. In some instances, it may not be possible to associate skeletons with a particular living descendant community.[10] When this occurs, you should follow our own cultural standards for treatment of remains. Never forget that each skeleton once belonged to a human being, someone who had a family, friends, hopes, and disappointments, just like you.

You should also ask yourself what the benefits are to doing your study. Is it merely "interesting," or will others benefit from the knowledge it generates? Will it contribute to scientific knowledge and its advancement? Will it rely on or contribute to current thought and ways of thinking? If your answer is "no" to any of these questions, then you need to seriously rethink your project. Science moves forward, not backward; and it does so by holding projects to the highest ethical standards. Each scientist is individually accountable for their own work in this regard, and the scientific community as a whole is responsible for setting the bar high. See White et al. (2012) for a comprehensive discussion on ethical considerations with regard to the study of human skeletal remains.

To summarize this section, thinking of an idea boils down to learning how to focus your thinking about skeletal biology and discovering which topics excite and interest you most in the field. Get comfortable with library research (see DiGangi [Chapter 17], this volume) and start to learn what makes projects feasible. Even the best skeletal biologist was a beginner at some point and had to learn how to do research. The process will become easier the more practice you have with it. Finally, take advantage of your advisor's knowledge. Their job is to guide you on your intellectual journey towards your degree and therefore they will be one of the best resources available to you. Refer to Figure 2.2 for a flowchart breakdown of how to think of and develop ideas.

---

[9]Public Law 101-601; 25 U.S.C. § 3001 et seq. See discussion in DiGangi and Moore (Chapter 1), this volume.

[10]See for example Owsley and Jantz (in press) about Kennewick Man.

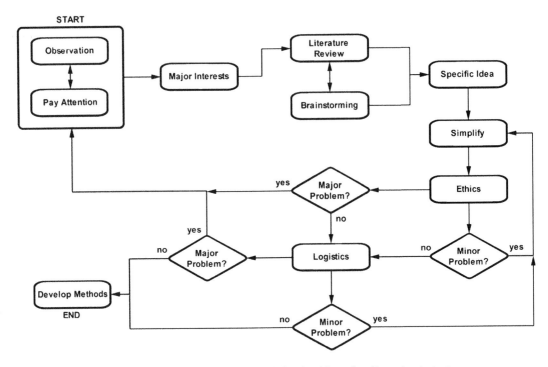

FIGURE 2.2   How to think of and develop ideas. See discussion in text.

CASE STUDY: THE DEVELOPMENT OF A DISSERTATION TOPIC

When I (MKM) was trying to discover my research passion in graduate school, I had not made a list of research interests as mentioned earlier in this chapter, but had written hundreds of questions in the margins of my notebooks throughout my undergraduate and graduate education. I decided to go back through each of the dozen or so notebooks and organize my scribbles. Fortunately, my little in-class epiphanies were often accompanied by excessive exclamation points, stars, or highlighter (I recommend you do the same). During my first course in archaeology at the Ohio State University, I remember the day I was introduced to the "Venus of Willendorf," the sculpture from the Upper Paleolithic period in what is now Austria dating to 26,000–24,000 BCE (Otte, 1990). See Figure 2.3. Not only was she beautifully sculpted, but something about her struck me as extraordinarily anatomically correct. The professor discussed the shape of her pubic triangle and voluptuous breasts as being anatomical exaggerations and labeled her a fertility goddess. I had spent many summers swimming with my own voluptuous grandmother, and there was nothing unnatural about the Venus' anatomy. The only exaggerations in my mind were her tiny arms and absent facial features, feet, and hands. Was it possible that someone who lived tens of thousands of years ago could have become obese? If so, how did they maintain a high body mass with a migratory lifestyle? This question among others was scribbled in the margins of that notebook a decade before I started working on my doctoral degree.

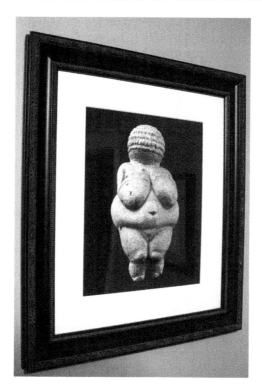

FIGURE 2.3   The Venus of Willendorf.

Throughout my graduate education, functional morphology (the interplay between form and function) continued to pique my interest. I was fortunate to have had the opportunity to work with the **William M. Bass Donated Skeletal Collection** at the University of Tennessee. With the increasing sample of obese individuals donated to the collection in recent years, I revisited this question posed by the Venus figurine. However, my first dissertation direction was a dead-end. I tried pursuing a forensic application thinking about facial reconstruction for obese individuals. Since I wanted to look at the relationship between bone and soft tissue, I began developing contacts at the University of Tennessee Medical Center, Department of Radiology. I applied for a graduate fellowship with an agency that had an interest in my research agenda, namely, facial reconstruction for obese and overweight people.

The project went unfunded, which forced me to reconsider my research question. I began to doubt its integrity and feared being pigeonholed in forensic anthropology (a possibility pointed out by my advisor). I also feared the research project might be perceived as pseudoscience, since much of facial reconstruction is more dependent upon the talent of the forensic artist than on the actual science of skeletal facial morphology (e.g., see Stephan and Henneberg, 2001). However, the original scientific problem proposed came back to the issue of body mass and the great effect it can have on the appearance of the face. I therefore expanded my original question to become the following: Is it possible to determine body mass from other parts of the skeleton? If so, would the markers imitate occupational markers of stress (see Smith [Chapter 7] and Kroman and Symes [Chapter 8], this volume) or would the bones themselves change shape? Do obese individuals have a specific pattern of skeletal pathology? Is there a difference in locomotion patterns between people of different body masses (underweight, normal, and overweight)? This ultimately led to my dissertation: *Body Mass Estimation from the Human Skeleton* (Moore, 2008).

To develop the necessary expertise for my dissertation, I took courses in the biomechanics and nutrition departments. The connections I had made previously at the Radiology Department of the University of Tennessee Medical Center also helped me to develop a research collaboration with the biomedical engineering department. The engineers were interested in designing joint prosthetics for an orthopedic company, for which they needed precise anatomical models of human bones to design the prosthetics correctly. I was able to negotiate a low price with the Radiology Department to conduct **computed tomographic (CT) scans** of the entire William M. Bass Donated Skeletal Collection. CT scans provide essentially three-dimensional X-rays of the skeleton. (For more information on medical imaging, see Moore [Chapter 14], this volume.)

I personally handled all the logistics of transporting the entire collection (approximately 500 individuals) to the medical center and supervised a team of anthropologists with scanning each skeleton in an assembly line fashion. The engineers were able to analyze the three-dimensional surface models of the bones, serving their needs for precise prosthetic creation; and I was able to use the data from the scans to look at shape changes in the femur between normal weight and obese subjects. This was a perfect symbiotic relationship for collecting massive amounts of data for multiple dissertations and publications in engineering and anthropology. The engineers benefitted from my collaboration with the radiologists and my access to the skeletal collection, and I did develop some expertise in biomechanics and functional morphology, but it was not necessary for me to become an engineer to write the computer code needed to complete the project.

The moral of this story is twofold. It can be valuable (and time consuming) to learn new skills, but do not let the lack of a specialized skill prevent you from pursing a particular research direction, especially if collaborating is a possibility. Collaborations can fulfill the need for diverse skill sets and provide new funding opportunities. Secondly, sometimes your project idea goes through several iterations before being finalized, so it is important to be flexible and creative as circumstances warrant.

FINAL THOUGHTS

"I have come to know that a problem does not belong to me, or to my team, ... or to my country; it belongs to the world." (Payne-Gaposchkin 1996:162)

You will be better prepared to embark on your research project if you heed the advice presented in this chapter. Once you do so, you will be able to count yourself among those trying to advance human knowledge of the natural world. Science indeed has noble goals, but never disregard that while noble, its practitioners are, after all, human. Science's noble goals can therefore be marred by the egos and personal ambitions of the scientists who practice it.

A particularly demonstrative example is that of the astronomer who discovered in 1925 that the most abundant element in stars was hydrogen—a stunning and monumental discovery rendered dubious and impossible almost immediately by leading scholars at the time, in all likelihood because this young PhD was a woman. Because Dr. Cecelia Payne-Gaposchkin allowed her male colleagues to push her into abandoning her thesis and into working on different problems, she is not credited for her discovery (Horn, 1998). Science should be practiced for science's sake, not solely for the sake of inflating one's pride or curriculum vitae. Do not allow your ego to interfere with the work of others, and conversely, do not allow the egos of others to interfere with your own work. While scientists will always be influenced by the prevailing thought and culture of the time, make the choice to be a student of science who fosters its goals through positive contributions and collegiality.

ACKNOWLEDGMENTS

We are grateful to Dr. Graciela Cabana whose thoughtful comments and suggestions on several drafts of this chapter helped us to vastly improve its contents and quality. Dr. Maria Smith had several useful comments as well. We thank Dr. Lyle Konigsberg for feedback that helped us with the hypothesis testing section of the chapter and Gregory Westerwick who provided interpretation of the Apollo Guidance Computer characteristics. Thanks are also due to Adriana Otero who formatted Figures 2.1 and 2.2. The first author would also like to thank Dr. Jonathan Bethard for his encyclopedic knowledge of references and other anthropological information and for being an excellent sounding board with helping her think through some of the concepts herein.

REFERENCES

Merriam-Webster's Collegiate Dictionary, 11th ed., 2003. Merriam-Webster, Springfield, Massachusetts.

Agresti, A., Finlay, B., 2009. Statistical Methods for the Social Sciences, 4th ed. Prentice-Hall, Upper Saddle River, New Jersey.

Bass, W.M., Jefferson, J., 2003. Death's Acre. G.P. Putnam & Sons, New York.

Bethard, J.D., 2013. Isotopes. In: DiGangi, E.A., Moore, M.K. (Eds.), Research Methods in Human Skeletal Biology. Academic Press, San Diego.

Buikstra, J.E., Ubelaker, D.H., 1994. Standards for Data Collection from Human Skeletal Remains. Arkansas Archaeological Survey, Fayetteville, Arkansas.

Darwin, C., 1859. On the Origin of Species By Means of Natural Selection. John Murray, London.

DiGangi, E.A., 2013. Library research, presenting, and publishing. In: DiGangi, E.A., Moore, M.K. (Eds.), Research Methods in Human Skeletal Biology. Academic Press, San Diego.

DiGangi, E.A., Hefner, J.T., 2013. Ancestry estimation. In: DiGangi, E.A., Moore, M.K. (Eds.), Research Methods in Human Skeletal Biology. Academic Press, San Diego.

DiGangi, E.A., Moore, M.K., 2013. Introduction to skeletal biology. In: DiGangi, E.A., Moore, M.K. (Eds.), Research Methods in Human Skeletal Biology. Academic Press, San Diego.

Gould, S.J., 1981a. Evolution as fact and theory. Discover 2, 34—37.

Gould, S.J., 1981b. The Mismeasure of Man. W.W. Norton & Company, New York.

Graziano, A.M., Raulin, M.L., 2000. Research Methods: A Process of Inquiry, 4th ed. Allyn & Bacon, Boston.

Hall, E.C., 1963. General Design Characteristics of the Apollo Guidance Computer. Report R-410. Massachusetts Institute of Technology, Cambridge.

Hammerl, E., 2013. Dental anthropology. In: DiGangi, E.A., Moore, M.K. (Eds.), Research Methods in Human Skeletal Biology. Academic Press, San Diego.

Horn, D., 1998. The shoulders of giants. Science 280 (5368), 1354–1355.

Huitema, B., 2011. The Analysis of Covariance and Alternatives: Statistical Methods for Experiments, Quasi-experiments, and Single-case Studies, 2nd ed. John Wiley & Sons, New Jersey.

Hutton, J., 1788. Theory of the Earth. Transactions of the Royal Society of Edinburgh 1, 209–304.

Kimmerle, E.H., Jantz, R.L., 2008. Variation as evidence: introduction to a symposium on international human identification. Journal of Forensic Sciences 53 (3), 521–523.

Konigsberg, L., Frankenberg, S., 2013. Demography. In: DiGangi, E.A., Moore, M.K. (Eds.), Research Methods in Human Skeletal Biology. Academic Press, San Diego.

Konigsberg, L., Frankenberg, S., Walker, R., 1997. Regress what on what: paleodemographic age estimation as a calibration problem. In: Payne, R. (Ed.), Integrating Archaeological Demography: Multidisciplinary Approaches to Prehistoric Population. Center for Archaeological Investigations, Southern Illinois University Carbondale, Occasional Paper No. 24, pp. 64–88.

Kroman, A.M., Symes, S.A., 2013. Skeletal trauma. In: DiGangi, E.A., Moore, M.K. (Eds.), Research Methods in Human Skeletal Biology. Academic Press, San Diego.

Langley-Shirley, N., Jantz, R.L., 2010. A Bayesian approach to age estimation in modern Americans from the clavicle. Journal of Forensic Sciences 55 (3), 571–583.

Lyell, C., 1830. Principles of Geology. John Murray, London.

Marden, K., Sorg, M., Haglund, W., 2013. Taphonomy. In: DiGangi, E.A., Moore, M.K. (Eds.), Research Methods in Human Skeletal Biology. Academic Press, San Diego.

Marder, M.P., 2011. Research Methods for Science. Cambridge University Press, Cambridge.

McKeown, A.H., Schmidt, R.W., 2013. Geometric morphometrics. In: DiGangi, E.A., Moore, M.K. (Eds.), Research Methods in Human Skeletal Biology. Academic Press, San Diego.

Moore, M.K., 2008. Body Mass Estimation from the Human Skeleton. Doctoral dissertation. The University of Tennessee, Knoxville.

Moore, M.K., 2013. Functional morphology and medical imaging. In: DiGangi, E.A., Moore, M.K. (Eds.), Research Methods in Human Skeletal Biology. Academic Press, San Diego.

Moore, M.K., Ross, A.H., 2013. Stature estimation. In: DiGangi, E.A., Moore, M.K. (Eds.), Research Methods in Human Skeletal Biology. Academic Press, San Diego.

National Academy of Sciences, 1992. Responsible Science, Vol. 1. Ensuring the Integrity of the Research Process. Panel on Scientific Responsibility and the Conduct of Research. National Academy of Sciences, National Academy of Engineering, Institute of Medicine.

Otte, M., 1990. Revision de la sequence du paleolithique superieur de Willendorf (Autriche). Bulletin de l'Institut Royal des Sciences Naturelles de Belgique 60, 219–228.

Owsley, D., Jantz, R.L., in press. Kennewick Man. A&M Press, College Station, Texas.

Payne-Gaposchkin, C., 1996. The dyer's hand: an autobiography. In: Haramundanis, K. (Ed.), Cecelia Payne-Gaposchkin: An Autobiography and Other Recollections, 2nd ed. Cambridge University Press, Cambridge.

Rojas, R., 2001. Encyclopedia of Computers and Computer History. Fitzroy Dearborn Publishers, Chicago.

Sang-Hun, C., 2009. Disgraced cloning expert convicted in South Korea. The New York Times (p. A12), New York.

Schmidt, C., Symes, S., 2008. The Analysis of Burned Human Remains. Academic Press, San Diego.

Shapere, D., 1974. Galileo: A Philosophical Study. The University of Chicago Press, Chicago.

Sharratt, M., 1994. Galileo: Decisive Innovator. Blackwell Publishers, Oxford.

Smith, M.O., 2003. Beyond palisades: The nature and frequency of late prehistoric deliberate violent trauma in the Chickamauga reservoir of East Tennessee. American Journal of Physical Anthropology 121 (4), 303–318.

Smith, M.O., 2013. Paleopathology. In: DiGangi, E.A., Moore, M.K. (Eds.), Research Methods in Human Skeletal Biology. Academic Press, San Diego.

Snieder, R., Larner, K., 2009. The Art of Being a Scientist: A Guide for Graduate Students and Their Mentors. Cambridge University Press, Cambridge.

Stephan, C., Henneberg, M., 2001. Building faces from dry skulls: are they recognized above chance rates? Journal of Forensic Sciences 46 (3), 432–440.

Todd, T., 1920. Age changes in the pubic bone: I. The male white pubis. American Journal of Physical Anthropology 3, 285–334.

Ubelaker, D., in press. Collections. In: Ubelaker, D., Blau, S., Fondebrider L. (Eds.), Bioarchaeology and human osteology. In Smith, C., Smith J. (Eds.), Encyclopedia of Global Archaeology. Springer, New York.

Ubelaker, D., De La Paz, J., 2012. Skeletal indicators of pregnancy and parturition: a historical perspective. Journal of Forensic Sciences 57, 866–872.

Uhl, N., 2013. Age-at-death estimation. In: DiGangi, E.A., Moore, M.K. (Eds.), Research Methods in Human Skeletal Biology. Academic Press, San Diego.

Usher, B.M., 2002. Reference samples: the first step in linking biology and age in the human skeleton. In: Hoppa, R.D., Vaupel, J.W. (Eds.), Paleodemography: Age Distributions from Skeletal Samples. Cambridge University Press, New York, pp. 29–47.

Walker, P.L., Johnson, J.R., Lambert, P.M., 1988. Age and sex biases in the preservation of human skeletal remains. American Journal of Physical Anthropology 76 (2), 183–188.

Walsh, A., Ollenburger, J., 2001. Essential Statistics for the Social and Behavioral Sciences: A Conceptual Approach. Prentice-Hall, Upper Saddle River, New Jersey.

Watson, J., Crick, F., 1953. A structure for deoxyribose nucleic acid. Nature 171, 737–738.

White, T.D., Ambrose, S.H., Suwa, G., Su, D.F., DeGusta, D., Bernor, R.L., Boisserie, J.-R., Brunet, M., Delson, E., Frost, S., Garcia, N., Giaourtsakis, I.X., Haile-Selassie, Y., Howell, F.C., Lehmann, T., Likius, A., Pehlevan, C., Saegusa, H., Semprebon, G., Teaford, M., Vrba, E., 2009. Macrovertebrate paleontology and the Pliocene habitat of Ardipithecus ramidus. Science 326, 87–93.

White, T.D., Black, M.T., Folkens, P.A., 2012. Human Osteology, 3rd ed. Academic Press, San Diego.

Wood, J.W., Milner, G.R., Harpending, H.C., Weiss, K.M., 1992. The osteological paradox: problems of inferring prehistoric health from skeletal samples. Current Anthropology 33, 343–358.

Zar, J., 2010. Biostatistical Analysis, 5th ed. Prentice-Hall, Upper Saddle River, New Jersey.

RECOMMENDED READING

Grene, M., Depew, D., 2004. The Philosophy of Biology: An Episodic History. Cambridge University Press, New York.

Mayr, E., 1989. Toward a New Philosophy of Biology: Observations of an Evolutionist. Harvard University Press, Cambridge.

PART II

RESEARCH ON ASPECTS OF THE BIOLOGICAL PROFILE

3

Age-at-Death Estimation

Natalie M. Uhl

INTRODUCTION

Estimation of age-at-death from human skeletal remains provides a crucial element of the biological profile. It typically is the first part of the biological profile to be assessed as the subsequent analyses (sex, ancestry, stature) are treated very differently for juveniles versus adults. The estimation of age-at-death from a human skeleton requires a thorough knowledge and understanding of biological and physiological processes—both developmental and degenerative—that affect the skeleton throughout life. It is assumed that the developmental processes are under a great deal of genetic control and thus are less susceptible to environmental influences. Populations exhibit differences in rate, timing, and duration of growth through time; these are referred to as **secular trends**[1] and are generally attributed to environmental factors like nutrition and exposure to disease agents. Degenerative processes inherently involve more variation because they are due in large part to the environment (nutrition, activity, occupation, etc.). For this reason, age-at-death estimates for adults require much broader age ranges, while estimates for juveniles can be narrower, more precise ranges.

When an anthropologist estimates "age," he or she is estimating *biological age*, that is, noting the biological changes in the skeleton associated with time and activity. However, *chronological age*, or calendar age, is the actual identifying feature of an individual. Chronological age is related to biological age, which allows us to use one to estimate the other, but this relationship is imperfect for many reasons. For example, even though the skeleton begins its development *in utero*, most societies exclude gestation from chronological age. Biological age is affected by activity and environment (e.g., nutrition, diet, disease load, stress), whereas chronological age steadily progresses as days, months, and years. The effects of environment and activity on biological but not chronological age make them gradually more different from each other and introduce error into any estimate of one from the other. Thus, age estimation for adults suffers from more error and less precision than age estimation for subadults (Nawrocki, 2010). This is particularly true for older adults—the variability inherent in age estimation increases with chronological age, so that estimated ranges for

[1]All bolded terms are defined in the glossary at the end of this volume.

someone who was in their twenties at death will be smaller than for someone who was in their sixties at death. This is why we refer to our analysis of age-at-death as an *estimation*, rather than as a *determination*.

Age estimation plays a large role in biological anthropology. In bioarchaeology and paleo-demography, age estimates for populations of skeletons can give us insight into the health of the population (see Smith [Chapter 7] and Konigsberg and Frankenberg [Chapter 11], this volume). They are indicative of growth processes as well as disease processes. Such inferences regarding health were previously made on the assumption of a simple relationship between the ages-at-death and the health of the living population. Wood and colleagues' (1992) seminal paper *The Osteological Paradox: Problems of Inferring Prehistoric Health from Skeletal Samples* ques-tions (among other things) the practice of using skeletal information to make inferences about the health of a population, given that the skeletons represent the individuals who *died*, not the individuals who were healthy and lived (or at least those able to fight off disease). Discussions of the **osteological paradox**[2] and resulting research have been a driving force of the major improvements in statistical techniques for age-at-death estimation over the past several decades (e.g., Boldsen et al., 2002). These techniques, namely **transition analysis** and various **multifactorial methods** (statistical combination of several age estimates), are discussed here.

In biological anthropology, age-at-death estimation is a critical part of the biological profile. At least a cursory estimation of age is required upon the initial examination of human remains to determine if the individual was an adult or a juvenile because methods for adults (assessing degenerative changes) differ from those used for juveniles (assessing develop-mental changes), as mentioned above. Several different areas of the skeleton demonstrating age-related changes have been utilized to create age-at-death estimation methods, although some have become much more ingrained in practice than others. Refining and improving techniques, as well as developing new and better methods, is still an area ripe for research.

Currently, most biological anthropologists use "phase" methods like Suchey–Brooks (1990) with means and standard deviations although the consensus seems to be that **Bayesian analysis** is a more appropriate way to estimate age-at-death. Bayesian analysis uses prior information (for example, the age distribution of a population) to provide more robust age-at-death estimates for particular individuals or populations. This kind of analysis is compatible with phase methods; it is merely a different way of approaching the calculation of the age-at-death estimate.

In this chapter I will introduce subadult age estimation, beginning with a review of bone growth, followed by a discussion of the methods used for estimating age from juveniles. Adult age estimation methods will be treated in depth, including consideration of multifac-torial methods (see Table 3.1), and the chapter will conclude with a case study illustrating the utility of Bayesian and transition analysis to the multifactorial age problem.

SUBADULT AGE-AT-DEATH ESTIMATION

Humans are characterized by a life history that includes altricial young and a distinctly prolonged postnatal ontogeny (Zeveloff and Boyce, 1982). This period of development, while

---

[2]See also DiGangi and Moore (Chapter 1) and Smith (Chapter 7), this volume.

TABLE 3.1 Common Age-at-Death Estimation Techniques

Indicator	Reference
JUVENILES	
Formation of Ossification Centers	Scheuer and Black, 2000
Epiphyseal Union	Scheuer and Black, 2000
Long Bone Length	Schaefer et al., 2009
Dental Development	See Hammerl (Chapter 10), this volume
ADULTS	
Pubic Symphysis	Brooks and Suchey, 1990
Auricular Surface	Lovejoy et al., 1985b
Fourth Rib	İşcan et al., 1984a,b
First Rib	DiGangi et al., 2009
Cranial Sutures	Meindl and Lovejoy, 1985; Nawrocki, 1998
Medial Clavicle (Older Adolescents, Young Adults)	Langley-Shirley and Jantz, 2010
Sacrum	Passalacqua, 2009
Dental Wear	Brothwell, 1989
Histology	Crowder and Pfeiffer, 2010
Multifactorial Method	Uhl et al., 2011

unique to humans compared to other species (Smith and Tompkins, 1995), is fairly predictable among human infants. Given this predictability we can utilize long bone length, dental development, or timing of epiphyseal appearance and union to estimate age-at-death for subadult remains, although the timing and extent of growth are known to vary, sometimes significantly, based on ancestral population and biological sex, and this variation increases with age (Stewart, 1979; Krogman and İşcan, 1986; Ubelaker, 1987; Humphrey, 1998).

Bone and Tooth Maturation and Growth

Formation of Ossification Centers

Human bone forms by two primary mechanisms—**intramembranous ossification** and **endochondral ossification**. Intramembranous ossification primarily occurs in the bones of the cranium, the facial bones, and the clavicle. The clavicle is the first bone in the body to begin ossification, commencing around 6 weeks' gestation, and the final bone to finish ossification in the late twenties (Scheuer and Black, 2000). Intramembranous ossification involves the direct mineralization of a membrane of mesenchyme (embryonic connective tissue) in a flat, spherical shape. The final product of intramembranous ossification is a layer of **diplöe** (spongy bone) in between two flat layers of compact bone, as in the parietal bone.

Most of the other bones in the body develop via endochondral ossification. This development does not initiate with a mesenchymal membrane but rather with a hyaline cartilage model of the bone. The diaphysis (shaft) of long bones begins formation first (called the *primary ossification center*) after vascularization of the cartilage. Ossification continues toward one or both ends of the diaphysis, but a layer of cartilage (the *metaphysis*) persists until elongation is finished (this timing differs within and between different bones; see the upcoming section on epiphyseal fusion). This plate of cartilage is often called the *growth plate*. The epiphyses (ends) of long bones begin ossification after the primary ossification center has formed so they are called *secondary ossification centers*. When elongation is complete the epiphyses fuse permanently to the diaphysis by replacement of the metaphyseal cartilage with bone. Scheuer and Black (2000) and Sadler (2004) provide detailed and authoritative accounts of bone development and growth.

The fragility of newly formed ossification centers makes them difficult to find in an archaeological context given taphonomic factors (see Marden et al. [Chapter 9], this volume); however, sometimes they are encountered in a medicolegal context. Biological anthropologists are recognized as experts not only in constructing a biological profile from skeletal remains but in the recovery of human remains and analysis of trauma to the skeleton. In these contexts, forensic anthropologists may be asked for an assessment of fetal or infant skeletal remains. Further, bioarchaeologists may have the opportunity to analyze fetal (rarely) or infant remains from archaeological sites (e.g., see Lewis, 2006; May et al., 2012).

Fazekas and Kósa (1978) were the first to address the utility of fetal remains in the forensic context. The next important tome to cover fetal and infant remains followed over 20 years later: *Developmental Juvenile Osteology* by Scheuer and Black (2000). The primary method of age-at-death estimation for fetal and infant remains is via assessment of the development of ossification centers because they begin formation *in utero* (Scheuer and Black, 2000). These ossification centers can be difficult to recover or identify without soft tissue or anatomical context, but standards do exist for age-at-death analysis, generally given in gestational months (Huxley, 2010).

Timing of Epiphyseal Union

Timing of epiphyseal union is preferred as a method over appearance of secondary ossification centers due to the fragility of newly formed ossification centers. Differential timing of epiphyseal fusion is found between bones and even within bones—for instance, bones with multiple epiphyses (e.g., proximal and distal) usually show fusion of those epiphyses at different times, such as the humerus and the femur. Some epiphyses, including many in the skull, fuse *in utero*, while others do not even begin to fuse until very late adolescence (Schaefer et al., 2009). The last epiphyses fuse in the early twenties; these include the medial clavicle (Langley-Shirley and Jantz, 2010) and the first sacral segment (Passalacqua, 2009).

Studies have consistently shown that epiphyseal union happens earlier in females than males (Flecker, 1942; Fishman, 1982; Krogman and İşcan, 1986). For example, Crowder and Austin (2005) analyzed a large contemporary sample (North Americans born after 1969 and as recently as 1991) for fusion of the distal tibia and fibula. Their overall results show some overlap, but even across varied ancestral populations females showed complete fusion of these epiphyses sometimes as early as 13 years of age. The youngest males with complete fusion were 15 years old. By 16 years old, all females showed complete fusion, regardless of ancestral group, but some males were as old as 19 years when fusion completed.

Schaefer and Black (2005) compared modern Bosnian males to the data of McKern and Stewart (1957), which include young North American males killed in the Korean conflict. They paint an interesting picture of populational differences for epiphyseal union. The American individuals in their study began epiphyseal union (the authors use the term "maturation") earlier than the Bosnian sample, but once the Bosnian sample began union they completed maturation (i.e., full union) faster than the Americans did. This example is a cautionary tale of the importance of using **population-specific standards** whenever possible, and in fact, the impetus for Schaefer and Black's (2005) study was the lack of agreement between anthropologically estimated ages and actual ages in this Bosnian sample (Komar, 2003). Population-specific standards are usually more effective because populations can differ in secular trends and/or environmental/occupation stresses that could affect the way skeletal changes correlate to chronological age.

In practice, most anthropologists continue to use the growth standards published in Ubelaker (1989) or Scheuer and Black (2000). However, Schaefer et al.'s (2009) *Juvenile Osteology: A Laboratory and Field Manual* provides a comprehensive collection of standards reproduced from multiple authors. Most beneficial about the presentation of the data in table format is that they indicate which population the study utilized and they include as much information as possible (i.e., if the authors provided ranges, those ranges are given). The manual is organized by body region (e.g., Lower Limb) and provides information on age-at-death related to epiphyseal appearance and union as well as long bone length. Because of its style as a manual, Schaefer and colleagues (2009) provide very little explanation of background, techniques, or application, so only an experienced anthropologist should use this information to estimate age-at-death. However, the more comprehensive (and hefty) Scheuer and Black (2000) volume is a main starting point for the reader wishing to learn more about bone growth and development.

Long Bone Length

Long bones, especially the large long bones that comprise the limbs, grow in both width and length; the latter provides the basis of another technique for estimating age-at-death from a juvenile skeleton.

Much of the work on the use of long bone length for estimating age for subadults comes from archaeology or large-scale longitudinal studies (Ogden et al., 2002). In archaeological contexts, there is no way to verify the actual age of the individual, but within a site or population long bone length can be correlated with dental development of associated remains (e.g., Johnston, 1962; Merchant and Ubelaker, 1977). Within a particular site or population this can be practical information for analyzing less complete sets of remains. However, in other populations or contexts the relationship between long bone length and dental development may differ for any number of genetic or environmental reasons (e.g., nutrition, disease).

Most biological anthropologists assign age estimates based on long bone lengths from ages published in Ubelaker (1989). These ages are aggregated from data from archaeological sites plus the Maresh (1955) measurements on radiographs of living children. The application of measurements from living individuals to dry bones introduces an (albeit small) source of error because bones shrink slightly as they dry (Hoffman, 1979).

Recently, Ousley et al. (2010) collected long bone length data on radiographs of known-age subadults at medical examiner offices and other clinical settings around the United States. This database (including formation and union of ossification centers, and long bone lengths) will soon be available for use by forensic anthropologists and other researchers. In the presentation, they cited the need for modern reference samples because modern North American children grow faster than those born in the 1950s (measured by Maresh and others) (Ousley et al., 2010). Most research points to a secular trend towards a faster and longer period of growth in Western populations, usually attributed to diet, because of either increased calories and/or nutrition (Danubio and Sanna, 2008), or chemicals and hormones (i.e., bovine growth hormone) used in Western livestock and agricultural practices (e.g., see Golub et al., 2003).

As mentioned earlier, Schaefer et al. (2009) have compiled the results of many studies on the relationship of age-at-death to diaphyseal length of long bones. Again, the authors provide information on the population used in each study, indicate number of males and females used, and report whether the measurements were taken on wet (via radiograph) or dry (forensic or archaeological) bones, as this could make a difference in the final calculation of size (Hoffman, 1979). For instruction on how to collect long bone measurements from juvenile remains, consult *Standards for Data Collection from Human Skeletal Remains* (Buikstra and Ubelaker, 1994), although Schaefer et al. (2009) should be consulted with regard to the analysis/interpretation of these measurements.

Dental Development

Dental development is the most accurate means for estimating age-at-death in subadults, probably because it is under fairly tight genetic regulation. Development of the dentition involves the formation, calcification, and eruption of the crown, as well as root growth and development. Refer to Hammerl (Chapter 10), this volume, for a review. Additionally, Hillson (1996) is an authoritative source on tooth development.

Schour and Massler (1941) and Ubelaker (1989) published charts illustrating 21 developmental stages from about 5 months *in utero* to 35 years old. Neither chart is sex-specific although many authors have noted sex differences (Schour and Massler, 1941; Smith, 1991; Smith, 2010). Ubelaker's impetus was to create a chart to be used in bioarchaeological contexts for prehistoric Native American remains, but the reproduction of his chart has made it popular for anthropological application to both prehistoric and modern remains.

Smith (2010) assessed both the Schour and Massler (1941) and Ubelaker (1989) charts on a modern clinical sample of living subadults using panoramic radiographs from a dentist. Her results show that each chart performs equally well, but that some of the stages, particularly those around ages 7–9, are significantly different for males and females. She also found that wider error intervals (age ranges) are needed for stages encompassing ages 6–14 years.

Again, Schaefer et al. (2009) have compiled the results of several dental analyses, including Ubelaker (1989), in their manual. One must have experience with examination of skeletal and dental remains to apply these charts in an age-at-death estimation. First, if the teeth were not fully formed, an experienced anthropologist (or dentist) would have to identify the individual teeth based on crown shape and development. Second, without knowledge of tooth formation and eruption processes, one could easily misapply information from the charts and tables in the analysis of subadult dental remains. Refer to Hammerl (Chapter 10), this volume, for more information on dental development and age estimation from the teeth.

STATISTICS AND ADULT AGE-AT-DEATH ESTIMATION

Traditional Statistical Methods

Many of the most popular methods for estimating age-at-death use phases for categorizing remains. Large skeletal samples (for example, the Suchey—Brooks method was initially developed on a sample of almost 800 individuals) are studied for trends in morphological change and then those changes are described and divided into phases. In other words, a particular bone will be chosen based on observations that a particular feature seems to demonstrate age-related change, and all the bones in the collection will be seriated based on **age cohorts** (15—20; 21—30; etc.) so that the changes can be easily described and grouped into phases.

Typically workers will publish the mean age of individuals in each stage, which is often used as the point estimate, along with the 95% confidence intervals for each phase for constructing an age range. Sometimes authors will instead include the standard deviation or **standard error** for each phase for use in constructing age ranges. Understanding the statistical theory underlying age-at-death estimates (mostly based on **regression analysis**) is very important for anthropologists employing these methods, especially in medicolegal cases that could require trial testimony. The Methods section of any age-at-death method paper will have a discussion of the statistical methods utilized, and therefore knowledge of statistics will facilitate comprehension.

Transition Analysis and Bayesian Theory

Transition analysis uses a "known" reference sample (skeletons for which sex, age-at-death, stature, etc. is known), preferably from the same human population as the individual being analyzed, and a **hazard model** (information that models survivorship) to estimate at what age those known individuals transition from one phase to another. This type of analysis provides a **highest posterior density distribution** (the probability after *a priori* (prior) information has been taken into account in Bayesian analysis) of age-at-transition; this information can be used for age-at-death estimation of an unknown individual. Because this analysis uses "prior" information (the reference sample) it is considered Bayesian in nature. Bayesian theory and the statistical methods developed from it use *a priori* information to alter the final probabilities.

In the context of age-at-death estimation the prior information includes the ages-at-transition of the known reference sample and a model of mortality for that population (see Konigsberg and Frankenberg [Chapter 11], this volume). To estimate an individual's age-at-death, one can calculate a percentage of the distribution (similar to a confidence interval, but it is distinct because the distribution is asymmetrical so this range is not centered on a mean), which gives a range. An anthropologist using a 95% estimate would report a larger (more conservative) age range, while an anthropologist using a 50% estimate would report a smaller range.

Accuracy and Precision

There has been much discussion as to the trade-off between *accuracy* and *precision* in reporting age-at-death estimates. In this context, an accurate age-at-death estimate refers to an estimate (range) that includes the actual age-at-death of the decedent. While

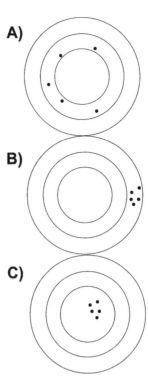

FIGURE 3.1 Schematic representation of accuracy and precision. **A.** Points that are accurate (approximating the bullseye) but not precise. **B.** Points that are precise (close together) but not accurate (far from the bullseye). **C.** Points that are both accurate (close to the bullseye) and precise (close together). An age-at-death estimate that is <u>accurate</u> includes the individual's age in the estimated range (although that range could be very large), while a <u>precise</u> estimate is close (in absolute units) to the actual age.

anthropologists strive to be accurate, an age range from 15 years to 100 years for most sets of remains is probably accurate but not very useful. A precise estimate is close to the actual age-at-death, but runs the risk of excluding the actual age-at-death. A common analogy to explain the relationship of accuracy to precision is a target with a bullseye. Hits that fall in a wide pattern all around the bullseye are accurate, but not precise. Hits that fall all in the same small area but far away from the bullseye are precise but not accurate. Accurate *and* precise hits (our goal) fall in a tight pattern near the bullseye. See Figure 3.1.

ADULT AGE-AT-DEATH ESTIMATION

Indicators of Adult Age-at-Death

The Pubic Symphysis

The pubic symphysis is the part of the skeleton where the two halves of the pelvis meet anteriorly. During life there is a thick pad of fibrocartilage between the bones and, commencing in early adulthood, the surface of the bone begins to change in predictable ways. It is unclear as to why the bone surface changes the way it does, but it has long been regarded as the most reliable skeletal indicator of age in adults (Krogman and İşcan, 1986). Its utility has been demonstrated for both paleodemography and forensic anthropology (Meindl and Lovejoy, 1989).

T. Wingate Todd first began studying and publishing on age changes in the pubic bones in 1920. He described ten morphological phases (categories) with associated age ranges. The early phases have very small age ranges (i.e., 2 or 3 year intervals) that gradually increase until phase X (10), which encompasses all individuals 50 years and older. Todd groups his phases into three stages: phases I–III, the postadolescent stages; phases IV–VI, during which the outline of the symphyseal surface is developed; and phases VII–X, during which there is a gradual decrease in bony buildup and finally a breakdown of bone.

Many authors have revised Todd's method on other skeletal samples (e.g., McKern and Stewart, 1957; Gilbert and McKern, 1973; Katz and Suchey, 1989). Although all of these generally agree with Todd's assessment of the age progression of the pubic symphysis, there is disagreement about how to quantify these changes and how this information should be transferred into an actual age estimate.

Rather than score the symphyseal surface as a whole, McKern and Stewart (1957) used a sample from the Korean War dead (i.e., many young men) to develop six stages (0–5) for each of three components: the dorsal demiface, the ventral demiface, and the whole surface of the pubic symphysis. In this way, there are no distinct phases with associated age ranges; rather, one can score all three components separately, sum the scores, and find the associated age range in a provided table. Their component method was designed to translate a large amount of morphological variation into a chronological age.

Gilbert and McKern (1973) later reworked this method for females based on observed differences between the sexes. They chose three components: the dorsal demiface, the ventral rampart, and the symphyseal rim. For each of these components there are five developmental phases that are scored; additionally a phase of "0" to denote absence is included.

Gilbert and McKern's (1973) analysis also includes a description of developmental differences between males and females. The dorsal demiface was found to be the first site of age-related changes, but the changes were accelerated in females. They also noted that the male symphyseal rim encloses the dorsal and ventral demifaces, but in females it separates the two because of the ventral rampart. Todd (1921) concluded that males and females differed by 2–3 years but Gilbert and McKern rather found a difference of 7–10 years in morphological age between the sexes. The authors also studied the effect of parity (birthing) on aging the female pubis. They could not articulate any concrete pattern, only cautioning that parity can cause the symphyseal face to look older than it actually is.

Meindl et al. (1985) were the first to statistically test the effect of ancestry and sex on pubic symphyseal aging. The results of the analysis of variance (ANOVA) were not significant for ancestry, sex, or any interactions between the three, but, not surprisingly, "age decade" was significant ($F = 3.86$, $p < 0.01$), indicating that age significantly affects the expression of pubic symphysis morphology.

Although the Todd method considers the entire surface of the pubic symphysis and therefore may fail to account sufficiently for the entire range of human variation, Meindl et al. (1985) believe that it better represents the chronological changes of the pubic symphysis.

They point out that an anomalous pubis may be incorrectly scored using McKern and Stewart's component method because the aging guidelines can be rather rigid. For example, if an anomalous pubic symphysis fails to form a ventral rampart it will not be aged at more than 29 years. If one understands the overall general chronological changes in the pubic symphysis, then Todd's stages can be applied more successfully than component methods.

Beginning in the late 1970s, much of the research on the pubic symphysis can be attributed, at least in part, to Judy Suchey (Suchey, 1979; Suchey et al., 1979, 1988; Katz and Suchey, 1989; Brooks and Suchey, 1990; Suchey and Katz, 1998). She used large samples of known individuals from California to test previous methods and develop new methods in an effort to increase the reliability of the pubic symphysis as an indicator of age-at-death.

In 1986, Katz and Suchey published the results of a large study of male pubic symphyses. They point out considerable problems with the samples and techniques of both Todd (1920, 1921) and McKern and Stewart (1957). For example, the actual ages of the sample originally used by Todd (now in the Hamann-Todd Human Osteological Collection[3]) were mostly estimated and rounded to the nearest 5 years while the cadavers were being prepared for dissection. Only three individuals had legal documentation of birth date, casting some doubt on real age information. Todd also removed certain individuals from the study if their morphology and age did not fit the chronological standard he had established, thus removing a great deal of variability. The McKern and Stewart method also does not encompass much human variation because it was developed on Korean War dead and thus consisted of mostly European American males in their early twenties who were born prior to World War II.

The sample used by Katz and Suchey consisted of 739 males autopsied at the Department of the Chief Medical Examiner-Coroner, County of Los Angeles. Age-at-death ranged from 14 to 92 years, with individuals from a diverse background (birthplaces in 32 countries). Suchey scored all of the pubic symphyses according to the Todd and the McKern and Stewart methods. Her observed ranges were much wider than those reported in the original studies. Her results support earlier studies (Brooks, 1955; Meindl et al., 1985) finding that the Todd system systematically over-ages, especially individuals under 40 years of age, and that neither the Todd nor the McKern and Stewart system can account for the sum total of human variation, especially in older phases. After a variety of analyses Katz and Suchey proposed a modified Todd method, where the ten phases were reduced to six phases (now referred to as the Suchey–Brooks[4] method, Figure 3.2).

Subsequently, Katz and Suchey (1989) focused on the question of whether or not ancestry differences exist in the morphology of the pubic symphysis. Todd (1921) noted minimal ancestral differences and Meindl et al. (1985) found ancestry to be insignificant in their analysis of pubic symphyseal aging. Katz and Suchey (1989), however, used their own large, multiancestral, known-age sample (n = 704) to test ancestral differences between "White," "Black," and "Mexican" groups. While the authors conceded that there was no morphological feature of the pubic symphysis that allowed the assessment of ancestry, they did find that

---

[3]This collection is curated by the Cleveland Museum of Natural History in Cleveland, Ohio.

[4]While the method is known as the Suchey–Brooks method, the publications are Katz and Suchey (1986) and Brooks and Suchey (1990).

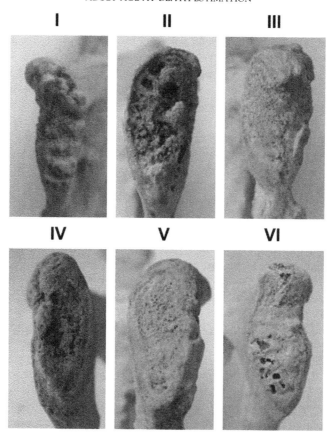

FIGURE 3.2 Pubic symphyses representing the six phases in the Suchey–Brooks method, from youngest (I) to oldest (VI).

individuals in different ancestral groups age differently.[5] New means and standard deviations were given for each revised Suchey–Brooks phase (I–VI) for the three populations, but sex differences are typically the only variable considered during application of the method.

Brooks and Suchey's (1990) revised Todd method rejects the three-component approach of McKern and Stewart (1957). They asserted that the three components do not vary independently and that an approach focusing on the entire pattern of morphological change (i.e., Todd's phase method) is easier to use. Therefore, Suchey and Brooks studied 1225 modern individuals from Los Angeles, including the 739 males that were previously analyzed by Katz and Suchey (1986). These individuals all had legally documented ages ranging from 14 to 99 years.

Brooks and Suchey (1990) used the Katz and Suchey (1986) analysis to refine the morphological descriptions for the modified Todd method. While the authors commended Todd for his accurate and comprehensive description of the aging of the pubic bone, modern statistical analyses on larger samples warranted combining several phases, resulting in a six phase

[5]As discussed earlier, this could be due to genetic factors, but is probably more influenced by environmental factors, like nutrition, access to medical care, disease load, activity level, stress, etc.

system. This method was first adopted for males (Katz and Suchey, 1986) and later for females (Brooks and Suchey, 1990). Brooks and Suchey (1990) reported that previous research (Todd, 1921; Gilbert and McKern, 1973) justified the need for a separate set of standards for females due to shape differences and pregnancy-related changes in the pelvis.

The mean, standard deviation, and a 95% confidence interval are reported for each phase for males and females. The 95% confidence interval is used as the predicted age range for a given unknown individual and is therefore more appropriately called a "prediction" interval (the term "confidence interval" has a different statistical meaning that does not apply here, strictly speaking).[6] Because of their large sample, detailed phase descriptions, and availability of corresponding casts,[7] the Suchey–Brooks method is the most widely used method today for aging the pubic symphysis (Figure 3.2).

Most forensic anthropologists, after scoring the pubic symphysis phase (I–VI), would report the mean of that phase as the "point estimate" for age-at-death for that individual, along with the provided ranges on either side of that point estimate (Garvin and Passalacqua, 2012). A few forensic anthropologists have pointed out statistical problems with this kind of reporting and instead advocate a more complex procedure called transition analysis (discussed earlier) (Boldsen at al., 2002) that can be used for any age-at-death indicator scored in ordinal phases (see DiGangi and Moore [Chapter 1], this volume) (e.g., pubic symphysis, auricular surface, sternal rib ends).

Studies continue on the pubic symphysis and the Suchey–Brooks method. For example, Berg (2008) reassessed this method for a modern American and modern Balkan sample and using transition analysis, added a seventh stage as well as a redefined stage V and VI. More recently, Hartnett (2010) found significant interobserver error with scoring (indicating improvements in training or phase descriptions are necessary) on a modern sample of autopsied individuals from Arizona and also described a phase VII for individuals in their seventies. It is clear that more validations should be done on this method for different populations.

The Auricular Surface

Lovejoy et al. (1985a) were the first to propose using the auricular surface of the ilium as an indicator of age-at-death. They had noted a high correlation between other skeletal age indicators and morphological changes of the auricular surface. The auricular surface is of great importance because it is more durable than other skeletal elements used for aging, and its morphology does not appear to be affected by sex or ancestry (Osborne et al., 2004). As with pubic symphyseal studies, Lovejoy et al. (1985a) stress the importance of understanding human aging as a process. They recommend eight phases with corresponding age ranges based on observations of morphological changes of the auricular surface. The first seven ranges are narrow, each only encompassing 5 years, while the final phase encompasses all individuals 60 years and older (see Figure 3.3). This method can be applied to either males

---

[6]Confidence intervals are 95% intervals of the distribution around a *mean*. An age-at-death estimate for an individual is not an estimate of a *mean*, it is the estimate of a single observation from a distribution and so involves much less confidence. The 95% intervals around a single observation are therefore referred to as "prediction intervals" and are much wider than confidence intervals.

[7]Casts are available from France Casting, www.francecasts.com.

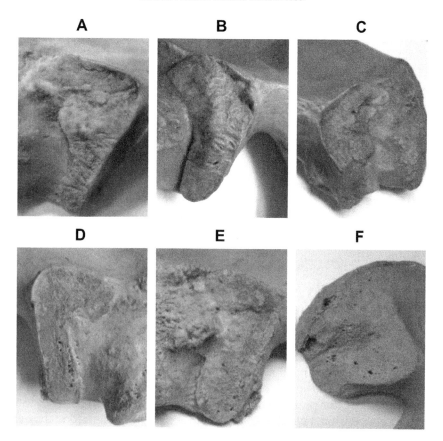

FIGURE 3.3 Auricular surface of the ilium, progressing from youngest (A) to oldest (F).

or females. Since their publication, this method has been widely used, but it has only recently been subjected to scientific scrutiny.

Buckberry and Chamberlain (2002) state that the rate of remodeling and degeneration of the auricular surface can be highly variable between individuals and populations because of the large effect *life history* has on the sacroiliac joint. They argued that the auricular surface aging technique had not undergone the same level of scrutiny as the pubic symphyseal aging technique. Therefore, in an attempt to accommodate more individual variation and make the method easier to apply, they devised a component system similar to the McKern and Stewart (1957) pubic symphysis method. Using the descriptions in Lovejoy et al. (1985a), Buckberry and Chamberlain devised progressive scores for transverse organization, surface texture, microporosity, macroporosity, and morphological changes of the auricular surface's apex. This study confirmed the applicability and reproducibility of the method and, upon cursory examination, the different components (with the exception of the retroauricular surface) showed a high correlation with true age.

The variable having the highest correlation with real age was the composite (sum) score of all five variables. No significant difference was found between males and females. The final scores were compressed into seven phases, each with a given range, mean, and median age (Buckberry and Chamberlain, 2002).

Shortly following the Buckberry and Chamberlain (2002) paper, Osborne et al. (2004) tested the Lovejoy et al. (1985a) method on a modern sample from the **Robert J. Terry Anatomical Skeletal Collection**[8] and **William M. Bass Donated Skeletal Collection**[9] and found that only 33% of the individuals were correctly aged using the original 5 year age ranges. An analysis of covariance (ANCOVA) found that age was the only significant influence on auricular surface morphology. Therefore, age assessment of the auricular surface does not need to account for different ancestral groups or sexes. "Collection" was included as a variable in the ANCOVA but was not significant, indicating that secular change (changes in morphology in populations over time) has not affected the morphological indicators of the auricular surface in the United States during the last century.[10] Osborne et al. (2004) advise that six phases (Figure 3.3), not the original eight (Lovejoy et al., 1985a) or revised seven (Buckberry and Chamberlain, 2002), should be used. However, Osborne et al.'s method has not caught on in practice (Garvin and Passalacqua, 2012), possibly because each phase is associated with large age ranges.

The Sternal Extremity of the Rib

While İşcan et al. (1984a,b) are most often credited with the development of aging of the sternal extremity of the rib, this indicator was actually noted earlier in print by Kerley (1970), Semine and Damon (1975), Ubelaker (1978), and McCormick (1980). McCormick was a pathologist and during his study of cadaver specimens, he noticed a positive relationship between the amount of mineralization in the costal cartilages on radiographs and known age-at-death. His study of over 200 cadavers confirmed this finding as a means to assess age-at-death broadly. However, this preliminary article only discussed broad changes and "does not allow the degree of precision that can be obtained by experts experienced in the evaluation of skeletal remains" (McCormick, 1980:740).

Currently, most anthropologists employ the technique described by İşcan et al. (1984a,b). Expanding on the work of Kerley (1970) and Ubelaker (1978), İşcan et al. (1984a,b) described changes in three components of rib morphology: (1) pit depth, (2) pit shape, and (3) rim wall and configurations of the ribs of European American males. İşcan and colleagues first analyzed the right fourth rib of 118 European American males autopsied at the Broward County Medical Examiner's Office, Fort Lauderdale, Florida. Eight phases were developed based on age-related changes, including the formation, depth, and shape of a pit, the configuration of the walls and rim around the pit, and the overall texture and quality of the bone. See Figure 3.4.

Based on observed sexual dimorphism in other studies of the ribs, İşcan et al. (1985) published different standards for European American females. Similar to their earlier study, ribs were seriated and eight phases were developed based on morphological changes. Unlike the male sample, where morphological changes did not occur until at least 17 years of age, the

---

[8]Curated by the National Museum of Natural History at the Smithsonian Institution, Washington, D.C.

[9]Curated by the Forensic Anthropology Center at the University of Tennessee, Knoxville, Tennessee.

[10]Refer to Moore and Ross (Chapter 6) and McKeown and Schmidt (Chapter 12), this volume for further discussion on secular change.

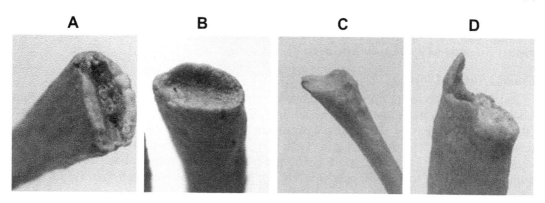

FIGURE 3.4 Sternal ends of the fourth rib, progressing from youngest (A) to oldest (D).

first signs of change appeared in females at 14 years. This determination, however, was based on one individual in the 10–15-year-old range. Any specimens younger than 14 years were scored as "0." The authors stated that morphological changes are so rapid between 14 and 28 years of age that phase differentiation could be made in 3 to 5 year intervals. As with the male sample, observed ranges for each phase were very large, but the age range estimates were reduced to 95% confidence intervals for the mean age of each stage.

Investigation into population differences in the morphology of the sternal extremity of the rib continued for several years, primarily by İşcan and colleagues (İşcan et al., 1985, 1987; İşcan, 1991). These studies found significant differences in the timing of morphological changes for different sexes, ancestry groups, and even occupations. İşcan et al. (1987) published new statistics and photos for ribs from African American males and females. While these studies are widely used and cited, the sample sizes were usually not sufficiently large to carry any statistical significance. For example, the African American female sample included 14 individuals. While population differences may exist, methods based on such small sample sizes cannot be used with confidence.

One of the most basic problems with the İşcan methods is the use of the fourth rib. Unless it is removed at autopsy or the entire rib cage is available, the fourth rib could be misidentified. Further, in archaeological or forensic contexts it could be missing or broken. Kunos et al. (1999) suggested the use of the first rib because it is easily identifiable and less prone to breaking. Their method not only focused on adult ribs, but included juvenile specimens as well. It is unique amongst other aging methods because of its flowchart process that walks the anthropologist through possibilities until the final use of a table to arrive at an age-at-death estimate.

Because the Kunos et al. (1999) method can be complicated to use and is of questionable utility in practice, DiGangi et al. (2009) devised a simpler method for assessing age-at-death from the first rib based on Kunos et al.'s (1999) observations of its morphological changes. These authors limited the method to two morphological features of the first rib and provided detailed descriptions and large color photographs of each phase. After scoring each feature, an anthropologist can use the provided reference table for posterior densities derived from transition analysis (given as 95% and 50% densities). The use and application of transition analysis to provide reference tables for age-at-death estimation is not free from some of the problems with age-at-death analysis, but it is the most statistically appropriate approach to this kind of analysis and it should be the future direction of research on morphological age-related changes, as previously discussed.

Cranial Suture Closure

Todd and Lyon began their extensive study of endocranial (interior skull) suture closure with European American males in 1924. They initiated this research because "the whole question of the relation of suture union to age remains an intricate and unsolved problem" (Todd and Lyon, 1924:329). Their study included over 300 crania of known ages ranging from 18 to 84 years of age. While the authors had access to larger numbers of crania, they eliminated individuals who did not have satisfactory documentation of age-at-death and individuals for whom the postcranial skeleton was not available for comparison. During the course of their research they also removed several crania that they deemed abnormal, thus critically reducing the amount of human variation in the sample.

The next year, Todd and Lyon (1925a) published their findings regarding ectocranial (exterior skull) suture closure for the same collection of 307 European American males. In this sample they found suture closure commences at the same time both endocranially and ectocranially. Once initiated, ectocranial fusion progresses more quickly and shows more individual variation. For these reasons Todd and Lyon concluded that cranial suture closure is not a very reliable aging indicator.

However, they also simultaneously published articles regarding both the endocranial and ectocranial closure of sutures in African American males (Todd and Lyon, 1925b,c). Although they only had 79 crania on which to base their conclusions, they believed that the establishment of their first standard could serve as a basis for comparison and offset the need for a larger sample. The results showed very little population difference in the closure of cranial sutures.

Several decades later, in the 1970s, osteologists began reconsidering cranial suture closure as a viable option for age determination (Johnson, 1976; Perizonius, 1984; Meindl and Lovejoy, 1985; Mann et al., 1987, 1991; Masset, 1989; Galera et al., 1998). Meindl and Lovejoy (1985) published a new method for age estimation from cranial suture closure. The authors claimed that "no studies exist in which suture closure has actually been *observed*" (Meindl and Lovejoy, 1985:57, their emphasis), and posited that Todd and Lyon's (1925a,b,c) practice of eliminating abnormal skulls from their studies is the reason for so much doubt as to the usefulness of cranial suture closure.

Meindl and Lovejoy's (1985) new method included observing one centimeter lengths of specific anatomical locations on sutures (to aid with repeatability) and a four-point scoring system: 0 = no observable closure, 1 = minimal closure (about 1–50%), 2 = significant closure (about 50–99%), and 3 = complete obliteration. Using the previous literature as a guide, the authors narrowed down ten specific sites for observation and limited their study to ectocranial sutures to increase the ease of use. These ten sites were divided into the "vault system" and the "lateral–anterior system," and modal patterns were investigated in each. The lateral–anterior system was more regular. Similar to the pubic symphyseal aging techniques of McKern and Stewart (1957) and Gilbert and McKern (1973), the authors produced a table of composite scores and a mean age and standard deviation for each score. However, as with other aging techniques, the standard deviations were rather large, as were the observed ranges. The authors noted that "the relationship between degree of closure and age is therefore only general" (Meindl and Lovejoy, 1985:62).

Meindl and Lovejoy also assessed the effect of ancestry and sex on the rate of suture closure. Using "error in prediction"[11] as the dependent variable, no independent variables or interactions were significant. Therefore, they concluded that sex and ancestry did not contribute a measurable bias in age estimation from cranial suture closure. Despite their moderately promising results, the authors still cautioned against the use of a single skeletal indicator of age-at-death and encouraged further development of cranial suture closure as an aging method.

Hershkovitz et al. (1997) published an article titled *Why Do We Fail in Aging the Skull from the Sagittal Suture?*, a scathing critique trying to put to rest this "traditional research obsession" of physical anthropologists (pp. 393−394). They quantified sagittal suture closure in 3636 skulls and found no useful age information after the age of 35 in addition to significant sex and ancestry differences. The authors postulated that cranial suture closure patterns are the result of a genetic predisposition for suture closure that differs between populations because of biological adaptation. They concluded that "Suture closure is neither a pathological phenomenon nor the result of [a] normal aging process" (Hershkovitz et al., 1997:398).

In 1998, Nawrocki expanded on the work of Meindl and Lovejoy (1985) and Mann et al. (1987, 1991) and developed a method of scoring 27 cranial landmarks along ectocranial, endocranial, and palatal sutures. Nawrocki used 100 crania from the Terry Collection including 50 females (25 European American and 25 African American) and 50 males (24 European American and 26 African American), ranging in age from 21 to 85 years with a mean age of 53.71 years. Importantly, no specimens were excluded from analysis for any reason except postmortem damage. Sutures on the vault were scored in one centimeter segments on a four-point scale, in accordance with Meindl and Lovejoy's method. Palatal sutures were observed along their entire length and are scored on the same scale.

Nawrocki's (1998) results revealed a moderate correlation between age and the summed cranial suture score for an individual. The results of an ANCOVA found definite variance resulting from sex, the interaction of ancestry and sex, and, of course, age. This interaction effect led Nawrocki (1998) to develop ancestry and sex-specific regression equations. A test of the equations on a different cadaver sample found that, as expected, the error rates and inaccuracy increased, but only to levels similar to other skeletal aging methods.

Zambrano (2005) reevaluated and tested Nawrocki's methods and found that the general "All Groups" equation outperformed the ancestry and sex-specific equations, based on the percentage of individuals whose actual age fell within the ± 2 standard error interval. He also reaffirmed that sex does in fact influence the rate and timing of cranial suture closure. Probably most importantly, his tests for secular trends found Nawrocki's equations (developed on the earlier Terry Collection) to be appropriate for modern, forensic collections.

---

[11]The authors define "error in prediction" as a linear combination of predicted minus actual age for each individual plus or minus another factor that is dependent on sex, ancestry, or decade of age (Meindl and Lovejoy, 1985).

Other Morphological Methods

Most anthropologists cite the Suchey–Brooks (1990) pubic symphyseal phases, Lovejoy et al. (1985a) auricular surface phases, İşcan et al. (1984a, b) sternal rib phases, and Meindl and Lovejoy (1985) cranial suture scores as their preferred methods for estimating age-at-death as previously discussed (Garvin and Passalacqua, 2012). However, specific cases can present situations that require the use of other parts of the skeleton and many additional age-at-death estimation techniques have been developed. For example, Passalacqua (2009) details a combined component/phase method of developmental and degenerative changes to the auricular surface of the sacrum. Langley-Shirley and Jantz (2010) presented five and three phase systems for estimating age-at-death from the clavicle. This method is based on epiphyseal fusion, but because the medial epiphysis of the clavicle is the last to fuse, this method applies mostly to young adults (those under 30). As with the DiGangi et al. (2009) first rib method they used transition analysis and provided reference tables with age ranges based on percentage of posterior density.

There are additional morphological (degenerative) changes in adult skeletons, many of which have not been evaluated or quantified in the same ways as the methods previously mentioned. Even with quantification and validation, many age-at-death methods exist but are not widely used in forensic anthropology casework (Garvin and Passalacqua, 2012). These include arthritic lipping and depth changes in the acetabulum (Rissech et al., 2006, 2007; Calce, 2012), and osteophytic lipping on vertebrae and other joints due to osteoarthritis (Van der Merwe et al., 2006; Zukowski et al., 2012). Often an anthropologist will not quantify arthritic changes as part of the formal age-at-death estimate, but that information is used to modify the final age-at-death estimate derived from more formal methods (Garvin and Passalacqua, 2012).

Dental Methods

In remains with adult dentition, age-at-death estimation techniques are limited to tooth features other than the development and eruption of teeth. Juveniles, of course, are aged based on their dental development (refer to Hammerl [Chapter 10], this volume). Some osteologists use the amount of wear on the occlusal surface of teeth as an age-at-death method, but modern diets are fairly soft, so forensic anthropologists generally do not use tooth wear in their estimates of age-at-death.[12] However, bioarchaeologists studying prehistoric remains may use tooth wear as part of their age estimation. Brothwell (1989) is one commonly used method.

Dental sclerosis is a process that results in progressive filling of the tooth dentin with transparent crystals beginning at the apex of the root and progressing toward the tooth crown (Beach et al., 2010). The utility of this process for estimating age-at-death has been recognized since the mid-twentieth century (Gustafson, 1947, 1950), but most anthropologists cite the technique of Lamendin et al. (1992). This technique only requires a light source and

---

[12]Incidentally, while forensic anthropologists do not generally use tooth wear for age-at-death estimations, they have used it as one of many cultural clues when trying to identify the country of origin of a decedent, i.e., to help with establishing whether unidentified individuals in Arizona are American citizens or undocumented border crossers (Birkby et al., 2008).

a measurement of the length of the transparent portion of the root. That measurement is then entered into a single regression formula regardless of sex or ancestry of the individual. Prince and Ubelaker (2002) validated the method's accuracy on a diverse skeletal sample, made adjustments, and found that although it was developed on a French population, it worked well for an American cadaveric sample, with mean errors around 8 years. When Prince and Ubelaker (2002) accounted for sex and ancestry the errors were further reduced to as low as 6.24 years for African American females. For more information on dentition, refer to Hammerl (Chapter 10), this volume.

Histology

Human bone is a dynamic tissue that constantly remodels in response to stressors in addition to being responsible for homeostasis of blood levels of minerals like calcium and phosphorus (Saladin, 2010). The basic organizational unit of cortical (compact) bone is the **osteon**. As a person ages, primary osteons are broken down (sometimes not completely) and replaced by new (secondary) osteons, presumably at a predictable rate. This turnover rate is the basis for histomorphological methods of age-at-death estimation (Stout, 1998). These methods are not widely used by anthropologists because of the need for both special-ized knowledge and specialized equipment to prepare and examine histological slides of the cortical bone (not to mention the destruction caused when obtaining the histological section), but when applied, these methods have potential to provide more precise age-at-death esti-mates for older individuals (Crowder and Pfeiffer, 2010).

Kerley (1965) was the first to publish an applicable method of age-at-death estimation based on histomorphology, but many have since followed with population-specific work, larger samples, and different bones (i.e., femur, rib, mandible, etc.), each leading to a different regression equation (e.g., Thompson, 1979; Stout and Paine, 1992; Cho et al., 2002). These methods still suffer from large age ranges, high interobserver error with osteon counts, and the possible impact of disease or metabolic changes that affect osteon turnover on an individual basis. For more information on histology, refer to Trammell and Kroman (Chapter 13), this volume.

Multifactorial Methods

Most biological anthropologists rely on multiple skeletal indicators of age-at-death when estimating age but lack a statistically sound method for combining individual indicators. Attempts at multifactorial aging (e.g., Brooks, 1955; Lovejoy et al., 1985a) have had generally disappointing results because they typically rely on either nonstatistical or linear statistical methods, creating problems with validity and applicability.

The first attempt at combining two or more skeletal aging methods was conducted by Brooks (1955), who utilized Todd's studies of cranial suture closure and changes of the pubic symphyseal surface in a skeletal population of prehistoric Native Ameri-cans and the Hamann Collection (now the Hamann-Todd Collection). She did not combine these two methods statistically but applied both methods to each individual in her sample. For the cadaveric Hamann Collection the correlation between pubic symphysis age and known age was acceptable in most cases but the correlation between cranial suture closure and known age was very low. In the prehistoric Native

American sample the mean age-at-death estimated from pubic symphyses differed by 10 years from the mean age-at-death estimate from cranial sutures. Her findings resulted in the caution that the skeleton was an entire unit during life so "no one age indicator is adequate" (Brooks, 1955:588).

Lovejoy et al. (1985b) presented the Multifactorial Summary Age method, which utilizes the pubic symphyseal face, auricular surface, radiographs of the proximal femur, dental wear, and suture closure. Their evaluation of skeletal aging methods summarizes that most methods are fairly inaccurate and can be gravely affected by interobserver error. This technique is intended for researchers engaged in paleodemography, so its applicability to individual specimens in forensic situations is questionable; however, it could be a plausible method in analysis of mass disasters or mass graves, although to this author's knowledge it is not used for such situations.

After the specimens are seriated according to Lovejoy et al. (1985b), each aging indicator is applied separately to each specimen and the scores are used to make an intercorrelation matrix,[13] which is then subjected to **principal components analysis** (a multivariate statistical procedure that combines several variables into a single variable for analysis). The correlation of each indicator with the first principal component is then taken as that variable's weight. Any factor with a correlation of at least $r = 0.70$ is incorporated into the model. The weighted average of each indicator then becomes the final age estimate (the "summary age") for each individual.

Over the past few decades a few more authors have attempted multifactorial methods (e.g., Saunders, 1992; Baccino and Zerilli, 1997; Baccino et al., 1999). It is clear from the literature that the use of multiple age indicators for the determination of age-at-death is ideal, but a scientific, quantitative, and easily applied method for combining the data is lacking. A comprehensive approach to aging is needed to simplify, and more importantly, standardize age-at-death estimation from skeletal remains. Further research is needed in this area.

Recently, paleodemographers have been at the forefront of multifactorial age-at-death estimation. Boldsen and colleagues (2002) developed a computer program (ADBOU) that collects data on multiple skeletal indicators scored as discrete ordinal phases and uses Bayesian inference to calculate the posterior probability density and estimate age-at-death. Unfortunately, tests of the ADBOU program have found it only moderately effective (Bethard, 2005; Uhl, 2008; Milner and Boldsen, 2012), in part because the trait scoring departs from the methods (e.g., Suchey–Brooks) to which many osteologists are accustomed. Without extensive practice, intra- and interobserver error can be problematic. Further, the ADBOU program comes with only a small choice of prior age-at-death distributions "hardwired" into the program. Bayesian analyses rely on these prior probabilities, together with the osteological data, to estimate ages at death for individual cases.

---

[13]The authors use the intercorrelation matrix as a means to generate the principal components, the first component of which is assumed to represent chronological age. The correlation of each indicator to that principal component is then used to weigh its contribution to a final multifactorial age estimate for an individual.

TABLE 3.2 Pubic Symphysis Reference Table

Stage	Mean Log Age	Median Age within Stage (exponentiated mean age)	Precision (1/var)
1	2.708094	15.00	10.932196
2	2.844875	17.20	8.625380
3	3.154550	23.44	10.341600
4	3.491685	32.84	8.948107
5	3.836729	46.37	9.964530
6	4.110183	60.96	13.583607

CASE STUDY: BAYESIAN THEORY APPLIED TO THE MULTIFACTORIAL AGE INDICATOR PROBLEM

Uhl et al. (2011) made use of a more diverse, and possibly more appropriate, reference sample and familiar skeletal scoring techniques to estimate age-at-death from multiple indicators when combined with an appropriate prior age-at-death distribution. Their data set consisted of age indicator scores for pubic symphysis (six phases; Brooks and Suchey, 1990), auricular surface (eight phases; Lovejoy et al., 1985a), and sternal rib end (eight phases; İşcan et al., 1984a, b, 1985) for 623 individuals from four modern collections: the Hamann-Todd Collection, the Bass Collection, the Terry Collection (all mentioned earlier), and the Pretoria Bone Collection.[14]

One initial issue addressed in studies employing transition analysis (DiGangi et al., 2009; Langley-Shirley and Jantz, 2010; Uhl et al., 2011) is whether the original scoring follows a particular transition model. A Lagrange multiplier test assesses these transition models by testing whether the addition of more variables improves the fit of the model. Uhl et al. (2011) found that the original six-phase pubic symphysis scoring and the eight-phase rib end scoring fit well in a cumulative log-probit model. The auricular surface scoring did not fit well, so the first four phases in the Lovejoy et al. (1985a) system were collapsed into a single phase. After making this collapse, the scoring did fit well in a cumulative log-probit model.

Following initial testing, Uhl and colleagues randomly sampled 100 individuals structured on age-at-death using a Gompertz hazard model of mortality estimated from the ages at death for Judy Suchey's Los Angeles County male forensic data. This Gompertz model was also used as the informative prior in estimating ages for the 100 individuals. After forming this "hold out" sample of 100, log-normal transition models (to normalize the data) were fit using the remaining 523 individuals, and the 95% highest posterior density region was found for each of the 240 morphological patterns (6 pubic symphyseal phases times 5 auricular surface phases times 8 rib phases) combined with the informative prior. The left and right boundaries of the distribution were placed in a reference table and then compared

---

[14]Curated by the Department of Anatomy at the University of Pretoria, Pretoria, South Africa.

TABLE 3.3 Auricular Surface Reference Table

Stage	Mean Log Age	Median Age within Stage (exponentiated mean age)	Precision (1/var)
1	2.708094	15.00	2.303171
2	3.638586	38.00	6.189976
3	3.837617	46.41	6.319739
4	3.971352	53.10	7.185791
5	4.096261	60.16	8.677416

TABLE 3.4 Fourth Sternal Rib End Reference Table

Stage	Mean Log Age	Median Age within Stage (exponentiated mean age)	Precision (1/var)
1	2.708094	15.00	10.477777
2	2.708094	15.00	5.379045
3	3.006817	20.22	8.140302
4	3.314185	27.50	8.380908
5	3.608466	36.90	7.923664
6	3.833493	46.22	8.702324
7	3.990612	54.10	10.427559
8	4.140792	62.85	12.749945

TABLE 3.5 Overall Mean Log Age and Precisions

Indicator	Mean Log Age	Precision (1/var)	Mean Log Age*Precision	Median Age within Stage (exponentiated mean log age)
Pubis Symphysis (Phase 3)	3.154550	3.154550	32.62300	23.44249
Auricular Surface (Phase 2)	3.638586	6.189976	22.52276	38.03801
Fourth Rib (Phase 5)	3.608466	7.923664	28.59227	36.90939
Sum Mean Log Ages			83.73803	
Sum Precision			24.45524	
Overall Mean Log Age			3.424138	30.69606

TABLE 3.6 Variances and Standard Deviation

Within-Indicator Variance	Between-Indicator Variance	Total Variance	Standard Deviation
0.040891	0.07354	0.114431	0.338276

to the actual ages for the hold out sample. Ninety-five of the 100 individuals had ages that fell within the 95% highest posterior density regions, indicating proper coverage. However, the widths of the 95% highest posterior density regions were sometimes quite considerable, reaching a maximum of 50 years for anyone in the final phase for all three indicators, reemphasizing the point that aging is variable, especially for older adults.

In practice, the reference tables (Tables 3.2–3.4) can be used to estimate ages on a case-by-case basis with age indicators assessed according to methods that anthropologists are already familiar with (i.e., Suchey–Brooks pubic symphysis phases, Lovejoy et al. auricular surface phases, and İşcan et al. sternal rib phases).

As an example, consider a set of remains that score as a Suchey–Brooks (pubic symphysis) phase 3, a Lovejoy et al. (auricular surface) phase 2, and an İşcan et al. (fourth sternal rib end) phase 5. Looking at the reference tables, the mean ages (on a log scale) are 3.154550, 3.638586, and 3.608466, respectively. The overall mean log age (across the three indicators) is found by summing the products of the individual mean log ages times the individual precisions (83.73803) and dividing by the sum of the individual precisions (24.45524). The mean log age in this case is 3.424138 years (Table 3.5). In order to integrate these separate estimates we need to know the within and between variance of the estimates. The precisions, given in the tables, are the inverse of the variance of each mean log age. If you sum the three precisions of each indicator for the scored phase (in this case, 10.341600, 6.189976, and 7.923664, respectively [Tables 3.2–3.4]) and take the inverse you have the within-indicator variance. The between-indicator variance is the variance of the three mean log ages for the indicators, and the total variance is the sum of the within-and between-indicator variance (Table 3.6). The standard deviation is the square root of the total variance; to obtain 95% confidence intervals for normally distributed data you multiply the standard deviation (calculated as 0.338276 for this case) by 1.96 (a standard scaling variable for how wide a curve will be when normally distributed) and add and subtract that from the overall mean log age. The final step is to exponentiate (convert from log numbers to regular numbers) the endpoints of the interval and the mean log age to convert it from log years to actual years. In this example, 3.424138 (mean log age) ± 0.663020 gives us a range of 2.761117–4.087159. When these numbers are exponentiated we have a final range of 15.81751 years to 59.57044 years with a mean of 30.69606.

CONCLUSION

The skeleton offers a wealth of information related to age-at-death in both juveniles and adults. Anthropologists continue to strive for a better understanding of skeletal development, including the influence of population and sex differences, so that epiphyseal fusion, long bone length, and dental development can be accurately applied to estimate age-at-death in juveniles. There are many challenges in the process of quantifying skeletal degeneration in adults and its relationship to chronological age, but research on modern skeletal collections is yielding more clues about this process, despite the effects of population history and individual variation in sex, health, activity levels, and disease.

A good deal of research is also needed to appropriately quantify both degeneration and variation and their relationship to chronological age to develop useful and practical methods. While the accuracy and precision with which we are realistically able to estimate age-at-death can sometimes be discouraging, it remains a fruitful ground for new research. This component of the biological profile is critical in both archaeological and forensic work, contributing to our understanding of past populations as well as helping to identify individuals in medicolegal contexts.

Students with an interest in age-at-death estimation should become well-versed in human osteology, including juvenile osteology, and basic statistical theory, especially theory related to regression. Many useful texts bring together different methods and perspectives on age-at-death estimation, including *Age Estimation of the Human Skeleton* (Latham and Finnegan, 2010), *Age Markers in the Human Skeleton* (İşcan, 1989), *The Human Skeleton in Forensic Medicine* (Krogman and İşcan, 1986), and *Paleodemography: Age Distributions from Skeletal Samples* (Hoppa and Vaupel, 2002). Students with access or resources to visit a skeletal collection have a variety of options: test the effectiveness of an existing method on that sample; try new statistical techniques for quantifying previously documented morphological changes; or devise new method(s) to quantify observed morphological changes suspected to be correlated with chronological age.

REFERENCES

Baccino, E., Zerilli, A., 1997. The two step strategy (TSS) or the right way to combine a dental (Lamendin) and an anthropological (Suchey–Brooks system) method for age determination. Proceedings of the American Academy of Forensic Sciences 3, 150.

Baccino, E., Ubelaker, D.H., Hayek, L.-A.C., Zerilli, A., 1999. Evaluation of seven methods of estimating age-at-death from mature human skeletal remains. Journal of Forensic Sciences 44 (5), 931–936.

Beach, J.J., Schmidt, C.W., Sharkey, R.A., 2010. Dental aging techniques: a review. In: Latham, K.E., Finnegan, M. (Eds.), Age Estimation of the Human Skeleton. Charles C. Thomas, Springfield IL, pp. 5–18.

Berg, G.E., 2008. Pubic bone age estimation in adult women. Journal of Forensic Sciences 53 (3), 569–577.

Bethard, J.D., 2005. A Test of the Transition Analysis Method for Estimation of Age-at-Death in Adult Human Skeleton Remains. M.A. thesis. University of Tennessee, Knoxville.

Birkby, W.H., Fenton, T.W., Anderson, B.E., 2008. Identifying Southwest Hispanics using nonmetric traits and the cultural profile. Journal of Forensic Sciences 53 (1), 29–33.

Boldsen, J.L., Milner, G.R., Konigsberg, L.W., Wood, J.W., 2002. Transition analysis: a new method for estimating age from skeletons. In: Hoppa, R., Vaupel, J. (Eds.), Paleodemography: Age Distributions from Skeletal Samples. Cambridge University Press, Cambridge, pp. 73–106.

Brooks, S.T., 1955. Skeletal age-at-death: the reliability of cranial and pubic age indicators. American Journal of Physical Anthropology 13 (4), 567–589.

Brooks, S.T., Suchey, J.M., 1990. Skeletal age determination based on the os pubis: a comparison of the Acsádi-Nemeskéri and Suchey–Brooks methods. Human Evolution 5, 227–238.

Brothwell, D.R., 1989. The relationship of tooth wear to ageing. In: Iscan, M.Y. (Ed.), Age Markers in the Human Skeleton. Charles C. Thomas, Springfield IL, pp. 303–316.

Buckberry, J.L., Chamberlain, A.T., 2002. Age estimation from the auricular surface of the ilium: a revised method. American Journal of Physical Anthropology 119 (3), 231—239.

Buikstra, J.E., Ubelaker, D.H., 1994. Standards for Data Collection from Human Skeletal Remains. Arkansas Archaeological Survey, Fayetteville, AR.

Calce, S.E., 2012. A new method to estimate adult age-at-death using the acetabulum. American Journal of Physical Anthropology 148 (1), 11—23.

Cho, H., Stout, S.D., Madsen, R.W., Streeter, M.A., 2002. Population-specific histological age-estimating method: a model for known African-American and European-American skeletal remains. Journal of Forensic Sciences 47 (1), 12—18.

Crowder, C., Austin, D., 2005. Age ranges of epiphyseal fusion in the distal tibia and fibula of contemporary males and females. Journal of Forensic Sciences 50 (5), 1001—1007.

Crowder, C., Pfeiffer, S., 2010. The application of cortical bone histomorphometry to estimate age-at-death. In: Latham, K.E., Finnegan, M. (Eds.), Age Estimation of the Human Skeleton. Charles C. Thomas, Springfield, IL, pp. 193—215.

Danubio, M.E., Sanna, E., 2008. Secular changes in human biological variables in Western countries: an updated review and synthesis. Journal of Anthropological Sciences 86, 91—112.

DiGangi, E.A., Bethard, J.D., Kimmerle, E.H., Konigsberg, L.W., 2009. A new method for estimating age-at-death from the first rib. American Journal of Physical Anthropology 138 (2), 164—176.

Fazekas, I.G., Kósa, F., 1978. Forensic Fetal Osteology. Akadémiai Kiadó, Budapest.

Fishman, L.S., 1982. Radiographic evaluation of skeletal maturation: a clinically oriented method based on hand-wrist films. Angle Orthodontist 52 (2), 88—112.

Flecker, H., 1942. Time of appearance and fusion of ossification centers as observed by roentogenographic methods. American Journal of Roentgenography 47, 95—159.

Galera, V., Ubelaker, D.H., Hayek, L.C., 1998. Comparison of macroscopic cranial methods of age estimation applied to skeletons from the Terry Collection. Journal of Forensic Sciences 43 (5), 933—939.

Garvin, H.M., Passalacqua, N.V., 2012. Current practices by forensic anthropologists in adult skeletal age estimation. Journal of Forensic Sciences 57 (2), 427—433.

Gilbert, B.M., McKern, T.W., 1973. A method for aging the female os pubis. American Journal of Physical Anthropology 38 (1), 31—38.

Golub, M.S., Hogrefe, C.E., Germann, S.L., Lasely, B.L., Natarajan, K., Tarantal, A.F., 2003. Effects of exogenous estrogenic agents on pubertal growth and reproductive system maturation in female rhesus monkeys. Toxicological Sciences 74 (1), 103—113.

Gustafson, G., 1947. Microscopic examination of teeth as a means of identification in forensic medicine. Journal of the American Dental Association 35 (10), 720—724.

Gustafson, G., 1950. Age determination on teeth. Journal of the American Dental Association 41 (1), 45—54.

Hammerl, E., 2013. Dental anthropology. In: DiGangi, E.A., Moore, M.K. (Eds.), Research Methods in Human Skeletal Biology. Academic Press, San Diego.

Hartnett, K.M., 2010. Analysis of age-at-death estimation using data from a new, modern autopsy sample—Part I: Pubic bone. Journal of Forensic Sciences 55 (5), 1145—1151.

Hoffman, J.M., 1979. Age estimations from diaphyseal lengths: two months to twelve years. Journal of Forensic Sciences 24 (2), 461—469.

Hershkovitz, I., Latimer, B., Dutour, O., Jellema, L.M., Wish-Baratz, S., Rothschild, C., Rothschild, B.M., 1997. Why do we fail in aging the skull from the sagittal suture? American Journal of Physical Anthropology 103 (3), 393—399.

Humphrey, L.T., 1998. Growth patterns in the modern human skeleton. American Journal of Physical Anthropology 105 (1), 57—72.

Huxley, A.K., 2010. Estimation of age from fetal remains. In: Latham, K.E., Finnegan, M. (Eds.), Age Estimation of the Human Skeleton. Charles C. Thomas, Springfield, IL, pp. 147—160.

İşcan, M.Y., 1991. The aging process in the rib: an analysis of sex- and race- related morphological variation. American Journal of Human Biology 3 (6), 617—623.

İşcan, M.Y., Loth, S.R., Wright, R.K., 1984a. Metamorphosis at the sternal rib end: a new method to estimate age-at-death in white males. American Journal of Physical Anthropology 65 (2), 147—156.

İşcan, M.Y., Loth, S.R., Wright, R.K., 1984b. Age estimation from the rib by phase analysis: white males. Journal of Forensic Sciences 29 (4), 1094—1104.

İşcan, M.Y., Loth, S.R., Wright, R.K., 1985. Age estimation from the rib by phase analysis: white females. Journal of Forensic Sciences 30 (3), 853–863.

İşcan, M.Y., Loth, S.R., Wright, R.K., 1987. Racial variation in the sternal extremity of the rib and its effect on age determination. Journal of Forensic Sciences 32 (2), 452–466.

Johnson, J.S., 1976. A comparison of age estimation using discriminant function analysis with some other age estimations of unknown skulls. Journal of Anatomy 121 (3), 475–484.

Johnston, F.E., 1962. Growth of the long bones of infants and young children at Indian Knoll. American Journal of Physical Anthropology 20 (5), 249–254.

Katz, D., Suchey, J.M., 1986. Age determination of the male os pubis. American Journal of Physical Anthropology 69 (4), 427–435.

Katz, D., Suchey, J.M., 1989. Race differences in pubic symphyseal aging patterns in the male. American Journal of Physical Anthropology 80 (2), 167–172.

Kerley, E.R., 1965. The microscopic determination of age in human bone. American Journal of Physical Anthropology 23 (2), 149–164.

Kerley, E.R., 1970. Estimation of skeletal age: after about age 30. In: Stewart, T.D. (Ed.), Personal Identification in Mass Disasters. National Museum of Natural History, Smithsonian Institution, Washington, D.C., pp. 57–70.

Komar, D.A., 2003. Lessons from Srebrenica: the contributions and limitations of physical anthropology in identifying victims of war crimes. Journal of Forensic Sciences 48 (4), 1–4.

Konigsberg, L.W., Frankenberg, S.R., 2013. Demography. In: DiGangi, E.A., Moore, M.K. (Eds.), Research Methods in Human Skeletal Biology. Academic Press, San Diego.

Krogman, W.M., İşcan, M.Y., 1986. The Human Skeleton in Forensic Medicine, 2nd ed. Charles C. Thomas, Springfield, IL.

Kunos, C.A., Simpson, S.W., Russell, K.F., Hershkovitz, I., 1999. First rib metamorphosis: its possible utility for human age-at-death estimation. American Journal of Physical Anthropology 110 (3), 303–323.

Lamendin, H., Baccino, E., Humbert, J.F., Tavernier, J.C., Nossintchouck, R.M., Zerilli, A., 1992. A simple technique for age estimation in adult corpses: the two criteria dental method. Journal of Forensic Sciences 37 (5), 1373–1379.

Langley-Shirley, N., Jantz, R.L., 2010. A Bayesian approach to age estimation in modern Americans from the clavicle. Journal of Forensic Sciences 55 (3), 571–583.

Lewis, M.E., 2006. The Bioarchaeology of Children: Perspectives from Biological and Forensic Anthropology. Cambridge University Press, Cambridge.

Lovejoy, C.O., Meindl, R.S., Pryzbeck, T.R., Mensforth, R.P., 1985a. Chronological metamorphosis of the auricular surface of the ilium: a new method for the determination of adult skeletal age-at-death. American Journal of Physical Anthropology 68 (1), 15–28.

Lovejoy, C.O., Meindl, R.S., Mensforth, R.P., Barton, T.J., 1985b. Multifactorial determination of skeletal age-at-death: a method and blind tests of its accuracy. American Journal of Physical Anthropology 68 (1), 1–14.

Mann, R.W., Symes, S.A., Bass, W.M., 1987. Maxillary suture obliteration: aging the human skeleton based on intact or fragmentary maxilla. Journal of Forensic Sciences 32 (1), 148–157.

Mann, R.W., Jantz, R.L., Bass, W.M., Willey, P.S., 1991. Maxillary suture obliteration: a visual method for estimating skeletal age. Journal of Forensic Sciences 36 (3), 781–791.

Marden, K., Sorg, M.H., Haglund, W.D., 2013. Taphonomy. In: DiGangi, E.A., Moore, M.K. (Eds.), Research Methods in Human Skeletal Biology. Academic Press, San Diego.

Maresh, M.M., 1955. Linear growth of long bones of extremities from infancy through adolescence. American Journal of Disabled Children 89 (6), 725–742.

Masset, C., 1989. Age estimation on the basis of cranial sutures. In: İşcan, M.Y. (Ed.), Age Markers in the Human Skeleton. C.C. Thomas, Springfield, IL, pp. 71–103.

May, S., Robson-Brown, K., Vincent, S., Eyers, J., King, H., Roberts, A., 2012. An infant femur bearing cut marks from Roman Hambleden, England. International Journal of Osteoarchaeology in press.

McCormick, W.F., 1980. Mineralization of the costal cartilages as an indicator of age: preliminary observations. Journal of Forensic Sciences 25 (4), 736–741.

McKeown, A.H., Schmidt, R.W., 2013. Geometric morphometrics. In: DiGangi, E.A., Moore, M.K. (Eds.), Research Methods in Human Skeletal Biology. Academic Press, San Diego.

McKern, T.W., Stewart, T.D., 1957. Skeletal age changes in young American males. Analysed from the standpoint of age identification. Environmental Protection Research Division. Quartermaster Research Development Center, U.S. Army, Natick, Massachusetts. Technical Report EP-45.

Meindl, R.S., Lovejoy, C.O., 1985. Ectocranial suture closure: a revised method for the determination of skeletal age-at-death based on the lateral—anterior sutures. American Journal of Physical Anthropology 68 (1), 57—66.

Meindl, R.S., Lovejoy, C.O., 1989. Age changes in the pelvis: implications for paleodemography. In: Işcan, M.Y. (Ed.), Age Markers in the Human Skeleton. Charles C. Thomas, Springfield, IL, pp. 137—168.

Meindl, R.S., Lovejoy, C.O., Mensforth, R.P., Walker, R.A., 1985. A revised method of age determination using the os pubis, with a review and tests of accuracy of other current methods of pubic symphyseal aging. American Journal of Physical Anthropology 68 (1), 29—45.

Merchant, V.L., Ubelaker, D.H., 1977. Skeletal growth of the protohistoric Arikara. American Journal of Physical Anthropology 46 (1), 61—72.

Milner, G.R., Boldsen, J.L., 2012. Transition analysis: a validation study with known-age modern American skeletons. American Journal of Physical Anthropology 148 (1), 98—110.

Nawrocki, S.P., 1998. Regression formulae for the estimation of age from cranial suture closure. In: Reichs, K. (Ed.), Forensic Osteology: Advances in the Identification of Human Remains, 2nd ed. C.C. Thomas, Springfield, IL, pp. 276—292.

Nawrocki, S.P., 2010. The nature and sources of error in the estimation of age-at-death from the skeleton. In: Latham, K.E., Finnegan, M. (Eds.), Age Estimation of the Human Skeleton. Charles C. Thomas, Springfield, IL, pp. 79—101.

Ogden, C.L., Kuczmarski, R.J., Flegal, K.M., Mei, Z., Shumei, G., Wei, R., Grummer-Strawn, L.M., Curtin, L.R., Roche, A.F., Johnson, C.L., 2002. Centers for Disease Control and Prevention 2000 Growth Charts for the United States: Improvements to the 1977 National Center for Health Statistics Version. Pediatrics 109 (1), 45—60.

Osborne, D.L., Simmons, T.L., Nawrocki, S.P., 2004. Reconsidering the auricular surface as an indicator of age-at-death. Journal of Forensic Sciences 49 (5), 1—7.

Ousley, S., Stull, K., Frazee, K., 2010. A radiographic database for forensic anthropology. Proceedings of the American Academy of Forensic Sciences 16, 389—390.

Passalacqua, N.V., 2009. Forensic age-at-death estimation from the human sacrum. Journal of Forensic Sciences 54 (2), 255—262.

Perizonius, W.R.K., 1984. Closing and non-closing sutures in 256 crania of known age and sex from Amsterdam (A.D. 1883—1909). Journal of Human Evolution 13, 201—216.

Prince, D., Ubelaker, D.H., 2002. Application of Lamendin's adult dental aging technique to a diverse skeletal sample. Journal of Forensic Sciences 47 (1), 107—116.

Rissech, C., Estabrook, G.F., Cunha, E., Malgosa, A., 2006. Using the acetabulum to estimate age-at-death of adult males. Journal of Forensic Sciences 51 (2), 213—229.

Rissech, C., Estabrook, G.F., Cunha, E., Malgosa, A., 2007. Estimation of age-at-death for adult males using the acetabulum, applied to four Western European populations. Journal of Forensic Sciences 52 (4), 774—778.

Sadler, T.W., 2004. Langman's Medical Embryology, 9th ed. Lippincott Williams & Wilkins, Baltimore.

Saladin, K., 2010. Anatomy & Physiology: The Unity of Form and Function, 5th ed. McGraw Hill, New York.

Saunders, S.R., Fitzgerald, C., Rogers, T., Dudar, C., McKillop, H., 1992. A test of several methods of skeletal age estimation using a documented archaeological sample. Canadian Society of Forensic Sciences Journal 25 (2), 97—118.

Schaefer, M.C., Black, S.M., 2005. Comparison of ages of epiphyseal union in North American and Bosnian skeletal material. Journal of Forensic Sciences 50 (4), 777—784.

Schaefer, M., Black, S., Scheuer, L., 2009. Juvenile Osteology: A Laboratory and Field Manual. Academic Press, San Diego.

Scheuer, L., Black, S.M., 2000. Developmental Juvenile Osteology. Academic Press, San Diego.

Schour, I., Massler, M., 1941. The development of the human dentition. Journal of the American Dental Association 28, 1153—1160.

Semine, A.A., Damon, A., 1975. Costochondral ossification and aging in five populations. Human Biology 47 (1), 101—116.

Smith, B.H., 1991. Standards of human tooth formation and dental age assessment. In: Kelley, M.A., Larson, C.S. (Eds.), Advances in Dental Anthropology. Wiley-Liss, New York, pp. 143—168.

Smith, B.H., Tompkins, R.L., 1995. Toward a life history of the Hominidae. Annual Review of Anthropology 24, 257—279.

Smith, E.L., 2010. Age estimation of subadult remains from the dentition. In: Latham, K.E., Finnegan, M. (Eds.), Age Estimation of the Human Skeleton. Charles C. Thomas, Springfield, IL, pp. 57—78.

Smith, M.O., 2013. Paleopathology. In: DiGangi, E.A., Moore, M.K. (Eds.), Research Methods in Human Skeletal Biology. Academic Press, San Diego.

Stewart, T.D., 1979. Essentials of Forensic Anthropology: Especially as Developed in the United States. Charles C. Thomas, Springfield, IL.

Stout, S.D., 1998. The application of histological techniques for age at death estimation. In: Reichs, K. (Ed.), Forensic Osteology: Advances in the Identification of Human Remains, 2nd ed. C.C. Thomas, Springfield, IL, pp. 237–252.

Stout, S.D., Paine, R.R., 1992. Brief Communication: Histological age estimation using rib and clavicle. American Journal of Physical Anthropology 87 (1), 111–115.

Suchey, J.M., 1979. Problems in the aging of females using the os pubis. American Journal of Physical Anthropology 51 (3), 467–470.

Suchey, J.M., Katz, D., 1998. Applications of pubic age determination in a forensic setting. In: Reichs, K. (Ed.), Forensic Osteology: Advances in the Identification of Human Remains, 2nd ed. C.C. Thomas, Springfield, IL, pp. 204–236.

Suchey, J.M., Wiseley, D.V., Green, R.F., Noguchi, T.T., 1979. Analysis of dorsal pitting in the os pubis in an extensive sample of modern American females. American Journal of Physical Anthropology 51 (4), 517–540.

Suchey, J.M., Brooks, S.T., Katz, D.M., 1988. Instructions for use of the Suchey–Brooks system for age determination for the female os pubis. Instructional materials accompanying female pubic symphyseal models of the Suchey–Brooks system. Distributed by France Casting, Fort Collins, Colorado.

Thompson, D.D., 1979. The core technique in the determination of age-at-death in skeletons. Journal of Forensic Sciences 24 (4), 902–915.

Todd, T.W., 1920. Age changes in the pubic bone. I: The male white pubis. American Journal of Physical Anthropology 3 (3), 285–334.

Todd, T.W., 1921. Age changes in the pubic bone. II: The pubis of the male Negro-White hybrid, III: The pubis of the White female. IV: The pubis of the female Negro-White hybrid. American Journal of Physical Anthropology 4 (1), 1–70.

Todd, T.W., Lyon, D.W., 1924. Endocranial suture closure, its progress and age relationship: Part I. Adult males of the white stock. American Journal of Physical Anthropology 7 (3), 325–384.

Todd, T.W., Lyon, D.W., 1925a. Cranial suture closure, its progress and age relationship: Part II. Ectocranial suture closure in adult males of the white stock. American Journal of Physical Anthropology 8 (1), 23–45.

Todd, T.W., Lyon, D.W., 1925b. Cranial suture closure, its progress and age relationship: Part III. Endocranial closure in adult males of the negro stock. American Journal of Physical Anthropology 8 (1), 47–71.

Todd, T.W., Lyon, D.W., 1925c. Cranial suture closure, its progress and age relationship: Part IV. Ectocranial closure in adult males of the negro stock. American Journal of Physical Anthropology 8 (1), 149–168.

Trammell, L.H., Kroman, A.M., 2013. Bone and Dental Histology. In: DiGangi, E.A., Moore, M.K. (Eds.), Research Methods in Human Skeletal Biology. Academic Press, San Diego.

Ubelaker, D.H., 1978. Human Skeletal Remains: Excavation, Analysis, Interpretation. Aldine Publishing Company, Chicago.

Ubelaker, D.H., 1987. Estimating age at death from immature human skeletons: an overview. Journal of Forensic Sciences 32 (5), 1254–1263.

Ubelaker, D.H., 1989. Human Skeletal Remains: Excavation, Analysis, Interpretation, 2nd ed. Aldine Publishing Company, Chicago.

Uhl, N.M., 2008. ADBOU estimation in South African populations. Proceedings of the American Association of Physical Anthropology Annual Meetings 135 (S46).

Uhl, N.M., Passalacqua, N.V., Konigsberg, L.W., 2011. A Bayesian approach to multifactorial age-at-death estimation. Proceedings of the American Academy of Forensic Sciences (AAFS) Annual Meetings 17, 339.

Van der Merwe, A.E., Işcan, M.Y., L'Abbè, E.N., 2006. The pattern of vertebral osteophyte development in a South African population. International Journal of Osteoarchaeology 16 (5), 459–464.

Wood, J.W., Milner, G.R., Harpending, H.C., Weiss, K.M., Cohen, M.N., Eisenberg, L.E., Hutchinson, D.L., Jankauskas, R., Česnys, G., Katzenberg, M.A., Lukacs, J.R., McGrath, J.W., Roth, E.A., Ubelaker, D.H., Wilkinson, R.G., 1992. The osteological paradox: problems of inferring prehistoric health from skeletal samples [and Comments and Reply]. Current Anthropology 33 (4), 343–370.

Zambrano, C.J., 2005. Evaluation of Regression Equations Used to Estimate Age-at-Death from Cranial Suture Closure. M.S. thesis. University of Indianapolis, Indianapolis.

Zeveloff, S.I., Boyce, M.S., 1982. Why human neonates are so altricial. American Naturalist 120 (4), 537–542.

Zukowski, L.A., Falsetti, A.B., Tillman, M.D., 2012. The influence of sex, age and BMI on the degeneration of the lumbar spine. Journal of Anatomy 220 (1), 57–66.

4

Sex Estimation and Assessment

Megan K. Moore

INTRODUCTION

This chapter discusses research methods in sex estimation and assessment of the adult and subadult skeletons, including a historical perspective of research methods over the last century. A distinction can be drawn between **sex estimation**[1] (typically metric with estimable error rates) and **sex assessment** (nonmetric and without estimable error rates). The causes of **sexual dimorphism** are presented, examining both intrinsic and extrinsic factors, which is essentially the reason why we can estimate or assess sex from the skeleton. When sexing of the skeleton was first undertaken, visual assessment of sexual characteristics on the skull and pelvis were the predominant methods. Today, metric sex estimation methods have replaced the more subjective visual sex assessment, despite the fact that it is much more tedious to measure the bones than to make a quick visual assessment. The accuracy of existing metric and nonmetric sexing methods is therefore presented for the various skeletal elements. In sex estimation research, subadult sex estimation poses the most difficulties, as many of the secondary sexual characteristics of the skeleton do no fully develop until after puberty. The conclusion of the chapter addresses some of the demographic approaches to quantitatively estimate the probability of a skeleton being one sex or another.[2] This chapter concludes with recommendations for research areas in sex estimation and assessment that require more attention.

Estimating the sex of a human skeleton is very important for the bioarchaeologist and forensic anthropologist when building a biological profile. In forensic cases, correctly sexing an unknown individual can reduce the number of possible matches to missing persons by fifty percent. In bioarchaeology, sex estimation and assessment can help to reveal questions of differential access to resources or cultural variation in behavior as preserved in the **functional adaptations** of the skeleton, that I will discuss later in Chapter 14, this volume.

[1]All bolded terms are defined in the glossary at the end of this volume.

[2]This is addressed further in the chapter on demography in this volume by Konigsberg and Frankenberg (Chapter 11).

SEX ASSESSMENT VERSUS SEX ESTIMATION

Spradley and Jantz (2011) draw a distinction between sex assessment and sex estimation (as per a previous communication with Stanley Rhine), which is worth emphasizing. *Sex assessment* refers to the traditional and more subjective visual method used by anthropologists when looking at elements such as the pelvis or skull. *Sex estimation*, in contrast, is the metric estimation of sex using estimable error rates (Spradley and Jantz, 2011). Stewart (1979) recommended using metric sex estimation *only* as a validation of the more subjective visual sex assessment. The current consensus in sexing research, however, is to focus on metric sex estimation. This is demonstrated by the vast proportion of recent papers based on **discriminant function analysis** of metric traits versus publications on descriptive, nonmetric traits.

Though many researchers may publish papers claiming sex determination (Berrizbeitia, 1989; Kemkes-Grottenthaler, 2005; Rogers, 2005; Barrio et al., 2006; Case and Ross, 2007; Gualdi-Russo, 2007; Mahfouz et al., 2007a; Albanese et al., 2008), I believe this term is incorrectly used and implies greater confidence than is warranted. Until accuracy rates consistently reach 100% (which will likely never happen due to human variation), it is better to consider this endeavor as estimation of sex.

Another common error in terminology made in some publications is the incorrect use of the term *gender* instead of *sex* (Gilsanz et al., 1997; Beck et al., 2000). **Gender** is a sociocultural construct, whereas **sex** is a biological distinction (Walker and Cook, 1998). The latter term reflects what can be discerned from analysis of the human skeleton, though culture inevitably plays a role, as will be discussed.

Anthropologists traditionally used visual inspection of sexual dimorphism of the pelvis and skull to distinguish a male skeleton from a female one. The adult female skeleton maintains prepubescent gracility (except in the pelvis), whereas the adult male skeleton shows more robusticity than the female skeleton (especially at muscle insertion sites) in most cranial and postcranial elements (Stewart, 1979; Krogman and İşcan, 1986; Bass, 1987). For the purpose of childbirth, the female pelvis continues to grow and change shape until the age of about 18, but the male pelvis maintains prepubescent characteristics (see discussion below) (Buikstra and Ubelaker, 1994; Bogin, 1999).

Brothwell considered the traits that are "sexed upon inspection" to be the most important, especially those on the pelvis and skull (Brothwell, 1963). Stewart (1979) considered the method of looking at observable sex details (e.g., subpubic angle, size of the mastoid process) to be the simplest indicator of sex. He considered it to be a waste of time to measure traits that can be verified very quickly by the naked eye. Rogers wrote that nonmetric traits were "of more immediate value" to the forensic anthropologist because they required less time and effort than metric sex estimation (Rogers, 1987). More recently, calls for higher standards in the legal system have caused a shift toward greater emphasis on validation studies and the use of estimable error rates within skeletal biology. Before reviewing the various methods for sex estimation and assessment, a discussion about the various causes for sexual dimorphism (both intrinsic and extrinsic) will help keep a focus on the etiology of the sexual dimorphism that we use to estimate and assess sex from the skeleton.

SEXUAL DIMORPHISM: INTRINSIC VERSUS EXTRINSIC FACTORS

Many factors are involved in the development of the adult human skeleton. Bones are extremely plastic throughout life and are constantly changing in response to **extrinsic factors**, such as the **biomechanical** effects of load bearing and muscle forces acting on bone. Other extrinsic factors that can leave a record on the skeleton (in addition to biomechanical responses to forces) include the effects of nutritional status, activity levels and even body mass. During growth and development, bone is additionally affected by **intrinsic** or systemic factors under genetic constraint, such as hormone levels. Our ultimate goal is to tease apart these confounding variables to develop methods that enable us as skeletal biologists to distinguish traits that reflect only biological sex.

Sexual dimorphism is the difference between males and females of a species in terms of body size, body shape, the rate/timing of development, or behavior. Sexual dimorphism is a combined result of genetic factors (e.g., hormone levels) and the environment (e.g., nutrition and cultural behaviors) (Stinson, 2012). For example, human males and females exhibit dimorphism in body composition (fat versus lean mass), tooth size, and distal femoral breadth (Kieser, 1990; Mahfouz et al., 2007b; Stinson, 2012). In terms of femur length, human male femora can be anywhere from 3.3% to 10.7% longer than female femora. Compare this to male gorilla femora, which are 20.9% longer than female gorilla femora (Frayer and Wolpoff, 1985).

In humans, the primary sexual characteristics of the genitalia begin to differentiate and develop early *in utero* (Ulijaszek et al., 1998; Bogin, 1999). The secondary sex characteristics begin to develop at puberty and include differences in body size and pelvic morphology, among other distinctions. These secondary sex characteristics are more affected by the environment than are the primary sexual characteristics (Frayer and Wolpoff, 1985). An example of this is the reduction in size dimorphism in humans when there are nutritional deficiencies. Males are more affected by nutritional deficits, which results in less sexual dimorphism in size (Stini, 1975, 1982; Bogin, 1999; Ross et al., 2003). Moore and Ross discuss female buffering to environmental stress later in this volume (Chapter 6). The following discussion will elaborate on the distinctions between intrinsic and extrinsic factors that play a role in sexual dimorphism.

Intrinsic Factors in Sexual Dimorphism

Intrinsic factors in sexual dimorphism are factors that arise from within the body systemically as mentioned, a prime example being those controlled by the gonadal or pituitary hormones. Before the age of 12, it is difficult to accurately estimate the sex of a juvenile skeleton, due to the fact that most sexually dimorphic skeletal characters do not develop until puberty, as already discussed. The onset of puberty is accompanied by high sex hormone levels and initiates the last major growth spurt in humans (Bogin, 1999; Scheuer and Black, 2004). It is this adolescent growth spurt that manifests the secondary sexual characteristics in the skeleton. Some traits of the skeleton, however, appear to be tightly genetically controlled and are highly dimorphic. These include the size of the secondary dentition, as well as the shape of the pelvis, both of which appear very early in development (Fazekas and Kósa, 1978; Kieser, 1990; Scheuer and Black, 2004). Traits that are under greater genetic control seem to appear earlier than those affected more by the environment. Interestingly, sexual dimorphism is present in the fetal pelvis, becomes indistinguishable during childhood and then reappears after adolescence. The adult shape of the pelvic inlet has obvious ramifications for childbirth, which is likely why it is under intrinsic genetic control.[3]

Extrinsic Factors in Sexual Dimorphism

Extrinsic factors in sexual dimorphism are those that are introduced typically from outside the body. Examples of extrinsic factors include nutrition and the biomechanics of activity and locomotion, both of which are combined into the additional extrinsic factor of body weight that acts on the skeleton. Nutrition, an extrinsic factor, has been shown to accelerate the process of maturation in both humans and nonhuman primates. For instance, high fat and high protein diets can speed up the age of maturation in humans (Bogin, 1999; Kaplowitz et al., 2001; Kaplowitz, 2006). Rate acceleration in maturation has been demonstrated in the worldwide decrease in the age of menarche (the age of a girl's first menstruation), which many researchers attribute to nutrition (Bogin, 1999; Kaplowitz et al., 2001; Onland-Moret et al., 2005; Kaplowitz, 2006; Cho et al., 2010). Conversely, delayed maturation and growth stunting in skeletal elements is also due to extrinsic environmental stresses (e.g., malnutrition, disease) and can reduce sexual dimorphism in body size. Females show buffering to these extrinsic factors of nutritional stress; thus, growth stunting is less severe in females than males in terms of rates of growth and development (Stini, 1975, 1982; Stinson, 2012; Bogin, 1999; Ross et al., 2003). The reason for this buffering in females is unknown, but hypotheses surround the role females must play in pregnancy and childbirth: females must be better buffered against environmental stressors, even beginning in childhood, for the species to survive.

Extrinsic factors in skeletal maturation can also be due to the biomechanical influence of different forces on the skeleton, such as locomotion and gravity. The plasticity of bones during growth and development enables our skeletal system to be designed specifically for our size/weight, activities, and behaviors. If it were not, our bones would simply fail (i.e., fracture). The load-bearing bones of the lower limb seem to show more plasticity during maturation, especially in the diaphysis, yielding a high correlation with body mass and activity levels (Ruff and Hayes, 1988; Moro et al., 1996; Larsen, 1997; Ruff, 2000; Lieberman et al., 2001).

Intrinsic and extrinsic factors begin to blur when we consider the bones of the pelvis and the femur. There are no inherent differences in the femora of boys and girls, but this begins to change with the onset of puberty. There are, however, subtle differences in the fetal pelvis that disappear in children and reappear in adolescence. As mentioned above, the pelvis is under genetic control for shape, but this pelvic shape may have biomechanical consequences for the femur, which can be compounded as a result of an individual's behavior. By looking at population variation in sexual dimorphism of the skeleton, we can start to discern whether a skeletal trait is the result of intrinsic or extrinsic agents. If consistent patterns of sexual

---

[3]Simultaneously, the pelvis plays a pivotal role (pun intended) in the biomechanics of the lower leg in locomotion, influenced by extrinsic factors as described below.

dimorphism are found in the femur across all populations with vastly different activity patterns, then confidence increases that the dimorphic traits are the result of universal sex differences in the shape of the pelvis and not the result of population-specific activity patterns.

The entire skeleton is under varying amounts of intrinsic and extrinsic influences. According to Ruff (1987), biological anthropologists have focused on statistical techniques for differentiating sexes, without considering these functional aspects. If we are able to recognize not only biological differences but biomechanical differences as well, we may learn to better understand sexual dimorphism in humans and improve sex discrimination from the skeleton. I explain the functional adaptations of the skeleton in greater detail in the later chapter on functional morphology in this volume (Chapter 14). The following discussion of the various methods of sex estimation and sex assessment is not meant to be exhaustive, but intended to be a starting point for young researchers to develop interest in sexing from the human skeleton.

SEX ASSESSMENT

Sex Assessment: Pelvis

The anatomical illustration by Edward Mitchell published in 1819[4] demonstrates an early understanding of sexual dimorphism in the human pelvis (Figure 4.1). Several aspects of the female pelvis begin to change shape at puberty to accommodate the birth of a human infant's relatively large skull. For example, the pubic bone broadens, the pubic ramus thins and lengthens, and the auricular surface becomes slightly raised. The angle of the sciatic notch and the subpubic angle become obtuse. While these traits are difficult to quantify metrically, the visual observations are immediate and require no equipment, only knowledge and experience. Many texts offer descriptions and diagrams for sex assessment from the pelvis (Brothwell, 1963; Stewart, 1979; Krogman and İşcan, 1986; Bass, 1987; Rogers, 1987; Buikstra and Ubelaker, 1994; White et al., 2012).

In general, the female pelvis develops at puberty to have a broader inlet, whereas the male pelvis follows the preadolescent pattern, as shown in Figure 4.2. Thus, if sexing a subadult pelvis (possibly as young as 12 or 13), if there are female traits present, the researcher can be confident that it is in fact female. If, however, the traits seem masculine, the juvenile could be either female or male (Buikstra and Ubelaker, 1994). In *Standards for Data Collection From Human Skeletal Remains* (Buikstra and Ubelaker, 1994), only three methods for sex assessment from the pelvis are recommended: (1) the **Phenice method** of subpubic morphology, (2) the morphology of the greater sciatic notch, and (3) the presence of the preauricular sulcus, all of which are combined into the study by Bruzek (2002), yielding high classification accuracy rates, as discussed below.

The Phenice method is a visual sex assessment method of the anterior os coxa that examines the traits of the *subpubic concavity*, the *medial ischiopubic ramus* and the *ventral arc*, with sexing accuracy rates in excess of 95% according to the author (Phenice, 1969). Phenice

[4]The Mitchell engraving is based on illustrations done by the early skeletal biologist and anatomist Jean Joseph Sue (1710–1792).

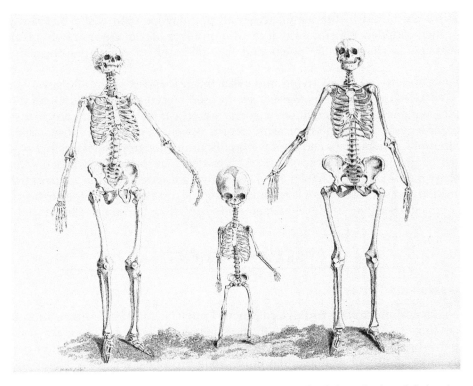

FIGURE 4.1   Edward Mitchell's 1819 illustration of sex differences in the skeleton (male on left, female on right), print based on J.J. Sue.

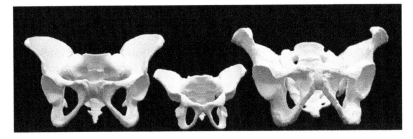

FIGURE 4.2   Pelvis of female on left, subadult in the center, and male on the right, depicting the similarities in a narrower subpubic angle in the subadult and adult male compared to the adult female.

(1969) determined that the ventral arc was the most sexually dimorphic and the ischiopubic ramus was the most ambiguous. The Phenice method can be extremely useful for the trained osteologist, with accuracy rates similar to those Phenice originally reported (96.5%) (Ubelaker and Volk, 2002). The method shows a high degree of subjectivity, however, it has much lower success when attempted by an untrained observer (accuracy rate of only 88.4%) (Ubelaker and Volk, 2002).

In order to improve upon the Phenice method and decrease its subjectivity, Bruzek (2002) used five measurements from the pelvis including a combination of the Phenice method, the preauricular sulcus, the greater sciatic notch, and inferior morphology including the ischio-pubic index. These characters were chosen to reflect more sex-specific functional adaptations of bipedality and the investigator achieved an accuracy rate of 95% (Bruzek, 2002). Future research could test whether this method has reduced subjectivity compared to the Phenice method alone. As mentioned above, most textbooks have extensive descriptions and lists of features established for sex assessment, sometimes having been ranked for their reliability. Studies are beginning to investigate error rates in sex assessment and this would be a possible area of future research (Rogers and Saunders, 1994; Konigsberg and Hens, 1998; Bruzek, 2002; Ubelaker and Volk, 2002; Walker, 2008).

Sex Assessment: Skull

The morphology of the skull has been the most studied part of the skeleton. Broca published the first scoring illustrations of sex assessment from the skull in 1875 (Walker, 2008). Visual sex assessment is relatively simple and does not require any anthropometric equipment; however, it can be difficult to measure the traits being visually assessed (e.g., the morphology of the brow ridge) (Walker, 2008). The chin of the male mandible is more square-shaped, whereas the female chin is more rounded. Male skulls are more robust, especially at muscle insertion sites. The female skull is typically more gracile, but analysis must be limited to adult ages between approximately 20 and 55 years,[5] as **masculinization** of the skull occurs with older age in females and younger males may not yet have developed secondary sex characteristics in the skull (Krogman and İşcan, 1986; Buikstra and Ubelaker, 1994).

It is important for a researcher to be very familiar with the pattern of variability within a population, because morphological features on the skull are population specific (Buikstra and Ubelaker, 1994). For example, one population may have males with very robust brow ridges, while another population may have males with relatively gracile brow ridges and less sexual dimorphism between males and females, as a result of human variation. For this reason, ordinal ranking of traits from 0 to 5 as per Buikstra and Ubelaker (1994) are recommended for discrimination (score of 0 as indeterminate, 1 as smallest or absent, 5 as largest). Walker (2008) preferred this ranked ordinal standard as opposed to the −2 to 2 system developed by Ascádi and Nemeskéri (1970). In this system in which 0 is intermediate between male traits and female traits, 0 in one population may not be a 0 in another population.

Comparative population studies are needed to investigate intrinsic and universal female or male traits versus those traits that are **population specific** or represent a continuum of expression between populations. Population variation in discrete and metric traits is discussed further in the chapter on ancestry estimation in this volume by DiGangi and Hefner (Chapter 5). As with sex assessment from the pelvis, current studies have been quantifying the visually assessed dimorphic traits of the skull (Rogers and Saunders, 1994; Konigsberg

---

[5]The younger age of this range approximates when masculine traits appear in adult males and the later age approximates when masculinization of the skull begins in females after menopause.

and Hens, 1998; Ubelaker and Volk, 2002; Walker, 2008), which has great potential for future research. Walker (2008) tested multiple types of discriminant function analysis using **ranked ordinal scores** of visually assessed features of the skull: mental eminence, orbit margin, glabellar region, nuchal area, and mastoid process. He found that logistic regression discriminant function analysis was the best statistical procedure to minimize misclassifications and sex biases of classification; he achieved 88% accuracy. This method is extremely population specific due to the aforementioned population variation in robusticity and gracility (Walker, 2008). Discriminant function analysis will be described later in this chapter under the section on metric sex estimation.

When beginning to test a new (or existing) trait for sex assessment, a useful process is to order all of the variation as a continuum, a process known as **seriation**. To seriate skulls (or any bones for that matter), you will select a specific trait of interest and then organize the skulls (that are clearly labelled with case numbers to preserve provenience) from those with absence or the least expression of the trait to those with greatest expression of the trait. "When sexing only skulls, always use the entire population under study" (White et al., 2012). White and colleagues state that the most accurate method of sex estimation is via the seriation method within a single population. Through training and experience, the seriation method yields correct sorting 80–90% of the time (White et al., 2012).

There is always overlap between males and females near the center of the distribution (often called the zone of overlap between the sexes), which makes sex estimation indeterminate within this middle range. Accuracy for those that are "certainly" one sex or the other (i.e., those outside the zone of overlap) is 100% in tests (Asala, 2002). See Figure 11.1 from Konigsberg and Frankenberg (Chapter 11) this volume, for a graphic depiction of this zone of overlap in sexual characters. If not using a sophisticated statistical analysis, this zone of overlap can unfortunately often include the majority of the population, which is why statistical analysis is preferred even for sex assessment of nonmetric traits. If the zone of overlap only includes a few individuals, the likelihood of the sex assessment can still be very high. One drawback is that this seriation method relies on a larger sample size. A situation in which there is more likely a sample large enough for seriation is found in archaeological samples, less so in forensic cases (White et al., 2012). However, large samples of individuals from a single population have also been recovered in forensic human rights investigations of mass graves, to which this technique could be applied for sex assessment.

METRIC SEX ESTIMATION

Metric sex estimation from the skeleton involves the quantitative analysis of measurable sexually dimorphic traits, such as the femoral head diameter or scapular height. Sex estimation using metric analysis has only recently become the standard in both forensic anthropology and bioarchaeology. Almost a century ago, Pearson (1915) first suggested that postcranial metrics be used for sex estimation. It has taken a long time for this to catch on, due to the speed and ease of visual sex assessment. Metric analysis, however, typically involves less subjectivity and lower inter- and intraobserver error (Adams and Byrd, 2002; Spradley and Jantz, 2011).

Over the last two decades, the scientific rigor of research methods within skeletal biology (as applied to forensic anthropology) has been called into question by important legal proceedings. As a result, there is now a need for more objectivity and standardization of approaches.[6] Expert witnesses giving court testimony in the United States must now demonstrate the reliability and relevance of the scientific methods implemented in order to analyze evidence according to the Federal Rules of Evidence (2001) and the ruling from the court case Daubert vs. Merrill-Dow Pharmaceuticals (1993). This reliability is determined by error rates that quantify observations and statistically report confidence levels (Adams and Byrd, 2002; Christensen, 2004). For example, Christensen (2004:2) stated, "scientific knowledge [must] be grounded in the methods and procedures of science" more than subjective opinion. This knowledge must be empirically tested, falsifiable, and subject to peer review through publication (Christensen, 2004). As many forensic anthropologists are also working in bioarchaeology, this has raised the standards across both specializations and has served to sharpen the skills of the researcher (Ubelaker, 2000). Most sex estimation research has since taken on a metric approach using discriminant function analysis or other multivariate quantitative methods.

Discriminant Function Analysis

Discriminant function analysis (DFA) is a statistical procedure that classifies unknown individuals and the probability of their classification into a certain group (such as sex or ancestry group). Discriminant function analysis makes the assumption that the sample is normally distributed for the trait. The **posterior probability** and **typicality probability** are applied to calculate the classification probabilities (Albanese et al., 2008).[7] The posterior probability is the probability that an unknown case belongs to a certain group based on relative **Mahalanobis' distances** measuring the distance to the center or **centroid** of each group. The typicality probability is how *likely* the unknown case belongs to a group based on variability within all groups. The discriminant function procedure has been programmed into most standard statistical packages for greater applicability.

Not all skeletal measurements are equally effective for sex estimation using DFA and the skill of the researcher plays an important role; practice and exposure to population variation are still crucial. Adams and Byrd (2002) compared 13 different measurements taken by 68 researchers. They discovered high interobserver variability in all measurements by researchers with less than 5 years of experience in osteometrics, but there was no significant improvement *after* 5 years of experience. Clearly, there is some level of subjectivity even within metric sex estimation, requiring some training by the researcher. This can be compared with the many years of training and experience necessary to become familiar with visual sexual dimorphism within a single population, especially to accurately assess sex from the cranial morphology (Buikstra and Ubelaker, 1994). Krogman explains the dichotomy between metric analysis versus descriptive analysis as "experience versus

---

[6]As further evidence of this, refer to the recently formed Scientific Working Group for Forensic Anthropology (SWGANTH), whose goals are setting best practices and minimum standards for forensic anthropology. See www.swganth.org.

[7]An excellent explanation for how to interpret the results from a discriminant function analysis is available in FORDISC 3.1 under the help menu (Ousley and Jantz, 2005:12).

statistical standardization" (Krogman and İşcan, 1986). The merits of metric sex estimation can be summarized with the famous quotation by Sir William Thomson Kelvin (1824–1907): "To measure is to know."

Sex Estimation: Cranial versus Postcranial

Many researchers have passed down the misconception to their students that the skull is the second best estimator of sex (for a discussion, see Spradley and Jantz, 2011). These authors compared craniometrics to postcranial metrics to evaluate accuracy in sexing across the skeleton. This study made use of positively identified individuals from the **Forensic Databank**[8] representing populations specific to the United States. Spradley and Jantz (2011) reported that correct classification rates by joint size alone (e.g., femur epicondylar breadth and tibia proximal epiphyseal breadth) achieved accuracy of 89–90% and multivariate analysis of joint size reached accuracy of 94%. This was compared to craniometric sex estimation, which only reached univariate classification rate of 78% for the bizygomatic breadth, though multivariate analysis did increase the classification rates for sexing. Thus, these authors concluded that postcranial metric sex estimation is preferable to craniometric sex estimation because of the higher accuracy rates, discrediting the view held for decades that the skull is superior to the long bones for sexing (Spradley and Jantz, 2011). Despite the lower classification rates for the skull compared to other postcranial elements, the following discussion of the skeletal elements will follow a top–down system of organization, starting with the skull.

Sex Estimation: Axial Skeleton

The Skull

Craniometric analysis applies a combination of both descriptive and metric approaches, sometimes quantifying observable descriptive traits that *are* measurable (e.g., length of the mastoid). An early study using discriminant function analysis of African Americans and European Americans by Giles (1970) reported rates of 83.2–88.4% accuracy using craniometrics. Hanihara (1959) measured Japanese skulls applying a discriminant function analysis for nine craniometric measurements, for which the best accuracy rates were 89.7%. Hanihara concluded thusly that the long bones performed better for sex estimation. Graw and colleagues (2005) even found sex differences in the angle of the course of the internal acoustic meatus of the temporal bone, but accuracy rates only reached 66% for sexing. Two separate studies have found bizygomatic breadth to be the best single sex discriminator of the cranium (85.5% and 78%, respectively) (Saini et al., 2011; Spradley and Jantz, 2011). Using a quadratic discriminant function analysis of 11 measurements from the Forensic Databank, multivariate craniometric sex estimation yielded accuracy rates of 82.7% (Konigsberg et al., 2009). Current research in multivariate analysis of the cranium is moving towards shape-based analysis, known as geometric morphometrics (Ross et al., 1999; Kimmerle et al., 2008), which is

---

[8]The Forensic Databank (FDB) is a database of metric information from forensic cases from around the world (mainly the United States) managed by the Forensic Anthropology Center at the University of Tennessee.

discussed more by McKeown and Schmidt (Chapter 12), this volume. Sex estimation using craniometrics from the Forensic Databank is available through the program FORDISC 3.1 (Ousley and Jantz, 2012). DiGangi and Hefner discuss FORDISC in more detail in the chapter on ancestry estimation in this volume (Chapter 5). Similar to visual methods of assessment discussed earlier, population specificity is equally important for craniometric studies.

Ribs and Vertebrae

For the most part, ribs have played a more central role in age estimation than sex estimation (refer to Uhl [Chapter 3], this volume). One study by İşcan and Loth (1986) demonstrated that the sternal rib ends do exhibit sexual dimorphism. This study used discriminant function analysis to compare the perpendicular measures of maximum superior—inferior height and maximum anterior—posterior breadth of the fourth sternal rib end in individuals with a rib phase between stages 1 and 7 (i.e., approximately 14—70 years). The average accuracy rate was 83% and the method worked better for females than for males. However, this method did not work for adults who were very young or very old (İşcan and Loth, 1986).

The vertebrae exhibit sexual dimorphism in size even before puberty. The developmental significance of this early sexual dimorphism is unknown, but this could be the result of either intrinsic hormone levels or extrinsic variables of population specific activity and/or body mass (Gilsanz et al., 1997). Male vertebrae are larger, especially the lumbar vertebrae. This study is discussed in further detail below under subadult sex estimation (Gilsanz et al., 1997). The atlas is significantly greater in breadth in males (Brothwell, 1963). A metric analysis of eight measurements of the articular surfaces and vertebral foramen area on the atlas provided sex estimation accuracy between 75% and 85% (Marino, 1995).

Sex Estimation: The Appendicular Skeleton

Upper Limb

SHOULDER GIRDLE

The upper arm and shoulder girdle may be one of the most sexually dimorphic areas of the skeleton (even better than the pelvis, see below), which is evident by the high rates of classification for the humerus, clavicle, and scapula. From the review of previous literature on sex estimation for this chapter, the highest single variable success rate was achieved from the humeral head diameter. This study by Frutos (2005) achieved 96% accuracy from univariate sexing of the humeral head diameter. This may be due to functional differences between males and females in population-specific behaviors, as well as intrinsic hormones that affect the bones and musculature of this region.

As previously discussed, Spradley and Jantz (2011) compared all of the cranial and postcranial elements from the Forensic Databank for sexing accuracy rates to create a hierarchy of effectiveness. The rankings of their univariate analysis with sexing accuracy rates for the upper limb were (1) scapula height (87%), (2) humeral head (86%), and (3) scapula width (86%). Multivariate discriminant function analysis from these measurements was able to achieve higher discrimination rates, up to 94%. The maximum length of the clavicle also shows high levels of sexual dimorphism with classification accuracy rates at 85%

(Spradley and Jantz, 2011). Frutos (2002) achieved sex estimation accuracy rates (86–95%) from discriminant function analysis for a Guatemalan sample, including the clavicle maximum length, clavicle midshaft circumference, and the height and width of the glenoid fossa.

RADIUS AND HAND

Berrizbeitia (1989) estimated sex from the head of the radius using multivariate discriminant function analysis on a sample of European and African Americans from the **Robert J. Terry Anatomical Skeletal Collection**.[9] The cross-validated results of the maximum and minimum head diameters combined yielded accuracy of 92% with the left side, 94% with the right, and 96% accuracy if both bones were used. Barrio and colleagues (2006) conducted univariate discriminant function analysis using the metacarpals for sex estimation. These researchers achieved accuracy of between 81% and 91%, with the best accuracy from the left second metacarpal. They found that the right hand is generally larger than the left and that the transverse dimensions are more dimorphic than the longitudinal measures (Barrio et al., 2006; Albanese et al., 2008). They concluded that this dimorphism is the result of extrinsic functional stress and physical activity, which will be highly population specific.

Lower Limb and Pelvic Girdle

PELVIS

The pelvis has had the reputation of having the best success for both sex estimation and sex assessment due the functional necessity of the female pelvic inlet to be wide for childbirth. A variety of indices and angles were developed decades ago for the purpose of sex estimation, but the earlier analyses lacked statistical rigor for successful application. The sexually dimorphic subpubic angle has been measured metrically and is acute in males and obtuse in females (Stewart, 1979). A study of anteroposterior radiographs (X-rays) of individuals from Uganda showed significant sexual dimorphism. In this study, the male subpubic angle mean was 93.86 degrees (SD=21.12 degrees) and 116.11 degrees (SD=17.79 degrees) for females, though sex discrimination accuracy rates did not exceed 71%, likely because they did not use a sophisticated statistical analysis (Igbigbi and Nanono-Igbigbi, 2003).

The **ischiopubic index** (length of pubis × 100/length of ischium) is lower in males and was hoped to be a replacement for the use of the subpubic angle in sex estimation accuracy (Brothwell, 1963). This index, however, includes the pubic length, the measurement that has the highest interobserver measurement error (Adams and Byrd, 2002). Another index is in the sacrum and has been used for sex estimation, called the **sacral corporobasal index** (S1 corpus width × 100/basal width), but there is extensive overlap between the sexes (Stewart, 1979). Some of these pelvic indices may provide better accuracy for sex estimation if discriminant function analysis is applied, as a suggestion for further study.

In the studies applying a univariate discriminant function approach, the success of the pelvis for sex estimation is surprisingly mediocre compared to many other postcranial elements. Patriquin and colleagues (2005) investigated metric sex estimation from the pelvis using discriminant function analysis on a sample of South African Blacks and Whites. The ischial length was

---

[9]This collection is curated by the National Museum of Natural History at the Smithsonian Institution in Washington, D.C.

the most sexually dimorphic trait (86% accuracy) followed by the diameter of the acetabulum (84% accuracy). For a multivariate discriminant function analysis of all the pelvic measurements, the accuracy for the first function was between 94% and 95.5% (Patriquin et al., 2005).

Spradley and Jantz (2011) report that the highest single variable from the pelvis for sex estimation accuracy was 85% for the os coxal height and 83% for the ischial length. The multivariate discriminant function analysis for the os coxa was between 89% and 90%, which ranked lower in accuracy rates than a multivariate analysis of the humerus, radius, clavicle, scapula, femur, tibia, ulna, and cranium (Spradley and Jantz, 2011).

One bioarchaeological study used semilandmark data to conduct geometric morphometric analysis to quantify the shape of the greater sciatic notch and ischiopubic region (González et al., 2007). The authors compared hunters and gatherers and early farmers from Argentina and concluded that the shape dimorphism in the pelvis was surprisingly not consistent between the populations. In a later study by some of the same authors, discriminant function analysis using the same geometric morphometric variables yielded success rates for the ischiopubic complex of 93% (González et al., 2009).

FEMUR

The Purkait method to estimate sex from the proximal femur was developed on a population from India (Purkait, 2005). The author suggests that the method is useful for sex estimation from fragmentary remains and that it may be more reflective of dimorphism due to the functional adaptations of the femur in response to the sexual dimorphism of body weight (Purkait, 2005). This method (shown in Figure 4.3) identifies a triangle on the posterior proximal femur that includes the apex of the lesser trochanter and greater trochanter and the most lateral point

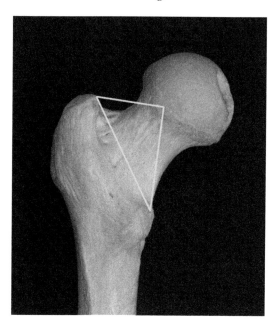

FIGURE 4.3   Purkait method of sex estimation from the proximal femur.

on the posterior femoral head (Purkait, 2005). The lengths of each of the sides of the triangle along with the three angles are included in the discriminant function analysis. The Purkait method achieved accuracy of between 81% and 87%, which is no better than sex estimation from a single measurement, such as the humeral or femoral head diameters (Purkait, 2005).

Brown and colleagues (2007) tested the Purkait triangle method on a population from the U.S. (Brown et al., 2007). Their results were comparable to those of Purkait (85.5%); and they achieved approximately the same accuracy using the femur head diameter alone (87%). When they combined one of the measures with the femoral head, the accuracy of the discriminant function analysis improved (90%) (Brown et al., 2007). They then used a threshold value or **sectioning point** (also known as a **demarking point**) for the length between the apices of the trochanters in conjunction with the femoral head diameter and the accuracy increased to 93.4% (Brown et al., 2007). A sectioning (or demarking) point is simply the average of both the male and female mean values (Bidmos and Asala, 2004).

A recent study by Albanese and colleagues (2008) hoped to improve upon the Purkait method by using an even more functional morphologic approach. These authors wanted to try to see if the proximal femur reflected the same functional adaptations for childbirth as the pelvis, assuming the pelvis is the best sex estimator (which is not true for metric methods as demonstrated earlier in this chapter). They added new measurements from the femur that were thought to reflect the sexual dimorphism that is seen in the pubic bone. Like the Purkait method, this method also creates a triangle by measuring between three points on the proximal femur: (1) the apex of the lesser trochanter, (2) the most lateral point on the greater trochanter, and (3) the most superior point on the fovea capitis on the head of the femur (see Figure 4.4).

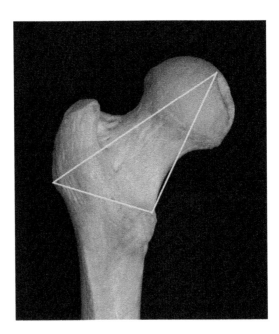

FIGURE 4.4   Albanese method of sex estimation from the proximal femur.

Unlike the Purkait (2005) method discussed above, the Albanese et al. method (2008) was developed to measure the size and angle of the femoral neck. This method was developed on more than 300 individuals from the Terry Collection and analyzed using the statistical method of logistic regression. The extremely high accuracy achieved using this method was between 95% and 97%. Albanese et al. (2008) claimed that their method is not population specific, but rather relies on biomechanical differences in males and females. The authors explain that they used logistic regression instead of the discriminant function approach for a number of reasons, with one being that logistic regression performs as well as discriminant function analysis, but has fewer assumptions (e.g., does not assume a normal distribution) (Albanese et al., 2008). A suggested research project could test the accuracy of the Albanese method on other population samples to determine the verity of the universal application of the approach.

One earlier study by İşcan and Miller-Shaivitz (1986) used discriminant function analysis to test whether the femur and tibia are equally dimorphic. They found that the femur and tibia are in fact equally effective for sex estimation in European Americans from the **Hamann-Todd Human Osteological Collection**,[10] but that only the femur was useful for estimation of sex in African Americans from that sample. İşcan and Miller-Shaivitz (1986) concluded that the epiphyses were better than the shaft for dimorphism due to the muscle insertion sites, with accuracy rates between 83% and 94%.

Using a traditional metric method, Asala tested the efficiency of the demarking point of the femoral head to estimate sex (Asala, 2001, 2002). The vertical and transverse diameters of the femoral head were measured and averaged for each sex. The average was then taken of the male and female averages to arrive at a demarking point (Bidmos and Dayal, 2004). The results revealed that the male femoral head diameters were significantly greater than those of the females. Using this simple method of sorting without discriminant function analysis can have very low overall success (only 32%) due to the zone of overlap between the sexes, but the accuracy for those that are "certainly" one sex or the other (i.e., those outside the zone of overlap) is 100% in tests (Asala, 2002). A sectioning point is based on the assumption that the standard deviations for both sexes is equal and that the sex ratio is exactly one to one, which is not necessarily the case. You need to first have an idea of the sex ratio. Without a sex ratio, you can estimate a ratio using the statistical procedure called **maximum likelihood estimation** (MLE). You can then use a **Bayesian analysis** to find the probability that an individual with a given measurement is male or female. For a more in depth explanation to this approach, refer to the chapter by Konigsberg and Frankenberg on demography in this volume (Chapter 11).

Asala and colleagues (2004) also conducted discriminant function analysis on 220 femora from South African Blacks using just the proximal and distal segments to calculate the sex estimation accuracy for fragmentary femora. They found multivariate analyses were better than univariate, with the proximal end of the femur (85.1%) more effective in sexing than the distal end (82.7%). These results were interpreted as potentially due to the role of the proximal femur in transmitting body weight. A more complex statistical analysis from three-dimensional computer models created from **computed tomographic (CT)** scans reveals an internal rotation of the distal femur in females, perhaps as a biomechanical means of

---

[10]This collection is curated by the Cleveland Museum of Natural History in Cleveland, Ohio.

returning the orientation of the knee along the sagittal plane (Mahfouz et al., 2007b). This latter three-dimensional study slightly contradicts the previous study (Asala et al., 2004) in terms of distal changes of the femur being more significant than proximal end changes. One reason may be that the three-dimensional analysis is likely more sensitive to the subtle shape changes, because it compares thousands of homologous points as opposed to just a few measurements with calipers. The results could be reflecting population variation in the shape of the femur.

PATELLA

The patella has had some success in terms of sex estimation. Kemkes-Grottenthaler (2005) and Mahfouz et al. (2007a) looked at sex differences in the patella and found significant sex differences in the maximum height and width of this bone. Introna and colleagues (1998) yielded 84% accuracy using multivariate discriminant function analysis of both maximum width and maximum height. Bidmos and colleagues (2005) had similar success in a South African sample, with better success for height (85%) compared to breadth (79%). A more complex method was used by Mahfouz and colleagues (2007a) that compared the three-dimensional shape from computer models developed using CT scans of modern individuals. This method achieved high success rates from a multivariate statistical analysis called *fuzzy clustering*, with testing accuracy rates as high as 93%.

TALUS AND CALCANEUS

Gualdi-Russo (2007) used discriminant function analysis to estimate sex from the talus and calcaneus in a northern Italian population. The author tested the method on an independent sample of 16 individuals that, despite a small sample size, had accuracy ranging from 87.9% to 95.7%, with the best accuracy achieved through a multivariate analysis of the talus. The accuracy was only 56.3% when tested on a sample of Italians from southern Italy, emphasizing the need for population-specific data (Gualdi-Russo, 2007).

Bidmos and colleagues measured the sexual dimorphism of the calcaneus and talus of South African populations and yielded similar results (Bidmos and Asala, 2004; Bidmos and Dayal, 2004). The calcaneus alone achieved accuracy of 85% when using the three most discriminating variables combined (Bidmos and Asala, 2004). Bidmos and Dayal also measured the talus of South African Blacks and achieved accuracy rates of 89.2% when three traits were combined (Bidmos and Dayal, 2004). The best single trait was the height of the talus head, which had an accuracy rate of 86.7%. When they tested this method using independent samples of South African Whites and Blacks, the accuracy for the more comparable population of other South African Blacks was high (70–90%), but the accuracy for the South African Whites was much lower (40–80%). The authors argued that this is further evidence of population specificity in sexually dimorphic skeletal dimensions (Bidmos and Dayal, 2004).

PROBLEMATIC AREAS OF SEX ESTIMATION

Subadult Sex Estimation

Subadult sex estimation has been perhaps the most problematic area of sex estimation for both forensic anthropologists and bioarchaeologists. According to Scheuer and Black (2004), morphological sex estimation on juveniles is "tentative at best." Komar and Buikstra (2009) caution that there are no reliable methods for sex estimation for subadults. There are two major obstacles to research attempts in this area: (1) there is a lack of large, known skeletal samples of subadults and (2) the smaller size of the bones increases the significance of measurement error. Due to the dearth of juvenile skeletal samples, many of the studies of sexual dimorphism in subadults have used radiographs, which do not necessarily compare well with dry bones (Bass, 1987).

With adult sex estimation, sexual dimorphism in size can be a useful means of discrimination within a single population (e.g., diameter of the humeral head). Size differences, however, are not useful in sex estimation of subadults because males and females mature at different rates and size dimorphism is not as substantial as in adults. For example, female infants and juveniles develop faster than males, but male subadults will be larger on average than females of the same age (Saunders, 2000; Scheuer and Black, 2004). Even by the twentieth week *in utero*, a female fetus is about 10% more developed than a male fetus (Saunders, 2000). Weaver explains that sexing a fetus by size can be a tautological exercise, as fetal age is never a certainty (Weaver, 1986).

Two potential research areas show promise in terms of sex estimation in subadults, but they must be considered simultaneously. These two research areas are (1) analysis of traits that show early signs of dimorphism and (2) analysis of the dimorphism in the rate/timing of development. Intrinsic sexual dimorphism develops early in life in the pelvis, cranium, and teeth. It is likely that only these traits will have any potential success (however limited) in subadult sex estimation and assessment. Dental development is more similar between the sexes, but skeletal development is somewhat dimorphic (Saunders, 2000). Hunt and Gleiser (1955) compared timing differences in dental and skeletal development using radiographs and achieved an accuracy rate of 81%. In another study of three diverse population samples, Franklin and colleagues found that the mandible is not sexually dimorphic in subadults, with an accuracy rate not much better than chance (59%) (Franklin et al., 2007). The accuracy of sex estimation is undoubtedly lower in juveniles than in adults. Thus, the goal for accuracy should be at least 75% (which is 50% better than chance) (Saunders, 2000). There are differences in the timing of skeletal and dental growth between subadult males and females, which, when compared to the few traits that are actually dimorphic could serve as a measure of sexual dimorphism. This is one area that could use further testing. There is still the problem of inter- and intraobserver error rates because the sex differences in metrics appear to be too small for reliable application (Scheuer and Black, 2004). Thus, methods that can increase measurement accuracy (e.g., 3-D digitization) are the goal for subadult sex estimation.

In subadults, the pelvis is the most sexually dimorphic bone in *infancy*, but the problem with sex estimation from the fetal pelvis is measurement error and the standardization of the position of the bone for measurement. Infant males have longer ilia, ischia, and femoral necks, whereas infant females have a longer pubis and a wider sciatic notch (Saunders, 2000). These differences mirror the later sexual dimorphism of the pelvis found in adults, according to Weaver (1980) and Fazekas and Kósa (1978). Weaver (1980) tested anthropologists' ability to estimate sex using the infant pelvis and found it to be unreliable. Holcomb and Konigsberg (1995) investigated the fetal sciatic notch shape and found significant sexual dimorphism, but the overlap was too great to be effective. Again, any methods that can capitalize on this existing early dimorphism by improving measurement accuracy are the goal for sexing infant and fetal remains.

Looking ahead to adolescent sex estimation, the pelvis of the male retains the more adolescent shape, whereas the female pelvis adapts for childbirth starting at puberty as previously stated. As explained above, this can give confidence to an assessment of sex in an early adolescent if there are female characteristics present (Buikstra and Ubelaker, 1994). If there are no female characteristics, this does not mean that it is the pelvis of a male; it could also be a female who has not begun to develop these secondary characteristics.

The vertebrae show some of the best opportunity for subadult sex estimation during the more problematic childhood to preadolescent phases (approximately 2–12 years). As mentioned previously, Gilsanz et al. (1997) found sexual dimorphism in children younger than 12 years in the lumbar vertebrae, most notably in the first lumbar vertebra (L1). In this study, the size of L1 was more highly correlated with sex than with body weight, the L1 being more than 11% smaller in girls. The authors concluded that sexual dimorphism in preadolescence might be due to a spike in testosterone levels of infant males during the first year of life (Gilsanz et al., 1997). Saunders explains that fetal testosterone from the testes present from the tenth week to the fifteenth week *in utero* is responsible for the major sex differentiation in infants (Saunders, 2000). After that time, the endocrine system contributes to sexual dimorphism, including size and weight dimorphism (Saunders, 2000). After this hormone peak *in utero*, hormone levels decrease and do not reach these peak levels again until puberty. This may explain why, for example, the fetal sciatic notch shows sexual dimorphism, but there is little dimorphism present during the rest of childhood in the shape of the sciatic notch.

Theoretically, dentition size should work for sexing subadults, as adult teeth begin development and eruption during childhood. As with measuring the fetal bones, however, the magnitude of this dimorphism may be too small to be significant (Saunders, 2000). Despite this, DeVito and Saunders (1990) employed a multivariate approach with deciduous tooth dimensions and achieved impressive sex estimation accuracy rates (75–90%), but there was considerable population variation. Hassett (2011) measured the buccolingual and mesiodistal diameters of the permanent canine teeth in adults and subadults and achieved 94% accuracy. This author suggested the measurements be taken at the tooth cervix to avoid problems with tooth wear. The sample size in this study was small and this method could be highly population specific, but this approach may provide a possible direction for future research. Molleson and colleagues (1998) were able to combine multiple features in juveniles from a Romano-British cemetery: the eye orbit, mandibular canine size, and the pelvic inlet. This method reached only 78% accuracy, but has good potential for sex discrimination considering the difficulty of sex estimation in subadults (Buikstra and Ubelaker, 1994). Despite all the disparaging comments about the potential to accurately estimate sex in subadults, there are at least some encouraging results published in this area.

DNA Analysis

One area that offers great potential for sex estimation in both subadults and fragmentary adults is DNA analysis. Molecular methods are one area in which the term *sex determination* could potentially be applied, due to alleles that only show up on the sex chromosomes. Some authors have suggested that if sex estimation is achieved with DNA, then sex can be treated as a known (Hummel and Herrmann, 1991; Saunders, 2000; Stone, 2000; Gibbon et al., 2009). Sex estimation from DNA ideally should work well because the X and Y chromosomes have distinct sequences (Saunders, 2000; Stone, 2000). However, there exist potential problems with sexing from DNA alone that are discussed further by Cabana and colleagues in this volume (Chapter 16). These authors point out the problem of false negatives. The absence of regions specific to the Y chromosome does not indicate a female necessarily, because the Y chromosome is already very small and genetic material is more easily degraded, especially in bioarchaeological samples.

Stone (2000) explains that there are two methods for sexing from DNA: repetitive sequences (which are chromosome specific) and single copy genes found on both the X and Y chromosomes (Stone, 2000). When using degraded ancient DNA, the repeat sequences are easier to amplify. The presence of a male product must indicate the subject is male, but the absence does not necessarily mean that the subject is female (Stone, 2000). In a comparison of molecular sex estimation to morphological estimation in subadults, there does not appear to be enough DNA left in the subadult skeleton to work successfully (depending on the age of the individual), though the molecular method may ultimately be more accurate when DNA is present (Saunders, 2000). Several problems with determining sex from DNA are contamination, DNA degradation, and the great time and financial investment (Buikstra and Ubelaker, 1994; Saunders, 2000) given that chemical/molecular approaches to sexing in subadults can be greatly biased taphonomically by burial environment (Stone, 2000). For a discussion of the problems of contamination and DNA degradation in genetic analysis, see Cabana et al. (Chapter 16), this volume.

Quantitative Sexing and Demography

In demography research, the estimation of sex involves calculating the probability that the sex is male or female. Konigsberg and Frankenberg include a comprehensive introduction to methods of calculating sex ratios in demography later in this volume (Chapter 11), but I will provide a brief overview. In order to calculate the probability that a skeleton belongs to one sex or another, there must be a sample of individuals of known sex from a similar population as the unknown to develop a sex ratio for that sample (number of males to number of females). This information is *prior* information,[11] which is then used in the calculation of the probability that the unknown is male. You calculate the probability that the individual is male, because the probability that it is female is one minus the probability of it being male. Developing a sex ratio for the sample in question is first accomplished by using a reliable osteological assessment of sex, such as the Phenice method described earlier, or with molecular methods. Ideally, multiple variables will indicate the sex of individuals in this sample, so that there is little ambiguity. This approach is very different from traditional sex estimation and assessment, which is described throughout this chapter. Instead of estimating sex, the question becomes, "What is the probability of sex given the observation of a certain feature?" Konigsberg and Frankenberg thoroughly explain this theoretical

[11]This approach is **Bayesian** in nature. Refer to Konigsberg and Frankenberg (Chapter 11) and Uhl (Chapter 3) for more information on Bayesian statistical approaches.

approach and statistical procedures involved in the chapter on demography in this volume (Chapter 11).

Sex Estimation and Pathology

Sex estimation from the presence of certain types of pathology can be an option if none of the above discussed methods is possible, though accuracy rates are **extremely low**. This method takes advantage of the fact that some diseases affect the sexes differentially (Reichs, 1986). For example, juvenile males are more prone to traumatic injury. As a result, the incidence of osteomyelitis (i.e. infection in the bone) occurs at a ratio of young males to females of 3:1 or 4:1, according to Reichs (1986). This ratio will be extremely population specific, depending on the sociocultural activities of children. Another skeletal pathology that occurs more in childhood is sporotrichosis (a type of fungal infection), which affects male juveniles three times more than female juveniles (Reichs, 1986). In adults, ankylosing spondylitis and gout both occur nine times more in males than females (Reichs, 1986). The timing of the onset of diseases can potentially be useful for sex differentiation. Osgood—Schlatter's disease is partial avulsion of the tibial tuberosity from overactivity in young adolescents and typically occurs earlier in females (DiGangi et al., 2010). These approaches should only be used as last resorts if all other methods have been exhausted, with the caveat that it does not allow you to obtain much more accuracy than the 50:50 probability you would get by guessing.

CASE STUDY: DEVELOPING POPULATION-SPECIFIC SEXING STANDARDS

As described in the Preface, this book's inspiration stemmed out of research courses held in Colombia. A massive osteological data collection effort by 34 scientists took place in Bogotá during February 2011. To collect data, the group split up into different data collection teams. I was personally in charge of the team collecting postcranial metrics. Each individual on the team was responsible for two to three bones (e.g., those of the forearm). Two other individuals on the team exclusively measured the entire skeleton of 30 individuals, to test for interobserver error. One goal of the postcranial metric team was to explore the best univariate indicators for sex estimation using measurements of the postcranial elements. As discussed previously, in a recent study of African and European Americans from the Forensic Database, the postcranial elements demonstrating the most effective sex discrimination were the femur, tibia, humerus, and scapula (Spradley and Jantz, 2011). Thus, the hypothesis for this project was that the population from Colombia would follow a similar pattern, with the femur, tibia, humerus, and scapula demonstrating the highest classification rates.

The sample that was studied is the Colombian Modern Skeletal Collection,[12] which is curated by the National Institute of Legal Medicine and Forensic Sciences in Bogotá, Colombia. The skeletal collection consists of individuals with known age, sex, and stature (cadaver or forensic) and is now one of the largest collections of known individuals in South America.

---

[12]Refer to the Preface in this volume for more information.

All of the individuals were born during the twentieth century and died in 2005 or 2006. The sample in this study consisted of 126 individuals (44 females, 81 males) with a mean age of 47 years. The statistical methods used included univariate discriminant function analysis with cross-validation and univariate analysis of variance (ANOVA) using the statistical software program SPSS®. In cross-validation, each case is classified by the functions derived from all cases other than that case. Only the bones of the left side of the body were included in the analysis in order to lessen the effect of handedness and potential occupational markers, especially in the upper limb.

The results of this study indicated the same general pattern of classification effectiveness as seen in the North American sample by Spradley and Jantz (2011) using the univariate ANOVA and cross-validated univariate discriminant function analysis. All of the variables, except for the humeral epicondylar breadth, showed statistically significant sexual dimorphism. The cross-validated univariate discriminant function analysis demonstrated that the best accuracy rates were for the scapular height and humeral head at 86% each. The scapular breadth came in third with an accuracy rate of 84.6%. Surprisingly, the accuracy rate for the femoral head (80.8%) was lower than that from the Spradley and Jantz (2011) study (86−88%), probably reflecting population specific behavior (Moore et al., 2012).

The results of this study could be extremely useful for identification, as the humerus is more resistant to taphonomic properties than many of the bones (Moore et al., 2012). Furthermore, the ability to achieve such a high degree of success from a single bone is more efficient and thus preferable for the fast-paced human identification laboratories in Colombia that see hundreds of cases each year. This research has the potential to play an important role in the development of population standards for Colombia and Latin America and may help provide a better standard of practice for forensic anthropology that can pass scrutiny by the Colombian judicial system and international criminal courts.

While our results were somewhat preliminary because of the relatively small sample size, the Colombian Modern Skeletal Collection has now more than tripled, enabling a reevaluation of this study. This case study illustrates that important research need not be those that are novel and unique. We used the Spradley and Jantz (2011) paper as a model and followed their methods to set up methods for our own study. This enabled us to generate the first population-specific metric sexing standards for a population. We recommend that the reader consider a similar option when contemplating a research project, be it in sex estimation or any other subject.

CONCLUSION

One way to develop a research project in sex estimation (or in any subject) is to test the results of a previously published research project. This is how science advances. This also makes developing the methodology easier, because you simply follow the same format in the original research project. This is extremely valuable when trying to develop population standards and serves to simplify (and demystify) the process for a young researcher. There is no need to reinvent the wheel. In order to begin your analysis of sex estimation, first determine whether there is a significant difference between males and females in the trait for which you are estimating. Seriation can help you better visualize the variation in the trait to develop an ordinal scoring system, if the trait is not easily measured metrically. Analysis of variation (ANOVA) is an acceptable statistical method to calculate whether the sexual dimorphism you observe is statistically significant. If the trait demonstrates significant sexual dimorphism, a discriminant function analysis is not as daunting as you might believe. In most statistical packages it is as simple as one click to conduct a discriminant function classification. Although these analyses may be much more feasible today, interpretation of the results requires a deeper understanding of statistics than is presented in this chapter. I recommend taking statistics courses through the math department of your university (including multivariate statistics) in addition to any courses that may be offered within the biological or social sciences. Most graduate programs in anthropology will have this same requirement. It would behoove you to take a course in osteometrics in addition to osteology and skeletal biology, if offered.

In some ways, research methods in sex estimation and assessment have changed a great deal in the last 50 years, yet many of the observations are still the same. Although a great deal of research has been conducted on the estimation and assessment of sex from the skeleton, there is still a need for a number of studies to be developed, as populations continue to evolve. Albanese and colleagues (2008:1283) state, "A widely accepted but erroneous view has been and continues to be that morphological methods can be applied across populations while metric methods are population specific." As demonstrated in nearly every study described in this chapter, population variation has a significant impact on the ability to estimate sex accurately from the skeleton. Metric standards must be population specific in both time and space (Buikstra and Ubelaker, 1994). Due to the scarcity of subadult skeletal collections, molecular methods could be used as the standard for sexing as explained above, against which metric sex estimation methods can then be validated. Molecular analyses could be used to develop a larger known sample of subadults in order to test and validate the use of new metric sex estimation methods in subadults. Other studies in subadults could compare skeletal and dental development to examine timing differences in growth and development that could be used to estimate sex.

Quantitative estimation of sex using the sex ratio in demography is yet another area that would be wise to pursue, in conjunction with other methods of sex estimation and assessment. Pathology is an area that has received very little attention, but will likely never provide accuracy for sex estimation that would be any better than chance. Sample sizes in this area are simply too small and confounding variables too large.

I encourage all new students of skeletal biology considering research in sex estimation to thoughtfully consider the etiology of sexual dimorphism. By investigating the intrinsic and extrinsic variables that ultimately cause sexual dimorphism, we may better select traits of importance and gain a deeper understanding of the biocultural variables involved in the development of the human skeleton.

REFERENCES

Adams, B.J., Byrd, J.E., 2002. Interobserver variation of selected postcranial skeletal measurements. Journal of Forensic Sciences 47 (6), 1193–1202.

Albanese, J., Eklics, G., Tuck, A., 2008. A metric method for sex determination using the proximal femur and fragmentary hipbone. Journal of Forensic Sciences 53 (6), 1283–1288.

Asala, S.A., 2001. Sex determination from the head of the femur of South African whites and blacks. Forensic Science International 117 (1–2), 15–22.

Asala, S.A., 2002. The efficiency of the demarking point of the femoral head as a sex determining parameter. Forensic Science International 127 (1–2), 114–118.

Asala, S.A., Bidmos, M.A., Dayal, M.R., 2004. Discriminant function sexing of fragmentary femur of South African blacks. Forensic Science International 145 (1), 25–29.

Acsádi, G., Nemeskéri, J., 1970. History of human life span and mortality. Akadémiai Kiadó, Budapest.

Barrio, P.A., Trancho, G.J., Sanchez, J.A., 2006. Metacarpal sexual determination in a Spanish population. Journal of Forensic Sciences 51 (5), 990–995.

Bass, W.M., 1987. Human osteology: a laboratory and field manual. Missouri Archaeological Society, Columbia, Mo.

Beck, T.J., Ruff, C.B., Shaffer, R.A., Betsinger, K., Trone, D.W., Brodine, S.K., 2000. Stress fracture in military recruits: gender differences in muscle and bone susceptibility factors. Bone 27 (3), 437–444.

Berrizbeitia, E.L., 1989. Sex determination with the head of the radius. Journal of Forensic Sciences 34 (5), 1206–1213.

Bidmos, M.A., Asala, S.A., 2004. Sexual dimorphism of the calcaneus of South African blacks. Journal of Forensic Sciences 49 (3), 446–450.

Bidmos, M.A., Dayal, M.R., 2004. Further evidence to show population specificity of discriminant function equations for sex determination using the talus of South African blacks. Journal of Forensic Sciences 49 (6), 1165–1170.

Bidmos, M.A., Steinberg, N., Kuykendall, K.L., 2005. Patella measurements of South African whites as sex assessors. Homo 56 (1), 69–74.

Bogin, B., 1999. Patterns of Human Growth. Cambridge University Press, Cambridge.

Brothwell, D.R., 1963. Digging up Bones; The Excavation, Treatment and Study of Human Skeletal Remains. British Museum, London.

Brown, R.P., Ubelaker, D.H., Schanfield, M.S., 2007. Evaluation of Purkait's triangle method for determining sexual dimorphism. Journal of Forensic Sciences 52 (3), 553–556.

Bruzek, J., 2002. A method for visual determination of sex, using the human hip bone. American Journal of Physical Anthropology 117, 157–168.

Buikstra, J.E., Ubelaker, D.H., 1994. Standards for data collection from human skeletal remains. Arkansas Archeological Survey, Fayetteville, AR.

DeVito, C., Saunders, S.R., 1990. A discriminant function analysis of deciduous teeth to determine sex. Journal of Forensic Sciences 35 (4), 845–858.

DiGangi, E.A., Bethard, J.D., Sullivan, L.P., 2010. Differential diagnosis of cartilaginous dysplasia and probable Osgood–Schlatter's disease in a Mississippian individual from East Tennessee. International Journal of Osteoarcheology 20 (4), 424–442.

Case, D.T., Ross, A.H., 2007. Sex determination from hand and foot bone lengths. Journal of Forensic Sciences 52 (2), 264–270.

Cho, G.J., Park, H.T., Shin, J.H., Hur, J.Y., Kim, Y.T., Kim, S.H., et al., 2010. Age at menarche in a Korean population: secular trends and influencing factors. European Journal of Pediatrics 169 (1), 89–94.

Christensen, A.M., 2004. The impact of Daubert: implications for testimony and research in forensic anthropology (and the use of frontal sinuses in personal identification). Journal of Forensic Sciences 49 (3), 427–430.

Fazekas, I.G., Kósa, F., 1978. Forensic Fetal Osteology. Akadémiai Kiadó, Budapest.

Franklin, D., Oxnard, C.E., O'Higgins, P., Dadour, I., 2007. Sexual dimorphism in the subadult mandible: quantification using geometric morphometrics. Journal of Forensic Sciences 52 (1), 6–10.

Frayer, D.W., Wolpoff, M.H., 1985. Sexual dimorphism. Annual Review of Anthropology 14, 429–473.

Frutos, L.R., 2002. Determination of sex from the clavicle and scapula in a Guatemalan contemporary rural indigenous population. American Journal of Forensic Medicine and Pathology 23, 284–288.

Frutos, L.R., 2005. Metric determination of sex from the humerus in a Guatemalan forensic sample. Forensic Science International 147 (2–3), 153–157.

Gibbon, V., Paximadis, M., Strkalj, G., Ruff, P., Penny, C., 2009. Novel methods of molecular sex identification from skeletal tissue using the amelogenin gene. Forensic Science International: Genetics 3 (2), 74–79.

Giles, E., 1970. Discriminant function sexing of the human skeleton. In: Stewart, T.D. (Ed.), Personal Identification in Mass Disasters. National Museum of Natural History, Washington, pp. 99–107.

Gilsanz, V., Kovanlikaya, A., Costin, G., Roe, T.F., Sayre, J., Kaufman, F., 1997. Differential effect of gender on the sizes of the bones in the axial and appendicular skeletons. Journal of Clinical Endocrinology and Metabolism 82 (5), 1603–1607.

Gonzalez, P.N., Bernal, V., Perez, S.I., Barrientos, G., 2007. Analysis of dimorphic structures of the human pelvis: its implications for sex estimation in samples without reference collections. Journal of Archaeological Science 34 (10), 1720–1730.

Gonzalez, P.N., Bernal, V., Perez, S.I., 2009. Geometric morphometric approach to sex estimation of human pelvis. Forensic Science International 189 (1–3), 68–74.

Graw, M., Wahl, J., Ahlbrecht, M., 2005. Course of the meatus acusticus internus as criterion for sex differentiation. Forensic Science International 147 (2–3), 113–117.

Gualdi-Russo, E., 2007. Sex determination from the talus and calcaneus measurements. Forensic Science International 171 (2–3), 151–156.

Hanihara, K., 1959. Sex diagnosis of Japanese skulls and scapulae by means of discriminant function. Journal of the Anthropological Society of Nippon 67, 191–197.

Hassett, B., 2011. Technical note: Estimating sex using cervical canine odontometrics: a test using a known sex sample. American Journal of Physical Anthropology 146 (3), 486–489.

Holcomb, S.M., Konigsberg, L.W., 1995. Statistical study of sexual dimorphism in the human fetal sciatic notch. American Journal of Physical Anthropology 97 (2), 113–125.

Hummel, S., Herrmann, B., 1991. Y-chromosome-specific DNA amplified in ancient human bone. Naturwissenschaften 78 (6), 266–267.

Hunt Jr., E.E., Gleiser, I., 1955. The estimation of age and sex of preadolescent children from bones and teeth. American Journal of Physical Anthropology 13 (3), 479–487.

Igbigbi, P.S., Nanono-Igbigbi, A.M., 2003. Determination of sex and race from the subpubic angle in Ugandan subjects. American Journal of Forensic Medicine and Pathology 24 (2), 168–172.

Introna Jr., F., Di Vella, G., Campobasso, C.P., 1998. Sex determination by discriminant analysis of patella measurements. Forensic Science International 95 (1), 39–45.

İşcan, M.Y., Loth, S., 1986. Estimation of age and determination of sex from the sternal rib. In: Reichs, K. (Ed.), Forensic Osteology: Advances in the Identification of Human Remains. Thomas, Springfield, IL, pp. 68–89.

İşcan, M.Y., Miller-Shaivitz, P., 1986. Sexual dimorphism in the femur and tibia. In: Reichs, K. (Ed.), Forensic Osteology: Advances in the Identification of Human Remains. Thomas, Springfield, IL, pp. 102–111.

Kaplowitz, P., 2006. Pubertal development in girls: secular trends. Current Opinion in Obstetrics and Gynecology 18 (5), 487–491.

Kaplowitz, P.B., Slora, E.J., Wasserman, R.C., Pedlow, S.E., Herman-Giddens, M.E., 2001. Earlier onset of puberty in girls: Relation to increased body mass index and race. Pediatrics 108 (2), 347–353.

Kemkes-Grottenthaler, A., 2005. Sex determination by discriminant analysis: an evaluation of the reliability of patella measurements. Forensic Science International 147 (2–3), 129–133.

Kieser, J.A., 1990. Human Adult Odontometrics: The Study of Variation in Adult Tooth Size. Cambridge University Press, Cambridge.

Kimmerle, E.H., Ross, A., Slice, D., 2008. Sexual dimorphism in America: geometric morphometric analysis of the craniofacial region. Journal of Forensic Sciences 53 (1), 54–57.

Komar, D., Buikstra, J., 2009. Forensic Anthropology. Contemporary Theory and Practice. Oxford University Press, Oxford, p. 132.

Konigsberg, L.W., Frankenberg, S.R., 2013. Demography. In: DiGangi, E.A., Moore, M.K. (Eds.), Research Methods in Human Skeletal Biology. Academic Press, San Diego.

Konigsberg, L.W., Hens, S.M., 1998. Use of ordinal categorical variables in skeletal assessment of sex from the cranium. American Journal of Physical Anthropology 107 (1), 97–112.

Konigsberg, L.W., Algee-Hewitt, B.F., Steadman, D.W., 2009. Estimation and evidence in forensic anthropology: sex and race. American Journal of Physical Anthropology 139 (1), 77–90.

Krogman, W.M., İşcan, M.Y., 1986. The Human Skeleton in Forensic Medicine. C.C. Thomas, Springfield, IL.

Larsen, C.S., 1997. Bioarchaeology: Interpreting Behavior from the Human Skeleton. Cambridge University Press, New York.

Lieberman, D.E., Devlin, M.J., Pearson, O.M., 2001. Articular area responses to mechanical loading: effects of exercise, age, and skeletal location. American Journal of Physical Anthropology 116 (4), 266–277.

Mahfouz, M., Badawi, A., Merkl, B., Fatah, E.E., Pritchard, E., Kesler, K., Moore, M., Jantz, R., 2007a. Patella sex determination by 3D statistical shape models and nonlinear classifiers. Forensic Science International 173 (2–3), 161–170.

Mahfouz, M., Merkl, B.C., Fatah, E.E., Booth Jr., R., Argenson, J.N., 2007b. Automatic methods for characterization of sexual dimorphism of adult femora: distal femur. Computer Methods in Biomechanics and Biomedical Engineering 10 (6), 447–456.

Marino, E.A., 1995. Sex estimation using the first cervical vertebra. American Journal of Physical Anthropology 97 (2), 127–133.

Molleson, T., Cruse, K., Mays, S., 1998. Some sexually dimorphic features of the human juvenile skull and their value in sex determination in immature skeletal remains. Journal of Archaeological Sciences 25 (8), 719–728.

Moore, M.K., Niño, F., Hidalgo, O., 2012. Univariate sex discrimination from the postcranial skeleton for a Colombian population. Proceedings of the American Academy of Forensic Sciences 18, 418–419.

Moro, M., van der Meulen, M.C., Kiratli, B.J., Marcus, R., Bachrach, L.K., Carter, D.R., 1996. Body mass is the primary determinant of midfemoral bone acquisition during adolescent growth. Bone 19 (5), 519–526.

Onland-Moret, N.C., Peeters, P.H., van Gils, C.H., Clavel-Chapelon, F., Key, T., Tjønneland, A., Trichopoulou, A., Kaaks, R., Manjer, J., Panico, S., Palli, D., Tehard, B., Stoikidou, M., Bueno-De-Mesquita, H.B., Boeing, H., Overvad, K., Lenner, P., Quirós, J.R., Chirlaque, M.D., Miller, A.B., Khaw, K.T., Riboli, E., 2005. Age at menarche in relation to adult height: the EPIC study. American Journal of Epidemiology 162 (7), 623–632.

Ousley, S.D., Jantz, R.L., 2012. FORDISC 3.1: Personal Computer Forensic Discriminant Functions. University of Tennessee.

Patriquin, M.L., Steyn, M., Loth, S.R., 2005. Metric analysis of sex differences in South African Black and White pelves. Forensic Science International 147 (2–3), 119–127.

Phenice, T.W., 1969. A newly developed visual method of sexing the os pubis. American Journal of Physical Anthropology 30 (2), 297–301.

Purkait, R., 2005. Triangle identified at the proximal end of femur: a new sex determinant. Forensic Science International 147 (2–3), 135–139.

Reichs, K., 1986. Forensic implications of skeletal pathology: sex. In: Reichs, K. (Ed.), Forensic Osteology: Advances in the Identification of Human Remains. Thomas, Springfield, IL, pp. 112–142.

Rogers, S., 1987. Personal Identification from Human Remains. Charles C. Thomas, Springfield, IL.

Rogers, T., 2005. Determining the sex of human remains through cranial morphology. Journal of Forensic Sciences 50 (3), 493–500.

Rogers, T., Saunders, S., 1994. Accuracy of sex determination using morphological traits of the human pelvis. Journal of Forensic Sciences 39 (4), 1047–1056.

Ross, A.H., McKeown, A.H., Konigsberg, L.W., 1999. Allocation of crania to groups via the new morphometry. Journal of Forensic Sciences 44 (3), 584–587.

Ross, A.H., Baker, L.E., Falsetti, A., 2003. Sexual dimorphism a proxy for environmental sensitivity? A multi-temporal view. Journal of the Washington Academy of Sciences 89 (1–2), 1–12.

Ruff, C.B., 2000. Body mass prediction from skeletal frame size in elite athletes. American Journal of Physical Anthropology 113 (4), 507–517.

Ruff, C.B., Hayes, W.C., 1988. Sex differences in age-related remodeling of the femur and tibia. Journal of Orthopedic Research 6 (6), 886–896.

Saini, V., Srivastava, R., Rai, R.K., Shamal, S.N., Singh, T.B., Tripathi, S.K., 2011. An osteometric study of northern Indian populations for sexual dimorphism in craniofacial region. Journal of Forensic Sciences 56 (3), 700–705.

Saunders, S.R., 2000. Subadult skeletons and growth-related studies. In: Katzenberg, M.A., Saunders, S.R. (Eds.), Biological Anthropology of the Human Skeleton. Wiley, New York, pp. 135–162.

Scheuer, L., Black, S.M., 2004. The Juvenile Skeleton. Elsevier Academic Press, San Diego.

Spradley, M.K., Jantz, R.L., 2011. Sex estimation in forensic anthropology: skull versus postcranial elements. Journal of Forensic Sciences 56 (2), 289–296.

Stewart, T.D., 1979. Essentials of Forensic Anthropology, Especially as Developed in the United States. Charles C. Thomas, Springfield, IL.

Stinson, S., Bogin, B., Huss-Ashmore, R., O'Rourke, D., 2012. Human Biology: An Evolutionary and Biocultural Perspective. Wiley-Blackwell, Hoboken, NJ.

Stini, W.A., 1975. Adaptive strategies of human populations under nutritional stress. In: Watts, E.S., Johnston, F.E., Lasker, G.W. (Eds.), Biosocial Interrelations in Population Adaptation. Mouton, The Hague, pp. 19–41.

Stini, W.A., 1982. Sexual dimorphism and nutrient reserves. In: Hall, R.L. (Ed.), Sexual Dimorphism in *Homo sapiens*. Praeger, New York, pp. 391–419.

Stone, A.C., 2000. Ancient DNA from skeletal remains. In: Katzenberg, M.A., Saunders, S.R. (Eds.), Biological Anthropology of the Human Skeleton. Wiley, New York, pp. 351–372.

Ubelaker, D.H., 2000. Methodological considerations in the forensic applications of human skeletal biology. In: Katzenberg, M.A., Saunders, S.R. (Eds.), Biological Anthropology of the Human Skeleton. Wiley, New York, pp. 41–68.

Ubelaker, D.H., Volk, C.G., 2002. A test of the phenice method for the estimation of sex. Journal of Forensic Sciences 47 (1), 19–24.

Walker, P.L., 2008. Sexing skulls using discriminant function analysis of visually assessed traits. American Journal of Physical Anthropology 136 (1), 39–50.

Walker, P.L., Cook, D.C., 1998. Brief communication: Gender and sex: vive la difference. American Journal of Physical Anthropology 106 (2), 255–259.

Weaver, D.S., 1980. Sex differences in the ilia of a known sex and age sample of fetal and infant skeletons. American Journal of Physical Anthropology 52 (2), 191–195.

Weaver, D.S., 1986. Forensic aspects of fetal and neonatal skeletons. In: Reichs, K. (Ed.), Forensic Osteology: Advances in the Identification of Human Remains. Charles C. Thomas, Springfield, IL, pp. 187–203.

White, T.D., Black, M.T., Folkens, P.A., 2012. Human Osteology. Academic Press, San Diego.

5

Ancestry Estimation

Elizabeth A. DiGangi, Joseph T. Hefner

INTRODUCTION

Why are biological anthropologists interested in studying ancestry when the topic is mired with controversy due to the ways race research has been used socially and politically? The answer is simple: anthropology is at its heart the study of humankind and all its aspects, both cultural and biological. Therefore, many early physical anthropologists were concerned with ordering or classifying human groups into categories, in part as a way to more fully understand humankind. As we will uncover in the pages ahead, much of this early effort was **typological,**[1] assuming that different groups of people conformed to types, and in many cases their research assumed a certain hierarchical arrangement of the various races. Current thought regarding ancestry conversely takes a population perspective and focuses on two primary objectives: (1) understanding the distribution of **human variation**; and (2) using that variation during human identification for medicolegal purposes.

As stated above, ancestry is arguably the most controversial topic we must contend with in biological anthropology in general, and more specifically, during the construction of the biological profile from human skeletal remains. While this controversy has existed for decades, we have only recently fully accepted that while race *does not* exist from a true biological standpoint, it *does* exist from a social standpoint, a realization that must be acknowledged. Further, while race is not biological *per se*, we are nevertheless able to estimate ancestry (given the social categories in use[2]) from a number of skeletal features, most notably from the skull.

---

[1]All bolded terms are defined in the glossary at the end of this volume.

[2]It is important to note that the social categories in use for race are *cultural* constructions and therefore arbitrary. Each culture will have its own unique system to categorize what it views as the different races. For example, the 2010 U.S. Census recognized 15 different categories (Humes et al., 2011), and technically six of those are nationalities (e.g., Japanese, Filipino). Conversely, the Brazilian census recognizes five categories in total (Instituto Brasileiro de Geografia e Estatistica, 2010). While the majority of these categories are arbitrary with no basis in biology, it nonetheless happens that we can estimate ancestral origin from the skull for four major categories (African, Asian, European, and Indigenous/Native American), as will be discussed in this chapter.

E.A. DiGangi and M.K. Moore: Research Methods in Human Skeletal Biology

You must be well versed on the history of race in anthropology before embarking on research in ancestry estimation. Therefore, this chapter will first review the different eras of thought and practice in anthropology regarding race and will demonstrate the social and political implications resulting from race research conducted by anthropologists and others in the past two centuries. A discussion of modern era ancestry estimation using robust statistics and a case study demonstrating a novel approach to ancestry estimation will be presented. After reading this chapter, you will have a better understanding of the history of race/ancestry estimation in anthropology as well as a modern scientific foundation upon which to base the exploration of your own questions.

A Note on Terminology

Throughout this chapter, the terms race and ancestry are used interchangeably. We will use the term "race" when discussing the history of the concept or when referring to how human groups have been classified, from either a supposedly biological or social standpoint. The term "ancestry" will be used in reference to modern thought about human variation. Additionally, we will only use the "-oid" terms (i.e., Caucasoid, Mongoloid, and Negroid) when referring to a specific taxonomic schemata used in the past. When talking about ancestry estimation today, the terms currently in vogue are European, Asian, and African, because these exclusively refer to a major geographic region of ancestral origin,[3] rather than to a taxonomic classification engorged with underlying social meaning.

(BRIEF) HISTORY OF RACE CONCEPT

This section is not meant to be an exhaustive review of the history of the race concept in anthropology and cannot mention every important player in the development of the concept. It will, however, set the basic background from which the reader can embark on further exploration of the topics raised. There are a number of books dedicated to the history of race in anthropology, notably *Man's Most Dangerous Myth* by Ashley Montagu, *The Mismeasure of Man* by Stephen J. Gould, and *"Race" is a Four-Letter Word* by C. Loring Brace, among many others. A recent dissertation by Algee-Hewitt (2011) comprehensively covers the subject as well. We encourage you to read these and others for a detailed background if you wish to embark on a study in ancestry estimation.

Further, the following sections will discuss several specifics from anthropology's history that may make many readers uncomfortable. It is important that you try to understand history within its own context—i.e., recognize that each scientist works within the boundaries and established viewpoints set by their own culture. Likewise, anthropologists today are confined by our own culture, even if we are self-aware of this fact and yet struggle to

---

[3]While these categories are still somewhat race-based (Mukhopadhyay and Moses, 1997) there is no consensus on what better alternative terminology would be.

break out of these imposed boundaries. Remember, every scientist (including you) is a product of his or her own time and culture.[4]

Beginnings

The practice of dividing humans into discrete groups dates back to the fifteenth century, when European explorers were encountering people who looked and acted very differently from themselves. The prevailing thought was that there must be a reason for these clear differences, and explaining them as distinct races made sense. Carolus Linnaeus is credited with creating the binomial nomenclature system of *Genus* and *species* still used today. He wrote in *Systema Naturae* (1759) that while humans represent one species, *Homo sapiens*, there are nevertheless subspecies of humans, which he subdivided based on geography and physical characteristics as well as personality characteristics. He called these subdivisions the *africanus, americanus, asiaticus*, and *europaeus* types. His classification of humans into subspecies effectively set the stage for the emphasis on classification and taxonomy that would dominate research on human differences for the next two centuries (Stanton, 1960).

Following Linnaeus, the German anatomist Johann Blumenbach was the first to lay out five different human races in the eighteenth century. As he saw them, the Caucasian, Mongolian, Ethiopian, American, and Malayan types captured the whole pattern of human races. He was the first to propose the use of the terms "Caucasoid" and "Mongoloid" with reference to the classification of peoples from Europe and Asia (Brace, 2005). While the categories proposed by Blumenbach were subject to change over the centuries to come, the terms Caucasoid and Mongoloid nevertheless continue to be used, albeit unadvisedly.

Monogenism and Polygenism

During this period in race research, there were attempts to explain the differences between the various races *and* to understand how these seemingly disparate races came to be. Two primary schools of thought existed: one group believed that that all human groups dated back to the Biblical Adam and Eve, and following that "perfect" coupling, environmental changes as well as population shifts occurred that led to the various races beyond Caucasoids (Brace, 2005). This **monogenistic** view stemmed from the belief in *The Great Chain of Being*, the idea first developed by ancient Greek philosophers and later revisited in Europe during medieval times. The Great Chain of Being posits that all living things are arranged in a hierarchy, with the Christian God at the top and human beings directly below (Lovejoy, 1936). This view fit well with the story of creation from Genesis, and therefore was compatible with a religious viewpoint that fit with the "scientific" view of the different races. It also hierarchically arranged the races in a way that provided religious support for their ordered placement.

Conversely, the **polygenists** believed that each race had its own unique origin. According to the polygenists, the Caucasoid race was oldest and therefore was the most evolved; conversely, the Negroid race was youngest and therefore was the least evolved. This viewpoint was popular in the nineteenth century, especially in the United States, which led

[4]For example, Kaszycka et al. (2009) demonstrated that the disparate views on race held by contemporary European anthropologists are both dependent on education and influenced by sociopolitical ideology.

European anthropologists to dub the anthropology in that country as "**The American School of Anthropology**" (Brace, 2005). Under this umbrella fits the research of Samuel George Morton.

Morton was an anatomist with an interest in craniometry working in Philadelphia. The movement towards an emphasis on skull measurement was an extension of typological theory, since it attempted to show from a biological and evolutionary standpoint the hierarchical arrangement of the races (Gould, 1981). Morton collected human skulls from around the world to measure. He was particularly interested in cranial (braincase) capacity, because he felt that particular measure would show unequivocally the correct racial hierarchical arrangement. His results demonstrated that Caucasoids had the highest cranial capacity; however, reanalysis of his data a century later by Gould demonstrated that Morton had either deliberately or subconsciously manipulated the data to fit his preconceived notions (Gould, 1978). Interestingly, Gould's work has recently been reanalyzed as well, and like Morton's, may have been inadvertently biased (Brace, 2005; Lewis et al., 2011).

Morton produced several volumes on craniometry describing in detail the relationship between the races as explicitly "proven" by science (e.g., Morton, 1839). Unsurprisingly based on his predetermined ideas, his results showed that white males were superior to others in terms of cranial capacity, with white females and people of other races lagging behind. His work not only was used as support for social policies of the time (e.g., justification of slavery in the United States), but also has been used by other researchers looking for biological justification for hierarchical classification of the races (e.g., Rushton, 1995). Another researcher doing similar work was Paul Broca, surgery professor and founder of the *Anthropology Society of Paris* in the mid-nineteenth century. He was interested in the physical weights of brains in order to establish a link between race, brain size, and intelligence (Gould, 1981). While his work was inconclusive, it has not stopped others from attempting similar comparisons, even up to the relative present day (i.e., Herrnstein and Murray, 1994).

HRDLIČKA, HOOTON, AND BOAS: THREE KEY FIGURES IN THE DEVELOPMENT OF THE DISCIPLINE

Three of the most important historical figures in the development of American physical anthropology are Aleš Hrdlička, Franz Boas, and Earnest Hooton. Their differing viewpoints on race continue to impact the field today. While Hrdlička and Hooton had similar views, Boas occupied a different camp entirely. Their scientific differences can be summed up into two opposite viewpoints on how to explain human variation: (1) as a result of separate evolutionary pathways leading to different races (Hrdlička and Hooton) versus (2) emphasis on the influence of environmental variables (i.e., culture, nutrition, stress, climate, etc.) on variation (Boas).

The former viewpoint is typological and focuses on creating categories based on arbitrary physical characteristics (skin color, facial features, etc.), which become linked to cultural characteristics. As such, typology inherently includes aspects of **biological determinism**—the concept that biology dictates not only physical traits, but sociocultural traits as well (e.g., "level" of civilization, language, intelligence, and so on). In other words, biological determinism states that an individual is destined for a certain fate socially and culturally depending on things such as country of birth, skin color, head shape and size, and other physical or cultural traits. It assumes *a priori* that categories exist and therefore attempts to classify each group and each physical and cultural characteristic. In contrast, the viewpoint emphasizing the importance of the environment is a holistic one that explores and tests the different processes leading to human variation (Caspari, 2009). Rather than making assumptions about the existence of discrete categories, it attempts to tease apart the complex environmental variables that have impacted the expression of biology (Caspari, 2009).

Aleš Hrdlička

Aleš Hrdlička immigrated to the United States from Eastern Europe as a child in the late nineteenth century. After training as a medical doctor, he went to France for a brief stay where he received his first formal instruction in anthropology (Brace, 2005). Following a position as a field anthropologist at the American Museum of Natural History in New York, he moved to the Smithsonian Institution where he would spend the bulk of his career as a physical anthropologist (Brace, 2005). Given his inspiration by Paul Broca's *Anthropology Society of Paris*, Hrdlička tried for years to set up a similar organization in the United States, which ultimately culminated in the creation of the *American Journal of Physical Anthropology* (AJPA) in 1918 and the later founding of the *American Association of Physical Anthropologists* (AAPA) in 1929 (Spencer, 1981; Brace, 2005). His position of authority within the museum, the journal, and the organization allowed Hrdlička to manage how anthropology could inform public discourse about race—the social meaning of race is implicit here (Caspari, 2009). For example, he personally played a role in influencing public policy on immigration in the United States by testifying before Congress in 1922 about his views on the hierarchical arrangement of the races and biological determinism (Oppenheim, 2010).

Hrdlička essentially viewed the different races as "stems of humanity" (as many of his contemporaries did) and focused his questions on the number of races that existed (Brace, 2005; Caspari, 2009; Oppenheim, 2010:93). Hrdlička defined physical anthropology as the study of comparative racial anatomy and emphasized a comparative, descriptive approach towards the study of the three main racial groups as he classified them (white, black, and yellow/brown); this emphasis was to best understand the white race (Blakey, 1987; Caspari, 2009; Oppenheim, 2010). Inherent in his thinking were elements of biological determinism. He believed that the social differences between the races were due to different evolutionary histories, and that the white race was superior (Blakey, 1987; Oppenheim, 2010). While Hrdlička did not produce students in his position at the Smithsonian, his founding of the two major organs of our discipline (the AJPA and AAPA) and his extensive scholarship solidified his status as one of the fathers of physical anthropology, deterministic views aside.

Franz Boas

Franz Boas held a PhD in physics from a German university but began practicing anthropology in the late nineteenth century. He took a full-time faculty position at Columbia University in New York in 1905 after spending several years at the American Museum of Natural History (Spencer, 1981; Caspari, 2009). Early on, he did ethnographic research with the Eskimo in the Canadian Arctic, an experience that provided him an understanding of the crucial role that culture plays in impacting biology and behavior, and not the other way around (Erickson, 2008). Rather than being based on typology and biological determinism, his thought system on human groups was geared instead toward investigating links between environment, culture, and the resulting biological variation (Erickson, 2008; Caspari, 2009). His experiences as an ethnographic fieldworker with different indigenous groups in Canada solidified his view that race is not a causal factor of cultural traits—i.e., that racial traits (skin color, head shape, etc.) do not cause or influence cultural features such as language (Erickson, 2008). Boas was an example of this: he was white, yet learned the language of the groups he studied in Canada and whenever possible even partook in their culture (Erickson, 2008).

Boas' landmark publication in 1910, *Changes in Bodily Form of Descendants of Immigrants,*[5] proposed that the cranial index of the children of immigrants born in the United States was different from the cranial index of their siblings born overseas.[6] His argument was that this biological change was due to the differing environments of the United States and the home countries of the immigrant parents. Perhaps nutrition had improved, or there was increased access to medical care for expectant mothers, but whatever the reason, his conclusions were evidence against biological determinist arguments. Even though Boas' conclusions have recently been modified (Sparks and Jantz, 2003; Jantz and Logan, 2010), his research was key in the early twentieth century towards undermining racial typologies and demonstrating that biological deterministic thinking has no scientific basis (Gravlee, 2003). Further, his emphasis on the importance of *testing* hypotheses about human variation rather than making broad assumptions about race is clear: "Nobody had tried to answer the questions *why* certain measurements were taken, *why* they were considered significant, [or] whether they were subject to other influences" (Boas, 1936; as quoted in Montagu, 1964a:16, emphasis added).

Boas' influence on the field in terms of his perspectives on race (rejecting types and embracing culture and environment as holding answers to human variation questions) and his stress on the importance of bringing an overall, holistic anthropological viewpoint to bear on problems in physical anthropology cannot be overstated (Caspari, 2009). In addition to being major professor of 20 students, many of whom went on to be influential in the field themselves (Erickson, 2008), his position on the importance of culture and environment in human variation research is the foundation for research questions today and it is clear that this emphasis will continue to shape the future of the discipline. In addition, his stress on the importance of metric traits to reveal **secular change**[7]—how time brings about changes in

---

[5]This publication was part of the Dillingham Commission, resulting in a 41-volume report on immigrant assimilation in the United States. See Lund (1994) for more information.

[6]At the time of Boas' publication, the United States was experiencing (and had been experiencing) an influx of immigrants from European countries and others. As a result, "native" born Americans—those white Americans already in the country for several generations—saw the Irish, the Italians, the Chinese, and others as different races from themselves. Immigrant groups with white skin did not start to be considered *socially* white until the 1920s (Jacobson, 1998). Immigrant groups with non-white skin of course today remain socially as non-white.

[7]See discussion on secular change in Moore and Ross (Chapter 6); and McKeown and Schmidt (Chapter 12), this volume.

biology due to changing variables in the environment—also continues today (e.g., Jantz and Jantz, 1999; Jantz and Jantz, 2000; Jantz, 2001).

Earnest Hooton

Earnest Hooton and Franz Boas, while personally cordial with each other, were professional adversaries, at least in terms of their very different philosophies in physical anthropology. Hooton was trained in the classics but became interested in anthropology during time spent at Oxford (as a Rhodes Scholar) prior to earning his PhD from the University of Wisconsin in 1911 (Spencer, 1981; Brace, 1982). In stark contrast to Boas, Hooton's ideas about race were polygenic and typological (Caspari, 2009). Furthermore, similar to Hrdlička, deterministic ideas were mired in his thoughts about race (Brace, 1982; Caspari, 2009).

Hooton was interested in the use of cranial nonmetric traits (e.g., presence/absence of the infraorbital suture) for classificatory purposes. He created the Harvard Blanks as a standard for recording of nonmetric traits, general cranial observations, and cranial measurements he deemed useful for answering his research interests about body form (Brues, 1990).

Many of his students shared his typological ideas, and several published books and articles that looked at race from a largely deterministic or typological point of view. Hooton's own publications ranged from the clearly typological (*On Certain Eskimoid Characters in Icelandic Skulls*—1918) to eccentric applications of typology and determinism (*Crime and the Man*[8]—1939). Ironically, Hooton seemingly was antiracist and participated in antiracism activities, e.g., attempting to create an antiracism group in anthropology (Caspari, 2003), yet his typological analyses supported a hierarchical arrangement of the races. From a historical perspective, even taking into account this history, Hooton is one of the most significant figures for the development of physical anthropology (Shapiro, 1954).

Hooton was incredibly influential in the growth of the field in large part because physical anthropology did not exist as an established discipline when he began at Harvard in 1913 and his program was the first to produce PhDs rapidly in the discipline (28 overall). Many of his students went on to lead physical anthropology programs in anthropology departments at major universities in the United States (Spencer, 1981; Giles, 1997). A large majority of currently practicing biological anthropologists (including both authors on this chapter) can trace their educational pedigree via thesis or dissertation committee members three or four steps back to Hooton, illustrating his overall impact on the field (Caspari, 2009).

SCIENTIFIC RACISM

Scientific racism is defined as the use of science to justify discrimination against groups of people based on perceived inherent differences. These inherent differences typically begin with skin color and other **phenotypic** traits that have been used to classify races and are expanded to include culture, intelligence, and morals (Nash, 1962; Blakey, 1999). Scientific

[8]This book in particular showcases Hooton's beliefs that people could be categorized almost *ad infinitum* (he has groups such as "native white" and "Old American," the difference between which depends upon how many generations their families have been in the United States) and that this typology determines one's propensity to commit certain types of crimes.

racism as a construct developed in the West over the past three centuries from two ideas: (1) scientific knowledge is authoritative; and (2) groups of people can be separated taxonomically on the basis of both physical and cultural characteristics (Marks, 2008). The history of taxonomically separating groups of people is mired with inquiry as to what defines or separates one group from another. Beginning with Linnaeus, groups were separated not just on the basis of obvious physical differences (skin color, hair color, etc.) but also on character traits (such as level of intelligence and culture) that were arbitrarily chosen to be definitive. With scientific racism, science is used to validate these co-associations. The problem is threefold: (1) as will be discussed later on, there is no biological basis for separating human groups on the basis of *race*; (2) character traits such as intelligence are complexly influenced by both genetics <u>and</u> environment and are not exclusive to one group of people versus another; and (3) given science's authority with the public, a scientific proclamation stating that physical and character differences are related is very difficult to retract.

Social Darwinism and *The Origin of Species*

The most famous publication in the nineteenth century was Charles Darwin's thesis on how species come into being (Darwin, 1859). While the concept of evolution was not new and several others had tried (and failed) to explain its mechanism, Darwin's explanation of **natural selection** was the first to logically elucidate a mechanism of **evolution**. Essentially natural selection states that those organisms having beneficial adaptations (beneficiality depends on the environment in which an organism lives) are more likely to survive, reproduce, and pass on those advantageous traits, while those organisms with nonbeneficial traits will not survive to reproduce, or at least not in significant numbers. The result is that advantageous traits will appear in organisms at a higher proportion than non-advantageous traits for a particular environment. Natural selection, along with other evolutionary forces (see Cabana et al. [Chapter 16], this volume) can lead to the formation of new species.

The book was revolutionary for the field of biology for obvious reasons, but it also spurred unforeseen effects in other fields and for society at large. While Darwin only briefly mentioned the implication of his theory for human beings in the last chapter of that volume,[9] other scholars latched onto the idea and extrapolated natural selection to include cultural achievement and development (Nash, 1962; Blakey, 1999; Graves, 2001). Each race, therefore, was believed to have its own specific level of intellect and culture by which it could be characterized (Nash, 1962; Blakey, 1999).

Herbert Spencer, a contemporary of Darwin, was the first to coin the now-famous phrase, "survival of the fittest" (Stanton, 1960; Shipman, 1994; Graves, 2001). When this phrase was applied to human beings, an individual's "fitness" was defined as intelligence, attractiveness, education, wealth, and cultural accomplishments, in addition to other characteristics.[10] Survival of the fittest was used to justify and rationalize social institutions like capitalism and

---

[9]Darwin discussed the origins of humans and the issue of race in a later publication, *The Descent of Man* (1871).

[10]It is important to point out that each of these categories is culturally bound, i.e., each culture has its own definition of intelligence, wealth, of what it means to be civilized and educated, and so on. In this case, it was the privileged sector of Western culture setting the categories and definitions.

colonialism, two systems that favor certain groups of people over others (Marks, 2008). It was considered that those not fit enough were simply not destined to survive and reproduce. This fate was not the fault of any person or institution, but through the destiny set forth by science. Evolution was therefore unfortunately used to explain and validate the differences between the classes, the races, and the sexes.

Eugenics

Social Darwinism also led to the belief that social and cultural traits (e.g., poverty, propensity to criminality) were inherited as were physical traits. Francis Galton (Darwin's cousin) coined the term "eugenics" in 1883 (from the Greek for "well born") to espouse his ideas of artificial selection for human beings (Shipman, 1994). In his view, "undesirable" traits were inherited, and therefore breeding programs for humans could be designed to combat the propagation of undesirable traits by allowing only "desirables"[11] to mate (Montagu, 1964b; Gould, 1981; Shipman, 1994:111; Graves, 2001; Paul, 2008). Galton argued that it was society's responsibility to control human reproduction so that the lower classes (including criminals and the poor) would be prevented from passing on their defects (Paul, 2008). Clearly, there was no consideration or even acknowledgment of any effect the environment had on the development of various "undesirable" characters. Of course, the environment in large part included the social conditions that the higher classes had imposed to create the lower classes.

Ernst Haeckel, who was a contemporary of Darwin's and a German biologist, further developed ideas such as these. He argued incorrectly that evolution was progressive and goal-directed leading to an ideal form (he argued for the Aryan type) and that social and cultural traits were freely inherited without influence from the environment (Graves, 2001). Similar to many of his contemporaries, Haeckel believed in a social hierarchy. For example, Haeckel wrote (disturbingly by today's standards) in 1905 (emphasis added), "These lower races ... are psychologically nearer to the mammals (apes or dogs) than to civilized Europeans; we must, therefore, *assign a totally different value* to their lives."

Charles Davenport, an influential American biologist in the early twentieth century, was responsible for introducing eugenics to the United States[12] (Shipman, 1994; Marks, 2008). His book, *Heredity in Relation to Eugenics* (1911), fed on the fears of the ruling class Americans, mainly that the influx of immigrants with certain undesirable traits (poverty, propensity towards criminality, homosexuality, chronic illness, etc.) would lead to the downfall of society (Davenport, 1911; Marks, 2008). Davenport's main thesis was that biology was behind the development or downfall of civilization. Five years later, Madison Grant used these ideas to argue that the answer to the problem lay in the sterilization of people deemed to be unfit (1916). This book, and other eugenic writings,[13] led to eugenics laws with 30

[11]One of the key dangers here is in who gets to decide which traits are "desirable" and which traits are not.

[12]Interestingly, while eugenic ideas spread worldwide, each country or region focused on one aspect more heavily than another (e.g., class differences in one country versus race differences in another) (Marks, 2008) thereby illustrating the pervasive nature of culture to even influence emphasis of racist thought.

[13]Not every scientist agreed with the tenets of eugenics, including Franz Boas (e.g., see Boas, 1918a), but few came out publicly to denounce it in the early days of the movement (Marks, 2008).

different states in the U.S. sterilizing people involuntarily over the next two decades (Suzuki and Knudtson, 1989; Marks, 2008). The state of California[14] alone for example forcibly sterilized 20,000 people before World War II on the basis of perceived mental disability, criminal history, or other undesirable traits[15] (Suzuki and Knudtson, 1989; Larson, 1996; Marks, 2008). Shamefully, these American laws helped to form the basis for genocidal practices in Nazi Germany (Suzuki and Knudtson, 1989), following a progression from forced sterilization to human extermination. The onset of the Great Depression in the United States redirected focus on domestic economic problems while eugenic ideas took hold and flourished in Germany during the same time period (Bozeman, 1997; Marks, 2008). While some involuntary sterilizations continued after WWII in the United States, the horror of the Holocaust and the fact that it was the end result of eugenic ideas discredited such programs. The laws were gradually removed, albeit quietly in many instances (Blakey, 1999; Marks, 2008).

Although it would seem that this should signal the end of the use of science to justify group inequality, recent examples of scientific racism continue to include proclamations that intelligence and race are linked, that athletes from certain groups are naturally better at particular sports than others, that different races are more prone to certain diseases than others, and that genes for different human behaviors are connected with race (see Gould, 1996; Armelagos and Goodman, 1998; Goodman, 2000; Graves, 2001; Smedley and Smedley, 2005; Sternberg et al., 2005; Marks, 2008; Gravlee, 2009). These beliefs persist in society at large regardless of the fact that none of these assertions can be or has been validated from a scientific standpoint. Furthermore, these stereotypes fail to account for socioeconomic and environmental factors (see for example discussion in Cartmill, 1999). In addition, the very existence of stereotypes that reinforce the popular view of race and biology act via culture to actually establish measurable differences in health between different racial groups (Gravlee, 2009). Gravlee (2009) has adapted Kuzawa's (2008) model of health inequalities to demonstrate how this occurs, in addition to a superb discussion. The reader is encouraged to refer to this paper for more information.

Obviously, scientific racism can have, and has had, very severe and tangible consequences. As a 21st century anthropologist contemplating an ancestry project, it is essential that you realize this discussion is <u>not</u> purely of academic interest. Our discipline has discarded the concept of biological race and with it the ideas that character traits are associated with physical traits. However, the fact remains that race is a social construct. Consequently, there is a societal cost especially for those perceived to be members of the so-called inferior races (Moses, 2004; Smedley and Smedley, 2005). Anthropology's past assertions have contributed to the solidification of societal ideas about race (Harrison, 1995, 1999) and therefore we need to decide how to manage the consequences. As Harrison notes, "… there is no theoretical, methodological, or political consensus shared across any of the subdisciplines on how to interpret and explicate the social realities that constitute race" (1999:610). Montagu described race as an "event" that is experienced (1964b:117) and our discipline has yet to systematically

---

[14]In early 2012, the state of North Carolina resolved to financially compensate its approximate 7500 living victims of involuntary sterilization, the first restitution for such cases in the United States (Severson, 2012).

[15]Feeblemindedness, alcoholism, and epilepsy were included as well (Suzuki and Knudtson, 1989).

examine the cost of this event socially or biologically (Armelagos and Goodman, 1998; Harrison, 1995, 1999; Lieberman and Kirk, 2004; Gravlee, 2009).

It is a reality that social race exists and that forensic anthropologists *can* estimate geographic ancestral origin from different bones. But this same reality makes ancestry estimation a delicate endeavor indeed. On the one hand, biological anthropologists say, "race does not exist biologically"; yet on the other, they say, "however, we can estimate ancestry from the skeleton." This contradictory message confuses the public, in part because they are not aware of the nuances of the evolutionary forces that have led to certain skeletal features, but also because such statements would seem to reinforce societal views about different race categories. Blakey refers to the conundrum of continued racial categorization as a "tangled web" (1999:42) and it is clear that untangling the web to move past categorization is an impossible task since we rely on traditional categories to estimate ancestry from skeletons. The point is that as anthropologists who estimate ancestry, it is our responsibility both to the discipline and to society to recognize the societal implications of doing ancestry estimation. We must consider two major interests of society: (1) victim/**decedent** identification, and (2) combating racism. How do we decide which interest is more important and how do we convincingly and clearly explain to the public the difference between social race categories and the characteristics of different geographic populations that we can see and measure from the skeleton?

MODERN THOUGHT ABOUT ANCESTRY

"To give up all general racial classifications would mean for anthropology freeing itself from blinkers it has too long worn, and focusing all its energy on its actual goal: the understanding of human variability, as it really is." *Jean Hiernaux (1964:43—44)*

One could argue that Franz Boas first laid the overall foundation for our current conception of ancestry just before the turn of the twentieth century (Caspari, 2009). His publications showcase his interest in human variation outside of race, rejecting both biological determinist and typological explanations (Caspari, 2009; and for example Boas, 1918b). He additionally focused on the concept of culture and the effect of the environment on human variation, perhaps being at least partially influenced by Edward Tylor's famous definition of "culture," still in use today: "that complex whole which includes knowledge, belief, art, law, morals, custom, and any other capabilities and habits acquired by man as a member of society" (Tylor, 1871; Caspari, 2009). During his career, he continued to publish on similar ideas; however, typological and racial determinist ideas continued to compete (Littlefield et al., 1982).

This began to change in 1951 with Sherwood Washburn's seminal paper, *The New Physical Anthropology*. In it, Washburn, a Hooton student, defined a new direction for the discipline: a movement away from applied typology and toward studies examining evolutionary change, population genetics, and human variation (1951). Essentially, this paper set up the framework for modern thought in biological anthropology, i.e., a focus on the **population** from an evolutionary perspective. The population in this sense can be defined as a group of contemporary human individuals living in relatively the same geographic area who have a shared culture that includes language, traditions, and belief systems and who tend to find mates from within the same group.[16] Several scholars contributed to this major shift in the discipline, including Ashley Montagu (a Boas student) and Frank Livingstone (a Harvard student who took classes from Hooton). These scholars argued that race does not exist because it does not explain the scope of human variation (Livingstone, 1962), it ignores evolutionary forces, and it is imbued with social meaning (Montagu, 1964; Washburn, 1964). Further, Comas (1961), in refute of biological determinism, additionally emphasized the importance that the environment plays in influencing trait expression.

While the discipline was changing focus, change nevertheless came slow. Littlefield et al. (1982) demonstrated that the majority of physical anthropology textbooks published between 1932 and 1969 took the position that human beings were divided into races. Interestingly, this trend began to decrease after 1970, with more texts arguing that races do not exist (Littlefield et al., 1982). Despite this gradual development over the past 40 years, Caspari (2003) contends that while the discipline may have discarded the race concept idea, certain aspects of racial thinking continue. This includes **essentialism** (viewing each racial taxonomic category as having certain essential features that define it which are due to a separate evolutionary history) and **cladistic thinking** (viewing the relationships between races as **clades**, with each race separate from the others having its own branch on a tree diagram) (Caspari, 2003).

While this is appropriate for illustrating evolutionary relationships between species, which by definition are reproductively isolated from each other, separating human groups into clades is not an appropriate way to explain human variation because (1) all modern humans belong to the same species and therefore we successfully mate with each other; and (2) it suggests that different human groups had separate evolutionary histories (evolving from separate ancestors), which is not the case. Today biological anthropologists study populations rather than races, but the definition of "population" still often incorporates these essentialist and cladistic aspects (Caspari, 2003). Future research should move beyond this type of antiquated thinking.

Human Variation

Recently, the *American Journal of Physical Anthropology* published a special issue on race and human variation (2009, 139(1): 1–107). The papers cover the range of agreement and disagreement regarding how the field currently conceptualizes human variation, in terms of its differences and patterns. The papers demonstrate that general agreement centers around several points: (1) variation exists within and between populations; (2) the environment, including culture and geography, has exerted considerable influence on variation; (3) race is neither a useful nor correct way to describe populations; and (4) research in human variation holds implications for society and fields such as forensics and medicine (Edgar and Hunley, 2009).

Conversely, disagreement centers on how the geographic patterns of variation are organized. One school of thought is that human variation is clinally distributed, and that more genetic variation exists *within* a population than *between* all populations (Livingstone, 1962; Lewontin, 1972; Edgar and Hunley, 2009). The concept of a **cline** was introduced by British

---

[16]This mate choice tendency is not absolute—all humans are members of the same species because there is, has been, and will continue to be **gene flow** between populations.

evolutionary biologist Sir Julian Huxley in 1938 and refers to a gradual change of a character or feature in a species over a geographical area (Lieberman, 2008). For example, Relethford (2009) argues that human phenotypic features such as skin color and craniometrics are patterned clinally (e.g., skin color being darkest near the equator and gradually lightening as latitude increases), and that natural selection controls traits such as expression of skin color from environmental pressure. Similarly, craniometrics are partially controlled by natural selection in some instances and selectively neutral in others, although craniometric differences still demonstrate more variation within local populations than between them. Relethford (2009) argues that while geographic patterning is evident in these traits, placing them into broad racial categories masks the true diversity of human variation.

The other school of thought explains variation as resulting from complex factors that contribute to evolutionary forces, such as migration, bottlenecks, and population divisions (e.g., Hunley et al., 2009). These complex factors interrupt gene flow as larger populations are split up. This leads to the **founder effect**, where the genes of a smaller segment of the larger population become overly representative of the parent population, resulting in **genetic drift**.[17] While workers such as Hunley and colleagues (2009) and Long and colleagues (2009) contend that the pattern of human variation is *nested* (the diversity in one population is a subset of the diversity found in another) rather than clinal, they come to the same conclusion as those in the cline camp: namely, that the traditional racial classification system is not adequate for explaining human variation.

Regardless of what the actual geographic pattern of variation turns out to be, the importance of the environment in expression of phenotypic traits cannot be overstated. There is a complex interplay between **genotype**, **phenotype**, and environment, which will never be fully teased apart. Remember that the environment consists of sociocultural and physical aspects to which an individual is exposed, beginning *in utero* and including but not limited to postnatal factors such as nutrition, diet, exposure to pathogens, climate, education, and physical and psychosocial stress. The environment essentially influences which traits will be beneficial, harmful, and neutral, factors that change as the environment changes.

Cartmill (1999) contends that culture also plays a strong role in how genes and the environment interact. The reader is encouraged to refer to that paper for an excellent discussion on the interplay between environment and heredity. Lieberman and Kirk (2004:137) further emphasize that one of the reasons the race concept has been rejected is due to the realization that cultures are "a dynamic expression of their history and ecology" *à la* Boas. Research that examines human variation must account for environmental factors and acknowledge that it is likely that not all of the different aspects of the environment's influence on trait expression will be uncovered.

Therefore, to restate the overall research problems currently under investigation: (1) What is the true nature of human **population history** that has led to the range of existing variation? (2) How can geographic patterns explain human variation? (3) How does geography and evolutionary forces contribute to the patterning of phenotypic and genotypic variation?

Many avenues are being used to address the numerous questions inherent to these problems, including from the field of **DNA** and from a **biological distance** perspective. Refer to

---

[17]See Cabana et al. (Chapter 16), this volume for further definition and discussion of evolutionary forces.

Cabana and colleagues (Chapter 16), this volume, for a discussion on what DNA analysis has revealed about human variation. Biological distance can be defined as how closely related or, alternatively, divergent populations are from one another. Given that one of the assumptions with biodistance analysis is that changes in allele frequencies due to evolutionary forces such as genetic drift and gene flow affect changes in phenotypic traits, including skeletal features (Stojanowski and Schillaci, 2006), studies of biological distance are relevant for the ancestry problem. Several workers have addressed the problem of human variation (especially within bioarchaeological studies) using biological distance models, with perhaps the work of Relethford and Blangero, and Konigsberg and colleagues being the most central (e.g., Relethford and Lees, 1982; Relethford and Blangero, 1990; Relethford, 1991; Konigsberg, 1990, 2000; Konigsberg et al., 1993; Konigsberg and Ousley, 1995). Refer to Konigsberg (2006) for a review and see McKeown and Schmidt (Chapter 12), this volume for more information on biodistance.

ANCESTRY AND FORENSIC ANTHROPOLOGY

Ancestry is the third component of the biological profile, after age-at-death and sex estimations. In any society with a diverse population like the United States, part of the recovery of decomposed, damaged, and/or skeletonized human remains from a medicolegal purview (e.g., from clandestine disposal to mass disaster) will often include questions by law enforcement regarding the race, or ancestry, of the victim.

When the skull (and more importantly the facial skeleton) is complete, the likelihood of estimating ancestry accurately is assumed to be high. We state this with a caveat however, as correct ancestry estimation depends on (1) the availability of an appropriate reference sample (discussed below), and (2) the analyst's ability and experience with the measurement techniques and his or her ability to correctly understand and visually assess the cranial nonmetric features associated with various ancestral groups.

However, as Sauer (1992:107) questioned, "If races don't exist, why are forensic anthropologists so good at identifying them?" The answer to this question lies in the fact that concordance exists between social race categories (i.e., Black, White) and cranial morphology (Ousley et al., 2009). Evolutionary forces (e.g., gene flow, genetic drift) have led to a discordance of skeletal traits (and other phenotypic traits) between populations enabling us to measure and analyze that data. This leads to ancestry estimations based on our knowledge of trait frequency in each major population group — e.g., variation in cranial morphology is structured by geography (Kennedy, 1995; Relethford, 2009). Sauer (1992) and Konigsberg et al. (2009) further reason that we must use the same terminology for ancestry categories used by the medicolegal community in order to make a contribution to the identification of remains.

There are two generally accepted methods of ancestry estimation in forensic anthropology: (1) metric analysis of cranial and postcranial measurements, and (2) nonmetric (morphoscopic) traits of the cranium. There are advantages and disadvantages to each of these approaches (outlined below). Prior to an in-depth look at each, a general comparison of the statistical treatment for each is warranted.

STATISTICAL APPROACHES

Metric traits are measured on a **continuous** scale (e.g., maximum cranial breadth can be, at least theoretically, any value between 0 and ∞) whereas **morphoscopic** traits are measured **categorically**. The statistical treatment of continuous data has several advantages over categorical data, which is assigned a value that is in one of several possible categories. Categorical variables do not always have a numerical meaning. In other words, variables like skin color (light, dark) and nasal aperture width (narrow, intermediate, wide) do not necessarily have an explicit numerical equivalent. Because of this feature, categorical data are not appropriately treated with the same statistical methods as their continuous (i.e., metric, numerical) counterparts. The statistical methods used to evaluate continuous data (see examples below) are more widely used and are generally better understood than those used for categorical methods. Therefore, we will briefly outline the methods used to treat continuous variables and spend the majority of our discussion on the treatment of categorical data. As stated, this is a brief overview and several statistical concepts will be introduced in the upcoming section. A certain knowledge of statistics is assumed—if any of these concepts are unfamiliar, we recommend taking graduate level statistics courses to catch up.

Metric Methods

Analyzing craniometric (and more recently postcranial metric) data to assess ancestry has a long history in anthropology. To analyze craniometric data, the first and therefore most important step is the proper collection of craniometric data. In the past, such data were collected using sliding and spreading calipers, craniofor, and mandibulometers, among other tools. However, a large number of laboratories are switching to three-dimensional digitizers for data collection (e.g., see McKeown and Schmidt [Chapter 12], this volume). No matter the method of data acquisition, the theoretical underpinnings are the same: the collection of landmark data and interlandmark distances for use in data analysis. The landmarks used by forensic anthropologists are rooted in the earlier work of several prominent (though often infamous) physical anthropologists—recall Morton's early craniometric data collection. However, Martin (1914) and Howells (1973, 1989, 1995) are considered the "gold standards" for landmark descriptions, illustrations, and definitions and should be consulted regularly by both inexperienced and experienced anthropologists. Of course, reading the literature and landmark definitions is no substitute for mentoring. Find an experienced anthropologist, pester them to no end and watch over their shoulder as they explain the nuances of data collection—it worked for us, it will work for you, as well. The interlandmark distances used in a final analysis (such as FORDISC—discussed below) are outlined in Martin (1914); Howells (1973, 1989, 1995) and Buikstra and Ubelaker (1994).

FORDISC and Discriminant Function Analysis

Once the data have been appropriately collected the next step is finding and using an appropriate known reference sample. In the United States, this is most often the **Forensic Anthropology Databank** (Jantz and Moore-Jansen, 1988) and the computer program

FORDISC 3.0 (FD3) (Jantz and Ousley, 2005). One part of properly utilizing FD3 is appreciating what, exactly, FD3 is doing. Fordisc uses **discriminant function analysis** (DFA) to classify an unknown individual into one of several reference populations and is, by and large, the most widely used classification statistic in forensic anthropology, particularly when the data are continuous.

Giles and Elliot (1962, 1963) first used a DFA on crania to determine sex and race for American White, American Black, and Amerindian[18] crania. Linear discriminant function analysis was developed as a means to classify a target individual (e.g., unknown crania) into one of several reference groups by incorporating a similar mathematical approach to regression analysis (Krzanowski, 2002). Whereas regression analysis uses a weighted combination of predictor variables to calculate some object's value (e.g., stature from measurements of the postcranial skeleton), DFA uses a weighted combination of those predictor variables to classify an unknown object into a reference group based on a distance statistic. The discriminant function score is a derived variable (Krzanowski, 2002), which is equal to the weighted sum of values for each variable.

The most common distance statistic employed in forensic anthropological research and classification is **Mahalanobis distance** (D^2), which is a distance measure similar in practice to Euclidean distance (the "ordinary" distance between two points as one would measure with a ruler), but that is not affected by scale or correlation (Krzanowski, 2002). Unlike Euclidean distance, D^2 is based on the covariance between variables and is used to measure the similarity (as the distance from a group **centroid**[19]) between unknown and known individuals. When interpreting the D^2 value, smaller distances equate to more similar individuals.

The statistical assumptions associated with DFA include *multivariate normality* and *homogeneity of variances/covariances*. Multivariate normality is one of the most common assumptions in statistics, as many tests and statistics are related to the normal distribution (think bell curve here). Generally, testing for multivariate normality is testing for univariate and bivariate normality, that is, testing to see that each variable is normally distributed and, likewise, that all pairs of variables are bivariate normal using one- and two-dimensional plots (i.e., histograms and scatterplots). In practice, this is generally sufficient for testing for multivariate normality, especially when using DFA as that method is relatively robust against deviations from multivariate normality. Other more robust methods to test for multivariate normality exist, but are beyond the scope of this work (cf., Mardia's statistic of multivariate skewness/kurtosis [Mardia, 1970] or the Doornik-Hansen multivariate normality test [Doornik-Hansen, 2008]).

The second assumption involves whether there is homogeneity of variances/covariances (or, testing that the level of variation in each group is relatively similar) and testing for this is also relatively straightforward. There are a variety of tests for homogeneity. In FD3, homogeneity among samples is tested using the Kullback (1959) test for homogeneity. If the level of

---

[18]These were the terms originally used by Giles and Elliot and also are terms used by FORDISC and the Forensic Databank. We will use the same terms when referring to FORDISC in this section to stay consistent with its terminology.

[19]The group centroid is the point that represents the mean for all variables in the multivariate space defined by the variables in the model.

heterogeneity within groups is high the analyst is encouraged to explore other statistical procedures, such as logistic regression (Jantz and Ousley, 2005).

Two additional considerations in DFA are **outliers** and *multicollinearity*. Discriminant function analysis is sensitive to the inclusion of outliers (individuals or measurements falling far outside the collective distribution of all other individuals or measurements). The researcher should carefully consider the data through graphs (plots) and descriptive statistics to identify potential outliers. If outliers are found, the cause for each should be identified, when possible. Remember, transcription errors (e.g., 24 entered as 42), incorrect data entry (entering maximum cranial breadth (XCB) for maximum cranial length (GOL)), and measurements that are just wrong (XCB measured as 145 when it is in fact 120) may lead to outliers. When these types of errors are identified the data should be corrected. If no explanation can be found, the individual may be dropped from the analysis unless there is good reason to suspect he or she is just an expression of the variation seen in that population.

Multicollinearity is the same as trait interdependence (correlation). When two variables are highly correlated (or one is the sum of other dependents) the parameter estimates behave erratically when the model (or the variables) undergoes even minute changes. While this does not affect the overall model, it does affect classifications based on that model. In other words, collinearity also means the standardized discriminant function coefficients cannot reliably assess the relative importance of the predictor variable(s), decreasing the overall strength of the final discriminant function for classification purposes. As with outliers, graphs (two-dimensional plots) of the variables will assist in identifying highly correlated variables.

Two additional statistics that can be obtained from the discriminant function analysis provide further information about the classification. The FORDISC 3.0 help file (Jantz and Ousley, 2005) goes into great detail about posterior and typicality probabilities, but a brief explanation will help the reader better understand some of the analyses described below. **Posterior probability** is the probability that the unknown belongs to any one of the populations selected for in the analysis and is based on the relative distances the unknown has (calculated using Mahalanobis distance, or D^2) to each population. Because it is the probability of belonging to any one of the populations used in the analysis, the posterior probability will always sum to 1. A major assumption (of classification statistics in general) is that the unknown individual truly belongs to one of the reference groups (hence the need for strict guidelines when selecting reference samples), because a DFA will always "force" a classification.

We can use another statistic, **typicality probability**, as a measure of how *likely* it is that the unknown does, in fact, belong to any one of those populations. Typicality probability is based on the absolute distances of the unknown from all groups, rather than the relative distances. Please note that the typicality probability is essentially equivalent to a univariate t-test. In other words, it is a measure of how many other individuals in a population would be expected to be as far or farther from that population's centroid than the unknown individual. As Jantz and Ousley (2005:np) point out "[typicality probabilities] below 0.05 (5%), or certainly 0.01 (1%) for a group … indicate questionable probability of membership in that group or the possibility of measurement error." This means that the typicality probability can essentially be ignored if the value is greater than 0.05, since such values do not indicate a statistically significant difference in the suite of measurements. When the value is less than

0.05, carefully consider the measurements entered and the populations (reference samples) included in the analysis.

Case Study: Using FORDISC

Identifying the appropriate reference sample is one of the more daunting aspects of ancestry assessment using FD3. FD3 has two major samples to which an unknown may be compared. The first is the Forensic Databank (FDB) (Jantz and Moore-Jansen, 1988), which had approximately 3400 cases and growing as of early 2011 (Ousley et al., 2011). The FDB consists of identified individuals from forensic cases originating predominantly from the United States. The second is the Howells database of 2504 individuals from 28 populations around the world compiled by W.W. Howells. When doing an analysis using FORDISC, the user chooses to which groups the unknown cranium should be compared. However, the challenge is in deciding at what point one group or another should be excluded from the comparison. The general consensus is to begin with a broad approach. In FD3, this would include all possible groups in the first analysis, and then, based on those results, removal of populations that are not probable. For example, if your results in the first analysis suggest a male individual, with all values being highest for males regardless of the population, then all females should be removed and the analysis processed again.

For the sake of example, let us assume that in the second analysis the values in Table 5.1 are obtained. Clearly, this individual is not a white male ($D^2 = 28.6$; Post. Prob. $= 0.000$). In fact, it is highly unlikely (improbable) that the cranium in the example above belongs to Hispanic males, Amerindians, or Black males, based on the low posterior and typicality probabilities. Once those groups are removed and the analysis is recalculated, we get the following results in Table 5.2.

Although the classification (Vietnamese male) has not changed, we have narrowed down the potential list of ancestral groups to four populations. Again, we could continue to narrow the populations down to just two groups (as suggested in the FD3 manual). However, for our purposes we can feel confident that this individual is most likely Vietnamese, though not to the exclusion of other reasonable possibilities. Wait a minute! That doesn't seem good enough. If you are like us, you will see that this is not enough information to make a final estimation of ancestry. Even if we reduce the number of variables (Table 5.3 using a stepwise selection — see the FD3 manual for a detailed discussion of this process) we are no closer to a final determination.

In fact, these results further muddy the issue because now the VM and GTM results are nearly identical. This is not an uncommon situation and it clearly demonstrates that a proper understanding of human variation, metric analysis, and nonmetric traits is necessary not only to correctly assess ancestry, but also to correctly interpret FD3 results and properly select reference samples.

So what are we to make of the example case described above? All of the assumptions for discriminant function are met, so the DFA appears to be performing well. Other chapters in this volume describe the importance of context when interpreting results from skeletal analyses. Perhaps the context (i.e., situation in which they were found) of these remains can assist in making our final decision.

This example was taken from the *FORDISC 3.0* help file (Jantz and Ousley, 2005) and is identified therein as Example 2. The measurements are from a University of Tennessee

TABLE 5.1   Multigroup Classification of Example 1 Using FD3

Group	Classified	Distance (D^2)	Post. Prob.	TypF
VM	**VM**	10.2	0.368	0.941
GTM		11	0.242	0.883
CHM		11.2	0.225	0.875
JM		12.7	0.107	0.783
HM		14.3	0.046	0.597
AM		17.5	0.010	0.648
BM		20.2	0.003	0.343
WM		28.6	0.000	0.036

Example 1 is closest to VMs.
VM = Vietnamese Males
GTM = Guatemalan Males
CHM = Chinese Males
JM = Japanese Males
HM = Hispanic Males
AM = Amerindian Males
BM = Black Males
WM = White Males

TABLE 5.2   Reduced Multigroup Classification of Example 1 Using FD3

Group	Classified	Distance (D^2)	Post. Prob.	TypF
VM	**VM**	10.7	0.669	0.927
GTM		13.5	0.164	0.769
CHM		14.5	0.101	0.716
JM		15.4	0.065	0.628

Example 1 is closest to VMs.

TABLE 5.3   Stepwise-Selected, Reduced Multigroup Classification of Example 1 Using FD3

Group	Classified	Distance (D^2)	Post. Prob.	TypF
VM	**VM**	2.4	0.465	0.82
GTM		2.6	0.433	0.791
CHM		6.8	0.051	0.288
JM		6.9	0.051	0.276

Example 1 is closest to VMs, however note that VM and GTM results here are nearly identical.

forensic case that was positively identified as a Laotian male. The reader is encouraged to utilize the help file and the tutorials within to further explore this example.[20] Of course, another approach is nonmetric (morphoscopic) data, which have been used to verify metric analyses or to refute their outcome. In the following section, we explore morphoscopic traits and their use in the assessment of ancestry.

Nonmetric Methods

Nonmetric traits have a long history in anthropology, particularly as they relate to ancestry assessment. However, there are two distinct types of cranial nonmetric traits: **epigenetic variants** and morphoscopic traits. While the focus of this chapter is on the latter, one should understand both types. Traditional cranial nonmetric, or discrete, traits ("epigenetic variants" following Hauser and DeStefano, 1989) are defined following Buikstra and Ubelaker (1994) as *"dichotomous, discontinuous, epigenetic traits*—non-pathological variations of skeletal tissues that can be better classified as present or absent (or as a point on a morphological gradient, e.g. small to large) rather than quantified by a measurement."

There are five major categories of epigenetic variants in the cranium: (1) extrasutural bone (e.g., Inca bone); (2) proliferative ossifications (e.g., pterygo-alar bridging); (3) ossification failure (e.g., septal aperture); (4) suture variation (e.g., metopic suture); and (5) foramina variation (e.g., zygomatico-facial foramen number) (Buikstra and Ubelaker, 1994). As discussed earlier, the roles played by the genome and the environment in the inheritance of cranial nonmetric traits (or any phenotypic traits) are poorly understood. However, these traits are routinely used in biological distance studies as a measure of relatedness within and between populations (i.e., Sjøvold 1977, 1984, 1986) and as a proxy for identifying familial relationships within cemeteries (Pilloud, 2009). In a forensic context, the traits used to assess ancestry are not necessarily the same characters as epigenetic variants, because of the unique history of morphoscopic traits in forensic anthropology (Hefner, 2009).

Morphoscopic Traits

Ousley and Hefner (2005) first used the term "macromorphoscopic" to describe the cranial nonmetric traits used in forensic anthropological research. They considered macromorphoscopic traits to be quasicontinuous variables of the cranium that can be reflected as soft-tissue differences in the living (cf., Brues' [1958]: second class of traits "due to the contour of bone in areas where it closely follows the surface … apparent in both skeleton and living"). Later, Hefner (2009) simplified the term to *morphoscopic* traits but maintained the original characterization of the variables. These traits fall into one of five classes: (1) assessing bone shape (e.g., nasal bone structure); (2) bony feature morphology (e.g., inferior nasal aperture morphology); (3) suture shape (e.g., zygomaticomaxillary suture); (4) presence/absence of data (e.g., post-bregmatic depression); and (5) feature prominence/protrusion (e.g., anterior nasal spine) (Hefner, 2009).

[20]FORDISC 3.0 is available from the Forensic Anthropology Center at the University of Tennessee <http://fac.utk.edu/fordisc.html>; additionally, any forensic anthropology laboratory in the U.S. and Canada will have a copy.

Morphoscopic traits are used to assess the ancestry of a single individual for the purpose of identification. The morphoscopic traits more commonly employed to assess ancestry can be found in Hefner (2009). These traits are drawn predominantly from trait lists found in Rhine (1990) and most introductory forensic anthropology textbooks. For an in-depth discussion on historical aspects of morphoscopic trait analysis not covered herein, see Hefner and colleagues' (2012) discussion of morphoscopic traits and the assessment of ancestry.

When assessing ancestry from an unknown set of skeletal remains we caution against the use of typological trait lists that supposedly typify the skull of an individual derived from a specific ancestral group, *sensu* Rhine (1990). A more methodologically sound approach involves focusing on individual traits (characters) and the *variable expression* of those traits (character states) within and between populations. Remember, no single trait is found exclusively in only one population, as with other phenotypic traits. As one of the authors has demonstrated elsewhere (Hefner et al., 2012), shovel-shaped incisors are often cited as an Asian-specific trait. While shoveling occurs in 70–85% of Asians worldwide (Scott and Turner, 1997) (not 100% as may be believed), the same trait is also found in almost all other populations, though in much lower frequencies (3–10% of Europeans; 8–11% of Africans [Scott and Turner, 1997]).

Nonmetric traits are not discrete or isolated within one population due to multiple factors. In fact, the variation results from very specific evolutionary mechanisms. Mechanisms such as the genetic effects of selective pressures from particular environments, the effects of gene flow between groups, and the random effects of drift and founding (Lahr, 1996) all play a role in the expression of variation within and between groups. Of course, by definition the different levels of gene flow, selection, and drift acting to establish this variation between groups is closely linked to geography (Lahr, 1996), and it is this geographic division that accounts for the high degree of variation observed among humans today.

Therefore, we need to understand the frequency of state expressions and meaningfully combine them into suites of significant traits using appropriate statistical methods. In that way we (anthropologists) can begin to see the necessary patterns of variation that permit valid assessments of ancestry using morphoscopic data. As with the craniometric data described earlier, this requires adequate reference data, standardized protocols for scoring the variables, and appropriate statistics for categorical data analysis.

To that end, Hefner (2003, 2007, 2009) collected data on the expression of a large number of morphoscopic traits from multiple skeletal populations and provided a series of simple, direct illustrations of each character state. The complete list of traits (characters and character states) and populations are fully described elsewhere (Hefner, 2009). By collecting such data, Hefner documented intergroup variation without making assumptions about so-called racial groups, and developed empirically supported methods for assessing ancestry.

How can these variables be combined to assess ancestry? The answer is via classification statistics appropriate for categorical data. A number of statistical approaches have proven useful to analyze morphoscopic data. Two of these are summarized below, and others (*k-nearest neighbor, canonical analysis of principal coordinates,* and *discriminant function analysis*) are discussed in Hefner et al. (2012) and Hefner (2013). Two additional methods are outlined below to give the reader a sense of the many ways this type of data can be used during forensic anthropological analysis.

Ordinal Regression

Ordinal regression analysis (ORA) measures the association of an ordinal response variable (a categorical variable with ordering—i.e., small, medium, large) to a set of predictor variables (a variable used to predict the value of another variable). In traditional linear regression, the sum-of-squared differences between a continuous dependent variable and the weighted combination of the independent variables are minimized prior to calculating regression coefficients. This is not the case when the dependent variable is ordinal. Ordinal regression calculates coefficients based on the assumption that the response variable is a categorical response with some underlying continuous distribution. In most cases, there is a valid theoretical basis for assuming this underlying distribution. However, even when this assumption is not met, the model can still theoretically produce valid results.

Rather than predicting the actual cumulative probabilities, an ORA predicts a function of those values using a process known as a link function. Simplistically, the link function links the model specified in the design matrix to the real parameters of the dataset. After initial model development, the predicted probability of each response category can be used to assign an unknown individual to a group. An ORA can be expressed as

$$\text{link}\,(\gamma_{ij}) = \theta_j - [\beta_1 \chi_{i1} + \beta_2 \chi_{i2} + \beta_p \chi_{ij}] \tag{5.1}$$

where link( ) is the link function for the current analysis, γ_{ij} is the cumulative probability of the jth category for the ith case, θ_j is the threshold for the jth category, p is the number of regression coefficients, $\chi_{i1} \ldots \chi_{ip}$ are the values of the predictors for the ith case, and $\beta_1 \ldots \beta_p$ are the regression coefficients. One of the benefits of ORA, and a similarity of ORA to analysis of variance (ANOVA), is the ability to assess the significance of individual response variables and to test for any interaction between all response variables. For example, ORAs allow one to determine if sex, ancestry, or the interaction of sex and ancestry significantly affect the expression of inferior nasal aperture morphology.

Ordinal regression analysis can be carried out using the PLUM function in SPSS®. The purpose of the ORA in ancestry research is twofold. First, as mentioned above, the ORA can be used to determine the significance of sex and ancestry, and the interaction of the two, on the expression of each morphoscopic trait. Significance is assessed at the $\alpha = 0.05$ level using the Wald statistic, a measure similar to the F-value in a traditional ANOVA. Each of these parameter estimates is then assessed for significance. As an example, the ORA parameter estimates for interorbital breadth are presented in Table 5.4. Once all significant traits are determined, we can apply the ORA with all significant traits set as the

TABLE 5.4 Parameter Estimates and Significance Levels for Interorbital Breadth

Ind. Variable	Estimate	Std. Error	Wald	df	Sig.
Ancestry	2.492	0.340	53.723	1	0.000
Sex	−1.113	1.250	0.792	1	0.373
Ancestry*Sex	0.929	1.299	0.512	1	0.420

TABLE 5.5 Classification Matrix for the ORA Two-Group Analysis

	Black	White	Total	% Correct
Black	203	15	218	93.12
White	22	124	146	84.93
Total	225	139	364	89.03

$\chi^2 = 190.709$; $p < 0.000$

TABLE 5.6 Classification Matrix for the ORA Three-Group Analysis

	Amerindian	Black	White	Total	% Correct
Amerindian	206	46	10	262	78.63
Black	59	130	29	218	59.63
White	10	33	103	146	70.55
Total	275	209	142	626	69.60

$\chi^2 = 287.765$; $p < 0.000$

predictor variables to assess ancestry for the entire sample. As Table 5.5 shows, the ORA works well, separating a sample of American Blacks and Whites (data collected by JTH) in a two-way analysis correctly nearly 90% of the time. Table 5.5 also presents the classification matrix for the two-group analysis.

Multiway ORAs are not as successful. In a three-way analysis the ORA correctly classified approximately 70% of the sample of American Whites, American Blacks, and Amerindians (Table 5.6). As more groups are added to the model the classification rate is drastically reduced. This may be because ORAs are somewhat sensitive to sample size. Yet the method is promising and merits further scrutiny and research.

Logistic Regression

Logistic regression (LR) is a statistical method similar to linear regression since LR finds an equation that predicts an outcome for a binary variable, Y, from one or more response variables, X. However, unlike linear regression the response variables can be categorical *or* continuous, as the model does not strictly require continuous data. To predict group membership, LR uses the log odds ratio rather than probabilities and an iterative **maximum likelihood** method rather than a least squares to fit the final model. This means the researcher has more freedom when using LR and the method may be more appropriate for nonnormally distributed data or when the samples have unequal covariance matrices. Logistic regression assumes independence among variables, which is not always met in morphoscopic datasets. However, as is often the case, the applicability of the method (and how well it works, e.g., the classification error) often trumps statistical assumptions. One drawback of LR is that the method cannot produce typicality probabilities (useful for forensic casework), but these values may be substituted with **nonparametric methods** such as ranked probabilities and ranked interindividual similarity measures (Ousley and Hefner, 2005).

TABLE 5.7   Likelihood Ratio Tests for the Two-Way Logistic Regression

Effect	Model Fitting Criteria	Likelihood Ratio Tests		
	−2 Log Likelihood of Reduced Model	Chi-Square	df	Sig.
Intercept	183.2665	0	0	—
INA	238.2002	54.9337	5	0.00000
IOB	207.4619	24.1953	2	0.00001
NAW	193.9302	10.6637	2	0.00484
NBS	199.0345	15.7680	4	0.00335
PBD	191.4299	8.1634	2	0.01688

INA = inferior nasal aperture
IOB = interorbital breadth
NAW = nasal aperture width
NBS = nasal bone structure
PBD = post-bregmatic depression

TABLE 5.8   Classification Matrix for Two-Way Logistic Regression

	Black	White	% Correct
Black	200	17	92.17
White	19	117	86.03
Total			89.80

Logistic regression analysis can also be carried out in SPSS® using the NOMREG procedure. We suggest a forward stepwise selection procedure. When we ran that analysis on a sample of data collected by JTH (2009) the LR stepwise selected five variables: (1) inferior nasal aperture, (2) interorbital breadth, (3) nasal aperture width, (4) nasal bone structure, and (5) post-bregmatic depression. The likelihood ratio test (Table 5.7) is significant and demonstrates that the reduced model is equivalent to the final LR model. The Cox and Snell pseudo R-squared statistics (not shown) (0.553) imply that approximately 56% of the variation in morphoscopic trait expression is explained by ancestry. This LR model is accurate for nearly 90% of the individuals in the sample (Table 5.8).

Each of these presented methods has advantages and disadvantages and each is suited to a particular task. We present these two statistics not to suggest they are the best or most appropriate methods but to demonstrate the flexibility of statistical methods to handle categorical data and to encourage the reader to explore these and other statistics for use in their own projects.

CASE STUDY: ASSESSING ANCESTRY FOR AN UNKNOWN

In statistical models morphoscopic traits perform as well as a metric analysis (Hefner 2007, 2009). The following section guides the reader through a typical analysis of morphoscopic traits, and presents reporting strategies to use following data analysis.

The first phase of morphoscopic trait analysis is the selection of the character states that best match the configuration exhibited by the unknown specimen (see example below). This is completed for each observable trait. Following this stage, appropriate classification statistics (e.g., ordinal regression, logistic regression, canonical analysis of principal coordinates (CAP), k-nearest neighbor (k-nn), discriminant function analysis) and suitable reference populations are selected. Once the statistical analysis has placed the unknown specimen into a population, the probability of group membership for the unknown specimen, and the overall error rate (misclassification rate or classification accuracy) of the model are reported along with the assigned group membership. This approach is likely familiar, as it is the same reporting strategy used in metric analyses.

The computer program *Macromorphoscopics*, designed specifically for the collection of morphoscopic trait data, is available from Hefner and Ousley (2005) and is also incorporated in the computer program **Osteoware** that is available at no charge from the Smithsonian Institution (https://osteoware.si.edu/). These programs facilitate data management and also standardize trait descriptions. To put the entire process in perspective the following example cranium is presented (Figure 5.1).

The morphoscopic traits for this cranium were scored following Hefner's (2009) illustrations and definitions. The following trait scores are noted: (1) the anterior nasal spine is well-developed and markedly protrudes from the face (ANS = 3); (2) the inferior nasal aperture is consistent with the straight morphology (INA = 3); (3) interorbital breadth is intermediate (INA = 2); (4) nasal aperture width is intermediate (NAW = 2); (5) the nasal bones exhibit steep lateral walls, with an accompanying broad surface plateau (NBC = 2); (6) nasal overgrowth is pronounced (NO = 1); and (7) no post-bregmatic depression is observed (PBD = 0). These visual observations alone are enough for the experienced forensic anthropologist to make an educated guess of ancestry.

However, recall that stopping at this point is unempirical and therefore not scientific. We must go a step further and apply a statistic to assess the overall classification. In this example, originally conducted for a medical examiner's office, I (JTH) used a novel classification

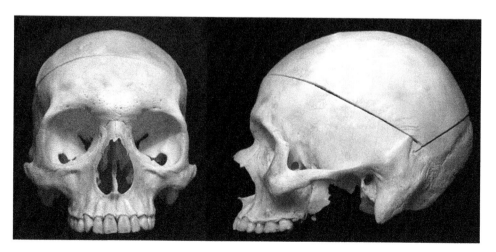

FIGURE 5.1   Cranium for case study: assessing ancestry for an unknown.

statistic soon to be published: an artificial neural network (aNN). The algorithm (and a graphical user interface) will be available in early 2013. Using the aNN, which contains data on over 1100 individuals collected by JTH (American Black, American White, Hispanic, East Asian, etc.), the cranium described above was correctly placed in the Hispanic category. This cranium, which originated along the U.S.—Mexico border, was later identified as a male from the northern Mexico state of Sonora who perished while crossing the border. Discussion of the problems inherent with the use of the category "Hispanic" is necessary here. See Box 5.1.

BOX 5.1

HISPANIC: WHAT'S IN A NAME?

The most recent census in the United States (2010) revealed that the group designated as Hispanic was the fastest growing minority group, with an increase in 15.2 million people over the last census in 2000. This has resulted in a total Hispanic population of 50.5 million, 16% of the total U.S. population (Humes et al., 2011). The census does not define "Hispanic" as a "race," considering that it is a separate concept from race. Therefore, individuals were able to self-report Hispanic origin and racial origin. Of those who identified as Hispanic, over half self-reported White as their race. About one third reported being in the category "some other race" alone while the rest reported being in other racial categories alone (e.g., Black, Asian (Humes et al., 2011).

These facts are telling of the problems inherent with ancestry estimation using a category designator such as "Hispanic." The fact that the Hispanic population has rapidly grown makes this an issue of importance for forensic anthropologists in the United States who must estimate the biological profile, as Spradley and colleagues (2008) have noted. The undocumented border crosser deaths issue in the

Southwestern United States has additionally highlighted the importance of this subject (Anderson, 2008; Anderson and Parks, 2008; Fulginiti, 2008; Birkby et al., 2008). Further, as several workers have discussed, "Hispanic" is a linguistic category, applied to individuals who speak Spanish as their native language (Slice and Ross, 2004; Ross et al., 2004; Spradley et al., 2008; Birkby et al., 2008; Hurst, 2012). The language being spoken has nothing to do with actual features measured from bones that may indicate ancestry; however, we persist in utilizing this category.

The 2010 U.S. Census defined Hispanic or Latino as "a person of Cuban, Mexican, Puerto Rican, South or Central American, or other Spanish culture or origin regardless of race" (Humes et al., 2011:2). The problem here is twofold: (1) we are using Hispanic as a racial category for forensic identification even in the face of evidence from sources such as the census data that individuals considering themselves to be Hispanic *also* consider themselves to be some other race; and (2) persons speaking Spanish as their native language (excluding Spain) originate from two continents and numerous countries, which include hundreds of millions of

(Continued)

BOX 5.1   *(cont'd)*

people. The existing diversity is therefore intrinsic. To illustrate this further, both Spradley and coworkers (2008) and Hurst (2012) have demonstrated that variability (in terms of skeletal features) in the Hispanic group is higher than was once thought.

Workers such as Ross et al. (2004) and Spradley et al. (2008) have noted the complexity of **population history** in Latin America leading to phenotypic heterogeneity. Each country in Latin America has its own particular history that in general began with indigenous groups, later conquest by Europeans, in several cases, importation of enslaved Africans, and later immigration of people from Europe and/or Asia. The extent to which these three latter events and their consequences (i.e., war, disease) affected each country's population history varies. Consequently, the majority of people in Latin America who speak Spanish as their native language do so as a result of European conquest but may ancestrally be European, African, indigenous, or a mixture of the three.

Therefore, Spradley et al. (2008) and Ross et al. (2004) both emphasized the need for population-specific standards with the latter authors especially stressing the necessity of regional studies to build metric and nonmetric trait information for Hispanics. As a brief example of such an attempt, López and colleagues (2012) recently presented results from a preliminary study in Colombia

to assess ancestry. As with many other South American countries, Colombia has a heterogeneous population as a result of European conquest, importation of enslaved Africans, and the resultant mating with the indigenous people. As ancestry has never been systematically studied in Colombia, López et al. (2012) used two modern samples of skeletons from different parts of the country (Bogotá and Medellín) to look at heterogeneity. Using craniometric interlandmark distances, biological distance plots revealed that the grouped Colombian data (Bogotá and Medellín) fell closest to the Hispanic group and far from the Guatemalan group from the Forensic Databank (FDB). However, when the Bogotá and Medellín samples were separated, Medellín fell closest to the FDB European-American group with Bogotá remaining close to the FDB Hispanics (López et al., 2012). This only begins to illustrate the heterogeneity within one country alone and underscores the need for more work in this area.

As the Hispanic population continues to grow in the United States, we predict that this issue will increasingly become a hot topic for research in forensic anthropology. We strongly suggest that students contemplating an ancestry project consider research on Hispanic populations and in particular travel to Latin American countries for data collection and analysis on modern samples.

FINAL THOUGHTS: THE FUTURE OF RESEARCH IN ANCESTRY ESTIMATION AND HUMAN VARIATION

To conclude, it seems that we have barely revealed the tip of the iceberg when it comes to the old race concept, modern thought on human variation, and ancestry estimation. There is much more to be explored. Allow the references herein to be points of departure.

There are numerous possibilities for research in this area. Biological distance studies have the potential to reveal more about the evolutionary forces and therefore unique population histories that have characterized *Homo sapiens* as a whole, both in the past and in the present. Increased and improved use of classification and exploratory statistics play a role in how we identify patterns of human variation and how we can use that variation to identify skeletonized remains. As Spradley and colleagues (2008:21) assert, "The formulae used by forensic anthropologists are only as good as the data that are used to derive them." Therefore, improving our datasets with craniometric and nonmetric data from modern populations all over the world will ultimately enhance our ability to estimate ancestry in addition to increasing our understanding of human variation.

Moreover, do not neglect to consider research regarding how race is culturally constructed (Gravlee, 2009) or how the race concept has affected individuals socially and biologically (Armelagos and Goodman, 1998; Harrison, 1995, 1999). Look to collaborate with anthropologists in other subdisciplines (Mukhopadhyay and Moses, 1997), as the sociocultural aspect of race is just as important as applying ancestry estimation to skeletons. We are holistic anthropologists first, united by the Culture concept with the other subdisciplines in anthropology. Remember, gone are the days of typology and biological determinism. Today, anthropologists must document human variation, its social consequences, and understand the global patterns of variation as they actually exist.

ACKNOWLEDGMENTS

We are grateful to Dr. Natalie Shirley, whose thoughtful comments and suggestions on a draft of this chapter improved its contents. We would also like to thank Dr. Bruce Anderson for providing and granting permission for the use of the cranium photographs in the case study. Thanks are further due to Dr. Jonathan Bethard for providing the results from the López and colleagues (2012) presentation.

REFERENCES

Algee-Hewitt, B.F.B., 2011. If and How Many 'Races'? The Application of Mixture Modeling to World-Wide Human Craniometric Variation. Unpublished PhD dissertation. The University of Tennessee, Knoxville, TN.

Anderson, B.E., 2008. Identifying the dead: Methods utilized by the Pima County (Arizona) Office of the Medical Examiner for undocumented border crossers: 2001–2006. Journal of Forensic Sciences 53 (1), 8–15.

Anderson, B.E., Parks, B.O., 2008. Symposium on border crosser deaths: introduction. Journal of Forensic Sciences 53 (1), 6–7.

Armelagos, G.L., Goodman, A.H., 1998. Race, racism, and anthropology. In: Goodman, A.H., Leatherman, T.L. (Eds.), Building a New Biocultural Synthesis. University of Michigan Press, Ann Arbor, pp. 359–377.

Birkby, W.H., Fenton, T.W., Anderson, B.E., 2008. Identifying southwest Hispanics using nonmetric traits and the cultural profile. Journal of Forensic Sciences 53 (1), 29–33.

Blakey, M.L., 1987. Skull doctors: intrinsic social and political bias in the history of American physical anthropology with special reference to the work of Ales Hrdlicka. Critique of Anthropology 7 (2), 7–35.

Blakey, M.L., 1999. Scientific racism and the biological concept of race. Literature and Psychology 45 (1/2), 29–43.

Boas, F., 1910. Changes in Bodily Form of Descendants of Immigrants. US Immigration Commission, Washington, DC. Senate Document No. 208, 61st Congress. US Government Printing Office.

Boas, F., 1918a. Review of The Passing of the Great Race; or The Racial Basis for European History by Madison Grant. American Journal of Physical Anthropology 1 (3), 363.

Boas, F., 1918b. Notes on the anthropology of Sweden. American Journal of Physical Anthropology 1, 415–426.

Bozeman, J., 1997. Technological Millenarianism in the United States. In: Robbins, T. (Ed.), Millenium, Messiahs, and Mayhem: Contemporary Apocalyptic Movements. Routledge, New York.

Brace, C.L., 1982. The roots of the race concept in American physical anthropology. In: Spencer, F. (Ed.), A History of American Physical Anthropology, 1930–1980. Academic Press, New York.

Brace, C.L., 2005. Race Is a Four Letter Word: The Genesis of the Concept. Oxford University Press, Oxford.

Brues, A.M., 1958. Identification of skeletal remains. Journal of Criminal Law, Criminology, and Police Science 48 (5), 551–563.

Brues, A.M., 1990. The once and future diagnosis of race. In: Gill, G.W., Rhine, S.J. (Eds.), Skeletal Attribution of Race. Maxwell Museum of Anthropology, Albuquerque, New Mexico, Anthropological Papers No. 4, pp. 1–8.

Buikstra, J.E., Ubelaker, D.H., 1994. Standards for Data Collection from Human Skeletal Remains. Arkansas Archeological Survey, Fayetteville, AR.

Cabana, G.S., Hulsey, B.I., Pack, F., 2013. Molecular methods. In: DiGangi, E.A., Moore, M.K. (Eds.), Research Methods in Human Skeletal Biology. Academic Press, San Diego.

Cartmill, M., 1999. The status of the race concept in physical anthropology. American Anthropologist 100 (3), 651–660.

Caspari, R., 2003. From types to populations: a century of race, physical anthropology, and the American Anthropological Association. American Anthropologist 105 (1), 65–76.

Caspari, R., 2009. 1918: Three perspectives in race and human variation. American Journal of Physical Anthropology 139, 5–15.

Comas, J., 1961. Scientific racism again? American Anthropologist 2 (4), 303–340.

Darwin, C., 1859. On the Origin of Species by Means of Natural Selection. John Murray, London.

Darwin, C., 1871. The Descent of Man, and Selection in Relation to Sex. John Murray, London.

Davenport, C., 1911. Heredity in Relation to Eugenics. H Holt & Company, New York.

Diamond, J., 1999. Guns, Germs, and Steel: The Fates of Human Societies. W.W. Norton & Co. New York.

Doornik, J.A., Hansen, H., 2008. An omnibus test for univariate and multivariate normality. Oxford Bulletin of Economics and Statistics 70, 927–939.

Edgar, H.J.H., Hunley, K.L., 2009. Race reconciled? How biological anthropologists view human variation. American Journal of Physical Anthropology 139, 1–4.

Erickson, P.A., 2008. Franz Boas. In: Moore, J. (Ed.), Encyclopedia of Race and Racism. Macmillan Reference USA, Detroit.

Fulginiti, L.C., 2008. Fatal footsteps: murder of undocumented border crossers in Maricopa County, Arizona. Journal of Forensic Sciences 53 (1), 41–45.

Galton, F., 1892. Hereditary Genius: An inquiry into its Laws and Consequences, 2nd ed. Macmillan, London.

Giles, E., 1997. Earnest Albert Hooton. In: Spencer, F. (Ed.), History of Physical Anthropology, Vol. I. Garland, New York, pp. 499–500.

Giles, E., Elliot, O., 1962. Race identification from cranial measurements. Journal of Forensic Sciences 7, 147–157.

Giles, E., Elliot, O., 1963. Sex determination by discriminant function analysis of crania. American Journal of Physical Anthropology 21, 53–68.

Goodman, A.H., 2000. Why genes don't count (for racial differences in health). American Journal of Public Health 90 (11), 1699–1702.

Gould, S.J., 1978. Morton's ranking of races by cranial capacity. Science 200, 503–509.

Gould, S.J., 1981. The Mismeasure of Man. W.W. Norton & Company, New York.

Gould, S.J., 1996. The Mismeasure of Man, Revised Edition. W.W. Norton & Company, New York.

Grant, M., 1916. The Passing of the Great Race. Scribner, New York.

Graves, J.L., 2001. The Emperor's New Clothes: Biological Theories of Race at the Millennium. Rutgers University Press, New Brunswick, New Jersey.

Gravlee, C.C., 2003. Boas's changes in bodily form: the immigrant study, cranial plasticity, and Boas's physical anthropology. American Anthropologist 105 (2), 326–332.

Gravlee, C.C., 2009. How race becomes biology: embodiment of social inequality. American Journal of Physical Anthropology 139, 47–57.

Haeckel, E., 1905. The Wonders of Life: A Popular Study of Biological Philosophy. Harper and Brothers Publishers, New York.

Hauser, G., De Stefano, G.F., 1989. Epigenetic Variants of the Human Skull. Schweizerbart, Stuttgart.

Harrison, F.V., 1995. The persistent power of race in the cultural and political economy of racism. Annual Review of Anthropology 24, 47–74.

Harrison, F.V., 1999. Introduction: Expanding the discourse on race. American Anthropologist 100 (3), 609–631.

Hefner, J.T., 2003. Assessing Nonmetric Cranial Traits Currently used in the Forensic Determination of Ancestry. Unpublished Master's thesis. The University of Florida, Gainesville, FL.

Hefner, J.T., 2007. The Statistical Determination of Ancestry Using Cranial Nonmetric Traits. Unpublished PhD dissertation, Department of Anthropology, The University of Florida, Gainesville, FL.

Hefner, J.T., 2009. Cranial nonmetric variation and estimating ancestry. Journal of Forensic Sciences 54 (5), 985–995.

Hefner, J.T., 2013. Cranial morphoscopic traits and the assessment of American Black, American White, and Hispanic. In: Berg, G.E., Ta'ala, S.C. (Eds.), Biological Affinity in Forensic Identification of Human Skeletal Remains: Beyond Black and White. Taylor and Francis, New York.

Hefner, J.T., Ousley, S.D., 2005. Macromorphoscopics [computer program]. Beta version. Hefner and Ousley, Kaneohe, HI.

Hefner, J.T., Ousley, S.D., Dirkmaat, D.C., 2012. Morphoscopic traits and the assessment of ancestry. In: Dirkmaat, D. (Ed.), A Companion to Forensic Anthropology. Wiley-Blackwell Hoboken, N.J., pp. 287–310.

Herrnstein, R., Murray, C., 1994. The Bell Curve. Free Press, New York.

Hiernaux, J., 1964. Concept of race and taxonomy of mankind. In: Montagu, A. (Ed.), The Concept of Race. The Free Press of Glencoe, Collier-Macmillan, London.

Hooton, E.A., 1918. On certain Eskimoid characters in Icelandic skulls. American Journal of Physical Anthropology 1, 53–76.

Hooton, E.A., 1939. Crime and the Man. Greenwood Press, New York.

Howells, W.W., 1973. Cranial variation in man: a study by multivariate analysis of patterns of difference among recent human populations. In: The Museum, Vol. 67. Papers of the Peabody Museum of Archaeology and Ethnology, Harvard University, Cambridge, MA.

Howells, W.W., 1989. Skull shapes and the map: Craniometric analyses in the dispersion of modern Homo. In: The Museum, Vol. 79. Papers of the Peabody Museum of Archaeology and Ethnology, Harvard University, Cambridge, MA.

Howells, W.W., 1995. Who's who in skulls: ethnic identification of crania from measurements. In: The Museum, Vol. 82. Papers of the Peabody Museum of Archaeology and Ethnology, Harvard University, Cambridge, MA.

Humes, K.R., Jones, N.A., Ramirez, R.R., 2011. Overview of Race and Hispanic Origin: 2010. US Department of Commerce, Economics and Statistics Administration, US Census Bureau.

Hunley, K.L., Healy, M.E., Long, J.C., 2009. The global pattern of gene identity variation reveals a history of long-range migrations, bottlenecks, and local mate exchange: implications for biological race. American Journal of Physical Anthropology 139, 35–46.

Hurst, C.V., 2012. Morphoscopic trait expressions used to identify southwest hispanics. Journal of Forensic Sciences 57 (4) 859–865.

Instituto Brasileiro de Geografia e Estatistica (2010). <http://www.censo2010.ibge.gov.br/resultados_do_censo2010.php>

Jacobson, M.F., 1998. Whiteness of a Different Color: European Immigrants and the Alchemy of Race. Harvard University Press, Cambridge.

Jantz, R.L., 2001. Cranial change in Americans. Journal of Forensic Sciences 46 (4), 784–787.

Jantz, L.M., Jantz, R.L., 1999. Secular changes in long bone length and proportion in the United States, 1800–1970. American Journal of Physical Anthropology 110, 57–67.

Jantz, R.L., Jantz, L.M., 2000. Secular change in craniofacial morphology. American Journal of Human Biology 12 (3), 327–338.

Jantz, R.L., Logan, M.H., 2010. Why does head form change in children of immigrants? A Reappraisal. American Journal of Human Biology 22, 702–707.

Jantz, R.L., Moore-Jansen, P., 1988. A Database for Forensic Anthropology: Structure, Content, and Analysis. Department of Anthropology, University of Tennessee. Report of Investigations No. 47.

Jantz, R.L., Ousley, S., 2005. FORDISC 3: Computerized Forensic Discriminant Functions. The University of Tennessee, Knoxville, TN.

Kaszycka, K.A., Strkalj, G., Strzalko, J., 2009. Current views of European anthropologists on race: Influence of educational and ideological background. American Anthropologist 111 (1), 43–56.

Kennedy, K.A.R., 1995. But professor, why teach race identification if races don't exist? Journal of Forensic Sciences 40 (5), 797–800.

Konigsberg, L.W., 1990. Analysis of prehistoric biological variation under a model of isolation by geographic and temporal distance. Human Biology 62, 49–70.

Konigsberg, L.W., 2000. Quantitative variation and genetics. In: Stinson, S., Bogin, B., Huss-Ashmore, R., O'Rourke, D. (Eds.), Human Biology: An Evolutionary and Biocultural Perspective. Wiley-Liss, Hoboken, NJ, pp. 135–162.

Konigsberg, L.W., 2006. A post-neumann history of biological and genetic distance studies in bioarchaeology. In: Buikstra, J.E., Beck, L.A. (Eds.), Bioarchaeology: The Contextual Analysis of Human Remains. Academic Press, San Diego, pp. 263–279.

Konigsberg, L.W., Ousley, S.D., 1995. Multivariate quantitative genetics of anthropomorphic traits from the Boas data. Human Biology 67, 481–498.

Konigsberg, L.W., Cheverud, J., Kohn, L.A.P., 1993. Cranial deformation and nonmetric trait variation. American Journal of Physical Anthropology 90, 35–48.

Konigsberg, L.W., Algee-Hewitt, B.F.B., Steadman, D.W., 2009. Estimation and evidence in forensic anthropology: sex and race. American Journal of Physical Anthropology 139, 77–90.

Krzanowski, W.J., 2002. Principles of Multivariate Analysis: A User's Perspective. Oxford University Press, London.

Kullback, S., 1959. Information Theory and Statistics. Wiley, New York.

Kuzawa, C.W., 2008. The developmental origins of adult health: Intergenerational inertia in adaptation and disease. In: Trevathan, W.R., McKenna, J.J. (Eds.), Evolutionary Medicine and Health: New Perspectives. Oxford University Press, New York.

Lahr, M.M., 1996. The Evolution of Modern Human Diversity: A Study of Cranial Variation. Cambridge University Press, Cambridge.

Larson, E., 1996. Sex, Race, and Science: Eugenics in the Deep South. Johns Hopkins University Press, Baltimore.

Lewis, J.E., DeGusta, D., Meyer, M.R., Monge, J.M., Mann, A.E., et al., 2011. The mismeasure of science: Stephen Jay Gould versus Samuel George Morton on skulls and bias. PLoS Biology 9 (6). http://dx.doi.org/10.1371/journal.pbio.1001071, e1001071.

Lewontin, R.C., 1972. The apportionment of human diversity. Evolutionary Biology 6, 381–398.

Lieberman, L., 2008. Clines and continuous variation. In: Moore, J. (Ed.), Encyclopedia of Race and Racism. Macmillan Reference USA, Detroit, pp. 341–346.

Lieberman, L., Kirk, R.C., 2004. What should we teach about the concept of race? Anthropology & Education Quarterly 35 (1), 137–145.

Linnaeus, C., 1758. Systema Naturae. 10th revised edition of 1758 [1956]. Laurentii Salvii, Stockholm.

Littlefield, A., Lieberman, L., Reynolds, L.T., 1982. Redefining race: the potential demise of a concept in physical anthropology. Current Anthropology 23 (6), 641–655.

Livingstone, F.B., 1962. On the non-existence of human races. Current Anthropology 3 (3), 279–281.

Long, J.C., Li, J., Healy, M.E., 2009. Human DNA sequences: More variation and less race. American Journal of Physical Anthropology 139, 23–34.

López, M.A., Casallas, D.A., Castellanos, D., Soto, F.V., Bethard, J.D., 2012. Unveiling ancestry in Colombia through morphometric analysis. Proceedings of the American Academy of Forensic Sciences 18, 418.

Lovejoy, A.O., 1936. The Great Chain of Being. Harvard University Press, Cambridge.

Lund, J., 1994. Boundaries of Restriction: The Dillingham Commission. University of Vermont History Review, Vol. 6. <http://www.uvm.edu/%7Ehag/histreview/vol6/lund.html>.

Mardia, K.V., 1970. Measures of multivariate skewness and kurtosis with applications. Biometrika 36, 519–530.

Marks, J., 2008. History of scientific racism. In: Moore, J. (Ed.), Encyclopedia of Race and Racism. Macmillan Reference USA, Detroit, Vol. 3, pp. 1–16.

Martin, V.R., 1914. Lehrbuch der Anthropologie in systematischer Darstellung mit besonderer Berücksichtigung der anthropologischen Methoden, für Studierende, Ärzte und Forschungsreisende. Textbook of anthropology systematically presented with special emphasis on anthropological methods. Gustav Fischer, Jena.

McKeown, A.H., Schmidt, R.W., 2013. Geometric morphometrics. In: DiGangi, E.A., Moore, M.K. (Eds.), Research Methods in Human Skeletal Biology. Academic Press, San Diego.

Mielke, J.H., Konigsberg, L.W., Relethford, J.H., 2011. Human Biological Variation, 2nd ed. Oxford University Press, New York.

Montagu, A., 1964a. The concept of race. In: Montagu, A. (Ed.), The Concept of Race. The Free Press of Glencoe, Collier-Macmillan, London, pp. 12–28.

Montagu, A., 1964b. Man's Most Dangerous Myth: The Fallacy of Race, 4th ed. The World Publishing Company, Cleveland and New York.

Moore, M.K., Ross, A.H., 2013. Stature estimation. In: DiGangi, E.A., Moore, M.K. (Eds.), Research Methods in Human Skeletal Biology. Academic Press, San Diego.

Morton, S.G., 1839. Crania Americana: Or, A Comparative View of the Skulls of Various Aboriginal Nations of North and South America; To Which is Prefixed an Essay on the Varieties of the Human Species. J Dobson, Philadelphia.

Moses, Y.T., 2004. The continuing power of the concept of race. Anthropology & Education Quarterly 35 (1), 146–148.

Mukhopadhyay, C.C., Moses, Y.T., 1997. Reestablishing race in anthropological discourse. American Anthropologist 99 (3), 517–533.

Nash, M., 1962. Race and the ideology of race. Current Anthropology 3 (3), 285–302.

Oppenheim, R., 2010. Revisting Hrdlicka and Boas: asymmetries of race and anti-imperialism in interwar anthropology. American Anthropologist 112 (1), 92–103.

Ousley, S.D., Hefner, J.T., 2005. Morphoscopic traits and the statistical determination of ancestry. Proceedings of the American Academy of Forensic Sciences 11, 291–292.

Ousley, S.D., Jantz, R.L., Fried, D., 2009. Understanding race and human variation: Why forensic anthropologists are good at identifying race. American Journal of Physical Anthropology 139, 68–76.

Ousley, S.D., Spradley, M.K., Jantz, R.L., 2011. Fordisc 3.1 Workshop February 2011, Chicago, IL.

Paul, D.B., 2008. History of eugenics. In: Moore, J. (Ed.), Encyclopedia of Race and Racism. Macmillan Reference USA, Detroit, pp. 441–447.

Pilloud, M.A., 2009. Community Structure at Neolithic Çatalhöyük: Biological Distance Analysis of Household, Neighborhood, and Settlement. Unpublished PhD dissertation. The Ohio State University, Columbus, Ohio.

Pounder, C., Adelman, L., Cheng, J., Herbes-Sommers, C., Strain, T., Smith, L., Ragazzi, C., 2003. Race: The Power of an Illusion. California Newsreel, San Francisco.

Relethford, J.H., 1991. Genetic drift and anthropomorphic variation in Ireland. Human Biology 63, 155–165.

Relethford, J.H., 2009. Race and global patterns of phenotypic variation. American Journal of Physical Anthropology 139, 16–22.

Relethford, J.H., Blangero, J., 1990. Detection of differential gene flow from patterns of quantitative variation. Human Biology 62, 5–25.

Relethford, J.H., Lees, F.C., 1982. The use of quantitative traits in the study of human population structure. American Journal of Physical Anthropology 25, 113–132.

Rhine, S., 1990. Non-metric skull racing. In: Gill, G.W., Rhine, S. (Eds.), Skeletal Attribution of Race: Methods for Forensic Anthropology Albuquerque: Maxwell Museum of Anthropology Anthropological Papers No. 4.

Ross, A.H., Slice, D.E., Ubelaker, D.H., Falsetti, A.B., 2004. Population affinities of 19th century Cuban crania: implications for identification criteria in South Florida Cuban Americans. Journal of Forensic Sciences 49 (1), 1–6.

Rushton, J.P., 1995. Race, Evolution, and Behavior: A Life History Perspective. Transaction, New Brunswick, NJ.

Sauer, N.J., 1992. Forensic anthropology and the concept of race: if races don't exist, why are forensic anthropologists so good at identifying them? Social Science & Medicine 34 (2), 107–111.

Scott, G.R., Turner II, C.G., 1997. The Anthropology of Modern Human Teeth: Dental Morphology and Its Variation in Recent Human Populations. Cambridge University Press, Cambridge.

Severson, K., 2012. Payment set for those sterilized in program. The New York Times (January 11 2012 p. A13), New York.

Shapiro, H., 1954. Earnest Albert Hooton 1887–1954. American Anthropologist 56, 1081–1084.

Shipman, P., 1994. The Evolution of Racism: Human Differences and the Use and Abuse of Science. Harvard University Press, Cambridge.

Sjøvold, T., 1977. Nonmetrical divergence between skeletal populations: the theoretical foundation and biological importance of C. A. B. Smith's mean measure of divergence. Ossa 4 (Suppl. 1), 1–133.

Sjøvold, T., 1984. A report on the heritability of some cranial measurements and nonmetric traits. In: van Vark, G.N., Howells, W.W. (Eds.), Multivariate Statistical Methods in Physical Anthropology. D. Reidel, Dordrecht, pp. 223–246.

Sjøvold, T., 1986. Infrapopulation distances and genetics of nonmetrical traits. In: Herrmann, B. (Ed.), Innovative Trends in der Prähistorischen Anthropologie: Mitteilungen der Berliner Geselhchaft für Anthropologie, Ethnologie und Urgeschichte. Verlag Marie Leidorf, Berlin, pp. 81–93.

Slice, D.E., Ross, A.H., 2004. Population affinities of Hispanic crania: Implications for forensic identification. Proceedings of the American Academy of Forensic Sciences 10, 280–281.

Smedley, A., Smedley, B.D., 2005. Race as biology is fiction, racism as a social problem is real. American Psychologist 60 (1), 16–26.

Sparks, C.S., Jantz, R.L., 2003. Changing times, changing faces: Franz Boas's immigrant study in modern perspective. American Anthropologist 105 (2), 333–337.

Spencer, F., 1981. The rise of academic physical anthropology in the United States (1880–1980): a historical overview. American Journal of Physical Anthropology 56, 353–364.

Spradley, M.K., Jantz, R.L., Robinson, A., Peccerelli, F., 2008. Demographic change and forensic identification: problems in metric identification of Hispanic skeletons. Journal of Forensic Sciences 53 (1), 21–28.

Stanton, W.R., 1960. The Leopard's Spots: Scientific Attitudes Toward Race in America, 1815–1859. University of Chicago Press, Chicago.

Sternberg, R.J., Grigorenko, E.L., Kidd, K.K., 2005. Intelligence, race, and genetics. American Psychologist 60 (1), 46–59.

Stojanowski, C.M., Schillaci, M.A., 2006. Phenotypic approaches for understanding patterns of intracemetery biological variation. Yearbook of Physical Anthropology 49, 49–88.

Suzuki, D., Knudtson, P., 1989. Genethics: The Clash Between the New Genetics and Human Values. Harvard University Press, Cambridge.

Tylor, E.B., 1871. Primitive Culture. Harper, New York. Reprinted 1958.

Washburn, S.L., 1951. The new physical anthropology. Transactions of the New York Academy of Sciences, Series II 13 (7), 298–304.

Washburn, S.L., 1964. The study of race. In: Montagu, A. (Ed.), The Concept of Race. The Free Press of Glencoe, Collier-Macmillan, London, pp. 242–260.

RECOMMENDED ADDITIONAL READINGS AND VIEWINGS

American Anthropological Association. Race—Are We So Different?® www.understandingrace.org.

Diamond, J., 1999. Guns, Germs, and Steel: The Fates of Human Societies. W.W. Norton & Co. New York.

Mielke, J.H., et al., 2011. Human Biological Variation, 2nd ed. Oxford University Press, New York.

Pounder, C., et al., 2003. Race: The Power of an Illusion (film series). California Newsreel, San Francisco.

6

Stature Estimation

Megan K. Moore, Ann H. Ross

INTRODUCTION

Living stature is defined as the maximum height attained during one's lifetime. Estimating stature can be important for individuation in forensic cases and mass disasters. It is one of the biological criteria that can assist in building the biological profile of an unidentified **decedent**[1] (a deceased individual) as well as support putative identifications (Konigsberg et al., 2006). For prehistoric studies, stature estimation can reveal developmental trends, environmental stress such as nutritional deficits, and evolutionary relationships. Several factors affect stature: sex, ancestry, age, **secular changes** from one generation to the next, and the environment. As with many measurements of humans, stature fits a bell curve distribution, meaning that most individuals will be about the same height, falling in the middle of the distribution. However, there will be individuals who are much shorter than average as well as individuals who are much taller than average, falling to the left and right extremes of the bell curve distribution, respectively. When considering stature estimation, the following generalizations can be made:

(1) Stature in humans increases until adulthood and then tends to decrease with advancing age after about 45 years (whether to compensate for age reduction in stature estimation is discussed later in this chapter) (Galloway, 1988; Giles and Hutchinson, 1991).
(2) Within a single population there is considerable variability.
(3) On average, male stature is greater than female stature, though a female in one population may be taller than a male in another population or within the same population.
(4) Population and twin studies have shown that anywhere from 65% to 90% of stature is due to inheritance (Li et al., 2004; Macgregor et al., 2006; Perola et al., 2007).
(5) Living stature may be estimated only *after* age, sex, and ancestry have been assessed, due to varying levels of sexual dimorphism, growth, skeletal degeneration, and population variation.

Hrdlička (1939) recognized that the correlations of long bones and stature would differ with sex, ancestry, and side of the body. From an attempt to use Pearson's stature equations

---

[1]All bolded terms are defined in the glossary at the end of this volume.

of Europeans on 48 Chinese males, Stevenson (1929) concluded that general equations are not feasible most likely as a result of variation in long bone proportions to stature. The influential work of Trotter and Gleser (1958) cautioned against combining formulae from different populations, investigators, generations, or geographic areas. Problems resulting from error in bone measurement (especially the tibia) (Jantz et al., 1995) and in the accuracy of the antemortem data have been discussed in several studies (Giles and Hutchinson, 1991; Willey and Falsetti, 1991; Ousley, 1995; Wilson et al., 2010). More recently, it has been noted that there is a high error when the reference sample and the estimated sample are genetically distinct, requiring modification of the statistical methods (Holliday and Ruff, 1997; Konigsberg et al., 1998; Hens et al., 2000; Ross and Konigsberg, 2002). Thus, despite numerous stature equations that have been developed for populations around the world, there is always the need for additional population-specific reference data. However, Komar and Buikstra (2009) argue for a more global approach and set of universal equations for stature estimation.

This chapter explores the history of stature estimation starting with the first mathematical attempts during the middle of the eighteenth century by Jean Joseph Sue (Stewart, 1979) using the ratio of the bone length to stature (also known as the **femur/stature ratio**). In 1899, the Englishman Carl Pearson developed the modern method of using **statistical regression** (Pearson, 1899). This is the predominant mathematical model used today (also known as **inverse calibration**), though it may be important to consider whether the individual's stature in question is likely from the population from which the formula was derived (Konigsberg et al., 1998).

As an alternative to early mathematical proportions, Dwight (1894) recommended an anatomical method of laying out the entire skeleton on an osteometric table to measure the postmortem stature (being careful to account for soft tissue thicknesses and spinal curvature). Fully (1956) proposed a similar but simpler method to estimate stature by measuring the height of each skeletal element individually, the sum of which is combined with a standardized soft-tissue estimate. More recent improvements to the anatomical method by Raxter and colleagues (2006) are included in this discussion. A method to estimate long bone length from fragmentary remains was first introduced by Müller (1935). This method was later improved by Steele and McKern (1969) and the process was then streamlined by Steele to directly estimate stature from the bone fragment (Steele, 1970). The prominent work of Trotter and Gleser (1952, 1958) utilized individuals from the **Robert J. Terry Anatomical Skeletal Collection,**[2] World War II dead, and Korean War dead. Their work produced regression equations still in use today, though often inappropriately, as they are based on historic anatomical collections that may not be appropriate for contemporary forensic casework.

The correlation of fetal bone length is important for the estimation of the age of the fetus and of the subadult (Fazekas and Kósa, 1966a, b; Scheuer and Black, 2004) but few studies have undertaken stature estimation in children (Telkka et al., 1962; Himes et al., 1977; Ruff, 2007; Smith, 2007; Abrahamyan et al., 2008; Cardoso, 2009). **Secular trends** show an increase in stature over the last few centuries, suggesting population-specific data must also be temporally specific (Trotter and Gleser, 1951b; Meadows and Jantz, 1995). Establishing population data for archaeological samples requires the anatomical method in addition to a mathematical method (Sciulli et al., 1990; Giannecchini and Moggi-Cecchi, 2008; Vercellotti

---

[2]Curated by the National Museum of Natural History at the Smithsonian Institution, Washington, D.C.

et al., 2009; Auerbach and Ruff, 2010). We will present the limitations of stature estimation to help you avoid common pitfalls. Finally, two case studies of stature estimation by the authors are presented to walk you through the process of how to conduct your own study.

METHODS IN STATURE ESTIMATION: THEN AND NOW

Dwight (1894) differentiated between two different methods for stature estimation: **mathematical** and **anatomical**. The mathematical methods calculated the proportion of each bone length to stature (e.g., femur/living stature ratio). However, the early mathematical methods were not reliable because body proportions vary from one population to another (Ruff and Walker, 1993). Dwight (1894) recommended using the mathematical method only if the anatomical method was not possible, due to the absence of various skeletal elements. The anatomical methods combine the measured height of each bone, accounting for spinal curvature and soft tissue thickness. Five years later, Pearson (1899) developed statistical regression. The femur/stature ratio was overshadowed by regression theory, which is the predominant method used today for two main reasons: (1) the ease of application (it requires only the length of a single element), (2) the common incompleteness of skeletons from archaeological sites and forensic cases, and (3) the relative accuracy of the stature estimations.

Mathematical Methods: Stature Ratio

Early mathematical models developed by French anatomists successfully explored **allometry** (differential growth of body parts) in body proportions of bone length and stature, but failed to coordinate amongst themselves a consistent measurement standard (e.g., metric vs. imperial measurements). In 1755, Jean Joseph Sue, a professor at the Louvre, published research comparing maximum imperial length of human bones, trunk length, and the complete length of both the upper and lower extremities to stature. Sue came to two conclusions. First, he found that trunk length is greater than lower extremity length until the age of 14. Second, Sue determined that the length of the upper limb exceeds the lower limb until birth. Unfortunately, Sue never specified how he took the measurements (maximum vs. physiologic length, etc.) (Stewart, 1979). Another French Professor of Legal Medicine in Paris, Matthieu Joseph Bonaventure Orfila, used the measurements of Sue and then took his own metric measurements from 51 cadavers and 20 skeletons. Orfila then used cadaver stature and attempted to estimate stature from the femur and/or the humerus. In 1823 in the United States, T. R. Beck used the Sue-Orfila method with feet and inches, but failed to convert the French imperial measurements to the Anglo-American feet and inches, which are not identical (Stewart, 1979).

Not long after Sue and Orfila, British anthropologists began their own mathematical attempts at stature estimation in bioarchaeological contexts. These anthropologists included John Thernam, Sir George Humphrey, and John Beddoe. Both the British and the French methods simply multiplied femur length by a constant number, which was the average proportion calculated from the femur/stature ratio (Dwight, 1894; Stewart, 1979). See Box 6.1 for the femur/stature ratio. Standardization of the measurement methodology was finally introduced by Paul Broca. Broca founded the Société d'Anthropologie de Paris in 1859 and developed the osteometric

---

BOX 6.1

EQUATIONS FOR THE FEMUR/STATURE RATIO

Equation 1. Stature Estimation Using Femur/Stature Ratio

$$\hat{x}_i = \frac{\bar{x}}{\bar{y}} y_i$$

ratio of mean stature to mean femur length multiplied by measured femur length

Equation 2. General Femur/Stature Ratio/Index

(femur length (cm)/stature) $\times$ 100 / 26.7

---

board. Paul Topinard, successor to Broca as head of the Société, recognized the need to accumulate larger samples and more skeletal data. In 1881, Topinard measured 141 skeletons and developed a constant ratio of the maximum length of the humerus, radius, femur, and tibia. Living stature was then achieved by adding a standardized 35 mm to account for soft tissues (Stewart, 1979). According to Stewart (1979), this was the first standardized formula to estimate stature. Not long after, Etienne Rollet (1888) was directed by his advisor to measure stature and long bones from cadavers for his doctoral thesis. He produced the first formal stature tables based on 50 males and 50 females, relating bone length to stature.

Manouvrier (1892) modified Rollet's tables (using the same data) by improving the table organization and taking additional measurements from fleshed bones. Manouvrier reduced Rollet's data by more than half, eliminating 26 males and 25 females because they were older than 60 years. One important improvement that Manouvrier made was to recommend that 2 mm be added to long bone length for dry bones and the addition of another 2 cm to the corresponding stature in the tables (Stewart, 1979). From 1898 to 1902, Hrdlička produced the first (nonregression) formulae for African Americans and European Americans; these consisted of long bone to stature ratios based on cadavers from dissecting rooms (Stewart, 1979).

Nearly a century later, Feldesman and colleagues (1988, 1990) rediscovered the femur/stature ratio when they were trying to determine if the *Australopithecus afarensis* specimen Lucy's (AL 288-1) femur was disproportionately short compared to that of modern humans. They compiled a sample of published data on modern humans from 13 different populations. The general femur/stature ratio yielded an average proportion for modern humans of 26.7% (i.e., the femur is on average 26.74% of stature), with a very low standard deviation of less than 1% (SD = 0.55%) for all 13 populations. More surprising was the finding that Lucy had nearly the same femur/stature ratio (Feldesman and Lundy, 1988). See Box 6.1.

Feldesman and colleagues (1990, 1996) continued to collect data from a total of 51 populations around the world to determine whether the femur/stature ratio was suitable and efficacious in modern and prehistoric human populations. The problem with the earlier study from 1990 (Feldesman et al., 1990) is that the samples were not all analyzed in the same way. For the latter study (Feldesman and Fountain, 1996), the authors used only samples in which the average population femur length and the average population stature were known. They revised their earlier hypothesis to be that there exists some population variation in the femur/stature ratio. The femur/stature ratio for Africans (27.25%) was significantly different than that for "Europeans" (26.64%) or "Asians" (26.31%), but there was much variation within the "African" samples. When they used an ancestry-specific ratio for a known specimen, however, the results were only slightly better than when using the generic formula (Feldesman and Fountain, 1996). If the population affinity was unknown, they recommended using the generic ratio. Ultimately, the femur/stature ratio works best for individuals around the mean (those individuals in the middle of the distribution) and does not perform well with outliers; it underestimates stature for shorter individuals and overestimates stature for taller individuals.

Mathematical Methods: Regression Theory

Manouvrier's earlier method from 1893 was quickly replaced by a mathematical method by the British biometrician Karl Pearson. Like Manouvrier, Pearson used Rollet's data (Rollet, 1888) to establish a new method based on regression theory (Pearson, 1899). Under regression theory, the independent and dependent variables are "fit" to the equation of a line:

$$y = mx + b \qquad (6.1)$$

where y is stature or the independent variable, m is the slope of the regression line, x is the bone length, and b is the intercept of the regression line.

If these variables are positively and closely correlated to each other, the data will plot along a line. See Figure 6.1. The regression line is the best estimation of the conditional mean for the **dependent variable** corresponding to each **independent variable** (Freedman, 1978). Regression theory uses **standard deviation** for the long bones and **coefficients of correlation** between the long bones and stature. **Least squares regression** is the resulting line that runs through the center of the population (Steele and McKern, 1969). Pearson set up the dependent variable to be stature and the independent variable to be bone length. The consequences of this early designation of stature as the dependent variable will be discussed later.

Pearson's regression was the first true "mathematical model." Unlike Manouvrier, Pearson did not omit any of the older aged individuals from his sample. He created two separate equations: one for cadaver (wet) and one for dry bones. From Rollet's data, Pearson subtracted the thickness of the cartilage and accounted for the increase in length when soaked in water (based on the dissertation of Heinrich Werner from 1897) (Pearson, 1899). Pearson came up with three rules for developing stature estimation equations. First, calculate the mean and standard deviation for the entire sample and determine the correlation with stature. Second, measure as many bones of the skeleton as possible. Third, there is an effect of time (i.e., secular change) and climate/environment on dimensions of body proportions (Krogman and İşcan, 1986). According to Pearson (1899), if stature correlations with a particular bone are high, then only 50—100 individuals may be needed to develop an equation. In other cases, several hundred individuals may be necessary. It is important to note that there are inherent errors in stature estimation when combining incongruent data of dry and fleshed specimens to living individuals (Krogman and İşcan, 1986).

In 1929, Paul Stevenson was the first researcher to test Pearson's statistical method of stature estimation on an independent sample. Stevenson worked as a professor in China

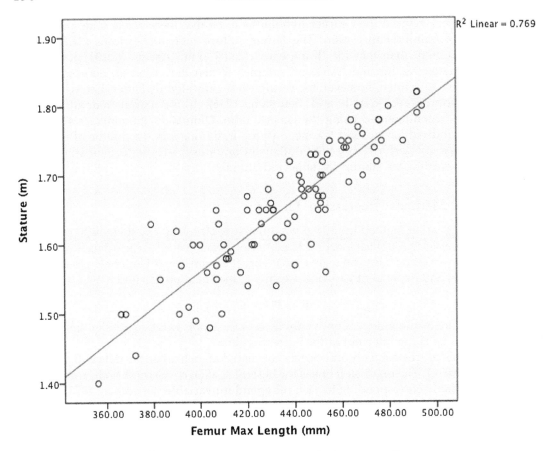

FIGURE 6.1   Statistical regression using the femur to predict stature.

where he measured 48 male cadavers, from which he developed regression equations. These did not compare well with Pearson's European data and Pearson's equations did not work successfully to estimate the stature of the Chinese individuals (Stevenson, 1929), indicating that population-specific equations are needed.

Through the early twentieth century, the mathematical methods of the Manouvrier tables and Pearson's equations became the standards for stature estimation. In 1948, Stewart recommended better equations and testing using the large Hamann–Todd cadaver sample from Case Western Reserve University in Cleveland, Ohio (Stewart, 1979). Two researchers independently embarked upon the challenge: Wesley Dupertuis and Mildred Trotter. In tests of the widespread applicability of Pearson's equations, Dupertuis and Hadden (1951) claimed that the population Pearson used was short and should not be used on tall populations. Their equations yielded stature estimates that were 8.5 cm taller than from Pearson's equations. They also did not think there was a difference between living and cadaver stature, but Trotter and Gleser disagreed (1952).

Dupertuis and Hadden (1951) had produced "general equations" for use on any population, despite the lessons learned from Stevenson that population-specific equations are necessary (Stevenson, 1929). They recommended using more than two bones to estimate stature (i.e., multiple regression) and that the lower limbs were better than the upper.

Trotter, on the other hand, echoed Pearson's recommendation for a representative sample from the same sex, age, ancestry, geographic area, and time period. Trotter and Gleser's formulae (1952, 1958) became more widely accepted than those of Dupertuis and Hadden (1951) because they used a larger sample of American World War II soldiers (including Asian data). They also provided a correction for age (Trotter and Gleser, 1951a). Trotter and Gleser altered Pearson's method in three ways. First, they used a combination of living stature and dry bones. Second, they introduced the first correction for age. Third, they *tested* the validity on a second sample of individuals who died during the Korean War (Trotter and Gleser, 1952, 1958).

Population-Specific Regression Formulae

From the mathematical model for the estimation of stature that was gaining acceptance in the field, it was becoming clear that population-specific data were needed. The study by Trotter and Gleser (1952) recognized some distinctions in limb proportion between African Americans and European Americans. Trotter and Gleser (1958) tested their formulae against data from the Korean War dead, and included new equations for Asian Americans and Mexican males. They concluded that, due to the different limb proportions, different equations are necessary for each population. Their results indicated that stature estimation for Puerto Ricans can be successful using equations for African Americans, but Mexicans differed from all groups, so separate equations were needed. The standard error of estimate (SEE)[3] was different for Korean War Europeans than for the WWII and Terry collections.

Further, Trotter and Gleser analyzed the longitudinal data compiled by Dr. Russell Newman in 1950 with the U.S. Army Quartermaster Research and Development Command of 48,685 records (Trotter and Gleser, 1958). From this, they concluded that the age for achieving maximum height had increased from the WWII dead (18 years) to the Korean War dead (full stature at 21–23 years)[4] (see discussion later in this chapter). They measured all of the long bones: humerus, radius, ulna, femur, tibia, and fibula. Trotter and Gleser determined that the lower limb is more reliable than the upper, so there is no reason to use the upper limb if the lower is present. They also recommended using the average of bone length of right and left sides if both sides are completely present (Trotter and Gleser, 1958). See Box 6.2 for lessons learned from Trotter and Gleser's research about what not to do in stature estimation.

Although the work of Trotter and Gleser has been used and respected by researchers around the world, one very serious error in their methodology has come to light. Jantz (1992) tested Trotter's and Gleser's female formulae using data from the **Forensic Databank**.[5] They found that for European Americans, the femur and tibia yielded stature estimates that differed by up to 3 cm between the bones, which led to further investigation of the Trotter and Gleser methods. Jantz and colleagues (1995) made an important discovery that Trotter had

---

[3]The standard error of estimate is used in regression analysis to examine how well a least squares line equation fits a data set.

[4]This secular change in the timing of growth is yet another reason why it is necessary to continually update stature formulae.

[5]This contains data from thousands of forensic cases curated by the University of Tennessee.

BOX 6.2

RULES LEARNED FROM TROTTER AND GLESER:
WHAT TO AVOID IN STATURE ESTIMATION

1. DO NOT combine formulae from
   different populations, investigators,
   geographic areas, or generations.

2. DO NOT determine the average from
   several equations, which are based on
   different bones or bone combinations.

3. DO NOT plot estimated stature to actual
   (observed) stature to test precision.

---

actually *mismeasured* the tibia for the 1952 publication (Trotter and Gleser, 1952) by excluding the medial malleolus, contrary to the published measurement description. Compounding the error, two different methods were used for the 1958 publication (Trotter and Gleser, 1958), which included the Korean War sample. Thus, any modern attempts to use the regression equations of Trotter and Gleser *must not rely on the 1958 formulae that include the tibia*.[6] If using the 1952 formulae, the *tibia should be measured without the malleolus* (Jantz et al., 1995).

Regression Formulae from Other Bones

After Pearson, stature studies using regression formulae sprang up for populations around the world. Researchers began to test other bones of the skeleton in addition to the long bones. The argument given for using other bones is the all too often scenario of poor preservation in both bioarchaeological and forensic contexts. It is important to point out that not all of the bones yield equally successful stature formulae. Musgrave and Haneja (1978) estimated stature from physiologic length of each metacarpal for European males and females using hand x-rays. The results from their equations were more variable for females ($r = 0.49-0.84$) than for males ($r = 0.53-0.67$). Giroux and Wescott (2008) provide excellent summary tables of previous studies for the sacrum, cranium, vertebrae, metacarpals, metatarsals, talus, and calcaneus. The best results for non-long bones are from the metatarsals, metacarpals, talus, and calcaneus, but no correlations exceeded $r = 0.89$. Pelvic dimensions provided no better stature estimates ($r < 0.77$) (Giroux and Wescott, 2008). Singh and Sohal (1952) and Olivier and Pineau (1957) created regression equations from the scapula and clavicle. Stature estimation using the clavicle does not seem to be a plausible option, because Jit and Singh (1956) reported errors of as much as 32 cm. Correlations of stature with craniometrics and **odontometrics** have the least success (not exceeding $r = 0.56$) (Kalia et al., 2008).

In 1960, Fully and Pineau published a mathematical method that regressed the entire length of the vertebral column on stature (Fully and Pineau, 1960). This method is a summation of the vertical body heights from the second cervical vertebra (C2) to the fifth lumbar vertebra (L5). They found that the combined heights of the fifth through seventh thoracic

---

[6]In other words, Trotter and Gleser (1952) measured the tibiae *without* the malleolus and Trotter and Gleser (1958) measured the Korean War sample tibiae *with* the malleolus (Jantz et al., 1995).

vertebrae (T5—7) and the first through third lumbar vertebrae (L1—3) best correlate with the overall spine length (r = 0.952). They concluded that this could be used if the entire vertebral column is not available. Fully and Pineau (1960) then compared different combinations of long bone and trunk lengths, developing equations for the femur and five lumbar vertebrae (r = 0.926) and for the tibia and five lumbar vertebrae (r = 0.908) (Fully and Pineau, 1960). Fully and Pineau measured the long bones differently from Trotter and Gleser, so comparative studies between the two are not possible. None of these regressions, except the combined vertebral lengths as per Fully and Pineau (1960), is as powerful as the formulae from the long bones. Tibbetts (1981) articulated the vertebral column to estimate stature, which is recommended only if the long bones are not available. However, any bones that do not represent a proportion of an individual's living stature should be avoided (Trotter and Gleser, 1958; Rathbun, 1984; Joyce and Stover, 1991).

Stature Regression for Non-U.S. Populations

Stature regression formulae have been calculated for populations all over the world. A number of studies have estimated the stature of Europeans. One early study measured the stature of 3000 living criminals in England from all over Great Britain (Macdonnel, 1901). This study measured head height, head breadth, third finger length, cubit length (elbow to the tip of the middle finger), and foot length. Brietinger (1937) measured the maximum lengths of long bones from 2400 German male skeletons, which estimated a taller stature than did Pearson's or Manouvrier's equations. Mendes-Correa (1932) measured the maximum lengths of the humerus, ulna, radius, femur, tibia, and fibula from a Portuguese sample. By studying the stature of both cadavers and living individuals, Mendes-Correa determined that living stature is 2 cm shorter than that of cadavers.

In 1950, Telkkä measured a Finnish sample of skeletons, which included 115 males and 39 females (Telkkä, 1950). Telkkä used the maximum length of the humerus, femur, tibia, and fibula and the physiologic lengths of the radius and ulna. He reported that supine cadaver stature is 2 cm greater than living stature. Furthermore, he recommended that if the bones are measured when wet, then 2 mm must be subtracted from the bone length before using the formulae due to shrinkage in drying (Telkkä, 1950). Allbrook (1961) measured the **percutaneous lengths** (i.e. via palpable landmarks on the skin) of the tibia and ulna from fleshed individuals with the limbs semi-flexed of British and East African ancestry. Černý and Komenda (1982) measured the humerus and femur of a Czech sample that included 148 males and 104 females.

Correctly or incorrectly, a common practice in stature estimation has been to develop regression formulae for populations from Asia lumped together with Native American populations. Stewart (1954) used the data from Trotter and Gleser (1952) and developed his own regression equations for Asians. Neumann (1967) prepared formulae for males and females from the femur and tibia for two Native American populations, but provided no standard error estimate. Not content with the accuracy of Trotter and Gleser formulae for Mesoamericans, Genovés (1967) produced stature regression formulae from 76 males and 59 females of Indigenous Mexican, *Mestizo*, and European ancestry using all of the long bones.[7] Genovés

---

[7]Try to pay attention to the size of the sample in each study. In the study by Genovés (1967), the number of males (76) and females (59) was further broken down into three ancestry groups, which is statistically problematic.

developed an elaborate system to "morphoscopically" distinguish the ancestry of individuals, to try to discern Indigenous from *Mestizo* from European (Genovés, 1967).[8] This elaborate system combined the phenotypic traits of hair color, eye color, skin color, dentition, body hair, and body form.

Asian populations were studied for stature estimation early on by Stevenson (1929), but other studies to develop Asian stature formulae did not follow for another half century. Yung-hao et al. (1979) measured 40 males from Chungking, a southwestern district of China and found that the femur and tibia formulae were the best indicators of stature. Shitai (1983) measured the radius, ulna, humerus, femur, and tibia from 50 Han Chinese from southern China. Shitai recommended using the same age corrections as Trotter and Gleser (1951a). Problems with age corrections will be discussed later in this chapter. Shulin and Fangwu (1983) published on stature estimation for 70 Southern Chinese males using bones other than the long bones of the limbs (cranial circumference, clavicle length, innominate length, and breadth of the scapula).

Many stature studies have been published on African populations, most using the Raymond Dart Collection[9] from South Africa. Allbrook (1961) measured the tibia and ulna of 429 living individuals and 53 skeletons from East Africa. Allbrook noted that the difference in percutaneous tibial length is not statistically significant from the dry bone length. Lundy (1983) measured 117 males and 125 females from the Dart Collection in South Africa. The actual stature was not known, so the Fully anatomical method was implemented first and used *in lieu* of actual stature. Bidmos studied stature in South Africans from the Dart Collection using the calcaneus and fragmentary long bones, along with an analysis of Fully's anatomical method, which is described below (Bidmos, 2005, 2006, 2008). More recently, the measurements of the skull were used to create regression formulae for indigenous South Africans (Ryan and Bidmos, 2007). For all the different populations around the world and the bones from which to estimate stature, the femur and tibia (if measured consistently) have yielded the most accurate results. The articulated vertebrae have also been successful, but researchers should avoid any bones that do not actually play a role in an individual's stature, with the lowest results for the estimation of stature from craniofacial bones or teeth.

Anatomical Methods

Dwight's Anatomical Method

Dwight (1894) preferred the anatomical method to the mathematical method despite it being extremely time consuming and requiring better expertise on the part of the researcher. Dwight developed a method made up of nine steps and used a long table as a giant osteometric board in order to reconstruct the skeleton. He made use of modeling clay to articulate the skeleton and to reconstruct the spinal curvature. His steps are listed in Box 6.3.

---

[8]It should be noted that Genovés measured the tibia without the malleolus in this study, similar to Trotter and Gleser (1952).

[9]The Raymond A. Dart Collection of Human Skeletons is curated at the University of the Witwatersrand, Johannesburg, South Africa.

Fully's Anatomical Method

Dwight's anatomical method was extremely laborious, so Fully (1956) decided to streamline the process. Fully (1956) was given the task of identifying French dead from German WWII era concentration camps in Austria. He developed his own anatomical method on a subset of 102 individuals with identification tags from the total 3165 individuals in his sample. The difference between his method and Dwight's method is that he used the individual bone measurements and not the length of the fully assembled skeleton. The steps of Fully's Anatomical Method are found in Box 6.4.

Fully came up with a single correction factor for all the soft tissue, depending on whether the individual was short, medium height, or tall. If the estimated stature is less than 153.5 cm, then 10 cm are added. If the estimated stature is between 153.6 and 165.4 cm, then 10.5 cm are added. Further, 11.5 cm are added to account for soft tissue thickness for any stature over 165.5 cm. Fully also stated that his method was specific to European populations (Fully, 1956).

Lundy (1988) conducted a validation study of stature estimation methods using three known European American soldiers killed during the Vietnam War. The study tested the reliability of the Fully method against Trotter and Gleser's formulae using the femur and tibia

---

BOX 6.3

DWIGHT'S ANATOMICAL METHOD

1. Place a metric scale along the length of the table.
2. Articulate the pelvis to L5 with the anterior superior iliac spine (ASIS) in the same horizontal plane as the pubic symphysis.
3. Check the accuracy of the spine segments with proportions of the cervical, thoracic, and lumbar vertebrae.
4. Place the femoral head in the acetabulum on one side with the distal condyles perpendicular to the table length.

5. Add the tibia with a space of 6 mm between it and the femur.
6. Add the talus with a space of 3 mm from the tibia and another 3 cm from the calcaneus.
7. Place the skull on clay 3 mm from the atlas.
8. Add 6 mm to account for scalp thickness.
9. In total, add 32 mm for soft tissue, which is similar to the 35 mm added for soft tissue as suggested by Topinard (1885).

BOX 6.4

FULLY'S ANATOMICAL METHOD

1. Skull height from basion to bregma
2. Vertebral body height C2–L5, S1
3. Femur physiological length
4. Tibia physiological length (with malleolus)

5. Talocalcaneal articulated height
6. Calculate skeletal stature
7. Add soft tissue correction factor of 10, 10.5 or 11.5 cm, depending on skeletal stature estimate.

---

for White males. For all three cases, the Fully method outperformed the Trotter and Gleser formulae. However, as mentioned previously, there is systematic bias of the Trotter and Gleser formulae as a result of mismeasurement of the tibia. Bidmos (2005) tested the Fully method on South African Blacks and Whites and found that it, too, had systematic bias when estimating the stature of South African Black individuals. According to Raxter and colleagues (2006), this bias might have been due to differences in the way in which the cadaver stature was originally measured (Raxter et al., 2006).

The Fully method has been consistently recognized as more precise than any of the mathematical methods and has therefore become the standard for testing mathematical models in bioarchaeological populations, for which a living stature is not known (Sciulli et al., 1990; Konigsberg et al., 1998; Bidmos, 2008; Auerbach and Ruff, 2010). Raxter et al. (2006) state, "Despite the sex/ancestry specificity of the regression formulae, there are always likely to be some individuals with unusual body proportions." Thus, by measuring every bone using the anatomical method (e.g., femur, tibia, vertebral bodies), stature is personalized for the proportions of each individual. This process is laborious and some researchers found the instructions by Fully were unclear for a few bones (Raxter et al., 2006).

Revised Fully Method

Raxter and colleagues (2006) revised the Fully method by providing better instructions for the measurements and by validating its accuracy and applicability. Like the Fully method, Raxter et al. (2006) recommended the addition of soft tissue corrections. One of the discrepancies of the Fully method is that average distance of the second cervical vertebra (C2) to basion is actually about 7 mm, but assumed by Fully to be null (Raxter et al., 2006). In addition, there is an average distance of 3.6 mm from the roof of the acetabulum to the first sacral segment (S1), again unaccounted for by Fully. There is also an overlap of the medial malleolus of the tibia by 1.5 cm, which counteracts part of the underestimation. Raxter and colleagues therefore recommend an average soft tissue correction of 12.4 cm while Fully had only recommended an average of 10.2 cm.

Further, Bidmos (2005) found the Fully method systematically underestimates living stature by 2.4 cm (Bidmos, 2005). The difference in the soft tissue correction recommended by Fully and that recommended by Raxter et al. (2006) may account for this 2.4 cm difference. Fully also used a Broca osteometric board (with a hole in the stationary end to place the intercondylar eminence through) to measure the tibia, which is not always available. Using a sample of African-American and European-American males and females from the Terry Collection, Raxter and colleagues accounted for the effects of sex, ancestry, and age. Ancestry and sex had no significant effect on the stature estimation, therefore Raxter and colleagues (2006) contend that *universal equations are possible*,[10] contrary to Fully's recommendations. Raxter et al. (2006) created regression equations (that included the correction factors) to better account for soft tissues and age. Using their equations, 95% of the estimated statures fall within 4.4 cm of actual stature. Refer to Box 6.5 for the revised Fully equations, as per Raxter et al. (2006).

---

[10]According to Raxter and colleagues (2006), universal stature equations (with soft tissue corrections) are possible when using the revised Fully method.

BOX 6.5

REVISED FULLY EQUATIONS AFTER RAXTER ET AL. (2006)

Revised Fully equation including age:
living stature = $1.009 \times$ skeletal height $-$ $0.0426 \times$ age $+ 12.1$ (for soft tissue)
($r = 0.956$, SEE $= 2.22$)

Revised Fully equation excluding age:
living stature = $0.996 \times$ skeletal height $+$ 11.7 (for soft tissue)
($r = 0.952$, SEE $= 2.31$)

Secular Change

Secular (or temporal) changes in stature from one generation to the next are caused by a combination of the environment, genetics, and evolutionary forces (Trotter and Gleser, 1951b). Secular trends are relevant for a number of biological traits in addition to stature, such as growth/maturity rates and morphology. For example, an increase/decrease in nutrition, exposure to infectious diseases, and access to medical care can all cause secular change from one generation to the next. See McKeown and Schmidt (Chapter 12), this volume, for further discussion of secular change. Trotter and Gleser (1951b) were the first to recognize secular changes in stature from the Terry and military collections using both bone lengths and reported stature (Trotter and Gleser, 1951b). The goal of their study was to detect irregular and cyclical patterns in stature across generations. They observed no secular trend from 1840 to 1895. A slight increase in stature occurred in African Americans between 1895 and 1905 and then a significant positive trend overall in the twentieth century. The results suggested that stature increase was not constant, but fluctuated from one decade to the next. Not all of the changes are positive; there can be small jumps with plateaus and small reductions (Trotter and Gleser, 1951b).

A comparable study by Meadows and Jantz (1995) used the **Huntington Collection,**[11] Terry Collection, and data from WWII casualties along with the Forensic Databank. They regressed long bone length on year-of-birth to show *allometric secular change*. This study found that secular change was greater in males, that the lower limb showed greater change than the upper limb, and that the distal elements are affected more than the proximal (Meadows and Jantz, 1995). All of the groups sampled exhibited an increase in femur length over time. These allometric secular changes are strongly dependent on environmental forces, showing that different bones respond more strongly to the environmental factors to reach genetic potential. Meadows and Jantz (1995) suggested that females were more resistant to environmental changes than were males (Meadows and Jantz, 1995). Other studies have shown that females are thought to be buffered in some way against environmental stressors due to their biological need to support pregnancy and lactation (Stini 1975, 1982; Ross et al. 2003; Bogin, 1988).

---

[11]The George Huntington Collection is curated by the National Museum of Natural History at the Smithsonian Institution, Washington, D.C.

PROBLEMS WITH STATURE ESTIMATION

Apples to Oranges: Data Comparison Problems between Antemortem and Postmortem Data

When estimating stature in skeletal biology, you are essentially comparing a dry bone length to the known stature of that individual. The way in which the living (or cadaver) stature was measured or reported can vary greatly. This creates a scenario of trying to compare apples (antemortem data) to oranges (postmortem data), which can be seriously fraught with error. Snow and Williams (1971) studied variations in living stature compared to skeletal remains. They found stature discrepancies from four sources of data: (1) self-reported, (2) measured with shoes, (3) not being fully erect, and (4) evening versus morning variation (Bass, 1979).

Ousley (1995) elaborated on the two different types of errors when dealing with stature estimation. Equations used can be flawed by incorrect measurement (postmortem) or incorrect antemortem data collection. All osteometric and anthropometric studies providing postmortem data are subject to inter- and intraobserver error. The antemortem data may also have systematic bias due to interobserver error in measuring stature, misreporting on ID cards, age changes in stature, and even due to such effects as the time of the day (you are taller in the morning). Ousley (1995) describes some data as more precise and other data as more accurate.[12] According to Ousley (1995), the greater the precision, the narrower the range of statures will be (i.e., there will be a low standard error), and the greater the accuracy, the more likely the actual stature will be included within the range of error, which may require widening that range. The goal for stature estimation ideally is both **precision** and **accuracy**.

Trotter and Gleser recommended broadening the error range to cover the 95% **confidence interval**, because this will increase accuracy as the range is more likely to include the actual stature, but the broader range will be less precise. Ousley recommends using what is called a **prediction interval** to increase precision because, unlike standard error (SE), it accounts for the sample size. This topic is discussed further in the chapter on age estimation by Uhl in this volume (Chapter 3). Suffice it to say that for the best possible estimate of stature, Ousley still suggests that the Fully method is the best estimator (Ousley, 1995).

Antemortem data can be recorded in two different ways that Ousley (1995) has defined as (1) **measured stature** (**MSTAT**) and (2) **forensic stature** (**FSTAT**). Medical or military records that include measurements of living stature (MSTAT) are extremely prone to interobserver error. Ousley (1995) noted that variation in MSTAT can be as much as 5 inches (12.7 cm) in some cases, depending on whether shoes were worn or even due to daily fluctuation in stature.[13] FSTAT is easier to obtain for missing persons, as it is the stature that is self-reported on the driver's license/identity card or as reported by a family member. FSTAT is subject to systematic bias due to age-related height reduction and misreporting discrepancies between males and females and between taller individuals and shorter individuals (Giles and Hutchinson, 1991; Willey and Falsetti, 1991). Giles and Hutchinson (1991) used data from a sample of 8000 military personnel and found that, depending on height, men overestimate

---

[12]See Uhl (Chapter 3), this volume for further explanation of accuracy versus precision.

[13]Stature taken early in the morning or immediately following a nap can be as much as two 2 cm taller (Ousley, 1995).

stature by about 2.5 cm, whereas women tend to over report their stature by only 1 cm.[14] Individuals who are extremely tall are actually more accurate in their self-reporting than shorter individuals.

In a comparable study by Willey and Falsetti (1991), 500 college students were measured for stature, which was then compared to self-reported stature on the individuals' driver's licenses. In this study, they found that reported stature for males is approximately one-half inch greater than measured stature. Females over-reported their stature by one-quarter inch, on average. There may also be an age bias if the driver's license reports stature before the cessation of growth, which is likely considering that the minimum age for driving in the U.S. and worldwide is mid to late teens (Willey and Falsetti, 1991).

To decrease the error with measured stature, Krogman and İşcan (1986) suggested measurement standards for living stature. They claim that it is necessary to keep the following landmarks in alignment with one another: (1) acromiale (most lateral shoulder girdle); (2) trochanterion (most lateral femur point in pelvis); and (3) malleolus lateralis (tip of the fibula) (Krogman and İşcan, 1986). Additionally, postural slumping should be avoided *or* the amount of **lordosis** (excessive inward curvature) and **kyphosis** (excessive outward curvature) should be recorded. A **stadiometer** is the most reliable, but it should be calibrated regularly.

It should be no surprise that we can become shorter after we reach our full adult stature, as a result of soft tissue compression, postural slumping, or even due to osteoporotic fracture. Age-related stature reduction begins around age 45 (Galloway, 1988; Giles and Hutchinson, 1991). This age onset differs from the estimate of 30 for stature decline by Trotter and Gleser (1951a). They arbitrarily chose the age of 30, because no longitudinal studies by 1951, to their knowledge, had confirmed the age-decline onset. Bertillon (1885) and Hooton (1947) found that decline commences at 25 years. Büchi (1950) claimed the stature decline began after the 40th year. Trotter and Gleser (1951a) argued that it is possible to distinguish secular change from the effects of aging in a cross-sectional study by measuring the length of the long bones against the reported stature.[15] They proposed an equation to correct for stature loss due to age to be subtracted from the estimated stature. See Box 6.6.

BOX 6.6

EQUATIONS FOR TOTAL LOSS OF STATURE DUE TO AGING

Trotter and Gleser equation for total loss of stature due to aging:

estimated stature − 0.06 (age − 30) = maximum stature estimate

Galloway equation for total loss of stature due to aging:

estimated stature − 0.16 (age − 45) = maximum stature estimate

---

[14]Interestingly, while men will overestimate their height, women tend to underestimate their weight.

[15]Stature reduction due to aging is independent of long bone length changes, as the reduction occurs in the soft tissues and possibly the vertebral bodies, discussed later in this chapter.

Trotter and Gleser (1951a) reevaluated Rollet's much earlier data and found similar average stature loss of about 1.2 cm over 20 years. This method does well until age 70 and then it begins to overestimate stature (Galloway, 1988). On a study of 8000 military personnel, Giles and Hutchinson (1991) recognized an age-related bias, in which stature begins to decrease between 40 and 44 years. They calculated that males lose on average 1 mm/year and females lose 1.25 mm/year. After the age of 75, the age decrease accelerates to 1.4 mm/year for males and 2.0 mm/year for females (Giles and Hutchinson, 1991). Galloway determined the age of stature reduction onset at 45 after surveying 550 individuals of older ages for maximum reported height when they were age 25 and measuring their current stature. There was a progressive loss in stature in both sexes, though her results had a relatively weak correlation. Galloway (1988) recommends using a revised correction factor for age to account for age-related stature decrease, as opposed to the one by Trotter and Gleser, (1951a). See both equations in Box 6.6.

Age-related decline in stature typically reflects compression of soft tissues and *not the length of the bones* (though osteoporotic fractures of the vertebrae can increase stature loss) (Galloway, 1988). Individuals are unlikely to change the initial stature on their driver's licenses, regardless of height increases or decreases (Galloway, 1988; Giles and Hutchinson, 1991; Willey and Falsetti, 1991). Thus, Ousley (1995) finds that FSTAT, as self-reported maximum stature on ID cards as a young adult, may more accurately reflect the calculated stature from the long bones, because the long bones do not change in length as a result of age. FSTAT is also more readily available than MSTAT.[16] To be conservative for forensic cases, Galloway (1988) recommends providing stature estimation both with and without age corrections.

Wilson and colleagues (2010) conducted an evaluation of stature estimation using the existing data in the Forensic Databank (FDB). When Ousley (1995) had used the same data 15 years earlier, there were fewer individuals in the FDB. With a larger sample size, Wilson and colleagues (2010) were able to test the accuracy of FSTAT and found that their **ASTAT** (or **Any Antemortem Stature Available**: cadaver, measured, or forensic) performed equally well as FSTAT. They used traditional inverse calibration and calculated prediction intervals and confidence intervals to compare precision and accuracy. The mean squared error represents differences between the actual/reported and the predicted stature, which was used to test the predictability power of the equations (Wilson et al., 2010).

Statistical Methods: Another Case of Apples to Oranges

Although most studies have used least squares regression, Konigsberg and colleagues (1998) point out that it is actually *inverse calibration* regression, because it solves for stature as the dependent variable (y = stature). When Pearson first introduced regression for stature estimation, he also set the trend for using the inverse calibration method (Pearson, 1899). In most other regression analyses in science, the independent variable x will have an effect on the dependent variable y. When stature is used as the y variable, it implies that the bone length measured *causes* stature, which is an improbable causal relationship. Depending on the context, other statistical methods may actually be better (Konigsberg et al., 1998). In allometry literature, stature *is explained by* the size of particular organs/bones (i.e. stature

---

[16]You have probably had your own stature measured many times and by many clinicians, but your driver's license stature is the most easily accessed stature.

is independent). But because stature is the more difficult variable, and bone length the more easily attainable measure, inverse calibration has become the norm for physical anthropology since first developed by Pearson (1899).

Konigsberg and colleagues (1998) point out that this inverse calibration is essentially a **Bayesian** statistical approach, in which an assumption is made that the stature distribution of the reference sample (that which was used to create the formula) is a reasonable prior. Another way to state this is as follows: it is reasonable to presume that the individual for whom we estimate stature likely is a member of the population used to pull the reference sample. If the goal is to estimate stature for an individual that likely comes from the same population, the inverse calibration regression performs with the least amount of bias. The inverse calibration equation shown below in Equation 6.2 does not look like the simple equation of a line presented earlier, because it explicitly includes the population means for femur length and stature, the covariance between stature and femur length, and the variance of femur length. The equation is as follows:

$$\hat{x}_i = \bar{x} + \beta_{xy}(y_i - \bar{y}) \tag{6.2}$$

In this equation, x is stature (the independent variable), $\hat{x}$ is the stature sought; $\bar{x}$ is the population mean, y is the bone length (the dependent variable), $\bar{y}$ is the population mean femur length in which β_{xy} is equal to $\text{cov}(x,y)/V_y$, and $\text{cov}(x,y)$ is the covariance between stature and femur length with V_y being the variance of femur length. Stature is essentially estimated by ordinary least squares.

According to this same statistical review (Konigsberg et al., 1998), classical calibration is the regression of bone length on stature, and then solving for stature or $x = (y-b)/m$. This statistical model is the approach taken in allometry studies and is shown below in Equation 6.3 below. Note that the only difference between equations 6.2 and 6.3 is the negative exponent, hence the "inversion" of the former:

$$\hat{x}_i = \bar{x} + \beta_{xy}^{-1}(y_i - \bar{y}) \tag{6.3}$$

Classical calibration works best when the case involves extrapolation beyond the reference sample limits (e.g., very tall, very short, or proportions different than the reference sample). An example of this might be estimating stature of a fossil hominid or a bioarchaeological specimen when there is not a sizeable or appropriate reference sample for comparison. This could also be necessary in a forensic case when the individual does not come from the reference sample and the proportions could be drastically different. For most forensic cases, however, we can make a strong Bayesian assumption that the stature likely falls within the distribution of some modern contemporary reference sample.

There are three other statistical models that can be used: **Major Axis** (MA), **Reduced Major Axis** (RMA) or a **long bone/stature ratio model**. Konigsberg and colleagues (Konigsberg et al., 1998; Hens et al., 2000) tested all of the above statistical models on a case with **extreme extrapolation**—estimating the stature of the *Australopithecus afarensis* fossil AL 288-1, also known as "Lucy." Lucy's stature was calculated using a modern human reference sample that included a sample of Mbutu Pygmies from West Africa. Lucy's "actual stature" was calculated from a reconstruction of the fossil, comparable to the Fully anatomical method. Konigsberg and colleagues (1998) stated, "The estimates from classical calibration, MA, and the ratio estimator are all fairly close to the anatomical reconstruction of 1,050 mm, while the inverse and RMA estimates are clearly too tall."

This extreme case of extrapolation beyond the mean worked well with classical calibration because it is the **maximum likelihood** estimator, in which the likelihood is proportional to the probability that an individual with a certain stature would have a long bone length that is identical to one existing in the actual population sample (Konigsberg et al., 1998). Therefore, the likelihood is proportional to the probability that the individual of stature x (Lucy) has a long bone equal to one that has already been measured. Konigsberg et al. (1998) make the argument that the femur/stature ratio, RMA, and MA can all be justified as the maximum likelihood estimator. Classical calibration performed the best, and thus is recommended in a case of extreme extrapolation. In most forensic cases, it is a fairly safe bet that it does not involve extrapolation beyond the mean, but this could serve as a good example for work in paleoanthropology or cases in which there is an individual with clear signs of extreme stature reduction or gigantism.

In mathematical stature estimation, one interesting discovery was that the slope or regression coefficient in stature estimation formulae does not seem to vary much between populations. Recall from above that the standard regression equation using inverse calibration is $y = mx + b$, where y = stature, x = bone length, m = slope or the regression coefficient, and b = the y-intercept.[17] Jantz (1992) raises the point that the regression coefficient varies little among populations and within populations, thus, you can use the regression coefficient established by Trotter and Gleser (1952), and then calculate new estimates for the y-intercept using the equation $b = \bar{y} - m\bar{x}$, where $\bar{y}$ and $\bar{x}$ are the population means. Jantz (1992) calculated the mean femur and tibia lengths from the Forensic Databank and inserted them into the above formula as $\bar{y}$ using the regression coefficient from Trotter and Gleser as b. The new calculated y-intercept could then be incorporated into the original Trotter and Gleser equation.

Fragmentary Remains

Incomplete bones are extremely commonplace in bioarchaeology and forensic studies. How then do you estimate stature? Some studies have investigated the proportion of different bone segments compared to the overall bone length; other studies directly compare the bone segment length to stature. To estimate stature from fragmentary remains, it is first necessary to determine which segments of the bones are the most reliable. Gertrude Müller (1935) of Vienna first defined bone segments of the tibia (n = 100), humerus (n = 100), and radius (n = 50), and calculated the proportion of each segment length compared to the entire bone. The bone length estimates were then applied to Manouvrier tables to calculate stature. This research paved the way for stature estimation from bone fragments by defining landmarks on the bones to standardize the bone segments.

Steele and McKern (1969) reworked the Müller method but used the femur, tibia, and humerus. They used the same model of standardized bone segments to estimate the length of long bones from bone fragments. With the landmarks defined, the distance from one

[17]In most statistical programs using statistical regression, the variables will be interpreted as stature = (constant × independent variable) + regression coefficient.

landmark to the next was measured to determine the segment length and the percentage of the total bone length. This research was carried out on a sample of Native American remains from Arkansas using ordinary least-squares regression to get the best possible line to estimate the total length of each bone. This could then be used to estimate stature by applying Trotter and Gleser (1958) and/or Genovés (1967) stature formulae.

Steele (1970) later presented formulae to estimate stature directly from each of the five to six segments, skipping over the step of estimating the length of each individual bone. Each of the bone segments is then regressed on stature using least-squares regression. These equations have a higher standard of error than when using a complete bone, but can be applied if whole bones are unavailable. Steele (1970) also provided age correction formulae.

Bass (1979) complained about the difficulty and inconsistency in finding the landmarks as described by Steele and McKern (1969). To address this concern and improve interobserver error, Simmons et al. (1990) developed a new method for stature estimation from fragmentary femora. They used Martin's measurements from 1957 for the femur (these are the same measurements listed in Buikstra and Ubelaker, 1994), but reduced the number of segments from 16 down to 9. The goal was to estimate the maximum length from each segment and to determine stature directly from the segment. It is more accurate to eliminate the middle step to estimate stature. Simmons et al. (1990) achieved means and standard deviations close to those of Trotter and Gleser (1952) and better than those of Steele and McKern (1969) due to a larger sample size. These revised measures by Simmons et al. (1990) are listed in Box 6.7; see also Figure 6.2.

Bidmos (2008) estimated stature using fragmentary femora of indigenous South Africans. He used 100 skeletons (50 male, 50 female) from the Raymond Dart Collection to create a calibration sample and then another 20 individuals as a test sample. Actual stature was calculated using the Fully method (Fully, 1956). He used only six measurements of the femur, along with maximum length, four of which were the same as those from Simmons et al. (1990), namely: vertical neck diameter (VND), upper breadth of femur (VHA), bicondylar breadth (BCB), and epicondylar breadth (EpB). He added medial condylar length (MCL) and lateral condylar length (LCL) because these two measures are highly reproducible and highly dimorphic. Ten centimeters were added to the stature calculations for "total skeletal height" to account for soft tissues. The resulting standard errors of estimate were only

---

BOX 6.7

SIMMONS ET AL. (1990) REVISED MEASUREMENTS FOR FRAGMENTARY FEMORA

- Maximum femoral length (FML)
- Vertical femoral head diameter (VHD)
- Vertical femoral neck diameter (VND)
- Upper breadth of the femur (VHA)
- Transverse diameter of the midshaft (WSD)

- Bicondylar breadth (BCB)
- Epicondylar breadth (EpB)
- Lateral condyle height (LCH)
- Medial condyle height (MCH)

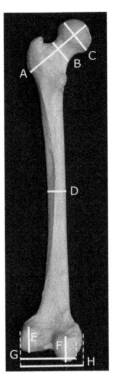

FIGURE 6.2   Bone segments used for stature estimation from fragmentary femora as per Simmons et al. (1990). A. VHA; B. VND; C.VHD; D. WSD; E. LCH; F. MCH; G. BCB; H. EpB. See Box 6.7 for explanation of these abbreviations.

slightly higher (SEE 3.72—4.38 cm) than estimating stature from intact femora (SEE 1.46—1.69 cm). The medial condyle height (MCL) had the highest correlation with total skeletal height in males (r = 0.74; SEE 3.72—4.36 cm). All of the dimensions in females had high correlations with total skeletal height (r = 0.80—0.85; SEE 3.82—4.18 cm) than those for males. Bidmos (2008) concluded that the distal femur measurements produce the best correlations with stature and femur length. Caution is recommended when considering use of these equations for populations other than the ones from which they were derived.

Estimating Stature in Children

Subadult stature estimation from long bones has not been as popular as subadult age estimation from long bones (or rather, diaphyses), for multiple reasons. One of the biggest obstacles when assessing stature is that sex and ancestry are next to impossible to assess in subadult skeletal remains. In addition, there are fortunately not many large samples of known subadult skeletal remains; however, radiographs can be substituted. The regression line in children is also not a straight line, as the bones do not all scale **isometrically** (at the same rate). There could, however, be circumstances in which stature estimation could become essential (as in a mass disaster) and the ability to estimate stature in subadults should not be ignored.

It is important to understand how bones grow in order to meaningfully measure the skeleton of subadults. **Endochondral bone growth** is the manner in which the long bones of the limbs grow from an original cartilage model. The bone first begins to develop *in utero* as a cartilage template of the bone. Primary centers of ossification begin at midshaft, with secondary mineralization occurring at the epiphyses (White and Folkens, 2000). Growth rates are extremely rapid in the first year after birth, decelerate gradually from 1 to 6 years and then are slow and uniform from 6 to 10 years (Bogin, 1988). Rates speed up again during puberty and then growth halts at adulthood when the long bones epiphyses fully fuse (any time between 19 and 25 years) (Bogin, 1988; Scheuer and Black, 2000). See also Uhl (Chapter 3), this volume.

When measuring subadults, the problem of stature estimation is similar to that brought up in the section above on fragmentary bones: What proportion of the whole bone length is the diaphysis versus the epiphysis? In the humerus, the proximal epiphysis is 1.3–2.2% of the total bone length (Seitz, 1923). In the tibia, the proximal epiphysis is 2.4–3.9% of the total bone length and the distal epiphysis makes up 1.8–2.9% of total length (Seitz, 1923). Balthazard and Dervieux (1921) and Smith and Moritz (1939) estimated fetal skeletal stature along with age. Olivier and Pineau (1958, 1960) recalculated these measurements and found that the estimates by Balthazard and Dervieux only worked postnatally, which is not necessarily a problem because we would only be interested in calculating stature or length for babies who have been born. This study also found that all the major long bones worked equally well and that the combining of two or more bones did not improve accuracy (Olivier and Pineau, 1958, 1960). Olivier (1969) estimated stature using the femoral diaphysis, with no account of population or sex. Telkkä et al. (1962) used radiographs of 3848 Finnish children (up to 15 years old) to measure the diaphyseal lengths. They realized the need to create separate age groups, as allometric growth is not consistent in each age group.

For children 10–15 years old, stature correlates linearly with all six long bones (humerus, radius, ulna, femur, tibia, fibula). For children aged 1–9 years, the correlation is linear with all of the bones, except for the femur, which requires a **logarithmic transformation**. The femur appears to be the exception (perhaps due to the evolutionary significance of bipedalism in our species) and does not scale isometrically to (at the same rate as) the other bones. If the regression of a bone length to stature is more of a curved line, transforming the line logarithmically can improve the correlation. For children under one year, all of the bones must be log transformed. Himes et al. (1977) found that the metacarpals correlate well with stature in children from rural Guatemala, using a least-squares regression method. In this study, 1597 radiographs of the left hand and wrist were studied longitudinally. Surprisingly (and fortunately), the growth of the metacarpals seemed to be unaffected by the environment, even when severe malnutrition had occurred.[18]

The more common use for long bone length in juveniles is to assess age (İşcan, 1988), which has been extensively studied in fetuses and subadults by Fazekas and Kósa (1966, 1978) and later by Scheuer and Black (2000, 2004). Fazekas and Kósa (1966, 1978) measured the remains of 138 Hungarian fetal skeletons of known age, sex, and height, 3–10 lunar months. They developed regression formulae for body height to bone length. Mehta and

---

[18]With chronic malnutrition, stature is significantly shorter from one generation to the next (Himes et al., 1977; Bogin, 1988).

Sing (1972) provided regression equations for crown–rump length from 50 fetuses. The age estimation of subadult remains is addressed by Uhl (Chapter 3), this volume.

CASE STUDIES: STATURE ESTIMATION

Case Study: Colombia

The forensic anthropologists in Colombia each see hundreds of cases each year; as a result, they have very little time to conduct independent research. There are currently no population standards in common use for stature, sex, or age estimation for modern Colombians. To estimate stature for forensic cases, Colombian scientists typically resort to the Trotter and Gleser (1952, 1958) "Mongoloid" or the Genovés (1967) Mesoamerican formulae for females. Neither of these population samples accurately reflects the population of modern Colombians who exhibit a high degree of mixed ancestry (Indigenous, European, African), and many of whom (particularly the population from which the majority of forensic cases are drawn) have environmental and sociocultural obstacles, such as proper nutrition and access to medical care.

Starting in 2009, a Colombian forensic anthropologist named Dr. César Sanabria decided to remedy this problem by developing a known modern Colombian skeletal collection. Working for the National Institute of Legal Medicine and Forensic Sciences in Bogotá, he contacted local cemeteries and received permission to curate those individuals unclaimed by family members after the standard 4-year burial period had elapsed. The alternative fate of unclaimed remains is cremation or the bones are placed in an ossuary (Sanabria and DiGangi, 2011). (Remains that are "claimed" in this sense are those for which family members continue to pay fees to the cemetery for burial.) This is a common practice in cemeteries around the world. Sanabria and the Institute were granted permission to curate the skeletal remains for use as a study collection (unless a family member were to come forward to claim the remains). This is one of the largest modern collections of identified human skeletal remains in South America and has the potential to provide a wealth of information about the modern Colombian population.

In February of 2011, a team of four American anthropologists and 30 Colombian forensic anthropologists, odontologists, and pathologists convened in Bogotá to conduct a massive research endeavor utilizing the new Colombian Modern Skeletal Collection. The researchers split into separate teams to collect the various types of skeletal data (i.e., craniometrics, **postcranial metrics**, sexing, aging, etc.). The first author of this chapter helped to organize the postcranial metrics team. All of the measurements were taken according to procedures outlined in Buikstra and Ubelaker's *Standards for Data Collection from Human Skeletal Remains* (1994). All of the descriptions had been translated into Spanish for this endeavor. Each of the seven researchers on the postcranial metrics team was responsible for a separate task. Two researchers measured all of the bones of a subset of 30 individuals, in order to provide an estimate of interobserver error, one researcher measured all of the tibiae and fibulae, another researcher measured the humeri, radii, and ulnae, etc. Each bone was measured three times by a single researcher and the average measurement was then recorded. At the end of each day, the handwritten measurements were entered into a spreadsheet, which was double-checked for accuracy in transcription.

Given that antemortem information is available about age, sex, stature (from ID cards), date of birth, place of birth, etc., this was a perfect opportunity to develop a set of stature formulae to serve as the reference sample for Colombian forensic cases. The sample consisted of 126 individuals (44 females, 81 males) with a mean age of 47 years. All of the long bones of the upper and lower limbs were included in univariate inverse regression formulae and the best multivariate regression equations were calculated using a stepwise procedure. The equation from the femur for males (Stature = (Femur*2.46) + 5.9004 +/− 3.760) has a high correlation ($r = 0.857$). The equation from the femur for females (Stature = (Femur*1.787) + 83.592 +/− 4.951) has a much lower correlation ($r = 0.692$). The best multivariate equation for males was from the femur and tibia combined (Stature = (Tibia*1.592) + (Femur*0.967) + 67.348 +/− 3.091; $r = 0.891$, adjusted $R2 = 0.784$). The best equation for the females was a univariate equation from the fibula (Stature = (Fibula*2.183) + 93.170 +/− 5.065; $r = 0.697$; adjusted $R2 = 0.460$). These results indicate that the sample size for the males is sufficient for reliable stature equations, but the sample size for the females should be larger to improve the correlations for reliability in forensic stature estimation. These results are still preliminary, due to the small sample size, especially of females. At this writing, the sample has grown to over 500 individuals and a second phase of data collection has been planned in order to increase the sample size for stature estimation, among other research endeavors.

Case Study: Chile

Sutphin and Ross (2011) compared stature estimates of modern Chilean juveniles to European American juvenile stature estimates derived using equations developed by Ruff (2007) and Smith (2007). Chileans are also an admixed population. However, the ethnohistorical origins are quite different exhibiting indigenous or native South American and European ancestries. The juvenile Chilean sample ($n = 38$) consists of known individuals from the Cementerio General with death dates between 1950 and 1970. Significant differences were observed for the teenage years for the femur (Figure 6.3), tibia (13−15 years), and humerus (16−17 years). This suggests that there is either a populational or nutritional difference in growth trajectories in the teenage years between Chilean and European American children. However, the younger or preteen age groups (4−6 and 7−9 years) showed no significant differences and thus, equations derived from American children can be utilized to predict stature in the younger age categories, but not for the teenage years.

FUTURE RESEARCH IN STATURE ESTIMATION

A recent meta-analysis on stature estimation for the last ten years found the most accurate predictors of stature continue to be the femur and tibia, the coefficient of correlation for which ranges from 0.82 to 0.93 (SEE 2.4−4.0 cm) for both males and females (Moore and Richter, 2012). Thirty of the cited studies in the meta-analysis compare the long bones of the upper and lower limbs. Fifteen of the studies compare the measurements of the hands or feet (fleshed, radiographic, tarsals, or metacarpals/metatarsals). The vertebrae are the next most commonly

6. STATURE ESTIMATION

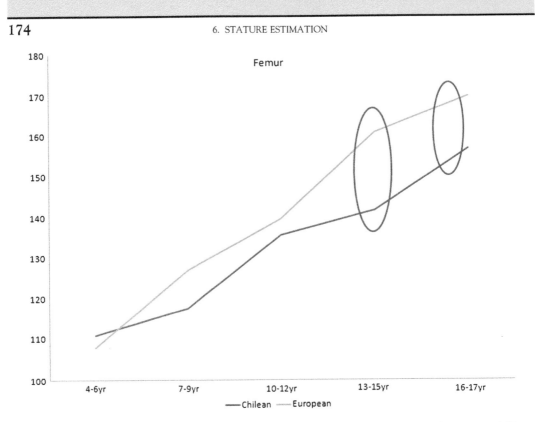

FIGURE 6.3 Difference in growth trajectories of the femur by year of age in Chilean and European children.

used elements to estimate stature. A handful of the studies in the meta-analysis look at measurements of the cranium, face, or dentition, but with little success ($r < 0.06$, SEE > 5.0 cm) and so should be avoided. Not surprisingly, the cranial sutures had the lowest success ($r = 0.09-0.363$) as there is no direct association between cranial sutures and living height! Multiple regression yields higher results than simple linear regression. Stature formulae for males tend to have higher correlations than those for females (Moore and Richter, 2012).

What Method Should You Use?

Bioarchaeology

The problem with prehistoric populations is that no known contemporary reference sample formulae are representative. Sciulli (1990) conducted a stature study for pre-Columbian populations from the Ohio River valley. They used the original Fully method as their actual stature on which they regressed the long bone lengths. They found that Trotter and Gleser overestimated stature due to different body proportions of their population sample (Sciulli et al., 1990). Auerbach and Ruff (2010) agreed with Sciulli et al. (1990) that the existing regression equations were not appropriate for the diversity of Indigenous North American populations. The designation of "Mongoloid" by Trotter and Gleser was not appropriate. They therefore sampled 967 skeletons from 75 archaeological sites and created three groupings to better differentiate the climatic and altitude allometric proportions. These groups include (1) high latitude/Arctic, (2) temperate, and (3) Great Plains. Auerbach and Ruff (2010) used the revised Fully method as a proxy for living stature, as it has shown to be successful universally. These formulae were then used to test their sex-specific regression equations based on single elements (Auerbach and Ruff, 2010).

Forensic Anthropology

In a forensic context, a Bayesian model or the use of informative or known priors should be the preferred model for stature estimation. Basically, Bayesian inference uses both *unconditional* (or the prior probability of a given stature being in the target sample) and *conditional* (the probability of obtaining the observed long bone length conditional on a given stature from the reference sample) probabilities to produce an informed parameter (Ross and Kimmerle, 2010). For example, Ross and Konigsberg (2002) used the knowledge that Eastern Europeans are taller than European Americans as a "known prior" in developing population-specific equations for the Balkans (Ross and Konigsberg, 2002).

CONCLUSION

There are many populations around the world in need of population-specific stature formulae, and thus, many opportunities for new research to be conducted in stature estimation. Accurate stature estimation requires that relevant formulae be developed that are population, age, sex, and temporally specific. Not only do body proportions vary around the world, but secular change can cause variations in stature and proportions from one generation to the next within a population. Most new research should focus on developing formulae for mathematical stature estimation from the long bones, vertebrae, or long bone fragments. Universal applicability of the revised Fully method (Raxter et al., 2006) has been demonstrated, but should be further tested in other populations.

Stature estimation is necessary in both bioarchaeological and forensic contexts. For a bioarchaeological researcher, if you have access to samples that are sufficiently large with skeletons intact, testing your new mathematical regression formulae against stature estimations based on the revised Fully method (Raxter et al., 2006) is the best option; however, this method is not very practical for forensic applications. When the entire skeleton is available, the revised Fully method is the most accurate method for stature estimation. In developing a mathematical method, the leg bones are the next best estimator of stature. If the leg bones are unavailable or fragmentary, try testing the Simmons et al. (1990) method to estimate stature from a fragment of the bone. If you only have smaller elements, the metacarpals have shown good success. For developing formulae for contemporary populations using known modern skeletal collections, use of a Bayesian statistical approach is advised. If there are only a few incomplete and isolated individuals that seem abnormally large or small, follow the advice for stature estimation with extreme extrapolation by Konigsberg and colleagues (1998).

Despite the seemingly overabundance of studies to estimate stature, new studies are always needed. Do your homework and investigate different collections around the U.S. or around the world that are available for study. Before jumping headfirst into your own research, try jumping at an opportunity to get involved in someone else's research, either in the field or in a lab. By getting involved in skeletal biology field and/or lab research, you can gain experience recognizing human variation, learn logistical and methodological skills for data collection/analysis, and make valuable connections with professors and graduate students. These field and lab research opportunities will help you open doors and gain the competence and confidence to pursue a research project of your own. As a student of anthropology, you probably have few reservations about travelling overseas to study a skeletal collection. Before you go off on a big research adventure domestically or abroad, it is better to have your project methodology outlined in terms of both data collection and statistical analysis. Will you measure every bone or just the left femora and tibiae? Will you include or exclude the malleolus in your tibial measurements? Will you be able to incorporate the revised Fully method to validate your new stature formulae? Developing new stature formulae and testing the validity of these formulae on independent samples will help improve our results for stature estimation to build the biological profile of unidentified human skeletal remains in both forensic and bioarchaeological contexts.

ACKNOWLEDGMENTS

I (MKM) would like to thank my husband and newborn infant son, along with all my students and colleagues for their patience throughout this long and grueling process. This project would not have happened without the motivation and inspiration from my collaborator and dear friend Dr. Elizabeth DiGangi.

REFERENCES

Abrahamyan, D.O., Gazarian, A., Braillon, P.M., 2008. Estimation of stature and length of limb segments in children and adolescents from whole-body dual-energy X-ray absorptiometry scans. Pediatric Radiology 38 (3), 311−315.

Allbrook, D., 1961. The estimation of stature in British and East African males. Based on tibial and ulnar bone lengths. Journal of Forensic Medicine 8, 15−28.

Auerbach, B.M., Ruff, C.B., 2010. Stature estimation formulae for indigenous North American populations. American Journal of Physical Anthropology 141 (2), 190−207.

Balthazard, I., Dervieux, A., 1921. [Anthropological study on the human fetus]. Annales de Médecine Légale 1, 37−42.

Bass, W.M., 1979. Developments in the identification of human skeletal material (1968−1978). American Journal of Physical Anthropology 51 (4), 555−562.

Bertillon, A., 1885. [Anthropometric Identification]. Melun, France, 65.

Bidmos, M., 2005. On the non-equivalence of documented cadaver lengths to living stature estimates based on Fully's method on bones in the Raymond A. Dart Collection. Journal of Forensic Sciences 50 (3), 501−506.

Bidmos, M., 2006. Adult stature reconstruction from the calcaneus of South Africans of European descent. Journal of Clinical Forensic Medicine 13 (5), 247−252.

Bidmos, M., 2008. Stature reconstruction using fragmentary femora in South Africans of European descent. Journal of Forensic Sciences 53 (5), 1044−1048.

Bogin, B., 1988. Patterns of Human Growth. Cambridge University Press, New York.

Breitinger, E., 1937. [Assessment of stature from the length of limb bones]. Anthropologischer Anzeiger 14, 249−274.

Büchi, E.C., 1950. [Changes in limb proportions of adult humans]. Anthropologische Forschungen 1, 1−44.

Buikstra, J.E., Ubelaker, D.H., 1994. Standards for data collection from human skeletal remains: Proceedings of a seminar at the Field Museum of Natural History, organized by Jonathan Haas. Arkansas Archeological Survey, Fayetteville, AR.

Cardoso, H.F., 2009. A test of three methods for estimating stature from immature skeletal remains using long bone lengths. Journal of Forensic Sciences 54 (1), 13–19.

Černý, M., Komenda, S., 1982. Reconstruction of body height based on humerus and femur lengths. Second Anthropological Congress of Ales Hrdlička, Universita Carolina Pragensis, 475–479.

Dupertuis, C.W., Hadden Jr., J.A., 1951. On the reconstruction of stature from long bones. American Journal of Physical Anthropology 9 (1), 15–53.

Dwight, T., 1894. Methods of estimating the height from parts of the skeleton. Medical Record N.Y. 46, 293–296.

Fazekas, I.G., Kósa, F., 1966a. [Current contribution and comparative studies of the determination of fetal body length on the basis of diaphyseal measurement of the bones of the extremities]. Deutsche Zeitschrift für die Gerichtliche Medizin 58 (2), 142–160.

Fazekas, I.G., Kósa, F., 1966b. Determination of the size of embryos from the dimension of the radius. Annales de Médine Légale, Criminologie, Police Scientifique et Toxicologie 46 (4), 262–272.

Feldesman, M.R., Fountain, R.L., 1996. Race specificity and the femur/stature ratio. American Journal of Physical Anthropology 100 (2), 207–224.

Feldesman, M.R., Lundy, J.K., 1988. Stature estimates for some Plio-Pleistocene fossil hominids. Journal of Human Evolution 17 (3), 583–596.

Feldesman, M.R., Kleckner, J.G., Lundy, J.K., 1990. Femur/stature ratio and estimates of stature in mid- and late-Pleistocene fossil hominids. American Journal of Physical Anthropology 83 (3), 359–372.

Freedman, B.J., 1978. Patterns of response to bronchodilators in asthma. British Journal of Diseases of the Chest 72 (2), 95–107.

Fully, G., 1956. [New method of determination of height]. Annales de Médine Légale, Criminologie, Police Scientifique et Toxicologie 36 (5), 266–273.

Fully, G., Pineau, H., 1960. [Determination of the height by means of the skeleton]. Annales de Médine Légale, Criminologie, Police Scientifique et Toxicologie 40, 145–153.

Galloway, A., 1988. Estimating actual height in the older individual. Journal of Forensic Sciences 33 (1), 126–136.

Genoves, S., 1967. Proportionality of the long bones and their relation to stature among Mesoamericans. American Journal of Physical Anthropology 26 (1), 67–77.

Giannecchini, M., Moggi-Cecchi, J., 2008. Stature in archeological samples from central Italy: methodological issues and diachronic changes. American Journal of Physical Anthropology 135 (3), 284–292.

Giles, E., Hutchinson, D.L., 1991. Stature- and age-related bias in self-reported stature. Journal of Forensic Sciences 36, 765–780.

Giroux, C.L., Wescott, D.J., 2008. Stature estimation based on dimensions of the bony pelvis and proximal femur. Journal of Forensic Sciences 53 (1), 65–68.

Hens, S.M., Konigsberg, L.W., Jungers, W.L., 2000. Estimating stature in fossil hominids: which regression model and reference sample to use? Journal of Human Evolution 38 (6), 767–784.

Himes, J.H., Yarbrough, C., Martorell, R., 1977. Estimation of stature in children from radiographically determined metacarpal length. Journal of Forensic Sciences 22 (2), 452–455.

Holliday, T.W., Ruff, C.B., 1997. Ecogeographical patterning and stature prediction in fossil hominids: Comment on M.R. Feldesman and R.L. Fountain, American Journal of Physical Anthropology (1996) 100:207–224. American Journal of Physical Anthropology 103 (1), 137–140.

Hooton, E.A., 1947. Up from the Ape (revised edition). MacMillan, New York.

Hrdlička, A., 1939. Practical Anthropometry. Wistar, Philadelphia, PA.

İşcan, M.Y., 1988. Wilton Marion Krogman, Ph.D. (1903-1987): the end of an era. Journal of Forensic Sciences 33 (6), 1473–1476.

Jantz, R.L., 1992. Modification of the Trotter and Gleser female stature estimation formulae. Journal of Forensic Sciences 37 (5), 1230–1235.

Jantz, R.L., Hunt, D.R., Meadows, L., 1995. The measure and mismeasure of the tibia: implications for stature estimation. Journal of Forensic Sciences 40 (5), 758–761.

Jit, I., Singh, S., 1956. Estimation of stature from clavicles. Indian Journal of Medical Research 44, 137–155.

Kalia, S., Shetty, S.K., Patil, K., Mahima, V.G., 2008. Stature estimation using odontometry and skull anthropometry. Indian Journal of Dental Research 19 (2), 150–154.

Komar, D., Buikstra, J., 2009. Forensic Anthropology. Contemporary Theory and Practice. Oxford University Press, Oxford, p.132.

Konigsberg, L.W., Hens, S.M., Jantz, L.M., Jungers, W.L., 1998. Stature estimation and calibration: Bayesian and maximum likelihood perspectives in physical anthropology. American Journal of Physical Anthropology (Suppl. 27), 65—92.

Konigsberg, L.W., Ross, A.H., Jungers, W.L., 2006. Estimation and evidence in forensic anthropology. Determining stature. In: Schmitt, A., Cunha, E., Pinheiro, J. (Eds.), Forensic Anthropology and Medicine. Complementary Sciences. From Recovery to Cause of Death. Humana Press, New Jersey, pp. 317—331.

Krogman, W.M., İşcan, M.Y., 1986. The Human Skeleton in Forensic Medicine. C.C. Thomas, Springfield, IL.

Li, M.X., Liu, P.Y., Li, Y.M., Qin, Y.J., Liu, Y.Z., Deng, H.W., 2004. A major gene model of adult height is suggested in Chinese. Journal of Human Genetics 49 (3), 148—153.

Lundy, J.K., 1983. Regression equations for estimating living stature from long limb bones in South African Negro. South African Journal of Science 779, 337—338.

Lundy, J.K., 1988. A report on the use of Fully's anatomical method to estimate stature in military skeletal remains. Journal of Forensic Sciences 33 (2), 534—539.

Macdonnel, W.R., 1901. On criminal anthropometry and the identification of criminals. Biometrika 1, 177—227.

Macgregor, S., Cornes, B.K., Martin, N.G., Visscher, P.M., 2006. Bias, precision and heritability of self-reported and clinically measured height in Australian twins. Human Genetics 120 (4), 571—580.

Manouvrier, L., 1892. [Determination of height from the long bones of the limbs]. Revue mensuelle de l'École d'Anthropologie 2, 227—233.

Meadows, L., Jantz, R.L., 1995. Allometric secular change in the long bones from the 1800s to the present. Journal of Forensic Sciences 40 (5), 762—767.

Mehta, L., Singh, H.M., 1972. Determination of crown—rump length from fetal long bones: Humerus and femur. American Journal of Physical Anthropology 36, 165—168.

Mendes-Correa, A.A., 1932. La taille des Portugais d'après les os longes. Anthropologie 10, 268—272.

Moore, M.K., Richter, S., 2012. Meta-analysis of forensic stature estimation. Published Abstract. American Journal of Physical Anthropology, 147 (S542), 217.

Müller, G., 1935. Zur bestimmung der Lange beschadigter extremitatenknochen. Anthropologisxher Anzeiger 12, 70—72.

Musgrave, J.H., Harneja, N.K., 1978. The estimation of adult stature from metacarpal bone length. American Journal of Physical Anthropology 48 (1), 113—119.

Olivier, G., 1969. Practical Anthropology. Charles C. Thomas, Springfield, IL.

Olivier, G., Pineau, H., 1958. [Determination of age from a fetus and from an embryo]. Archives d'Anatomie (La Semaine des Hôpitaux) 6, 21—28.

Olivier, G., Pineau, H., 1960. [New determination of fetal length from the diaphyses of the long bones]. Annales de Médecine Legale 40, 141—144.

Ousley, S., 1995. Should we estimate biological or forensic stature? Journal of Forensic Sciences 40 (5), 768—773.

Pearson, K., 1899. Mathematical contributions to the theory of evolution: on the reconstruction of stature of prehistoric races. Philosophical Transactions A 192, 169—244.

Perola, M., Sammalisto, S., Hiekkalinna, T., Martin, N.G., Visscher, P.M., Montgomery, G.W., et al., 2007. Combined genome scans for body stature in 6,602 European twins: evidence for common Caucasian loci. PLoS Genetics 3 (6), e97.

Raxter, M.H., Auerbach, B.M., Ruff, C.B., 2006. Revision of the Fully technique for estimating statures. American Journal of Physical Anthropology 130 (3), 374—384.

Rollet, E., 1888. [On the measurement of the long bones of the limbs]. Thèses pour le doctorat en médecine, lière series, Université de Lyon, 1—128.

Ross, A.H., Kimmerle, E.H., 2010. Contribution of quantitative methods in forensic anthropology: a new era. In: Blau, S., Ubelaker, D. (Eds.), Handbook of Forensic Anthropology and Archaeology. Left Coast Press, Walnut Creek, pp. 479—489.

Ross, A.H., Konigsberg, L.W., 2002. New formulae for estimating stature in the Balkans. Journal of Forensic Sciences 47 (1), 165—167.

Ross, A.H., Baker, L.E., Falsetti, A., 2003. Sexual dimorphism a proxy for environmental sensitivity? A multi-temporal view. Journal of the Washington Academy of Science 89, 1—12.

Ruff, C.B., 2007. Body size prediction from juvenile skeletal remains. American Journal of Physical Anthropology 133, 698—716.

Ruff, C.B., Walker, A., 1993. Body size and body shape. In: Walker, A., Leakey, R.E. (Eds.), The Nariokotome Homo erectus skeleton. Harvard University Press, Cambridge, MA, pp. 234—265.

Ryan, I., Bidmos, M.A., 2007. Skeletal height reconstruction from measurements of the skull in indigenous South Africans. Forensic Science International 167 (1), 16–21.

Scheuer, L., Black, S.M., 2000. Developmental Juvenile Osteology. Academic Press, San Diego.

Scheuer, L., Black, S.M., 2004. The Juvenile Skeleton. Elsevier Academic Press, London.

Sciulli, P.W., Schneider, K.N., Mahaney, M.C., 1990. Stature estimation in prehistoric Native Americans of Ohio. American Journal of Physical Anthropology 83 (3), 275–280.

Shulin, P., Fangwu, Z., 1983. Estimation of stature from skull, clavicle, scapula and os coxa of male adult of Southern China. Acta Anthropologica Sinica 2, 253–259.

Seitz, R.P., 1923. Relation of epiphyseal length to bone length. American Journal of Physical Anthropology 6, 37–49.

Simmons, T., Jantz, R.L., Bass, W.M., 1990. Stature estimation from fragmentary femora: a revision of the Steele method. Journal of Forensic Sciences 35 (3), 628–636.

Singh, B., Sohal, H.S., 1952. Estimation of stature from clavicles in Punjabis. A preliminary report. Indian Journal of Medical Research 40, 67–71.

Smith, S., Moritz, A.R., 1939. Forensic Medicine, 2nd Edition. Little, Brown and Company, Boston.

Smith, S.L., 2007. Stature estimation of 3–10-year-old children from long bone lengths. Journal of Forensic Sciences 52 (3), 538–546.

Snow, C.C., Williams, J., 1971. Variation in premortem statural measurements compared to statural estimates of skeletal remains. Journal of Forensic Sciences 16, 455–464.

Steele, D.G., 1970. Estimation of stature from fragments of long limb bones. In: Stewart, T.D. (Ed.), Personal Identification in Mass Disasters. Smithsonian Institution, Washington, DC, pp. 85–97.

Steele, D.G., McKern, T.W., 1969. A method for assessment of maximum long bone length and living stature from fragmentary long bones. American Journal of Physical Anthropology 31 (2), 215–227.

Stevenson, P., 1929. On racial differences in stature long bone regression formulae, with special reference to stature reconstruction formulae for the Chinese. Biometrika 21, 303–318.

Stewart, T.D., 1979. Essentials of Forensic Anthropology, Especially as Developed in the United States. Charles C. Thomas, Springfield, IL.

Stini, W.A., 1975. Adaptive strategies of human populations under nutritional stress. In: Watts, E.S., Johnston, F.E., Lasker, G.W. (Eds.), Biosocial Interrelations in Population Adaptation. Mouton, The Hague, pp. 19–42.

Sutphin, R., Ross, A.H., 2011. Juvenile stature estimation: a Chilean perspective. In: Ross, A.H., Abel, S. (Eds.), The Juvenile Skeleton in Forensic Abuse Investigations. Springer, New York, pp. 167–177.

Telkka, A., 1950. On the prediction of human stature from the long bones. Acta Anatomica (Basel) 9 (1-2), 103–117.

Telkka, A., Palkama, A., Virtama, P., 1962. Estimation of stature from radiographs of long bones in children. Annales Medicinae Experimentalis et Biologiae Fenniae 40, 91–96.

Trotter, M., Gleser, G., 1951a. The effect of ageing on stature. American Journal of Physical Anthropology 9 (3), 311–324.

Trotter, M., Gleser, G.C., 1951b. Trends in stature of American whites and Negroes born between 1840 and 1924. American Journal of Physical Anthropology 9 (4), 427–440.

Trotter, M., Gleser, G.C., 1952. Estimation of stature from long bones of American Whites and Negroes. American Journal of Physical Anthropology 10 (4), 463–514.

Trotter, M., Gleser, G.C., 1958. A re-evaluation of estimation of stature based on measurements of stature taken during life and of long bones after death. American Journal of Physical Anthropology 16 (1), 79–123.

Vercellotti, G., Agnew, A.M., Justus, H.M., Sciulli, P.W., 2009. Stature estimation in an early medieval (XI–XII c.) Polish population: testing the accuracy of regression equations in a bioarcheological sample. American Journal of Physical Anthropology 140 (1), 135–142.

White, T.D., Folkens, P.A., 2000. Human Osteology. Academic Press, San Diego.

Willey, P., Falsetti, T., 1991. Inaccuracy of height information on driver's licenses. Journal of Forensic Sciences 36 (3), 813–819.

Wilson, R.J., Herrmann, N.P., Jantz, L.M., 2010. Evaluation of stature estimation from the database for forensic anthropology. Journal of Forensic Sciences 55 (3), 684–689.

Yung-hao, W., Chia-ying, Ping-Cheng, H., 1979. [Estimation of stature from long bones of Chinese male adults in South-west District]. Acta Anatomica Sinica 10, 1–6.

7

Paleopathology

Maria Ostendorf Smith

INTRODUCTION

The study of disease, nutritional deprivation, and mechanical stress in human remains recovered from archaeological contexts is called **paleopathology**.[1] It includes the examination of mummified remains as well as skeletonized material. Paleopathology has a long history of scholarly interest, but not a very long history as an investigative tool. This use is a phenomenon of the late twentieth century. It developed very quickly out of a constellation of **paradigm** shifts that occurred after 1950 that reflected a maturing of anthropology as a discipline (Washburn, 1951; Armelagos, 1997, 2011; Buikstra, 1977a; Buikstra and Cook, 1980; Angel, 1981; Armelagos et al., 1982; Armelagos and Van Gerven, 2003; Cook and Powell, 2006; Marks, 2010; Relethford, 2010). These shifts included the abandonment of **racial typology** as a primary, if not exclusive, tool of skeletal analysis (Armelagos and Van Gerven, 2003; Cook and Powell, 2006; also see DiGangi and Moore [Chapter 1] and DiGangi and Hefner [Chapter 5], this volume). This abandonment of the physical "type" or discrete "race" logically redirected physical anthropological research of human biological diversity in the direction of the role of **plasticity** (e.g., growth, maturation, and malnutrition) in determining apparent physiological differences between ethnic groups (Hulse, 1981; Marks, 2000; Roberts, 1995). This information provided support for the causative role of **physiological stressors** such as nutritional deprivation, culture (e.g., weaning practices, sex roles, slavery), chronic disease, and the various kinds of reactive bone that had long been observed on human skeletal material (known collectively as the **biocultural approach**) (Goodman et al., 1988; DiGangi and Moore [Chapter 1], this volume). Determining the causal or **synergistic** connection of bone pathology to stressors has been an active part of skeletal analysis since the late 1960s (e.g., Carlson et al., 1974; Mensforth et al., 1978; Stuart-Macadam, 1992; Wapler et al., 2004; Walker et al., 2009).

The co-association of pathological conditions with life stressors acquired an interpretive context in the late 1960s with the development of **processual archaeology** (Binford and Binford, 1968; Willey and Phillips, 1958). This paradigm shift directed archaeological analysis away from cataloging and creating cultural chronologies (timelines) toward reconstructing human societies using the material archaeological record to engage in hypothesis testing.

---

[1] All bolded terms are defined in the glossary at the end of this volume.

Dubbed the "New Archaeology," it emerged during a time of fundamental methodological reassessment within the small community of scholars interested in assessing skeletal pathology (e.g., Goldstein, 1963; Jarcho, 1966; Putschar, 1966; Stewart, 1966; Stewart and Quade, 1969).These scholars argued for a shift towards skeletal sample-based (i.e., rather than individual case-based) analysis, better bone-based criteria for **differential diagnosis** (defined later on), and greater visibility of paleopathological research (as it was consistently buried in the appendix of site reports).

A directional shift was already underway as (1) the study of disease was analytically being linked with culture history (e.g., Angel, 1966), (2) diagnostic texts such as D.R. Brothwell's *Digging up Bones* (1963), Calvin Wells' *Bones, Bodies, and Disease* (1964), and D.R. Brothwell and A.T. Sandison's *Diseases in Antiquity* (1967) were published, and (3) skeletal sample-based analysis was being conducted (e.g., Angel, 1981; Armelagos, 1968). By 1970, the methodological merging of processual archaeology, **analytical paleopathology,** and the biocultural approach had redefined skeletal analysis.

A pivotal decade for skeletal analysis was 1970—1980. Within this decade, a number of key studies revealed unexpected co-associations of subsistence strategy and the health prevalence of certain pathologies (e.g., **porotic hyperostosis, cribra orbitalia, linear enamel hypoplasia,** and **nonspecific infection**), which indicated that the transition to agriculture was not the presumed surplus-producing, population increase facilitating, cost—benefit basis for civilization as had been thought (e.g., Armelagos, 1968; Armelagos and Dewey, 1970; Lallo 1972; Cassidy, 1972; Cook, 1976; Lallo et al., 1977, 1978; Buikstra, 1977b; Lallo and Rose, 1979; Buikstra and Cook, 1980; Diamond, 1987). Indeed, this first generation research culminated in must-read titles such as *Disease and Death at Dr. Dickson's Mounds* (Goodman and Armelagos, 1985) and *Paleopathology at the Origins of Agriculture* (Cohen and Armelagos, 1984). By the end of the decade, analytical paleopathology had been subsumed under a new label: **bioarchaeology** (Buikstra, 1977b). Paleopathology as currently defined focuses on disease diagnostics, quantification, and antiquity; analytical paleopathology (in addition to paleodemography, mortuary analysis, trace element analysis, etc.) is part of bioarchaeology.

The growth of bioarchaeology in the ensuing decades has been exponential (Larsen, 1997; Steckel and Rose, 2005; Buikstra and Beck, 2006; Grauer, 2012). Every year new studies build piecemeal toward a more comprehensive socioeconomic and temporal picture of various regional historic and prehistoric human populations. For most cultural contexts, this is an ongoing research trajectory that has not yet reached, much less exceeded, its probative limits.

The Osteological Paradox

There are several interpretive cautions in analytical paleopathology with respect to the community health implications, social meaning, and economic context of any given pathology. The first of these cautions is outlined in a publication entitled *"The osteological paradox: Problems of inferring prehistoric health from skeletal samples"* (Wood et al., 1992) and addressed in subsequent discussions (Wood et al., 1992; Jackes, 1993; Byers, 1994; Cohen et al., 1994; Mendonça de Souza et al., 2003; Wright and Yoder, 2003). Wood and colleagues outline three issues: (1) the demographic meaning of the skeletal sample (Konigsberg and Frankenberg [Chapter 11], this volume); (2) congruence of the pathological state of the dead and the population they derive from; and (3) the differential vulnerability—frailty of individuals. The age-at-death distribution is the framework upon which pathologies are evaluated. Certainly age estimates must be robustly determined, but cemeteries are an accumulation of the dead and pathology prevalence in these individuals may not reflect the prevalence of health stress in the living population.

With regard to the second point, the scholar must be mindful that conclusive statements about community health are relative (between samples, between subsistence strategies, between **age cohorts**, between the sexes) and not necessarily indicative. Along these lines, the health status of an individual may also be misleading. The individual who lives long enough for a disease process to disseminate to bone may demonstrate resiliency in contrast to an individual who, without osteological evidence of illness, dies at the acute stage. The latter may give a false impression of good community health. Therefore it is necessary to control for age-at-death, that is, compare by same skeletal age cohorts. If it is possible, the disease process should be identified as active or healed at death. The scholar must be aware of when the health status marker manifests itself. For example, **cribra orbitalia** is a marker of childhood stress (Stuart-Macadam, 1985; Stuart-Macadam and Kent, 1992). Adults with cribra are therefore survivors of this childhood stress.

Differential vulnerability to disease (frailty), the third point, is difficult to identify or quantify. There are, however, nonpathological data variables that can be marshaled to provide the extenuating circumstances that synergistically increase the likelihood of frailty. These include evidence of a poor-quality diet (e.g., through trace element analysis, isotope analysis, see Bethard [Chapter 15], this volume) and compromised growth (rate of long bone growth) (see Wright and Yoder, 2003; Uhl [Chapter 3], this volume). Certainly multiple stress indicators should be assessed together to address the issues raised by the osteological paradox. But if for whatever reason(s) this is not possible, analytical paleopathology should always consider alternative explanations and suggest avenues for future research.

Post-processualism and Agency Theory

Bioarchaeology as a research methodology is certainly an offshoot of (the New) processual archaeology, as already discussed. However, since the 1980s, there have been criticisms of its essentially exclusive adherence to external or environmental causal variables (e.g., climate, agricultural intensification; population growth) and systems theory (variables are interconnected components that create a system) to explain culture change (e.g., Hodder and Hudson, 2003; Trigger, 2006). This approach certainly limited the avenues of explanation and, among other things, negated the social role(s) individuals play in self-determination. This reaction has come to be known as **post-processualism**. In turn post-processualism has been criticized as being cross-disciplinary social-science rhetoric, nonscientific, and devoid of method (e.g., Bintliff, 1993; Arnold and Wilkens, 2001).

Bioarchaeology has essentially sidestepped the theoretical criticisms of processualism for three main reasons: (1) because of its medical underpinnings; (2) because it draws data and explanation from multiple disciplines; and (3) probably because skeletal analysis remains peripheral to problem solving within archaeology (e.g., Bentley et al., 2009). However, there are more measured assessments of processualism and post-processualism (e.g., Kosso, 1991; Huffman, 2004; Trigger, 2006; Bentley et al., 2009) and what has positively emerged are multiple lenses through which material culture and, by extension, health stress indicators may be evaluated. This includes **agency theory** (see Dobres and Robb, 2000; Dornan, 2002) as well as **gender archaeology** and **feminist archaeology** (see Gero and Conkey, 1991; Hays-Gilpin, 2000; Wilkie and Hayes, 2006; Wylie, 2007).

Agency, Gender, and Osteobiography

The analytical paleopathology of the twenty-first century is increasingly reflecting the vocabulary and theoretical issues of post-processual archaeology (Buikstra and Scott, 2009; Baadsgaard et al., 2012). This includes gender and feminism (Geller, 2008, 2009; Agarwal and Glencross, 2011) and conceptualization of the body (corporeality) (Hamilakis et al., 2002; Sofaer, 2006; Knudson and Stojanowski, 2008, 2009; Buikstra and Scott, 2009; Agarwal and Glencross, 2011). Recent interpretive trends have broadened to consider cultural variables (e.g., disease equated with sin or punishment, pathology seen as transformative blessing) for the prevalence and patterns of paleopathology (e.g., Little and Papadopoulos, 1998; Roberts, 2000; Waldron, 2007a; Duncan and Hofling, 2011; Marsteller et al., 2011; Smith et al., 2011). Topics adopted from post-processualist perspectives include social identity, age-related changes in role or identity, the social meaning or context of personal life history, and gender (i.e., social role). Social identity reflects cultural membership (ethnic identity) and self-conceptualization (Waldron, 2007a; Knudson and Stojanowski, 2008, 2009) and, to date, has been paleopathologically addressed in studies of deliberate cranial modification (i.e., head binding) (Blom, 2005; Duncan, 2009; Torres-Rouff, 2009). Changes in social roles or identities may also occur over the lifespan of an individual. These may be marked by events or rites-of-passage which may not be congruent with age-at-death categories (e.g., Gilchrist, 2000; Glencross, 2011; Sofaer, 2011). In other words, the post-processual perspective reminds the researcher that a biological child may be a social adult (e.g., Lewis, 2007; Halcrow and Tayles, 2011; Mays and Eyers, 2011).

A broader role of the individual (**osteobiography**) is emerging, whether as a methodology (Saul and Saul, 1989) or as a vehicle to address the contextual meaning of an individual's particular life as a member of a particular culture who shaped and is shaped by it (Robb, 2002). That is, the individual (or few individuals) need not be part of a sample to have an explanatory or interpretive role (e.g., Saul and Saul, 1989; Robb, 2002; Rosado and Vernacchio-Wilson, 2006; Renschler, 2007; Stodder and Palkovich, 2012).

A fundamental bioarchaeological analytical tool is the biological sex of an individual. As a research tool, it provides a **control** the same way comparisons by age, subsistence economy, or temporal context are utilized. Although colloquially sex may be equated with gender, sex (biology) in bioarchaeology is not the same as gender (role) and never has been (see Walker and Cook, 1998). Biological sex may predicate on certain behaviors or abilities, but it carries with it no social agenda or exclusive power to classify by social identity. However, sex can be used to test for social role and sex-based health vulnerabilities in a given cultural context (e.g., Grauer and Stuart-Macadam, 1998).

The interpretive frameworks a scholar adopts may vary, but the supportive pathological data must be invariably accurately identified and quantified. This is particularly true if the skeletal material is only temporarily available for study and the information collected becomes the sole record. What follows is a practical guide to paleopathology and an introduction to the analytical process.

SKELETAL STRESS MARKERS OF BIOARCHAEOLOGICAL VALUE

An effective pathological condition for directed sample-based analytical problem solving is one that is relatively common in skeletal material. Therefore, pathologies that occur as isolated cases (e.g., cancer, Paget's disease, ankylosing spondylitis), however critical they may be for establishing temporal and spatial distribution of the disease in question or as useful bases for particular osteobiographies, are generally not effective directed-research tools. The pathological conditions should certainly have behavioral or health corollaries that can be used to reconstruct some aspect of community life.

The presence of these relatively common pathological conditions indicates a chronic, perhaps long-standing, process. Therefore, the bioarchaeological value is not just the raw frequency of cases, but the age-at-death of the affected individuals. There is a suite of pathological conditions utilized in the first generation of bioarchaeological inquiry that have behavioral or health status corollaries that are still routinely and effectively utilized. These conditions, often simply referred to as **stress markers**, can be investigated separately or collectively depending on the research question or the scope of the research project.

Porotic Hyperostosis and Cribra Orbitalia

There are two places on the cortical surface of the cranium that often exhibit discrete areas of small, penpoint diameter (circa 1 mm) pitting. Porotic hyperostosis (also referred to as cribra cranii) is the pitting on the **cortex** of both upper parietal bones (Figure 7.1a). It is accompanied by **cancellous (diploic)** bone expansion (i.e., **hyperostosis**) (Figure 7.1b). A similar but independent phenomenon is cribra orbitalia, a usually bilaterally expressed sieve-like pitting in

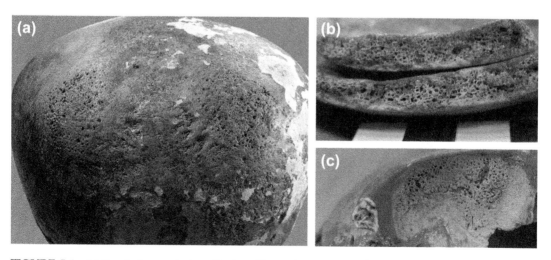

FIGURE 7.1   (a) Porotic hyperostosis as illustrated by surface pitting on the left and right parietals. (b) Porotic hyperostosis as illustrated by expansion of the cancellous (i.e., diploic) bone. Normal adult mid-parietal thickness ranges from 0.4 to 0.8 mm. (c) A remodeled example of cribra orbitalia.

the roof of the eye orbits (Figure 7.1c). These are pathologies of childhood that have been differentially linked to anemia, scurvy, parasite load, inflammation, genetic conditions (e.g., sicklemia, thallasemia), and vitamin deficiency (Angel, 1966; Stuart-Macadam, 1987, 1992; Stuart-Macadam and Kent, 1992; Ortner and Erickson, 1997; Ortner, 2003; Wapler et al., 2004; Walker et al., 2009; Oxenham and Cavill, 2010). Both pathological conditions are routinely used as measures of stress that are compared between subsistence economies, sociopolitical circumstances, and ecological circumstances (e.g., Kent, 1986; Hirata, 1990; Mittler and Van Gerven, 1994; Robledo et al., 1995; Larsen and Sering, 2000; Fairgreve and Molto, 2000; Salvadei et al., 2001; Facchini et al., 2004; Sullivan, 2005; Buzon, 2006; Keenleyside and Panayotova, 2006). Indeed, when nothing is known about a particular osteological sample, cribra orbitalia and porotic hyperostosis are invariably part of the first wave of information collected.

Reactive Changes on Bone

Equally fundamental health status information that is routinely collected in analytical paleopathology is the reactive changes visible on the cortical surface of bone that flag chronic infection or inflammation (caused by traumatic injury, burns, physical or chemical irritant, etc.) (Lallo et al., 1978; Rogers and Waldron, 1989). See Figure 7.2a and 7.2b. The morphology of these reactive changes is similar, if not identical, in many pathological processes (Weston, 2008). As a result, and although inflammation is also a likely cause, the presence of this generic reactive change is bioarchaeologically referred to as nonspecific infection. Often this is discriminated as cortical change (**periostitis**) or internal spongy bone change (**osteomyelitis**) that additionally displays with dead (necrotic) bone (sequestrum) and a drain (cloaca) for exuded pus as well as a shell of new bone growth (involucrum).

Certain disease processes are known as **specific diseases** because they differentially affect certain bones or are manifested by particular types of lesions. A number of specific diseases such as tuberculosis, treponemal disease, leprosy, and brucellosis have epidemiological and

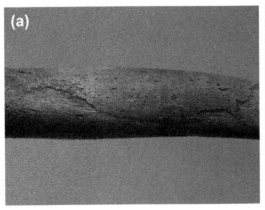 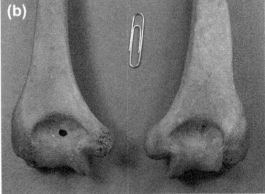

FIGURE 7.2   (a) Periostitis as new (woven) bone plaque deposited superior to the cortical surface. (b) Periostitis as the resultant shaft (diaphyseal) expansion of mature (lamellar) bone. Note the shaft of the humerus on the left compared to the one on the right.

community health correlates that merit their being assessed separately (e.g., Roberts et al., 2002; Roberts and Buikstra, 2003; Powell and Cook, 2005; Mutolo et al., 2012).

Like (1) porotic hyperostosis and (2) cribra orbitalia (both too often generically referred to as anemia), (3) nonspecific infection has been a useful measure of comparative community or social group stress. These three conditions are often collectively evaluated with subadult long bone length (reflective of compromised growth), the dental enamel defects referred to as **linear enamel hypoplasia** (or LEH), which flag health stressors affecting the integrity of dental enamel (Hammerl [Chapter 10], this volume), and, of course, age-at-death (Uhl [Chapter 3], this volume) and sex (Moore [Chapter 4], this volume). Other stress markers that have been effectively used include radiographically detected subadult growth interruptions (Harris lines) (e.g., Mays, 1995; Ameen et al., 2005; Papageorgopoulou et al., 2011) and rickets/osteomalacia (Ortner and Mays, 1998; Mays et al., 2005; Pinhasi et al., 2006; Brickley et al., 2007; Brickley and Ives, 2008).

Degenerative Joint Disease and Occupational Stress Markers

The joints of the body are mechanical constructs that permit or constrain movement at the juncture of two or more bones. They fundamentally consist of a circumscribed area of cushioned bone-to-bone contact surrounded by tissues that stabilize the juncture and tissues that enable movement. There are three types of pathological changes at the joint that have been the focus of paleopathological interest. The first is the reactive change visible on the joint (articular) surface that is often generically referred to as degenerative joint disease (DJD). The type of change varies with the nature of the joint surface and includes **osteoarthritis** (Figure 7.3a), vertebral osteophytosis, Schmorl's nodes, necrotic foci, and osteochondritis dissecans (see Aufderheide and Rodríguez-Martín, 1998; Ortner, 2003 for definitions and descriptions). The second type of reactive change is extra-articular and consists of small smooth-planed cortical surface remodeling due to bone-to-bone pressure (i.e., a facet)

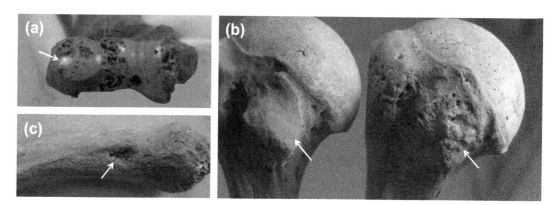

FIGURE 7.3   (a) Osteoarthritis of the distal humeral joint with porotic pitting and eburnation (polish) of the joint surface. (b) Left image of the humeral head illustrates the normal area of insertion of the subscapularis muscle (arrow) and the right image illustrates the area (arrow) with mechanical damage (enthesopathy). (c) On a clavicle, a deep lesion (syndesmosis) (arrow) is evident at the insertion of the costoclavicular ligament.

consequential to habitual postural habits (e.g., squatting facets, Poirier's facet, Charles's facet) (see Kennedy, 1989). The third type reflects circumarticular changes in areas of ligament or tendon attachment (e.g., enthesopathies, syndesmoses [Figure 7.3b, 7.3c], Osgood-Schlatter syndrome) (Kennedy, 1989; Benjamin et al., 2006; DiGangi et al., 2010). These have traditionally been labeled musculoskeletal stress markers (MSM) but, more recently, Robert Jurmain and Sébastien Villotte (2010) have advocated a different, less cause-presumptive label: entheseal changes (EC), which will be used here.

The primary bioarchaeological value of DJD, pressure facets, and EC changes is the presumptive co-association of these reactive changes with repetitive labor-intensive activity which arguably predicts, among other things, subsistence, skilled labor, or sexual division of labor. Such activities include grain-grinding or nut pounding (use of the quern, mortar and pestle, mano and metate), burden bearing (tump line, balancing on the head), labor skill (weaver, blacksmith, archer), and transport (canoe, kayak, rickshaw, horseback). Many activity-specific stress markers have been identified (Kennedy, 1989). However, there are a wide range of extraneous factors that affect whether DJD and EC are skeletally expressed. These include trauma/microtrauma (see Kroman and Symes [Chapter 8], this volume), body size or weight, genetic predisposition, age, and ergonomically incorrect activity patterns (e.g., heavy lifting with the spine and not the legs, poor posture). Sometimes joint damage is simply idiopathic (i.e., no known cause) (Jurmain, 1999; Weiss, 2003, 2004, 2007; Benjamin et al., 2006).

Many studies have indeed linked differential prevalence and severity of stress markers with subsistence change or sexual division of labor (e.g., Bridges, 1991; Chapman, 1997; Lai and Lovell 1992; Molleson, 1994; Hawkey and Merbs, 1995; Robb, 1998; Steen and Lane, 1998; Jurmain, 1990, 1999; Lovell and Dublenko, 1999; Eshed et al., 2004; Fornaciari et al., 2007; Molnar, 2006, 2011; Villotte et al., 2010; Niinimäki, 2011). However, these pathologies have had a mixed history of behavior-associated explanatory power primarily relating to difficulties of quantification (e.g., if it is hypertrophy or damage) and primary cause (Stirland, 1998; Wilczak, 1998; Jurmain, 1999; Weiss, 2007; Cardoso and Henderson, 2010; Jurmain and Villotte, 2010; Villotte et al., 2010; Jurmain et al., 2012; Weiss et al., 2012). It is clear from research conducted thus far that age and body size play a strong role in prevalence and severity of EC and must be controlled for if differences in activity patterns within and between skeletal samples are to be diagnosed correctly. As greater analytical control over the range of causative variables (e.g., age, robusticity) and more precise quantification occurs (e.g., Stirland, 1998; Wilczak, 1998; Weiss, 2003; Molleson, 2007; Jurmain and Villotte, 2010; Jurmain et al., 2012; Milella et al., 2012; Niinimäki, 2012; Weiss et al., 2012), more bioarchaeological studies of DJD and EC will be conducted. This is a promising area for future research.

IDENTIFYING A PATHOLOGY

Experience is the best teacher. This begins with familiarization with the texture and contours of normal bone. This may sound fundamental but be mindful that postmortem damage (e.g., root marks, mechanical or chemical exfoliation of the outer cortex, exposure of cancellous bone) can be mistaken for pathological conditions (White and Folkens, 2005:49−66 and Marden et al. [Chapter 9], this volume). When in doubt, do not dismiss the observation but record it for later comparative evaluation. No one ever regrets being too comprehensive. Know where muscle tendons and ligaments are located, particularly those on the shaft (diaphysis) of long bones (e.g., linea aspera of the femur, deltoid tuberosity of the humerus, popliteal line of the tibia, and ankle ligaments). The novice scholar often misinterprets the exuberant bone growth of mechanical stress (called *enthesopathies* at tendon insertions and *syndesmoses* at ligament insertions) for infectious reaction.

Recommended Reference Materials

Have on hand an osteology text (e.g., Steele and Bramblett, 1988; White and Folkens, 1999; Juurlink, 2009; White et al., 2012) in order to help identify fragmentary material. If material is particularly fragmentary, have reference bones available. For some identifications (e.g., phalanges of hands and feet), models are essential. A prudent scholar always has access to at least one encyclopedia of bone pathology. The paleopathology "bibles" are Donald Ortner's *Identification of Pathological Conditions in Human Skeletal Remains* (2003) and *The Cambridge Encyclopedia of Human Paleopathology* by Arthur C. Aufderheide and Conrado Rodríguez-Martín (1998). There are also other available resources, including image-rich paleopathological resource books (e.g., Steinbock, 1976; Zimmerman and Kelly, 1982; Ortner and Putschar, 1985;[2] Mann and Hunt, 2005; Waldron, 2007b, 2008), course texts (e.g., Mays, 1998; Cox and Mays, 2000; Roberts and Manchester, 2007; Pinhasi and Mays, 2008; Katzenberg and Saunders, 2008; Waldron, 2008; Pinhasi and Stock, 2011), the Global History of Health Project *Data Collection Codebook*,[3] the *Guidelines to the Standards for Recording Human Remains*[4] (Brickley and McKinley, 2004) and the *Standards for Data Collection from Human Skeletal Remains* by Buikstra and Ubelaker (1994).[5]

Differential Diagnosis

Diagnostic skill also comes with experience. The scholar should be mindful that an **acute** pathological process (e.g., measles, typhus, plague) does not leave a macroscopic reactive bone signature on the skeleton; however, a **chronic** process disseminates to bone in later stages. Bone also has a limited spectrum of reactive responses to disease, inflammation, deprivation, and trauma (Aufderheide and Rodríguez-Martín, 1998; Ortner, 2003). This means that a particular suite of reactive changes may have one or more causes (e.g., vitamin deficiency or parasite load), and one or more mediating factors (e.g., frailty, body size, age), or be caused by one or another specific disease that may not or cannot be teased apart (e.g.,

---

[2]An earlier version of this book (Ortner and Putschar, 1981) is downloadable at http://www.sil.si.edu/smithsoniancontributions/Anthropology/pdf_hi/SCtA-0028.pdf (all Internet links current as of publication).

[3]http://global.sbs.ohio-state.edu/new_docs/Codebook-01-24-11-em.pdf

[4]http://www.babao.org.uk/HumanremainsFINAL.pdf

[5]Online image catalogs are available at http://www.museumoflondon.org.uk/Collections-Research/LAARC/Centre-for-Human-Bioarchaeology/Resources/Photographs/Default.htm and, courtesy of Donald Ortner, at http://global.sbs.ohio-state.edu/cd-contents/Ortner-slides/Book%20001-jpg/.

ankylosing spondylitis versus DISH,[6] treponemal disease: yaws versus bejel[7]). However, under certain contextual circumstances (based on information from archaeology or ecology), the causes or factors can be differentially weighed. With respect to similarly presenting diseases, there may be particular reactive changes that distinguish one from another. In order to identify a particular pathology or mediating factor, the scholar must therefore be aware of the total range of bone change associated with the progress of that pathology and the other disease processes that might mimic such responses (i.e., differential diagnosis).

This does not mean that other reactive responses are not possible. Other, and likely ever-present, stress circumstances (e.g., malnutrition, osteoporosis, or endemic disease process) may impact a particular pathology (i.e., a synergistic response) that could complicate the bone's repair process. Therefore, the scholar should fully describe all the changes and their distribution throughout the skeleton because (1) pathologies may interact synergistically, (2) detail would help discriminate between pathologies and support a particular differential diagnosis, and (3) potentially disease-discriminating minor changes may exist which might previously have been overlooked. However, in the end, a diagnosis is always a probability statement and the prudent scholar always considers (and reports) alternative identifications.

There is a set vocabulary utilized in differential diagnosis that the scholar should know and utilize. If reactive changes are categorized as **pathognomonic** (often misspelled as "pathognomic"), they are unique to the disease described and reflect the highest level of diagnostic confidence. Pathological indicators that are labeled **diagnostic** also indicate a high level of diagnostic confidence, but the reactive changes may not be exclusive to the disease process. If a reactive change is labeled as "consistent with" or a similar descriptor (e.g., "indicative"), the changes are generic but the particular disease cannot be diagnostically excluded. This final category is useful if a disease process has been identified in a given archaeological sample by pathognomonic or diagnostic cases and other cases are suspected. Adjectives for "consistent with" are often metaphorically used (e.g., "probable," "possible") to suggest the confidence with which pathological cases are diagnosed. In many osteological samples, most cases fall into the "consistent with" category. This does not necessarily reflect the diagnostic shortcomings of the observer. Rather, it reflects the inherent complexity of disease progress in individuals who differ in vulnerability (i.e., frailty) and the significant overlap in reactive changes (Weston, 2008). It also emphasizes the analytical utility of the category of nonspecific infection to suggest stress.

---

[6]Ankylosing spondylitis (AS) and diffuse idiopathic skeletal hyperostosis (DISH) describe bone overgrowth of the ligamentous sheaths of vertebral bodies. Ideally they can be distinguished by the predilection of location and pattern of reactive change. That is, AS is described as "bamboo-spine" and DISH is often described as resembling "dripping candle wax." Many particularly advanced cases when overgrowth is morphologically complex and bilateral on the vertebral body are difficult to distinguish. This can be particularly problematic in archaeological contexts as cases may be incomplete or poorly preserved. See Rogers et al. (1985), Aufderheide and Rodríguez-Martín (1998:96−105), and Ortner (2003:558−560, 571−577).

[7]Osteologically indistinguishable syndromes of an endemic pre-Columbian disease. See Cook and Powell (2005).

Cranial and Orbital Roof Porosis and Differential Diagnosis

The reactive conditions of childhood that have become the mainstay of analytical paleo-pathology are porotic hyperostosis and cribra orbitalia. These are descriptive labels and not diagnoses. Some of the causes of porotic hyperostosis (vault) and cribra orbitalia (orbital roof) are shared (Walker et al., 2009; Oxenham and Cavill, 2010). Which factor is the more likely explanation for the porotic pitting seen in a skeletal sample depends on the origin of the collection and the cultural and sociopolitical circumstance. For example, there is no hereditary anemia in the Americas, but it should be considered when evaluating skeletal samples where malaria is/was endemic (e.g., circum-Mediterranean or Southeast Asia) (e.g., Borza, 1979; Hershkovitz et al., 1991; Sallares et al., 2004; Keenleyside and Panayotova, 2006). However, the other causes should be carefully (and synergistically) assessed as stresses such as folic acid deficiency during pregnancy, the ubiquity of common intestinal worm infections (Farid et al., 1969; Weiss and Goodnough, 2005), and protein or calorie malnutrition (Stuart-Macadam and Kent, 1992) can be differentially prevalent between the sexes, between social classes, and between subsistence strategies (e.g., Vercellotti et al., 2010).

Vitamin C Deficiency and Scurvy

Parietal pitting and cribra orbitalia are part of a suite of cranial and postcranial reactive changes that also occur in subadult scurvy (chronic vitamin C deficiency) and rickets (chronic vitamin D deficiency). Therefore, the entire cranium as well as the postcranial skeleton should be examined as these metabolic diseases can be differentially diagnosed. Vitamin C (ascorbic acid), acquired solely from the diet (citrus fruits and cruciferous vegetables), is an essential nutrient which, among other things, maintains cartilage and blood vessels, acts as an antioxidant, fortifies the immune system, and facilitates iron absorption (Stuart-Macadam, 1989; Brickley and Ives, 2008).

Chronic deficiency results in scurvy that in advanced clinical stages displays with subcu-taneous hemorrhaging, open wounds, and loss of teeth, and, without metabolic intervention, can result in death (Brickley and Ives, 2008). Scurvy has been differentially diagnosed in several archaeological contexts (Stuart-Macadam, 1989; Ortner and Erickson, 1997; Ortner et al., 1999a, b, 2001; Brickley and Ives, 2006). Features to look for to distinguish a case of scurvy include cortex-penetrating pinpoint to penpoint sized pores (circa 0.5—1 mm) on the greater wing of the sphenoid bone, the lateral zygomatic arches, alveolar area of the maxilla, and/or the lambdoidal area of the occipital bone (Ortner and Erickson, 1997; Ortner et al., 1999a, b, 2001) and scapulae (Brickley and Ives, 2006).

Vitamin D Deficiency and Rickets

In addition to parietal pitting and cribra orbitalia, rickets differentially displays with abnormalities consistent with insufficient calcium that individually are nondiagnostic, but collectively make a supportable case. The suite of characteristics consists of long bone shaft deformities (bowing, flaring at the metaphyses), long bone growth plate deformities (rough-ness, porosity, concavity or "cupping" of distal plates) and rib abnormalities (deformity, porosity, and flaring at the costochondral joint) (Ortner and Mays, 1998; Mays et al., 2006). Although rickets has been identified archaeologically (Ortner et al., 2001; Blondiaux et al.,

2002; Pfeiffer and Crowder, 2004; Pinhasi et al., 2006), it is only recently that osteomalacia (i.e., adult vitamin D deficiency) has (e.g., Brickley et al., 2005, 2007).

Periostitis and Differential Diagnosis

Reactive bone indicative of infection, trauma, or inflammation can occur anywhere on the skeleton. On the long bones it displays as shaft thickening, as rough striated exterior surface, and/or new bone deposition (**woven bone**). It can also occur as discrete pitted lesions or areas of pitting. Sometimes this reactive change is localized, that is, restricted to one bone. Periostitis can also occur on multiple bones, often bilaterally. Most cases of periostitis are non-diagnostic (meaning that a nonspecific infection is indicated). However, certain specific diseases have predilections to certain bones and/or additionally display with pathogno-monic or diagnostic features. These include diseases of bioarchaeological significance such as tuberculosis, leprosy, treponemal disease, and brucellosis.

Tuberculosis

Tuberculosis is an infectious respiratory disease indigenous to both the Old and New Worlds caused by a bacterium of the genus *Mycobacterium*. The paleopathological interest in the disease stems from its association with concentrated aggregate living and poor community health as well as its reputed high mortality and morbidity (Roberts and Buikstra, 2003; Stone et al., 2009). It also has an epidemiological history that includes an inexplicable pre-antibiotics drop in prevalence in Europe after the nineteenth century (Roberts and Buik-stra, 2003). Although a chronic respiratory disease, it disseminates via the bloodstream throughout the body with a predilection for the visceral surface of the ribs, the broad ends of long bones (i.e., metaphyses), certain joints (knee, hip, elbow), and bones of the hands and feet.

For the most part, the reactive changes are nondiagnostic. However, the disease is most characteristically evident in the spine. Cavitating (hole-forming) lesions on the anterior verte-bral body are a precursor to the diagnostic sharply angled vertebral column collapse (referred to as a kyphosis or gibbus) known as Pott's disease (Aufderheide and Rodríguez-Martín, 1998; Ortner, 2003). However, this same pattern of vertebral destruction occurs in the fungal infections blastomycosis (North America) and actinomycosis (worldwide) except that the former differentially displays cavitations on the dorsal surface and the latter differ-entially involves more vertebral surfaces (articular facets, transverse and spinous processes) (Kelly and Eisenberg, 1987; Mann and Hunt, 2005).

Brucellosis

An Old World disease with a predilection for vertebral bodies of bioarchaeological interest is brucellosis. It is a disease associated with the consumption of dairy products or meat (cattle, horses, sheep, goats) and has a considerable antiquity (Capasso, 1999; D'Anastasio et al., 2011; Mutolo et al., 2012). Ideally it is distinguishable from tuberculosis by the lack of vertebral collapse and cavitating lesions that exhibit reparative reactive bone (Zimmerman and Kelly, 1982).

But, despite the existence of nuanced differences between these pathologies that predilect the vertebrae, the perennial problem of poor preservation can prevent confident diagnosis (e.g., Mays et al., 2001), a frustration that all diagnosticians encounter. Fortunately, genetic

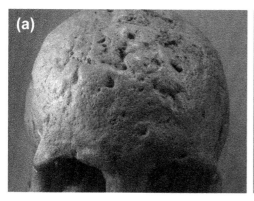 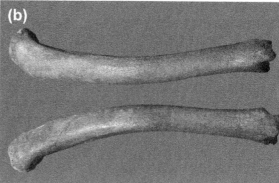

FIGURE 7.4 (a) Pathognomonic caries sicca of treponemal disease. (b) Diagnostic sabre tibiae of treponemal disease.

screening is now possible and the genetic markers for brucellosis have bridged this diagnostic gap (Mutolo et al., 2012). Indeed, genetic data have confirmed tuberculosis and plague (*Yersinia pestis*) in other circumstances (e.g., Crubézy et al., 1998; Mays et al., 2001; Verena et al., 2011) and may become a more common paleopathologic diagnostic tool in the future.

Non-venereal Treponemal Disease

Non-venereal treponemal disease[8] is a chronic infectious cutaneous disease of childhood transmitted by skin-to-skin contact. It has an antiquity of 3000+ years (as yaws and/or treponarid) in North America (Powell et al., 2005). Like tuberculosis, it is a disease of aggregate living and poor community hygiene that became pervasive in North American skeletal samples with the intensification of agriculture (Powell and Cook, 2005).

Treponemal disease often presents as nondiagnostic periostitis, but it also has distinctive reactive changes that are pathognomonic for the disease (Hackett, 1975). These include cavitating lesions on the cranium that heal in a star-shaped (stellate) pattern and, in an advanced state, coalesce to a nodular (coral or cauliflower textured) cranial surface (known as caries sicca) (Figure 7.4a). Diagnostic of treponemal disease is a marked anterior bowing of the tibia (sabre shins) (Figure 7.4b). Nasopalatal damage is also characteristic of non-venereal and venereal (i.e., syphilis) treponemal disease.

This type of damage is also characteristic of leprosy (or Hansen's disease) (Cook, 2002), an illness of considerable antiquity and profound social stigma (Zias, 2002; Roberts, 2002; Robbins et al., 2009; Stone et al., 2009). However, leprosy is not indigenous to the New World. Distinguishing leprosy from syphilis rests diagnostically on the former's predilection for distal body elements (hands and feet). These display as contracted and atrophied (claw hand appearance) or atrophy of the distal fingers and toes (pencil point appearance) (Aufderheide and Rodríguez-Martín, 1998; Ortner, 2003).

The more observations that can be marshaled, the greater the likelihood a deduced diagnosis is the correct one. That is, zeroing-in on the primary or most extensive pathological condition is

[8]The venereal form, syphilis, is not unequivocally evident in pre-Columbian Europe and apparently of North American origin but of unclear antiquity (Powell and Cook, 2005).

insufficient. To repeat, the entire skeleton should be inventoried for any and all pathological changes and, if feasible, include radiographic or **CT** (computed tomography) imaging and molecular data (e.g., **DNA** identification of the pathogen). Comprehensive paleopathological inventorying certainly demands an objective, non-biased scoring and quantification protocol. Scoring criteria are available but note that there are still unresolved problems of reproducibility (e.g., Waldron and Rogers, 1991; Jacobi and Danforth, 2002; Grauer, 2008; Stodder, 2012).

Quantification

If the reader is interested in undertaking a paleopathological study, understanding how to quantify the data will be essential as the strategy here differs from that of other areas in skeletal biology. As a result, the most difficult aspect of diagnostics is probably quantification. Pathologies are not necessarily a simple presence—absence phenomenon. There will likely be a continuous grade from normal to abnormal and often it is difficult to determine the threshold of abnormal. This is certainly true of EC (entheseal change). Even if a threshold for abnormal is determined, severity will also be manifested on a progressive continuum. It is admittedly difficult to force a continuous phenomenon into discrete categories. Additionally, severity may vary between populations and may fundamentally affect the quantification of disease prevalence. For example, an observer's characterization of severity as mild in one sample may be characterized by another observer in a second sample as being at a threshold-normal level. This difference in scoring criteria is called **observer error.** It may reflect the differences between multiple observers (interobserver error) or within a single observer over a large skeletal sample (**criteria drift**).

Observers must particularly be vigilant against criteria drift occurring throughout the process of data collection as one gradually (almost subconsciously) changes their decision-making process with application of the scoring protocol as the number of skeletons (and therefore variety of features/pathologies) they have seen increases. One way to minimize observer error is to do a blind study in which two observers independently score a given pathology and compare the results. Even if scoring is equivalent, it should be spot-checked periodically for criteria drift. Single observers should rescore the first twenty or so cases at a later date to test for criteria drift. If changes in the threshold of presence or severity are detected, the sample should be spot-checked until no discrepancy occurs.

Scoring Protocol

There are several standards and protocols available complete with exemplary images. These include the aforementioned resources in the earlier section on reference materials. There are also software programs such as **Osteoware,**[9] a data-entry program that was developed by the Smithsonian Institution that helpfully includes an image module to facilitate scoring (http://osteoware.si.edu/guide/pathology-module). However, this does not mean that ambiguities will not occur (e.g., Jacobi and Danforth, 2002). Therefore, before undertaking any given project, it is always a good idea to survey the literature for precise and reproducible scoring criteria. Publications and reports will contain a Materials and Methods

[9]Downloadable free standardized skeletal documentation software from the Smithsonian Institution: https://osteoware.si.edu/

section that describes the diagnostic criteria and scoring protocols. Detailed studies (e.g., monographs, theses, and dissertations) will invariably provide more exemplary illustrations or images of the severity categories.

Description

Vocabulary for particular bare bone pathology will become evident from reading background bioarchaeological and paleopathological literature. For analytical paleopathology, the goal of pathological identification is the underlying biocultural meaning that the pathology had for the person and their society. Disease descriptors should be simple and to the point, particularly as most bioarchaeologists do not have a medical background (e.g., Buikstra and Ubelaker, 1994:114–115; Ortner, 2003:50–51). For nonspecific periostitis, it is appropriate to simply describe and distinguish active new bone (woven bone) that is deposited on the cortical surface (plaque) from cortex-integrated/integrating (healed/healing) mature bone (**lamellar bone**). Particularly dense bone is often distinguished (**sclerosis**) and descriptors are often used to clarify the dimension and topography of the reactive change (e.g., terms often used are: striated, exuberant, spiculated, moth-eaten, nodular, endosteal expansion, **lytic**, and/or **blastic**). Often for want of a better label, certain metaphorical descriptors have been used (e.g., tree bark, orange-peel, pin-prick, honey-comb, furry, velvety, vermiculate, and/or labyrinth-like). Word choice will depend on the diagnostic value of the descriptor and whether detail is fundamental to the research question.

The basic value of quantification for any study is to have objective well-substantiated information in order to assess a skeletal sample for specific research questions. The process may initially seem daunting or intimidating but consider first and foremost that it is a tool for problem solving, not an exercise in right or wrong. However, the more detailed a description, the easier it will be for others to evaluate the differential diagnosis made.

HOW TO COLLECT PATHOLOGICAL DATA

The Tool Kit

If skeletal pathological assessment is undertaken on collections that are not in-house, particularly if work will be undertaken in the field, the researcher should create a kit of essential tools. This kit should minimally include a good hand lens, a good quality sliding caliper, a metric scale measuring tape, a mini goose-neck flashlight, nonhardening clay, various pens, a soft bristle paint brush or a mini dust pan set (for cleaning and clean up), pencils (certainly graphite and ideally a small box of colored ones), highlighter and permanent markers, self-stick notes in several sizes, a photographic scale (in millimeters), and, if reconstruction is permitted, contact cement and (temporarily and judiciously used) painter's (or other easily removable) tape. It would also be a good idea to have archival quality small zip-lock bags on hand to segregate the pathological bone for future reassessment or consultation. The work kit would also benefit from office essentials such as paper clips, a mini-stapler, and a ruler (a 6-inch one is adequate). For robust transport (particularly for the calipers), consider housing it all in a small, hinged plastic box. Since laptop computers are indispensable, other practical items include a power strip and an extension cord or two. If research takes the scholar abroad, adapter plugs or converters may dictate whether cords or power strips should be purchased in the country where the research is conducted.

The amount or variety of drawing/sketching tools included in the kit will depend on whether pathological information will be immediately entered into a computer database or first drawn on score sheets. The use of a computer database implies that the scoring protocols and the severity scales have already been established. However, with ever-changing repatriation laws, consider the possibility that the current project may become the only record for the sample. If that may indeed be the case, a nonsubjective, project-independent visual record may be preferred. This might simply consist of standard size sheets of paper with two-dimensional outline drawings of the bones printed on it. Buikstra and Ubelaker (1994) as well as Internet sources[10] have ready-made score sheets of the whole skeleton as well as larger versions of the individual bones. If other aspects are needed, personal score sheets can be cobbled by downloading copyright-free images[11] from the web and resizing or organizing them with an image editing computer program.

Initial Data Collection

Be sure to inventory all skeletons for completeness. To determine the frequency of a pathological condition, note that the total sample is not the total number of individuals available; rather, it is the number of individuals that preserve enough of the body elements necessary to determine the presence or absence of the pathology being assessed. For example, nasal bones are fragile and often display extensive postmortem damage. The nasal margin is also subject to reactive change due to (for example) chronic treponemal disease infection (i.e., goundou). In an assessment of pre-Columbian treponemal disease that included determining the presence and prevalence of reactive bone at the nasal margin (Smith, 2006), this author created a score sheet with several rows and columns of the mid-face (adapted from Buikstra and Ubelaker, 1994:203). The preserved nasal margins were simply outlined on the drawing in pencil. The inventory was quickly accomplished and sample size was later determined by separating out the cases with nasal margins deemed too incomplete for presence/absence categorization. The benefit of such a technique is that it enables the inventory to be undertaken by others but keeps the determination of inclusion or exclusion under the control of the researcher.

Before recording any pathology, certainly shade or cross-hatch on the data sheet the parts of the skeleton or bone that are missing. This need not be precise, just enough to answer basic questions about skeletal or bone completeness. Use another color or medium (e.g., colored pencil, highlighter pen) to draw where the bone exhibits reactive change(s). If the pathology is complex (e.g., periostitis and trauma), consider assigning a color to each pathological condition. Remember, clarity is important if this is to become archived information.

If the permanent storage of a paper record is impractical or problematic, scan the sheets. If a totally paperless route is preferred, consider using scanned images in a computer or

---

[10]Such as http://www.statemuseum.arizona.edu/crservices/burial/hum_rem_inventory.pdf.

[11]For example, for public domain text see Gray, Henry. Anatomy of the Human Body. Philadelphia: Lea & Febiger, 1918; Bartleby.com, 2000, www.bartleby.com/107/.

graphics pad and enter the pathological information on the screen[12] with a stylus, light pen, or other pointing device. This may take longer than drawing by hand or be impractical without sources of electrical power, so project completion deadlines or field circumstances may ultimately dictate the recording method. Although three-dimensional imaging is the gold standard for recording information, the current reality is that this technology remains expensive or inaccessible for many researchers (see Moore [Chapter 14], this volume).

Observations are most effectively recorded if the bone under examination is not rolling or pitching on the table. Many laboratories have cloth-covered tables (usually ticking fabric or duck cloth), c. 8" x 8" square bean bags, or bean-filled cloth "donuts" for steadying such material. These are usually homemade. However, if there are none available or to spare, an easy ersatz solution is a sturdy zip-lock plastic bag or a tied-off tube sock filled with pea gravel, dried rice, or dried beans. These bean bags are also effective for propping bones under photo cloths when photographing.

THE PHOTO KIT AND PHOTOGRAPHS/OTHER IMAGES

Photograph all pathologies, even suspected ones. Scoring or severity protocols may change or be refined over time. Without an objective photo record of the condition, scored data may become unusable, particularly for intersite or interobserver comparisons. This means a photographic tool kit is necessary. This includes a digital camera with a battery system that allows nonstop photographing either by maintaining a cache of spare batteries or alternately using a second rechargeable battery (the charger then being a photo kit essential), a millimeter scale, a soft brush (for keeping the lens dust free), a photographic background, a mini tripod, a large capacity image storage system (i.e., an external hard drive or an Internet file hosting service), and perhaps extra (swing arm) lights. The camera must be capable of good close-up photographs (a macro lens), have manual functions, and preferably have a large tiltable LCD view screen.

Good photographs are a function not just of the camera, but of the patience and expertise of the photographer. Practice close-up shots BEFORE the project is undertaken and remember to always use a (millimeter) scale or scalable object (e.g., a coin, a standard paper clip) in the photo. Learn how the camera performs with and without the flash in low-light, indirect lighting, or fluorescent versus incandescent lighting circumstances. This will enable you to adjust the shoot location to meet the needs of the camera. If even breath-holding does not eliminate camera shake (and the resultant fuzzy photo), use a small tripod. It may be necessary to take several shots of the same view or position to get a sharp, crisp image. Do not depend on the digital camera's LCD screen to verify that this was accomplished. Periodically download the camera images to a computer and confirm the in-focus shots on the computer screen. Note that the camera assigns a number to each image. Either keep a log of the photo numbers for each case or as an alternative, make your first photo of each case the place on the bone where the site and burial numbers have been permanently inked. Should the skeletal material not have been so inventoried, use a small self-stick note (ready and available in the tool box) to identify the individual (site number and burial

---

[12]For example, Adobe Illustrator or freeware such as Paint.net.

number) in the first photo frame. The frugal scholar will get at least four cases (one label per side) per self-stick note. These little sticky notes are also very useful for inserting personal opinions or queries in the photo to later facilitate differential diagnosis or other follow-up for example.

If the work area is windowless or has high ceiling lights, lighting may need to be augmented in order to obtain sharp photo images. Many institutions have photo workstations with adjustable lighting available for visiting scholars. However, if this is not the case, inexpensive small tabletop swing arm lamps are invaluable (and can be totally dismantled for portability). Depending on the available light, as few as two and as many as four lamps may be needed. Set up the camera so it makes larger megapixel images to avoid pixelation so they can be used in journal publications or if photos should need cropping. Larger size photo files will require sufficient storage capabilities and a backup (e.g., an external hard drive AND a file hosting service).

If a personal photo workstation needs to be created, consider what the most effective background color and texture should be to showcase the bone features. The background should not reflect light, cast a harsh shadow, have a texture that draws the focus of the camera lens, or be a distraction for the viewer. Three types of portable backgrounds are the most effective: (1) cloth, (2) sand, or (3) translucent plastic windowpane or photo-frame glass.[13] The most portable option is the fabric remnant. The cloth should be at least one square meter to allow folding or bunching to prop an unstable bone fragment. The color value should also contrast enough with the object so that grayscale photos are not monochromatic. Therefore, having several background cloths of different colors and textures will meet all contingencies.

A shallow pan with very small diameter craft sand is an inexpensive and extremely effective method for photographing small bones or loose teeth. Of course the only shortcoming here is stray sand grains, but keeping a mini dust pan set handy as well as lining the photo station with a shower curtain liner will catch errant grains. A method of virtually eliminating object shadow is a photo background composed of a piece of sturdy plastic photo-frame or window pane that is either already etched or frosted, or clear but covered on one side with translucent self-adhesive shelf liner paper. Support the plastic pane at the corners (low-tech options include small paper cups or toy blocks) a few inches above the tabletop. Placing colored paper or cloth on the table underneath the pane provides a diffused background color. Blue is particularly pleasing as the effect mimics the sky. This translucent background also enables greater maneuverability with light (e.g., enabling back lighting) and camera angles. See DiGangi and Moore (Chapter 2), this volume, for further recommendations regarding photographs.

When circumstances permit, pathologies should be radiographed or CT scanned. This documentation may be a critical factor in differential diagnosis as cortical thickness, obliteration of the medullary cavity, endosteal lytic or tumorous lesions, bone density, and traumatic injury are not always evident from macroscopic examination, particularly if the bone is intact. It is also important as comparative medical data are often exclusively radiographic.

[13]Products include Plexiglas. Most hardware stores sell small plastic windowpanes and many photo or poster frames use plastic instead of plate glass.

CHOOSING A COLLECTION: NOT IN A VACUUM

Context

For bioarchaeological problem solving, the skeletal samples need a context (temporal, cultural, and subsistence), ideally a large enough sample size for simple statistical analysis (e.g., **chi square** or **Fisher's exact test**), and minimal sampling bias.[14] The premise of bioarchaeology is that chronic and developmental pathology reflects the stresses of lifestyle (e.g., status, sex, affluence, enslavement), subsistence (e.g., hunter–gatherer, intensive agriculturalist, horticulturalist), settlement pattern (e.g., hamlet, urban area, farmstead, ephemeral campsite), and environment (e.g., endemic malaria, desert, Little Ice Age). This means having a comprehensive understanding of the archaeological context both temporally and spatially. In order for site samples to be effectively evaluated or compared, the scholar needs to know the factors that may have affected the prevalence or pattern of a pathology. For example, if the sample is from a nonmalarial environment, then porotic hyperostosis would not be the consequence of a genetic anemia, such as sickle cell. It is also important to recognize that disease contexts change over time, such as the unequivocal presence of endemic malaria in the Apennine (i.e., Italian) Peninsula and the southern Balkan Peninsula in classical Greek and Roman antiquity (Soren et al., 1995; Sallares et al., 1999; Sallares, 2002).

Excavation History

It is important to know the excavation history of the site or sites being examined. If the mortuary context of the culture was differential, that is if social status, age, or family affiliation dictated where an individual was buried, then it is important to know if the sample was archaeologically derived from one area or context or recovered from various contexts. For example, if the sample was exclusively recovered from well-constructed mausoleums or central plazas, the sample may be exclusively composed of persons of status and affluence. If the comparative sample was recovered from a cemetery of enslaved persons, then an explanation of health status difference needs to begin with analysis of how the social factor of enslavement affected health, rather than how a broader variable such as settlement pattern did. Cultures that differentially excluded fetuses or neonates from communal cemeteries will exhibit an underrepresentation of infant mortality. The opposite may be true if in a different cultural context infants are interred in house floors and archaeological recovery protocols are biased in favor of domestic structures over cemeteries. Therefore, the scholar should be aware of the mortuary context (e.g., grave goods, interment location) of the sample and the recovery priorities of the excavation.

Sampling Bias

Sampling bias also extends to differential bone preservation within and between excavated sites. Acids in the soil may differentially dissolve infant bones and those of

---

[14]For example, by burial treatment or burial location. See upcoming discussion and further discussion of bias in DiGangi and Moore (Chapter 2), this volume.

osteoporotic senior adults. Attention to the integrity of the bone surface (e.g., flaked, cracked, or peeled cortical bone), bone completeness (e.g., missing distal or proximal ends of long bones, missing ribs), or bone element absence (e.g., no phalanges) will alert the scholar to question the representativeness of the age-at-death profile as well as to the possibility of **pseudopathologies**. For example, an eroded outer cortex that exposes the normal internal cancellous bone may easily be mistaken for a pathological condition. Awareness of preservation problems, use of a hand lens, and a thorough photographic record are key factors in the gathering of objective and accurate biocultural information.

Sample Size and Statistical Analysis

The size of the skeletal sample will determine the method of bioarchaeological inquiry. If the objective is to compare the prevalence of pathological conditions between samples, between the sexes, between statuses, or between subsistence for significant difference, then the samples should be large enough to enable simple statistical tests. See DiGangi and Moore (Chapter 2), this volume, for a discussion on sample size. Two commonly, but not exclusively, used statistical tests are chi-square and Fisher's exact test. Conventional wisdom indicates that the former is used when the expected number in any cell of a contingency table (for example, two rows by two columns) is greater than five. Otherwise, and preferentially, Fisher's exact test is used. Both statistics test the hypothesis of no difference (i.e., a **null hypothesis**) between the samples' prevalence. Both statistics generate a calculated value (p) which, if less than 0.05 (i.e., a confidence interval of 95%) rejects the null hypothesis.[15] Besides statistical software packages that can be purchased or are available through educational institutions, there are a number of free statistical programs on the Internet that calculate a wide variety of tests. There are many ways to pose health status questions and, with advice from statistics experts, information can be segregated and tested to answer specific questions (exemplified below).

If the sample consists of less than (say) a dozen individuals, the analysis is primarily descriptive. This does not mean that the individual is simply inventoried and assessed for the presence of pathologies as well as other particular information (e.g., **discrete traits** and metric data). Assessment requires more contextual information (osteobiography) about the individual such as mode of interment, grave accompaniments, and burial location within the bonded cemetery area and within the community.

This information, in turn, is compared to and contrasted with in two ways. First, if available, the osteobiographic information is compared to prevalence patterns generated from bioarchaeological ("population"-based) assessments of larger skeletal samples drawn from the same archaeological context (e.g., another local site from the same time period or cultural phase) as the small sample. This would help ascertain how typical the individuals are relative to the health patterns of the comparative sample. For example, if the study is a single case of a high-status individual who happens to be the only case of rickets in the entire cultural phase, a closer examination of the individual's social role is merited. The second way a small

---

[15]The null hypothesis is the default condition or expectation of any given test. It can be either supported or not supported by the outcome of a statistical test. Refer to DiGangi and Moore (Chapter 2), this volume.

sample or single individual (like the hypothetical lone rickets case) may be assessed is through extensive *post hoc* historical, ethnographic, archaeological, and archival research to contextualize the life experience(s) of the individual(s). To maintain scientific rigor, interpretation about the personhood of the skeleton requires more than *a priori* interpretations; it should require the sociocultural equivalent of the differential diagnosis.

PALEOPATHOLOGICAL INFORMATION AS A PROBLEM-SOLVING TOOL

Being able to organize data to answer questions is a fundamental research skill. It involves being able to identify pathological conditions that are useful, the ability to identify and quantify the conditions on the skeleton, the ability to segregate or aggregate the information into meaningful testing units, and the use of statistical methods to test whether observations are spurious or serendipitous, or have cultural meaning. This is fundamentally different from the basic term paper that is a literature review or an argumentative paper that uses published research to marshal an argument. Bioarchaeological inquiry at its fundamental level is based on new information that is comparatively analyzed using basic demographic information (e.g., age-at-death, sex) and some form of statistical testing. The results may often be unexpected, challenge conventional wisdom, and generate further questions and analysis. Frankly, that is where the fun begins. The reader interested in analytical paleopathology can develop their research skills in this area by becoming intimately familiar with general paleopathological literature (e.g., Ortner 2003, mentioned earlier) and the literature specific to the temporal and cultural context in which they wish to focus their efforts.

Case Studies in Bioarchaeological Problem Solving: The Osteobiography

Many small samples or single cases speak eloquently about community health, social position, and life choices faced and made within the lifespan of those individuals represented. The best examples of culture context-illuminating case studies are the various mummified remains that may or may not have a high public profile. Remains of soft tissue have a wider range of information potential, are not necessarily easier to obtain (i.e., require high-tech data-collecting strategies, such as CT scans), and certainly necessitate a team effort from medical and biochemical experts.

Case Study: The Egyptian Mummy Asru

A particularly demonstrative example of the utility of agency (e.g., action of the individual within society) in an osteobiography is the case of the Manchester Museum's (United Kingdom) Egyptian mummy #1777. According to her sarcophagus, she was Asru, the Chantress of the Amun temple in Karnak who lived during the eighth century B.C. (Third Intermediate Period) (David and Garner, 2003; Booth, 2007; David, 2008).

Multifaceted medical and biochemical analysis of her remains revealed that the 50–60-year-old high-status woman had pneumoconiosis (desert lung) from inhaling sand, mechanical injuries (vertebral fractures, slipped disc, osteoarthritis), septic arthritis of the hands, and several parasitic infestations. These parasites were Guinea worm (which causes fever, severe diarrhea, intestinal bleeding and anemia), schistosomiasis or bilharzia (bladder wall flatworm parasite), and a hydatid (tapeworm) cyst in the lung. From a cultural contextual viewpoint, her high status evidently did not buffer her from life's maladies, particularly as the parasitic involvement evident in her body is clinically associated with poor community hygiene. Among her discomforts, she would have had a particularly difficult time breathing. This would have been a difficult professional burden as she apparently was an esteemed chantress, that is, a professional singer.

Case Studies in Bioarchaeological Problem Solving: The Large Sample

Case Study: The Sudanese Nubia

The best way to explain the process is by example. A fitting beginning is to illustrate how a single measure of health stress, cribra orbitalia, functions as a tool of inquiry. Equally fitting is a case study from the archaeological context that generated much of the pioneer bioarchaeological research (Mittler and Van Gerven, 1994).

Nubia, or the Kingdom of Kush, is a culture from classical antiquity that straddled the Nile River between what is now Aswan in modern Egypt and Khartoum in Sudan. Nubians from the site of Kulubnarti (Figure 7.5a) were sedentary small-scale agro-pastoralists characterized by a high-carbohydrate (millet, sorghum, vegetables) and low-protein (domesticated goats) diet (Turner et al., 2006). The sample at the time of this study (Adams et al., 1999) was divided into two temporal groups: Early Christian (~550–750 A.D.) (170 crania) characterized by centralized political authority and Late or Terminal Christian (~750–1500 A.D.) (164 crania) characterized by local political autonomy. The two temporal samples were compared to each other as well as by age and sex.

Mittler and Van Gerven scored cribra orbitalia as present–absent and active (porotic, sieve-like) or healed (smooth lamellar texture, pores bridged by bone). The authors had a large sample and opted to divide the sample into six subadult age categories by years (0–1, 2–3, 4–6, 7–9, 10–12, 13–15) and five sexable adult categories (16–20, 21–30, 31–40, 41–50, 51+). Studies with smaller sample sizes may need to collapse age categories. If that is necessary, care should be taken to not obscure the weaning age (circa 2–5) as it is associated epidemiologically with high mortality.[16]

---

[16]During this critical stage in life, small children are increasingly reliant on foods that may be raw, undercooked, and bacteria-laden. They are also more socially and physically independent, which increases the likelihood of physical contact with unhygienic objects or places. With a still immature immune system, reactive responses to toxins or pathogens may be inflammatory or purgative (weanling diarrhea) resulting in dehydration, malnutrition, and early death. In many marginal subsistence contexts, acute weanling diarrhea is endemic (Scrimshaw et al., 1968). Identifying chronic illness in this age-at-death category speaks volumes about community health stress. Chronic conditions also strongly co-associate with adult age-at-death. That is, severity increases with age. Adult age categories should have a firm upper age limit for the easiest category to age: the young adult. There is a lot of living between 18 years and 35 years of age; a sample biased in the 18–26 years age-at-death category may indeed have a different disease prevalence than one biased between 25 and 35 years of age. Perceived subsistence or settlement differences may actually be sample differences in median age-at-death. Always acknowledge the possibility of sampling error, particularly if the sample size is small, less than 75 or 50 for example.

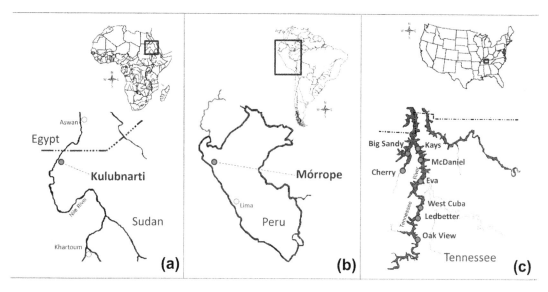

FIGURE 7.5 Maps of (a) Sudanese Nubia, Sudan, (b) Mórrope in the Lambayeque region of Peru, and (c) west-central Tennessee, United States.

As cribra orbitalia is a childhood condition (Stuart-Macadam, 1985; Stuart-Macadam and Kent, 1992), the authors examined the prevalence across all the subadults. There was a steep increase in frequency across the infant (0–1 year, 7/41 or 17.07%) and weaning (2–3 years, 17/34 or 50%) categories with prevalence peaking (75–78%) across the next three categories (4–6 years, 7–9 years, and 10–12 years) and dropping to 50% in the 13–15-year-old category. The prevalence across age categories can be tested for significance using a simple 2×2 contingency table (e.g., Fisher's exact test). For example, the proportion of weanlings with cribra (17 with, 17 without) relative to the 4–6-year-old age category (42 with, 15 without) is statistically significant ($p < 0.05$ [$p = 0.0257$]) (see above).

Because of small sample sizes, sex differences could only be addressed in the collective sample, not by temporal unit. Despite the sample being pooled, sample size segregated by sex across five adult age categories dramatically reduced the number of individuals in each age group. For example, there were only 6 males and 11 females in the 16–20 adult age category and 11 males and 14 females in the 21–30 adult age category. The interpretive question would be: Are 3/6 cribra (50%) cases in the young males compared to 3/9 (33%) cases in females spurious results or culturally significant? Rather than speculating about the meaning of what in all likelihood could be mathematical sampling error, Mittler and Van Gerven, exemplifying the analytical effectiveness of using multiple stress indicators, marshaled previous research on the Kulubnarti samples on subadult long bone growth (Moore et al., 1986) and linear enamel hypoplasia data (Van Gerven et al., 1990) to argue that young males are demonstrably stressed, therefore the results in this study are probably not spurious. Had they pooled the young adult sample to a 16–30 years age-at-death category, the sex differences (6/17 male cases, 7/23 female cases) would not have been statistically significant ($p = 1.0000$) and the authors would not have probed further. This demonstrates the importance of proper methods construction and critical analysis (see DiGangi and Moore [Chapter 2], this volume). Scholars undertaking studies on small samples should always prudently acknowledge, despite favorable results, that sampling error (e.g., sample size, median age-at-death) may color or obscure results.

Multiple parameters that were tested across the temporal difference consistently pointed to the Early Christian period as more stressed. Age-at-death patterns indicated that the Early Christian sample experienced cribra orbitalia at an earlier age, sustained higher subadult frequencies longer, and through the age category of 10–12 years, had higher frequencies of unhealed lesions ($p < 0.05$). Based on their assessment of the temporal context, political autonomy was better for community health than an overarching civil authority. These results corroborated previous research (Van Gerven et al., 1981, 1990). Considerable and varied bio-archaeological research has also been conducted on the Kulubnarti and other Sudanese Nubian material since the publication of this study (e.g., Adams et al., 1999; Buzon, 2006; Prendergast et al., 1986; Turner et al., 2006).

Case Study: Pre- and Post-Spanish Contact in Peru

An example of how multiple stress indicators can be marshaled to assess differential health stress is a multiple site assessment (a **meta-analysis**) of the post-Columbian consequences of Spanish contact in the Lambayeque Valley in northern coastal Peru (Figure 7.5b) (Klaus and Tam, 2009). This particular study illustrates how analysis can still be effectively undertaken despite the (perennial) problem of small sample size or uneven between-sample sizes. The goal of the study was simple: determine if there were negative health consequences to Spanish contact (Farnum, 2002; Klaus, 2008). This is not simply confirming the obvious as there is ample evidence of differential stress in pre-Hispanic Peru across subsistence and political change (e.g., Elzay et al., 1977; Toyne, 2002; Blom et al., 2005; Grace, 2011).

The Spanish entrada into the Lambayeque Valley occurred in 1532 but wide-reaching sociocultural transformation apparently did not occur until the 1590s when several other things happened: a settlement shift (dispersed communities to aggregate settlement), an economic shift (subsistence agriculture to mono-crop [sugar cane or alfalfa] plantations), and political subjugation (from a socioeconomic reciprocity system). This study compared a late pre-Hispanic (900–1532 A.D.) multiple-site skeletal sample (n = 272) with Early–Middle Colonial era (1536–1640 A.D.) (n = 386) and Middle–Late Colonial era (1640–1750 A.D.) (n = 485) skeletal samples from a single cemetery in the town Mórrope (north-west of the regional capital of Chiclaya).

Measures of systemic stress included (1) longitudinal growth stunting, (2) reduced female fertility, (3) linear enamel hypoplasia (LEH),[17] (4) periostitis, and (5) porotic hyperostosis.

Growth stunting as measured by growth rate[18] (i.e., change in femoral length across age categories) as an investigative tool derives from the observation that long bone lengths

---

[17]See Hammerl (Chapter 10), this volume, for a discussion of linear enamel hypoplasia.

[18]Growth rates have been effectively used as another way of assessing the synergism (causal interplay) of cribra orbitalia and mortality (age-at-death) in the Sudanese Nubian material (Hummert and Van Gerven, 1983).

(not rate of change) plotted by age have limited explanatory power (Lovejoy et al., 1990; Saunders and Hoppa, 1993). Klaus and Tam (2009) determined that after age five, the post-contact children did indeed display a slower rate of growth that was statistically significantly different.

A way of measuring population growth (fertility) is to comparatively assess the ratio of surviving reproductive age women (30+ years of age) to subadults who survived infancy and weaning (5+ years of age) (Buikstra et al., 1986). Females who are undernour-ished and overworked have difficulties conceiving and carrying pregnancies to term (Ellison and O'Rourke, 2000). In this study, small adult total sample sizes made a separate assessment of female health problematic so Klaus and Tam utilized the fertility ratio D_{30+}/D_{5+} as a proxy for the health status of adult females (2009). A ratio was generated for each time period and a straightforward statistical test (z-ratio[19]) did indeed indicate a statistically significant drop in fertility with Spanish contact.

Klaus and Tam had extensive problems with sample size within and between the temporal groups necessitating broad age categories. Nevertheless, for LEH assessment in the 15–24.9 years age-at-death category (males and females) there were 55/69 pre-contact (79.7%) individuals versus 4/9 (44%) post-contact individuals. The total sample size for assessing periostitis prevalence for the pre- AND post-contact horizons in the 35–44.9 (males and females) age-at-death category was small, only 11 individuals. How should analysis proceed?

The authors opted to use a method not affected by sample size that is infrequently adopted bioarchaeologically but is often utilized in health-related studies (and horse racing): the odds ratio (Waldron, 1994; McHugh, 2009). This statistic assesses the ratio of two outcomes (e.g., presence versus absence), not the raw frequency (percent of a particular outcome), between two groups. The odds ratio (OR) statistic performs a comparison between two samples (e.g., pre- versus post-contact) of the quotient of the outcomes of two events or conditions (e.g., compare pre-contact presence ÷ absence with post-contact presence ÷ absence). The authors utilized a statistical package (SAS 9.1) to test for a significant difference between all of the paired comparisons.[20] The OR results were porotic hyperostosis and (particularly) periostitis expectedly increased in prevalence in the post-contact period but LEH showed a decline. The authors consider three plausible explanations for the LEH decline: sampling bias, the shorter duration tooth development within which to document enamel-damaging stress episodes, and (most likely) a historically documented epidemiological shift to acute rather than chronic health problems.

Case Study: Treponemal Disease and Sedentism

Most **specific infections** are recognized by no more than a few cases in any one skeletal sample. However, if a multiple site sample in close geographic proximity and similar social and economic contexts can be generated (a meta-analysis), a specific disease can become a tool of bioarchaeological inquiry. One of these circumstances is the prevalence of trepo-nemal disease in an eight-site sample (n = 581) that straddles the Late Archaic (circa 3000

---

[19]This can be calculated at websites such as http://faculty.vassar.edu/lowry/propdiff_ind.html.

[20]The odds ratio can be easily calculated using free software available online. For example: http://www.hutchon.net/ConfidOR.htm.

B.C. to 1000–500 B.C.) and an Early Woodland (~500 B.C. to 0 A.D.) period in west-central Tennessee (Smith, 2006) (Figure 7.5c).

Endemic treponemal disease is epidemiologically associated with poor community hygiene and archaeologically co-associates with sedentism and aggregate (village) settlement pattern (Aufderheide and Rodríguez-Martín, 1998; Ortner, 2003; Cook and Powell, 2005). It is present in low case frequencies (circa 2–4%) in the hunter–gatherer Archaic period of the Eastern United States (Kelly, 1980; Cook and Powell, 2005; Powell et al., 2005). The disease, not surprisingly, dramatically increased to circa 10% after 1000 A.D. (Mississippian period) as maize cultivation and village settlement patterning intensified (Aufderheide and Rodrí-guez-Martín, 1998; Ortner, 2003; Hutchinson et al., 2005; Cook and Powell, 2005; Powell et al., 2005). The question generated from this observation is whether treponemal disease ALSO dramatically increased to a higher frequency in emergent horticulturists of the Early Woodland period.

The Woodland period (1000 B.C. to 1000 A.D.) in the Eastern United States is characterized by several subsistence-settlement changes: sedentism, widespread adoption of pottery, and horticulture (Anderson and Mainfort, 2002). A convenient marker for the emergence of the Woodland period (1000 B.C.) is the presence of pottery (Farnsworth and Emerson, 1986; Sassaman, 2004) as some degree of settlement (i.e., kilns) is presumed (Brown, 1986, 1989). However, the earliest potters in the Southeastern United States are archaeologically characterized as hunter–gatherers (Farnsworth and Emerson, 1986; Anderson and Mainfort, 2002). In the Tennessee sample, the only material culture difference between the Archaic and the Early Woodland horizons is the presence of fishhooks and pottery (Bowen, 1975, 1977). Therefore, there is little to argue that there is a change in subsistence-settlement pattern. But if a sedentism-sensitive health parameter is demonstrably different between the temporal horizons, then you have effectively utilized bioarchaeology as an archaeological problem-solving tool.

The results from the Tennessee meta-analysis (barring sampling error) were nothing less than striking: 0.5–1% (n = 378) in the Late Archaic to 9.1% (n = 88) in the Early Woodland (Smith, 2006). These results corroborate earlier studies suggesting that ecology and site density matter in the visibility of treponemal disease (Cook and Powell, 2005; Hutchinson et al., 2005). Clearly knowing the archaeological context and the unanswered sociopolitical, subsistence, and settlement questions enables the bioarchaeologist to address issues that the material culture remains cannot.

CONCLUSION: PALEOPATHOLOGY AS AN INVESTIGATIVE TOOL

In the decades since the adoption of the biocultural approach, the problem-solving abilities of paleopathological data have certainly not been fully exploited or exhausted. The appeal of bioarchaeology is that for every question answered, several new ones are formulated. Unexpected results are particularly exciting. Arguably, as long as there are questions to be posed and data that can be marshaled to address them, analytical paleopathology will continue to be a vibrant research tool. It should be noted that it cannot be said that analysis of a skeletal sample is "finished" or that all the data are collected. To argue so is to equate termination with completion.

Successful research projects effectively begin with familiarity with the human skeleton and the look and texture of normal bone. Knowing the morphology and the diagnostic features of common conditions is the next step. When the unfamiliar is encountered, the paleopathological diagnostic texts are essential (e.g., Aufderheide and Rodríguez-Martín, 1998; Ortner, 2003), as are journal article searches (for example, *American Journal of Physical Anthropology*, (the new) *International Journal of Paleopathology*, and *International Journal of Osteoarchaeology*). Further, do not neglect a search of the medical literature. General disease encyclopedias are a good place to start. Thorough description is necessary for reliable diagnosis, particularly if the study sample is not local or only temporarily available. Therefore time and effort should be devoted to determining methods of observation (score sheets, photographs, computer data entry, radiographs) and quantification (presence/absence, severity scale). Analytical success includes familiarity with the recovery and cultural context of the sample. Always consider soliciting advice or help with statistical analysis. Above all, read.

There will always be impediments to effective analytical paleopathology. These include problems of skeletal sample context such as preservation and recovery bias and an incomplete temporal sequence. Other problems relate to differential diagnosis, quantification, and the osteological paradox. The strength of analytical paleopathology is that it has a multidisciplinary methodology. It cannot be effectively undertaken without the approaches, analytical tools, and datasets that are reflected in the other chapters in this volume.

REFERENCES

Adams, W., Van Gerven, D.P., Guise, D., 1999. Kulubnarti III: The Cemeteries. Archaeopress, Oxford.

Agarwal, S.C., Glencross, B.A., 2011. Social Bioarchaeology. John Wiley & Sons, Malden.

Ameen, S., Staub, L., Ulrich, S., Vock, P., Ballmer, F., Anderson, S.E., 2005. Harris lines of the tibia across centuries: A comparison of two populations, medieval and contemporary in Central Europe. Skeletal Radiology 34 (5), 279—284.

Anderson, D.G., Mainfort, R.C. (Eds.), 2002. The Woodland Southeast. University of Alabama Press, Tuscaloosa.

Angel, J.L., 1966. Porotic hyperostosis, anemias, malarias, and the marshes in the prehistoric Eastern Mediterranean. Science 12 (3737), 760—763.

Angel, J.L., 1981. History and development of paleopathology. American Journal of Physical Anthropology 56 (4), 509—515.

Armelagos, G.J., 1968. Paleopathology of Three Archaeological Populations from Sudanese Nubia. Unpublished PhD dissertation. University of Colorado, Boulder.

Armelagos, G.J., 1997. Paleopathology. In: Spencer, F. (Ed.), History of Physical Anthropology: An Encyclopedia, Vol. 2. Garland Publishing, New York, 790—796.

Armelagos, G.J., 2011. Histories of scholars, ideas, and disciplines of biological anthropology and archaeology. Reviews in Anthropology 40 (2), 107—133.

Armelagos, G.J., Dewey, J., 1970. Evolutionary response to human infectious disease. Bioscience 20 (5), 271—275.

Armelagos, G.J., Van Gerven, D.P., 2003. A century of skeletal biology and paleopathology: contrast, contradictions, and conflict. American Anthropologist 105 (1), 51—62.

Armelagos, G.J., Carlson, D.S., Van Gerven, D.P., 1982. The theoretical foundations and development of skeletal biology. In: Spencer, F. (Ed.), A History of Physical Anthropology, 1930—1980. Academic Press, New York, 305—328.

Arnold, P.J., Wilkens, B.S., 2001. On the Vanpool's 'scientific' postprocessualism. American Antiquity 66 (2), 361—366.

Aufderheide, A.C., Rodriguez-Martin, C., 1998. The Cambridge Encyclopedia of Human Paleopathology. Cambridge University Press, New York.

Baadsgaard, A., Boutin, A.T., Buikstra, J.E. (Eds.), 2012. Breathing New Life into the Evidence of Death: Contemporary Approaches to Bioarchaeology. SAR Publication, Santa Fe, NM.

Benjamin, M., Toumi, H., Ralphs, J.R., Bydder, G., Best, T.M., Milz, S., 2006. Where tendons and ligaments meet bone: attachment sites ("entheses") in relation to exercise and/or mechanical load. Journal of Anatomy 208 (4), 471–490.

Bentley, R.A., Maschner, H.D.G., Chippendale, C. (Eds.), 2009. Handbook of Archaeological Theories. AltaMira Press, Lanham, MD.

Bethard, J.D., 2013. Isotopes. In: DiGangi, E.A., Moore, M.K. (Eds.), Research Methods in Human Skeletal Biology. Academic Press, San Diego.

Binford, S.R., Binford, L., 1968. New Perspectives in Archaeology. Aldine Press, Chicago.

Bintliff, J., 1993. Why Indiana Jones is smarter than the post-processualists. Norweigan Archaeological Review 26 (2), 91–100.

Blom, D., 2005. Embodying borders: human body modification and diversity in Tiwanaku society. Journal of Anthropological Archaeology 24 (1), 1–24.

Blom, D.E., Buikstra, J.E., Keng, L., Tomczak, P.D., Shoreman, E., Stevens-Tuttle, D., 2005. Anemia and childhood mortality: latitudinal patterning along the coast of pre-Columbian Peru. American Journal of Physical Anthropology 127 (2), 152–169.

Booth, C., 2007. People of Ancient Egypt. Tempus, Gloucestershire.

Borza, E., 1979. Some observations on malaria and the ecology of central Macedonia in antiquity. American Journal of Ancient History 4, 102–124.

Bowen, W.R., 1975. Late Archaic Subsistence and Settlement in the Western Tennessee Valley. M.A. thesis. University of Tennessee, Knoxville.

Bowen, W.R., 1977. A reevaluation of late Archaic subsistence and settlement patterns in the western Tennessee Valley. Tennessee Anthropology 2, 101–120.

Brickley, M., Ives, R., 2006. Skeletal manifestations of infantile scurvy. American Journal of Physical Anthropology 129 (2), 163–172.

Brickley, M., Ives, R., 2008. The Bioarchaeology of Metabolic Bone Disease. Academic Press, Oxford.

Brickley, M., McKinley, J. (Eds.), 2004. Guidelines to the Standards for Recording Human Remains. BABAO, Department of Archaeology, University of Southampton, & the Institute of Field Archaeologists, SHES, University of Reading From http://www.babao.org.uk/HumanremainsFINAL.pdf.

Brickley, M., Mays, S., Ives, R., 2007. An investigation of skeletal indicators of vitamin D deficiency in adults: effective markers for interpreting past living conditions and pollution levels in 18th- and 19th-century Birmingham, England. American Journal of Physical Anthropology 132 (1), 67–79.

Bridges, P.S., 1991. Degenerative joint disease in hunter-gatherers and agriculturalists from the Southeastern United States. American Journal of Physical Anthropology 85 (4), 379–391.

Brothwell, D.R., 1963. Digging up Bones: the Excavation, Treatment and Study of Human Skeletal Remains, 3rd ed. British Museum of Natural History, London [1981].

Brothwell, D.R., Sandison, A.T., 1967. Diseases in Antiquity: A Survey of the Diseases, Injuries, and Surgery of Early Populations. C.C. Thomas, Springfield, IL.

Brown, J.A., 1986. Early ceramics and culture: a review of interpretations. In: Farnsworth, K.B., Emerson, T.E. (Eds.), Early Woodland Archaeology. Center for American Archaeology Press, Kampsville, IL, pp. 598–608.

Brown, J.A., 1989. The beginnings of pottery as an economic process. In: van der Leeuw, S.E., Torrence, R. (Eds.), What's New? A Closer Look at the Process of Innovation. Unwin Hyman, London, pp. 203–224.

Buikstra, J.E., 1977a. Biocultural dimensions of archeological study: a regional perspective. In: Blakely, R.L. (Ed.), Biocultural Adaptation in Prehistoric America, Southern Anthropological Society Proceedings, 11(6), pp. 67–84.

Buikstra, J.E., 1977b. Differential diagnosis: an epidemiological model. Yearbook of Physical Anthropology 20, 316–328.

Buikstra, J., Beck, L., 2006. Bioarchaeology: The Contextual Study of Human Remains. Elsevier, New York.

Buikstra, J.E., Cook, D.C., 1980. Paleopathology: an American account. Annual Review of Anthropology 9, 433–470.

Buikstra, J.E., Scott, R.E., 2009. Identity formation: Communities and individuals. In: Knudson, K., Stojanowski, C. (Eds.), Bioarchaeology and Identity. University Press of Florida, Gainesville FL, pp. 24–55.

Buikstra, J.E., Ubelaker, D. (Eds.), 1994. Standards for Data Collection from Human Skeletal Remains: Proceedings of a Seminar at the Field Museum of Natural History. Arkansas Archaeological Survey Press, Fayetteville, AR.

Buikstra, J.E., Konigsberg, L.W., Bullington, J., 1986. Fertility and the development of agriculture in the prehistoric Midwest. American Antiquity 51, 528–546.

Buzon, M.R., 2006. Health of the non-elites at Tombos: Nutritional and disease stress in New Kingdom Nubia. American Journal of Physical Anthropology 130 (1), 26–37.

Byers, S.N., 1994. On stress and stature in the osteological paradox. Current Anthropology 35 (3), 282–284.

Cardoso, F.A., Henderson, C.Y., 2010. Enthesopathy formation in the humerus: Data from known age-at-death and known occupation skeletal collections. American Journal of Physical Anthropology 141 (4), 550–560.

Carlson, D.S., Armelagos, G.J., Van Gerven, D.P., 1974. Factors influencing the etiology of cribra orbitalia in prehistoric Nubia. Journal of Human Evolution 3 (5), 405–410.

Cassidy, C.M., 1972. A Comparison of Nutrition and Health in Pre-agricultural and Agricultural Amerindian Skeletal Populations. Unpublished PhD dissertation. University of Wisconsin.

Chapman, N.E., 1997. Evidence for Spanish influence on activity induced musculoskeletal stress markers at Pecos Pueblo. International Journal of Osteoarchaeology 7 (5), 497–506.

Cohen, M.N., Armelagos, G.J. (Eds.), 1984. Paleopathology at the Origins of Agriculture. Academic Press, New York.

Cohen, M.N., Wood, J.W., Milner, G.R., 1994. The osteological paradox reconsidered. Current Anthropology 35 (5), 629–637.

Cook, D.C., 1976. Pathologic States and Disease Process in Illinois Woodland Populations: An Epidemiologic Approach. Unpublished PhD dissertation. University of Chicago.

Cook, D.C., 2002. Rhinomaxillary syndrome in the absence of leprosy: an exercise in differential diagnosis. In: Roberts, C.A., Lewis, M.E., Manchester, K. (Eds.), The Past and Present of Leprosy. Archaeopress, Oxford, pp. 85–92.

Cook, D.C., Powell, M.L., 2005. Piecing the puzzle together: North American treponematosis in overview. In: Powell, M.L., Cook, D.C. (Eds.), The Myth of Syphilis: The Natural History of Treponematosis in North America. University of Florida Press, Gainesville, pp. 442–479.

Cook, D.C., Powell, M.L., 2006. The evolution of American paleopathology. In: Buikstra, J.E., Beck, L.A. (Eds.), Bioarchaeology: The Contextual Analysis of Human Remains. Academic Press, San Diego, pp. 281–322.

Cox, M., Mays, S. (Eds.), 2000. Human Osteology in Archaeology and Forensic Science. Greenwich Medical Media, London.

Crubézy, E., Ludes, B., Poveda, J.D., Clayton, J., Crouau-Roy, B., Montagnon, D., 1998. Identification of Mycobacterium DNA in an Egyptian Pott's disease of 5,400 years old. Comptes Rendus de l'Académie des Sciences—Serie III, Sciences de la Vie 321 (11), 941–951.

D'Anastasio, R., Staniscia, T., Milia, M.L., Manzoli, L., Capasso, L., 2011. Origin, evolution and paleoepidemiology of brucellosis. Epidemiology and Infection 139 (1), 149–156.

David, A.R., 2008. Egyptian Mummies and Modern Science. Cambridge University Press, New York.

David, A.R., Garner, V., 2003. Asru, an Ancient Egyptian temple chantress: modern spectrometric studies as part of the Manchester Egyptian Mummy Research Project. Molecular and Structural Archaeology: Cosmetic and Therapeutic Chemicals, NATO Science Series 117, 153–162.

Diamond, J., 1987. The worst mistake in the history of the human race. Discover Magazine 1987, 64–66.

DiGangi, E.A., Hefner, J.T., 2013. Ancestry estimation. In: DiGangi, E.A., Moore, M.K. (Eds.), Research Methods in Human Skeletal Biology. Academic Press, San Diego.

DiGangi, E.A., Moore, M.K., 2013. Application of the scientific method to skeletal biology. In: DiGangi, E.A., Moore, M.K. (Eds.), Research Methods in Human Skeletal Biology. Academic Press, San Diego.

DiGangi, E.A., Moore, M.K., 2013. Introduction to Research in Skeletal Biology. In: DiGangi, E.A., Moore, M.K. (Eds.), Research Methods in Human Skeletal Biology. Academic Press, San Diego.

DiGangi, E.A., Bethard, J.D., Sullivan, L.P., 2010. Differential diagnosis of cartilaginous dysplasia and probable Osgood–Schlatter's disease in a Mississippian individual from East Tennessee. International Journal of Osteoarchaeology 20 (4), 424–442.

Dobres, M., Robb, J., 2000. Agency in Archaeology. Routledge, New York.

Dornan, J.L., 2002. Agency and archaeology: past, present, and future directions. Journal of Archaeological Method and Theory 9 (4), 303–329.

Duncan, W.N., 2009. Cranial modification among the Maya: absence of evidence or evidence of absence? In: Knudson, K.J., Stojanowski, C.M. (Eds.), Bioarchaeology and Identity in the Americas. University Press of Florida, Gainesville, pp. 177–193.

Duncan, W.N., Hofling, C.A., 2011. Why the head? Cranial modification as protection and ensoulment among the Maya. Ancient Mesoamerica 22, 109–210.

Ellison, P.T., O'Rourke, M.T., 2000. Population growth and fertility regulation. In: Stinson, S., Bogin, B., Huss-Ashmore, R., O'Rourke, D. (Eds.), Human Biology: An Evolutionary and Biocultural Perspective. Wiley, New York, pp. 553–586.

Elzay, R.P., Allison, M.J., Pezzia, A., 1977. A comparative study on the dental health status of five Precolumbian Peruvian cultures. American Journal of Physical Anthropology 46 (1), 135–140.

Eshed, V., Gopher, A., Galili, E., Hershkovitz, I., 2004. Musculoskeletal stress markers in Natufian hunter-gatherers and Neolithic farmers in the Levant: the upper limb. American Journal of Physical Anthropology 123 (4), 303–315.

Facchini, F., Rastelli, E., Brasili, P., 2004. Cribra orbitalia and cribra crania in Roman skeletal remains from the Ravenna area and Rimini (I–IV century AD). International Journal of Osteoarchaeology 14 (2), 136–146.

Fairgrieve, S.I., Molto, J.E., 2000. Cribra orbitalia in two temporally disjunct population samples from the Dakhleh Oasis, Egypt. American Journal of Physical Anthropology 111 (3), 319–331.

Farid, Z., Patwardhan, V.N., Darby, W.J., 1969. Parasitism and anemia. American Journal of Clinical Nutrition 22 (5), 498–503.

Farnsworth, K.B., Emerson, T.E. (Eds.), 1986. Early Woodland Archaeology. Center for American Archaeology Press, Kampsville, IL.

Farnum, J.F., 2002. Biological Consequences of Social Inequalities in Prehistoric Peru. Unpublished PhD dissertation. University of Missouri-Columbia.

Fornaciari, G., Brier, B., Fornaciari, A., 2007. Secrets of the Medici. In: Parker, M.P., Angeloni, E. (Eds.), Annual Editions: Archaeology. McGraw-Hill Contemporary Learning Series, Dubuque, pp. 120–122.

Geller, P.L., 2008. Conceiving sex: fomenting a feminist bioarchaeology. Journal of Social Archaeology 8 (1), 113–138.

Geller, P.L., 2009. Bodyscapes, biology, and heteronormativity. American Anthropologist 111 (4), 504–516.

Gero, J.M., Conkey, M.W. (Eds.), 1991. Engendering Archaeology: Women and Prehistory. Wiley-Blackwell, Oxford.

Gilchrist, R., 2000. Archaeological biographies: realizing human lifecyles, -courses, and -histories. World Archaeology 31 (3), 325–328.

Glencross, B.A., 2011. Skeletal injury across the life course: towards understanding social agency. In: Agarwal, S.C., Glencross, B.A. (Eds.), Social Bioarchaeology. John Wiley & Sons, Malden, MA, pp. 390–409.

Goldstein, M.S., 1963. Human paleopathology. Journal of the National Medical Association 55 (2), 100–106.

Goodman, A.H., Armelagos, G.J., 1985. Disease and death at Dr. Dickson's Mounds. History 9 (85), 12–18.

Goodman, A.H., Thomas, R.B., Swedlund, A.C., Armelagos, G.J., 1988. Biocultural perspectives on stress in prehistoric, historical, and contemporary population research. Yearbook of Physical Anthropology 31 (Suppl. 9), 169–202.

Grace, E., 2011. Demography, paleopathology, and Health status of the Moche Remains. In: Huambacho, Peru: A Comprehensive Osteological Analysis. M.A. thesis. Louisiana State University, Eunice.

Grauer, A.L., 2008. Macroscopic analysis and data collection in paleopathology. In: Pinhasi, R., Mays, S. (Eds.), Advances in Human Paleopathology. Wiley Liss, New York, pp. 57–76.

Grauer, A.L., 2012. A Companion to Paleopathology. Blackwell Companions to Anthropology. Wiley-Blackwell, New York.

Grauer, A.L., Stuart-Macadam, P., 1998. Sex and Gender in Paleopathological Perspective. Cambridge University Press, New York.

Hackett, C.J., 1975. An introduction to diagnostic criteria of syphilis, treponarid and yaws (treponematoses) in dry bones, and some implications. Virchows Archive A Pathology, Anatomy, and Histology 368 (3), 229–241.

Halcrow, S.E., Tayles, N., 2011. The bioarchaeological investigation of children and childhood. In: Agarwal, S.C., Glencross, B.A. (Eds.), Social Bioarchaeology. Wiley-Blackwell, New York, pp. 333–360.

Hamilakis, Y., Pluciennik, M., Tarlow, S. (Eds.), 2002. Thinking through the Body: Archaeologies of Corporeality. Kluwer Academic/Plenum Publishers, New York.

Hammerl, E., 2013. Dental anthropology. In: DiGangi, E.A., Moore, M.K. (Eds.), Research Methods in Human Skeletal Biology. Academic Press, San Diego.

Hawkey, D.E., Merbs, C.F., 1995. Activity-induced musculoskeletal stress markers (MSM) and subsistence strategy changes among ancient Hudson Bay Eskimos. International Journal of Osteoarchaeology 5 (4), 324–338.

Hays-Gilpin, K., 2000. Feminist scholarship in archaeology. Annals of the American Academy of Political and Social Science 571 (1), 89–106.

Hershkovitz, I., Ring, B., Speirs, M., Galili, E., Kislev, M., Edelson, G., Hershkovitz, A., 1991. Possible congenital hemolytic anemia in prehistoric coastal inhabitants of Israel. American Journal of Physical Anthropology 85 (1), 7–13.

Hirata, K., 1990. Secular trend and age distribution of cribra orbitalia in Japanese. Human Evolution 5 (4), 375–385.

Hodder, I., Hutson, S., 2003. Reading the Past: Current Approaches to Interpretation in Archaeology, 3rd ed. Cambridge University Press, Cambridge.

Huffman, T.N., 2004. Beyond data: the aim and practice of archaeology. South African Archaeological Bulletin 59 (180), 66–69.

Hulse, F.H., 1981. Habits, habitats, and heredity: a brief history of studies in human plasticity. American Journal of Physical Anthropology 56 (4), 495–501.

Hummert, J.R., Van Gerven, D.P., 1983. Skeletal growth in a Medieval population from Sudanese Nubia. American Journal of Physical Anthropology 60 (4), 471–478.

Hutchinson, D., Larsen, C.S., Williamson, M., Green-Clow, V.D., 2005. Temporal and spatial variation in the patterns of treponematosis in Georgia and Florida. In: Powell, M.L., Cook, D.C. (Eds.), The myth of syphilis: the natural history of treponematosis in North America. University of Florida Press, Gainesville, pp. 92–116.

Jackes, M., 1993. On paradox and osteology. Current Anthropology 34 (4), 434–439.

Jacobi, K.P., Danforth, M.E., 2002. Analysis of interobserver scoring patterns in porotic hyperostosis and cribra orbitalia. International Journal of Osteoarchaeology 12 (4), 248–258.

Jarcho, S., 1966. Human Palaeopathology. Yale University Press, New Haven.

Jurmain, R., 1990. Paleoepidemiology of a central California prehistoric population from CA-ALA-329: II. Degenerative disease. American Journal of Physical Anthropology 83 (1), 83–94.

Jurmain, R., 1999. Stories from the Skeleton: Behavioral Reconstruction in Human Osteology. Taylor and Francis, London.

Jurmain, R., Vilotte, S., 2010. Report from Workshop in Musculoskeletal Stress Markers (MSM): limitations and achievements in the reconstruction of past activity patterns. University of Coimbra. July 2–3, 2009. Coimbra, CIAS — Centro de Investigação em Antropologia e Saúde. Terminology. Entheses in medical literature and physical anthropology: a brief review. From: http://www.uc.pt/en/cia/msm/MSM_terminology3.

Jurmain, R., Alves Cardoso, F., Henderson, C., Vilotte, S., 2012. Bioarchaeology's Holy Grail: The reconstruction of activity. In: Grauer, A.L. (Ed.), Companion to Paleopathology. Wiley-Blackwell, New York, pp. 531–552.

Juurlink, B.H., 2009. Human Osteology & Skeletal Radiology: An Atlas and Guide. CRC Press, New York.

Katzenberg, M.A., Saunders, S.R., 2008. Biological Anthropology of the Human Skeleton, 2nd ed. Wiley-Liss, New York.

Keenleyside, A., Panayotova, K., 2006. Cribra orbitalia and porotic hyperostosis in a Greek colonial population (5th to 3rd centuries BC) from the Black Sea. Journal of Osteoarchaeology 16 (5), 373–384.

Kelley, M.A., 1980. Disease and Environment: A Comparative Analysis of Three Early American Indian Skeletal Collections. Unpublished PhD dissertation. Case Western Reserve University, Cleveland.

Kelley, M.A., Eisenberg, L.E., 1987. Blastomycosis and tuberculosis in early American Indians: a biocultural view. Midcontinental Journal of Archaeology 12 (1), 89–116.

Kennedy, K.A.R., 1989. Skeletal markers of occupational stress. In: Iscan, M., Kennedy, K. (Eds.), Reconstruction of Life from the Skeleton. Alan R. Liss, New York, pp. 129–160.

Kent, S., 1986. The influence of sedentism and aggregation on porotic hyperostosis and anaemia: a case study. Man, New Series 21 (4), 605–636.

Klaus, H.D., 2008. Bioarchaeology of Life and Death in Colonial South America: Systemic Stress, Adaptation, and Ethnogenesis in the Lambayeque Valley, Peru AD 900–1750. Unpublished PhD dissertation. The Ohio State University.

Klaus, H.D., Tam, M.E., 2009. Contact in the Andes: bioarchaeology of systemic stress in colonial Mórrope, Peru. American Journal of Physical Anthropology 138 (3), 356–368.

Knudson, K.J., Stojanowski, C.M., 2008. New directions in bioarchaeology: recent contributions to the study of human social identities. Journal of Archaeological Research 16, 397–432.

Knudson, K.J., Stojanowski, C.M., 2009. Bioarchaeology and Identity in the Americas. University Press of Florida, Tallahassee.

Konigsberg, L.W., Frankenberg, S.R., 2013. Demography. In: DiGangi, E.A., Moore, M.K. (Eds.), Research Methods in Human Skeletal Biology. Academic Press, San Diego.

Kosso, P., 1991. Method in archaeology: middle-range theory as hermeneutics. American Antiquity 56 (4), 621–627.

Kroman, A.M., 2013. Skeletal trauma. In: DiGangi, E.A., Moore, M.K. (Eds.), Research Methods in Human Skeletal Biology. Academic Press, San Diego.

Lai, P., Lovell, N.C., 1992. Skeletal markers of occupational stress in the fur trade: a case study from a Hudson's Bay Company fur trade post. International Journal of Osteoarchaeology 2 (3), 221–234.

Lallo, J.W., 1972. Skeletal Biology of 3 Prehistoric American Indian Populations from Dickson Mounds. PhD. dissertation. University of Massachusetts, Amherst.

Lallo, J.W., Rose, J.C., 1979. Patterns of stress, diseases, and mortality in two prehistoric populations from North America. Journal of Human Evolution 8 (3), 323–334.

Lallo, J.W., Armelagos, G.J., Mensforth, R., 1977. The role of diet, diseases and physiology in the origin of porotic hyperostosis. Human Biology 49, 471–483.

Lallo, J.W., Armelagos, G.J., Rose, J.C., 1978. Paleoepidemiology of infectious disease in the Dickson Mounds population. Medical College of Virginia Quarterly 14 (1), 17–23.

Larsen, C.S., 1997. Bioarchaeology: Interpreting Behavior from the Human Skeleton. Cambridge University Press, New York.

Larsen, C.S., Sering, L., 2000. Inferring iron deficiency anemia from human skeletal remains: the case of the Georgia Bight. In: Lambert, P. (Ed.), Bioarchaeological Studies in Life in the Age of Agriculture. University of Alabama Press, Tuscaloosa, pp. 116–133.

Lewis, M.E., 2007. The Bioarchaeology of Children: Perspectives from Biological and Forensic Anthropology. Cambridge University Press, Cambridge.

Little, L.M., Papadopoulos, J.K., 1998. A social outcast in Early Iron Age Athens. Hesperia: The Journal of the American School of Classical Studies at Athens 67 (4), 375–404.

Lovejoy, C.O., Russell, K.F., Harrison, M.L., 1990. Long bone growth velocity in the Libben population. American Journal of Human Biology 2 (5), 533–541.

Lovell, N.C., Dublenko, A.A., 1999. Further aspects of fur trade life depicted in the skeleton. International Journal of Osteoarchaeology 9 (4), 248–256.

Mann, R.W., Hunt, D.R., 2005. Photographic Regional Atlas of Bone Disease: A Guide to Pathologic and Normal Variation in the Human Skeleton. Charles C. Thomas, Springfield, IL.

Marden, K., Sorg, M.H., Haglund, W.D., 2013. Taphonomy. In: DiGangi, E.A., Moore, M.K. (Eds.), Research Methods in Human Skeletal Biology. Academic Press, San Diego.

Marks, J., 2000. Human biodiversity as a central theme of biological anthropology: then and now. In: Marks, J. (Ed.), Racial Anthropology: Retrospective on Carleton Coon's The Origin of Races (1962). University of California, pp. 1–10. Kroeber Anthropological Society Papers, No. 84.

Marks, J., 2010. the two 20th-century crises of racial anthropology. In: Little, M.A., Kennedy, K.A.R. (Eds.), Histories of American Physical Anthropology in the Twentieth Century. Lexington Books, Lanham, pp. 187–206.

Marsteller, S.J., Torres-Rouff, C., Knudson, K.J., 2011. Pre-Columbian Andean sickness ideology and the social experience of leishmaniasis: a contextualized analysis of bioarchaeological and paleopathological data from San Pedro de Atacama, Chile. International Journal of Paleopathology 1 (1), 24–34.

Mays, S., 1995. The relationship between Harris lines and other aspects of skeletal development in adults and juveniles. Journal of Archaeological Science 22 (4), 511–520.

Mays, S., 1998. The Archaeology of Human Bones. Routledge, London.

Mays, S., Eyers, J., 2011. Prenatal infant death at the Roman Villa site at Hambledon, Buckinghamshire, England. Journal of Archaeological Science 38 (8), 1931–1938.

Mays, S., Taylor, G.M., Legge, A.J., Young, D.B., Turner-Walker, G., 2001. Paleopathological and biomolecular study of tuberculosis in a medieval skeletal collection from England. American Journal of Physical Anthropology 114 (4), 298–311.

Mays, S., Turner-Walker, G., Syversen, U., 2006. Osteoporosis in a population from Medieval Norway. American Journal of Physical Anthropology 131 (3), 343–351.

McHugh, M.L., 2009. The odds ratio: calculation, usage, and interpretation. Biochemia Medica 19 (2), 120–126.

Mendonça de Souza, S., Maul de Carvalho, D., Lessa, S., 2003. Paleoepidemiology: is there a case to answer? Memorias do Instituto Oswaldo Cruz Volume 98 (1), 21–27.

Mensforth, R.P., Lovejoy, C.O., Lallo, J.W., Armelagos, G.J., 1978. The role of constitutional factors, diet, and infectious disease in the etiology of porotic hyperostosis and periosteal reactions in prehistoric infants and children. Medical Anthropology 2 (1), 1–59.

Milella, M., Belcastro, M.G., Zollikofer, C.P.E., Mariotti, V., 2012. The effect of age, sex, and physical activity on entheseal morphology in a contemporary Italian skeletal collection. American Journal of Physical Anthropology. http://dx.doi.org/10.1002/ajpa.22060.

Mittler, D.M., Van Gerven, D.P., 1994. Developmental, diachronic, and demographic analysis of cribra orbitalia in the Medieval Christian populations of Kulubnarti. American Journal of Physical Anthropology 93 (3) 287–297.

Molleson, T., 1994. The eloquent bones of Abu Hureyra. Scientific American, 70–75. August 1994.

Molleson, T., 2007. A method for the study of activity related skeletal morphologies. Bioarchaeology of the Near East 1, 5–33.

Molnar, P., 2011. Osteoarthritis and activity — an analysis of the relationship between eburnation, musculoskeletal stress markers (MSM) and age in two Neolithic hunter-gatherer populations from Gotland, Sweden. International Journal of Osteoarchaeology 21 (3), 283–291.

Molnar, P., 2006. Tracing prehistoric activities: Musculoskeletal stress marker analysis of a stone-age population on the Island of Gotland in the Baltic Sea. American Journal of Physical Anthropology 129 (1), 12–23.

Moore, M.K., 2013. Functional morphology and medical imaging. In: DiGangi, E.A., Moore, M.K. (Eds.), Research Methods in Human Skeletal Biology. Academic Press, San Diego.

Moore, M.K., 2013. Sex estimation and assessment. In: DiGangi, E.A., Moore, M.K. (Eds.), Research Methods in Human Skeletal Biology. Academic Press, San Diego.

Mutolo, M.J., Jenny, L.L., Buszek, A.R., Fenton, T.W., Foran, D.R., 2012. Osteological and molecular identification of brucellosis in Ancient Butrint, Albania. American Journal of Physical Anthropology 147 (2), 254–263.

Niinimäki, S., 2011. What do muscle marker ruggedness scores actually tell us? International Journal of Osteoarchaeology 21 (3), 292–299.

Niinimäki, S., 2012. The relationship between musculoskeletal stress markers and biomechanical properties of the humeral diaphysis. American Journal of Physical Anthropology 147 (4), 618–628.

Ortner, D.J., 2003. Identification of Pathological Conditions in Human Skeletal Remains. Academic Press, New York.

Ortner, D.J., Erickson, M.F., 1997. Bone changes in the human skull probably resulting from scurvy in infancy and childhood. International Journal of Osteoarchaeology 7 (3), 212–220.

Ortner, D.J., Mays, S.A., 1998. Dry bone manifestations of rickets in infancy and childhood. International Journal of Osteoarchaeology 8 (1), 45–55.

Ortner, D.J., Putschar, W.G.J., 1985. Identification of Pathological Conditions in Human Skeletal Remains. Smithsonian Institution Press, Washington, D.C.

Ortner, D.J., Butler, W., Cafarella, J., Milligan, L., 1999a. Evidence of probable scurvy in subadults from archaeological sites in North America. American Journal of Physical Anthropology 114 (4), 343–351.

Ortner, D.J., Kimmerle, E., Diez, M., 1999b. Skeletal evidence of scurvy in archaeological skeletal samples from Peru. American Journal of Physical Anthropology 108, 321–331.

Ortner, D.J., Butler, W., Cafarella, J., Milligan, L., 2001. Evidence of probable scurvy in subadults from archaeological sites in North America. American Journal of Physical Anthropology 114 (4), 343–351.

Oxenham, M.F., Cavill, I., 2010. Porotic hyperostosis and cribra orbitalia: the erythropoietic response to iron-deficiency anaemia. Anthropological Science 118 (3), 199–200.

Papageorgopoulou, C., Suter, S.K., Rühli, F.J., Siegmund, F., 2011. Harris lines revisited: prevalence, comorbidities, and possible etiologies. American Journal of Human Biology 23 (3), 381–391.

Pfeiffer, S., Crowder, C., 2004. An ill child among mid-Holocene foragers of southern Africa. American Journal of Physical Anthropology 123 (1), 23–29.

Pinhasi, R., Mays, S., 2008. Advances in Human Paleopathology. Wiley Liss, New York.

Pinhasi, R., Stock, J.T., 2011. Human Bioarchaeology of the Transition to Agriculture. Wiley Liss, New York.

Pinhasi, R., Shaw, P., White, B., Ogden, A.R., 2006. Morbidity, rickets, and long-bone growth in post-Medieval Britain—a cross-population analysis. Annals of Human Biology 33 (3), 372–389.

Powell, M.L., Cook, D.C. (Eds.), 2005. The Myth of Syphilis: The Natural History of Treponematosis in North America. University Press of Florida, Gainesville.

Powell, M.L., Bogdan, G., Cook, D.C., Sandford, M.K., Smith, M.O., Weaver, D.S., 2005. Treponematosis before 1000 B.C.? The skeletal evidence. In: Powell, M.L., Cook, D.C. (Eds.), The Myth of Syphilis: The Natural History of Treponematosis in North America. University of Florida Press, Gainesville, pp. 418—441.

Prendergast, M.K., Thorp, S., Van Gerven, D.P., 1986. Pattern of dental eruption, skeletal maturation, and stress in a Medieval population from Sudanese Nubia. Human Evolution 1 (4), 325—330.

Putschar, W.G.J., 1966. Problems in the pathology and paleopathology of bone. In: Jarcho, S. (Ed.), Human Paleopathology. Yale University Press, New Haven, pp. 57—65.

Relethford, J.H., 2010. Race and the conflicts within the profession of physical anthropology during the 1950s and 1960s. In: Little, M.A., Kennedy, K.A.R. (Eds.), Histories of American Physical Anthropology in the Twentieth Century. Lexington Books, Lanham, pp. 207—220.

Renschler, E., 2007. An Osteobiography of an African Diasporic Skeletal Sample Integrating Skeletal and Historical Information. Dissertation. University of Pennsylvania.

Robb, J.E., 1998. The interpretation of skeletal muscle sites: a statistical approach. International Journal of Osteoarchaeology 8 (5), 363—377.

Robb, J.E., 2002. Time and biography: Osteobiography of the Italian neolithic lifespan. In: Hamilakis, Y., Pluciennik, M., Tarlow, S. (Eds.), Thinking through the Body: Archaeologies of Corporeality. Kluwer Academic/Plenum Publishers, New York, pp. 153—172.

Robbins, G., Mushrif-Tripathy, V., Misra, V.N., Mohanty, R.K., Shinde, V.S., Gray, K.M., Schug, M.D., 2009. Ancient skeletal evidence for leprosy in India (2000 B.C.). PLoS ONE 4 (5), e5669. http://dx.doi.org/5610.1371/journal.pone.0005669.

Roberts, C.A., 2000. Did they take sugar: the use of skeletal evidence in the study of disability in past populations. In: Hubert, J. (Ed.), Madness, Disability, and Social Exclusion: The Archaeology and Anthropology of Difference. Routledge, London, pp. 46—59.

Roberts, C.A., Buikstra, J.E., 2003. The Bioarchaeology of Tuberculosis: A Global View on a Re-emerging Disease. University Press of Florida, Gainesville.

Roberts, C.A., Manchester, K., 2007. The Archaeology of Disease. Cornell University Press, Ithaca, NY.

Roberts, C.A., Lewis, M.E., Manchester, K. (Eds.), 2002. The Past and Present of Leprosy: Archaeological, Historical, Palaeopathological and Clinical Approaches. Proceedings of the 3rd International Congress on the Evolution and Palaeoepidemiology of the Infectious Diseases (ICEPID). British Archaeological Reports. International Series. Archaeopress, Oxford.

Roberts, D.F., 1995. The pervasiveness of plasticity. In: Mascie-Taylor, C.G.N., Bogin, B. (Eds.), Human Variability and Plasticity. Cambridge Studies in Biological and Evolutionary Anthropology. Cambridge University Press, New York, pp. 18—45.

Robledo, B., Trancho, G.J., Brothwell, D., 1995. Cribra orbitalia: health indicator in the late Roman population of Cannington (Somerset, Great Britain). Journal of Paleopathology 7 (3), 185—193.

Rogers, J., Waldron, T., 1989. Infections in palaeopathology: the basis of classification according to most probable cause. Journal of Archaeological Science 16 (6), 611—625.

Rosado, M.A., Vernacchio-Wilson, J., 2006. Paleopathology and osteobiography of the people of Peñuelas, Chile's semiarid north. Memorias do Instituto Oswaldo Cruz 101 (Suppl. II), 85—95.

Sallares, R., 2002. Malaria and Rome: A History of Malaria in Ancient Italy. Oxford University Press, New York.

Sallares, R., Gomzi, S., Bouwman, A., Anderung, C., Brown, T., 1999. Identification of a malaria epidemic in antiquity using ancient DNA. In: Robson Brown, K. (Ed.), Archaeological Sciences 1999. Proceedings of the Archaeological Sciences Conference, University of Bristol, 1999. Archaeopress, Oxford, pp. 120—125.

Sallares, R., Bouwman, A., Anderung, C., 2004. The spread of malaria to Southern Europe in antiquity: new approaches to old problems. Medical History 48 (3), 311—328.

Salvadei, L., Ricci, F., Manzi, G., 2001. Porotic hyperostosis as a marker of health and nutritional conditions during childhood: studies at the transition between Imperial Rome and the Early Middle Ages. American Journal of Human Biology 13 (6), 709—717.

Sassaman, K.E., 2004. Complex hunter-gatherers in evolution and history: a North American perspective. Journal of Archaeological Research 12 (3), 227—280.

Saul, F., Saul, J., 1989. Osteobiography: a Maya example. In: Iscan, M.Y., Kennedy, K.A.R. (Eds.), Reconstruction of Life from the Skeleton. Alan R. Liss, New York, 287–302.

Saunders, S.R., Hoppa, R.D., 1993. Growth deficit in survivors and non-survivors: biological mortality bias in subadult skeletal samples. Yearbook of Physical Anthropology 36 (17), 127–151.

Scrimshaw, N., Taylor, C.E., Gordon, J.E., 1968. Interactions of Nutrition and Infection. World Health Organization Monograph #57.

Smith, M.O., 2006. Treponemal disease in the Middle Archaic to Early Woodland periods of the Western Tennessee River Valley. American Journal of Physical Anthropology 131 (2), 205–217.

Smith, M.O., Betsinger, T.K., Williams, L.L., 2011. Differential visibility of treponemal disease in pre-Columbian stratified societies: does rank matter? American Journal of Physical Anthropology 144 (2), 185–195.

Sofaer, J.R., 2006. The Body as Material Culture: A Theoretical Osteoarchaeology. Cambridge University Press, New York.

Sofaer, J.R., 2011. Bodies and encounters. Seeing invisible children in archaeology. In: Coskunsu, G., Biehl, P. (Eds.), Children as Archaeological Enigma: Are Children Visible or Invisible in the Archaeological Record? SUNY Press, Dulles, VA.

Soren, D., Fenton, T., Birkby, W., 1995. The late Roman infant cemetery near Lugnano in Teverina, Italy: some implications. Journal of Paleopathology 7, 13–42.

Steckel, R.H., Rose, J.C., 2005. The Backbone of History: Health and Nutrition in the Western Hemisphere. Cambridge University Press, New York.

Steele, D.G., Bramblett, C.A., 1988. The Anatomy and Biology of the Human Skeleton. Texas A&M Press, College Station.

Steen, S.L., Lane, R.W., 1998. Evaluation of habitual activities among two Alaskan Eskimo populations based on musculoskeletal stress markers. International Journal of Osteoarchaeology 8 (5), 341–353.

Steinbock, R.T., 1976. Paleopathological Diagnosis and Interpretation: Bone Diseases in Ancient Human Populations. C.C. Thomas, Springfield, IL.

Stewart, T.D., 1966. Some problems in human paleopathology. In: Jarcho, S. (Ed.), Human Paleopathology. Yale University Press, New Haven, pp. 43–55.

Stewart, T.D., Quade, L.G., 1969. Lesions of the frontal bone in American Indians. American Journal of Physical Anthropology 30 (1), 89–110.

Stirland, A.J., 1998. Musculoskeletal evidence for activity: problems of evaluation. International Journal of Osteoarchaeology 8 (5), 354–362.

Stodder, A.L., 2012. Data and data analysis issues in paleopathology. In: Grauer, A. (Ed.), A Companion to Paleopathology. Wiley-Blackwell, New York, pp. 339–356.

Stodder, A.L., Palkovich, A.M., 2012. The Bioarchaeology of Individuals. University Press of Florida, Gainesville.

Stone, A.C., Wilbur, A.K., Buikstra, J.E., Roberts, C.A., 2009. Tuberculosis and leprosy in perspective. American Journal of Physical Anthropology 40 (Suppl. 49), 66–94.

Stuart-Macadam, P.L., 1985. Porotic hyperostosis: representative of a childhood condition. American Journal of Physical Anthropology 66 (4), 391–398.

Stuart-Macadam, P.L., 1987. Porotic hyperostosis: new evidence to support the anemia theory. American Journal of Physical Anthropology 74 (4), 521–526.

Stuart-Macadam, P.L., 1989. Nutritional deficiency diseases; a survey of scurvy, rickets and iron deficiency anaemia. In: Iscan, M.Y., Kennedy, K.A.R. (Eds.), Reconstruction of Life from the Skeleton. Alan R. Liss, New York, pp. 201–222.

Stuart-Macadam, P.L., 1992. Porotic hyperostosis: a new perspective. American Journal of Physical Anthropology 87 (1), 39–47.

Stuart-Macadam, P.L., Kent, S. (Eds.), 1992. Diet, Demography, and Disease: Changing Perspectives on Anemia. Aldine, Chicago.

Sullivan, A., 2005. Prevalence and etiology of acquired anemia in Medieval York, England. American Journal of Physical Anthropology 128 (2), 252–272.

Torres-Rouff, C., 2009. The bodily expression of ethnic identity: head shaping in the Chilean Atacama. In: Knudson, K.J., Stojanowski, C.M. (Eds.), Bioarchaeology and Identity in the Americas. University Press of Florida, Gainesville, 212–227.

Toyne, J.M., 2002. Tales Woven in their Bones: The Osteological Examination of the Human Skeletal Remains from the Stone Temple at Tú Cume, Peru. M.A. thesis. University of Western Ontario, London, Ontario.

Trigger, B.G., 2006. A History of Archaeological Thought, 2nd ed. Cambridge University Press, New York.

Turner, B.L., Edwards, J.L., Quinn, E.A., Kingston, J.D., Van Gerven, D.P., 2006. Age-related variation in isotopic indicators of diet at medieval Kulubnarti, Sudanese Nubia. International Journal of Osteoarchaeology 17 (1), 1–25.

Uhl, N.M., 2013. Age-at-death estimation. In: DiGangi, E.A., Moore, M.K. (Eds.), Research Methods in Human Skeletal Biology. Academic Press, San Diego.

Van Gerven, D.P., Sandford, M.K., Hummert, J.R., 1981. Mortality and culture change in Nubia's Butn el Hujur. Journal of Human Evolution 10, 395–408.

Van Gerven, D.P., Hummert, J.R., Moore, K.P., Sandford, M.K., 1990. Nutrition, disease, and the human life cycle: a bioethnography of a medieval Nubian community. In: DeRousseau, C.J. (Ed.), Primate Life History and Evolution. Monographs in Primatology, Vol. 14. Wiley-Liss, New York, pp. 297–323.

Vercellotti, G., Caramella, D., Formicola, V., Fornaciari, G., Larsen, C.S., 2010. Porotic hyperostosis in a Late Upper Palaeolithic skeleton (Villabruna 1, Italy). International Journal of Osteoarchaeology 20 (3), 358–368.

Verena, J., Schuenemann, K.B., DeWitte, S., Schmedes, S., Jamieson, J., Mittnik, A., Forrest, S., Coombes, B.K., Wood, J.W., Earn, D.J.D., White, W., Krause, J., Poinar, H.N., 2011. Targeted enrichment of ancient pathogens yielding the pPCP1 plasmid of *Yersinia pestis* from victims of the Black Death. Proceedings of the National Academy of Sciences, USA 108 (38), E746–E752.

Villotte, S., Castex, D., Couallier, V., Dutour, O., Knusel, C.J., Henry-Gambier, D., 2010. Enthesopathies as occupational stress markers: evidence from the upper limb. American Journal of Physical Anthropology 142 (2), 224–234.

Waldron, T., 1994. Counting the Dead: The Epidemiology of Skeletal Populations. John Wiley & Sons, New York.

Waldron, T., 2007a. Hidden or overlooked: where are the disadvantaged in the skeletal record? In: Insoll, T. (Ed.), The Archaeology of Identities: A Reader. Routledge, London.

Waldron, T., 2007b. Palaeoepidemiology: The Measure of Disease in the Human Past. Left Coast Press, Walnut Creek, CA.

Waldron, A., 2008. Paleopathology. Cambridge University Press, New York.

Waldron, T., Rogers, J., 1991. Inter-observer variation in coding osteoarthritis in human skeletal remains. International Journal of Osteoarchaeology 1 (1), 49–56.

Walker, P.L., Cook, D.C., 1998. Gender and sex: vive la difference. American Journal of Physical Anthropology 106 (2), 255–259.

Walker, P.L., Bathurst, R.R., Richman, R., Gjerdrum, T., Andrushko, V., 2009. The causes of porotic hyperostosis and cribra orbitalia: a reappraisal of the iron-deficiency-anemia hypothesis. American Journal of Physical Anthropology 139 (2), 109–125.

Wapler, I., Crubézy, E., Schultz, M., 2004. Is cribra orbitalia synonymous with anemia? Analysis and interpretation of cranial pathology in Sudan. American Journal of Physical Anthropology 123 (4), 333–339.

Washburn, S.L., 1951. The new physical anthropology. Transactions of the New York Academy of Science 13 (2), 298–304.

Weiss, E., 2003. Understanding muscle markers: aggregation and construct validity. American Journal of Physical Anthropology 121 (3), 230–240.

Weiss, E., 2004. Understanding muscle markers: lower limbs. American Journal of Physical Anthropology 125 (3), 232–238.

Weiss, E., 2007. Muscle markers revisited: activity pattern reconstruction with controls in a central California Amerind Population. American Journal of Physical Anthropology 133 (3), 931–940.

Weiss, E., Corona, L., Schultz, B., 2012. Sex differences in musculoskeletal stress markers: problems with activity pattern reconstructions. International Journal of Osteoarchaeology 22 (1), 70–80.

Weiss, G., Goodnough, L.T., 2005. Anemia of chronic disease. New England Journal of Medicine 352 (10), 1011–1023.

Wells, C., 1964. Bones, bodies, and disease: Evidence of disease and abnormality in early man. In: Ancient Peoples and Places, Vol. 37. Thames and Hudson, London.

Weston, D.A., 2008. Investigating the specificity of periosteal reactions in pathology museum specimens. American Journal of Physical Anthropology 137 (1), 48–59.

White, T.D., Black, M.T., Folkens, P.A., 2012. Human Osteology. Academic Press, San Diego, CA.

White, T.D., Folkens, P.A., 1999. Human Osteology, 2nd ed. Academic Press, New York.

White, T.D., Folkens, P.A., 2005. The Human Bone Manual. Academic Press, New York.

Wilczak, C.A., 1998. Consideration of sexual dimorphism, age, and asymmetry in quantitative measurements of muscle insertion sites. International Journal of Osteoarchaeology 8 (5), 311–325.

Wilkie, L.A., Hayes, K.H., 2006. Engendered and feminist archaeologies of the recent and documented pasts. Journal of Archaeological Research 14 (3), 243–264.

Willey, G.R., Phillips, P., 1958. Method and Theory in American Archaeology. University of Chicago Press, Chicago.

Wood, J.W., Milner, G.R., Harpending, H.C., Weiss, K.M., 1992. The osteological paradox: Problems of inferring prehistoric health from skeletal samples. Current Anthropology 33 (4), 343–370.

Wright, L.E., Yoder, C.J., 2003. Recent progress in bioarchaeology: approaches to the osteological paradox. Journal of Archaeological Research 11 (1), 43–70.

Wylie, A., 2007. Doing archaeology as a feminist: introduction. Journal of Archaeology Method and Theory 14, 209–216.

Zias, J., 2002. New evidence for the history of leprosy in the ancient Near East: an overview. In: Roberts, C.A., Lewis, M.E., Manchester, K. (Eds.), The Past and Present of Leprosy: Archaeological, Historical, and Clinical Approaches. British Archaeological Reports, Oxford, pp. 259–268.

Zimmerman, M.R., Kelley, M.A., 1982. Atlas of Human Paleopathology. Praeger, New York.

Investigation of Skeletal Trauma

Anne M. Kroman, Steven A. Symes

INTRODUCTION

As the fields of biological and forensic anthropology have grown, bone trauma has become an increasingly vital component in the analysis of skeletal remains. Biological anthropologists require a correct understanding of skeletal trauma and injury biomechanics for the assessment of remains from both the recent and distant past to help tell many things about the population being studied. For example, **acute injury**[1] patterns help determine the circumstances that may have surrounded the death of an individual. **Chronic injury** patterns may contribute to an increased awareness regarding the overall health and welfare of the individual as well as the rate of survivable trauma. Just as physicians and medical researchers examine medical records to study health in contemporary populations, skeletal evidence provides us with our best glimpse into injury and pathology in past populations.

In the forensic arena, anthropologists are working close at hand with forensic pathologists in increasing numbers, and are being called on to examine skeletal trauma to help with the diagnosis of cause (e.g., gunshot wound) or manner of death (e.g., homicide). In the analysis of skeletal trauma, the interpretation of fractures plays a critical role. Correct fracture pattern interpretation is useful in determining such things as the type of trauma (i.e., **blunt trauma**, **ballistic trauma**, or **sharp trauma**), number of impacts or blows to the body, location of these impacts, and amount of force that was used, just to name a few. The forensic anthropologist, along with the forensic pathologist, is able to reach these conclusions by understanding the science of physics and knowledge of the material properties of bone to correctly "read" fractures.

While the analysis of skeletal trauma is not a new concept to biological or forensic anthropology, there has been a recent expansion of the methodology used in trauma research. Historically, trauma and injury has always been studied from a retrospective approach by looking at collections from the archaeological record or case samples retained from forensic

---

[1]All bolded terms are defined in the glossary at the end of this volume.

autopsy. While these collections and samples certainly provide anthropologists with invaluable information, and the majority of this work is exceptional, research using case studies is inherently limited. Often, there is little or no information as to the exact circumstances of the death, or the cause of the injury being studied.[2]

In recent years, there has been an increase in experimental or prospective research into skeletal trauma using both animal models and human cadavers. While difficult and costly, experimental research offers the opportunity to address specific questions in a very controlled environment. There is also the ability to create replicable results over multiple experiments. The best approach to understanding skeletal trauma from an anthropological perspective is a combination of these two approaches: cases of known cause of death are used to illustrate the biomechanics of bone trauma, while prospective research helps to validate these examples. Each research modality offers a chance to explore different types of questions in the field of skeletal biology.

BASIC CONCEPTS IN BONE TRAUMA

To be able to understand skeletal trauma, it is of paramount importance that anthropologists understand the fundamental basics of bone biology and biomechanics. A brief overview is provided here to introduce key concepts, while the more comprehensive and in-depth overviews provided by Brinckmann et al. (2002), Cowin (1989), Evans (1970), Frost (1967), Low and Reed (1996), and Roark and Young (1975) are recommended for further study.

Biomechanics is the application of the biological science of forces and energies to a living tissue. An understanding of biomechanics, as well as the biological and material properties of bone, lends critical insight into the mechanics of fracture creation and propagation. It is important for an anthropologist to recognize that the creation of injuries and fractures is dependent on several factors. First, there are the **extrinsic factors**, which include all variables involved with how the injuries occur. It is best to conceptualize the extrinsic variables as those that are "outside" of the body. Examples of extrinsic factors commonly studied in the context of trauma and injury include the type of **load** or **force** (defined in the next section) including their magnitude and rate of application (Gonza, 1982).

Secondly, there are **intrinsic factors** that shape the way the body and bone respond to injury. These can be conceptualized as variables that are "within" the body. These intrinsic dynamics deal with the material properties of human bone, as well as other related tissues in the body. The material and structural properties of bone influence the creation and propagation of fractures (Gonza, 1982). Examples of intrinsic factors include bone geometry, bone mineralization, and bone remodeling.

---

[2]The Crow Creek Massacre, occurring around 1350 A.D. in what is now South Dakota, is a notable exception. A Native American raiding party slaughtered almost 500 rival villagers and dumped the bodies in a mass grave (Zimmerman et al., 1981). In this case, contextual analysis of the remains disposition allowed inferences about the cause and manner of death, even though death had occurred over six centuries before the remains were analyzed.

Definitions and Basic Principles of Biomechanics

Force

The impacting force or type of applied load plays a key role in fracture creation and propagation. Force is defined as an "action or influence" that is "applied to a free body" (Turner and Burr, 1993). In other words, a force is anything that alters the state of motion of an object (Low and Reed, 1996). A force simply pushes or pulls on an object. Newton's first law of motion states that a force must be applied to change the velocity or direction of movement of an object. Newton's second law of motion states that the resulting change in momentum of the object is proportional to the force applied (Low and Reed, 1996). As an example, the more force that is applied in hitting a baseball with a bat, the faster the ball will travel. **Force** (F) is calculated as mass (m) times **acceleration** (a):

$$F = ma$$

Force is measured in newtons (N) or pounds (lb). Force is a "vector quantity," meaning that it has direction or magnitude. This is an important concept for understanding skeletal trauma biomechanics, where the direction of the force applied to the bone becomes an important variable, as will be explained later.

Load

A **load** is a force, or combination of forces that is sustained by an object (Low and Reed, 1996; Frost, 1967). For example, the weight of the human body creates a load on the feet.

Stress

When examining load type, the most common term used is "**stress**." Stress is defined as "force per unit area" (Turner and Burr, 1993), thus calculated:

$$Stress = force/area$$

Stress is calculated by newtons per square meter. The unit of 1 newton per square meter (N/m^2) is 1 pascal. Stress is reported in pascals.

Stress is further subdivided into three areas: **compressive stress**, **tensile stress**, and **shear stress** (Alms, 1961; Nordin and Frankel, 1989; Turner and Burr, 1993). Compressive stress is developed when a load acts to make the material shorter. Likewise, tensile stress is formed when a load works to stretch the material. Shear stress results when one area of material slides across another area of material. These three types of stress do not exist in isolation. No matter how simple the loading scheme, compressive, tensile, and shear stress are always occurring in combination.

Strain

The magnitude of load is referred to in terms of **strain**. Strain is defined as "percentage change in length, or relative deformation" (Turner and Burr, 1993):

$$Strain = increased\ length/original\ length$$

Since strain is ratio derived, there are no units of measure used for strain. You can think of strain as the percent of length change from a start length with a known applied load. For example, aluminum with a set axial applied load (a load applied to the long axis of a beam) will stretch to perhaps 1.5 times its original length but steel subjected to the same axially applied load may not stretch at all. Therefore, steel can handle more axial strain then aluminum.

Poisson's Ratio

Poisson's ratio describes the ratio of change from an applied strain in the object's length and width (Turner and Burr, 1993). Ashman et al. (1984) report a range in Poisson's ratio between 0.28 and 0.45. To summarize, if 1% strain is applied to a human femur in the longitudinal direction, a corresponding strain in the horizontal dimension will be between 28% and 45% (Turner and Burr, 1993). Therefore, if the femur is subjected to a compressive load on each end, the femur shaft diameter will increase in dimension by 28% to 45% of the original diameter.

Young's Modulus

The ratio of stress to strain in a material is known as **Young's modulus**, denoted with the variable E with units of pressure in pascal or N/m^2 (Low and Reed, 1996). Young's modulus calculates the change in dimension of an elastic material under compressive or tensile force, and is often used to depict how brittle or stiff the material is. Young's modulus can be used to predict the elongation or compression of a material under a given load so long as the load is less than the yield load for the material. If the material is subjected to a load greater than the yield load then the material will either crumple under compression or plastically stretch under tensile load. This brings up the topic of deformation.

Deformation

Materials under stress pass through two main stages before failure. These are **elastic deformation** and **plastic deformation** (Low and Reed, 1996). Elastic deformation is a state when a material can return to its original form, once pressure is released. An example of elastic deformation is a sponge that changes shape when squeezed then returns to its original form when released. Another example of elastic deformation is a spring with one end attached to the ceiling and a weight attached to the other end. The spring will stretch with the load lowering toward the ground. When the weight is released the spring will rebound and coil back toward the ceiling. This exemplifies the elastic nature of the spring to coil back to its original shape and length.

Plastic deformation is a level of deformation from which the material will never recover its original form. An example is a paper clip: once unfolded, it will never exactly be the same. You can also imagine the spring mentioned before and add additional weight. If too much weight is added, the spring will stretch toward the floor but once the weight is released the spring will no longer recoil to its exact original shape or length.

Fracture

In bone trauma, fracture is the term used for failure of bone. A fracture occurs when there is a complete separation of molecules and loss of structure and function (Low and Reed,

1996). Fractures often begin at either the weakest area in the bone, or the area where the force applied first overcomes the strength of the bone. Fractures can be large and noticeable or as small as being visible only under a microscope.

Biomechanics and Biomaterials of Human Bone

It is just as important to understand the properties of bone as a tissue as it is to understand basic biomechanics.

Bone Tissue Structure

Vertebrate skeletal systems contain two types of bone, **cortical** or compact and **cancellous** or spongy (Harkess et al., 1984). Cortical bone is stiff and more dense, while cancellous bone is porous and lightweight with a characteristic fragile honeycomb appearance. While the makeup of each type of bone is identical, cortical and cancellous bone differ greatly in reaction to force due to their construction. Cortical bone has a higher Young's modulus, indicating greater stiffness (Nordin and Frankel, 1989). It can withstand a greater amount of axial compression than tension before failure. Cancellous bone is less stiff and can withstand a greater amount of axial tension than cortical bone can. Cortical bone fails when strain exceeds 2%, while cancellous bone can withstand up to 7% axial tensile load (Nordin and Frankel, 1989).

Bone Histology

A basic understanding of histology is important in order to understand how bone responds to stress, even on a microscopic level. Bone is composed of cells and an extracellular matrix. Bone cells include **osteoblasts**, **osteoclasts**, and **osteocytes** (Bouvier, 1989). Osteoblasts are cuboidal cells that are responsible for the secretion of bone matrix. Osteoclasts are larger, multinucleated cells responsible for the absorption of bone. Osteocytes are osteoblasts that have finished their function of secreting bone matrix and have become trapped within hardened matrix, and are now responsible for bone maintenance. The circular structures that house the osteocytes are known as **osteons**. While most trauma studies deal mainly with the macroscopic response of bone to trauma, a good foundation in bone histology can deepen the understanding of bone's response to trauma. Refer to Trammell and Kroman (Chapter 13), this volume for more information on histology; and for a more comprehensive overview of bone histology see Crowder and Stout (2012).

Bone's Response to Chronic Stress

Another unique aspect of bone is its ability to remodel in response to chronic stress. These patterns are referred to as *musculoskeletal markers of stress* (MSM) and are often utilized by anthropologists to investigate activity patterns. The theory behind stress markers involves the physiology driving muscle and bone interaction (Weiss, 2004). As muscles in the body are more frequently used, overused, or used in unusual ways, increased stress is put on the periosteum (nutritive fibrous covering of bone where muscle tendons initially attach) and the bony cortex. As per Wolff's law (Wolff, 1892), bone is a living responsive material and therefore it remodels in response to stress, forming larger, rougher areas of muscle attachment (Woo et al., 1981). While the type of stress that induces increased muscle markers is different from the acute stress that creates injury and fractures, it is still another example of how an applied understanding of biomechanics can aid an anthropologist in gathering information from a skeleton. Kennedy (1989) is an authoritative reference on musculoskeletal markers of stress, especially those considered to be correlated with certain occupations. Smith (Chapter 7), this volume, also includes a discussion of MSM.

Material Properties of Bone

Both cortical and cancellous bones are **anisotropic** materials (for a review see Antich, 1993; Bonfield et al., 1985; Evans, 1973; Johnson, 1985; Keaveny and Hayes, 1993; Nordin and Frankel, 1989; Turner and Burr, 1993). Characteristically, anisotropic materials have different material properties based on the different directions or axes of the bone (i.e., long axis, short axis, etc.). For example, the human femur is designed to withstand the stress of weight bearing. The femur is therefore much stronger and more resistant to an axial load, or a force along the long axis of the bone, than a force that is applied perpendicularly. This differs from **isotropic** materials that are more homogeneous, having the same material properties in all directions.

Human cortical bone has a particular type of anisotropy referred to as **transverse isotropy**, because it has the same resistance to force in all transverse directions, and a higher resistance in the longitudinal direction (Keaveny and Hayes, 1993). For example, a femur shaft has the same properties in all transverse or cross sections, but these properties are different from the longitudinal axis. The histology of bone contributes to its anisotropy. Human bone is stronger in the longitudinal dimension (the direction in which the osteons run) than in the transverse direction. Human bone is also stronger under compression than under tension or shear in most cases. Human limbs and bone have adapted to constant compressive stress from daily activity and therefore have a higher resistance to compression than tension.

Human bone is also a **viscoelastic** material (for a review see Bonfield et al., 1985; Piekarski, 1970; Turner and Burr, 1993). The term viscoelastic means that the material can behave either as an elastic material or as a more resistant material depending on the rate of strain applied. A viscoelastic material behaves in different ways depending on the rate and the duration of loading. Cortical bone is extremely sensitive to strain. Cortical bone absorbs a large amount of energy from a normal activity such as running a mile. However, if less energy is applied all at once, such as landing from a high fall, the failure level is reached and a fracture results. Histologically, fractures induced by low load rate follow the interstitial bone around the osteons, while at a higher load they travel indiscriminately through the bone (Piekarski, 1970).

The viscoelastic properties of bone also play an important role in trauma interpretation. While the same basic principles of biomechanics and physics operate for both ballistic trauma and blunt force trauma (i.e., when bone is impacted by another object) the resulting fracture patterns are quite different (Berryman and Symes, 1998). This difference is due to the rate of loading. Blunt force trauma impacts bone at *miles per hour* while a ballistic projectile impacts bone at *feet per second* (Symes et al., 1989, 2012). Keaveny and Hayes (1993) state that at high rates of loading, bone will behave like a brittle material (such as glass) and therefore will skip the stage of plastic deformation and will fail quickly under sufficient applied force.

Bone Deformation

Bone under stress and strain reacts in a predictable manner, as outlined extensively by Keaveny and Hayes (1993), Nordin and Frankel (1989), and Turner and Burr (1993). The deformation of the material has a direct relationship to the force of the load exerted upon it. This relationship is depicted as a stress–strain or load–deformation curve (Figure 8.1). Load–deformation curves depict the stages that bone undergoes throughout loading until complete failure. The elastic deformation region is the first area of the load–deformation curve. When bone is in elastic deformation and the load is removed the bone will return to its former shape with no visual structural alteration. Bone enters the plastic deformation stage when a tolerance threshold has been reached. After release of the force, bone in the plastic deformation stage cannot return to its original shape even though visible fracture may not be evident.

Load–deformation curves provide information on the amount of energy absorbed, load sustained, and deformation achieved before failure (Nordin and Frankel, 1989). The amount of energy absorbed is calculated by the area underneath the curve, and by the load and deformation sustained at failure.

The overall structure stiffness is demonstrated by the slope of the curve. Stiffness is calculated by using the modulus of elasticity or Young's modulus. The stiffer the material, the higher the moduli value. Young's modulus is important in bone fracture mechanics to demonstrate stiffness or ductility (ability to bend or deform), which has a great influence on fracture mechanics. Brittle materials (glass) deform very little before failure, while ductile materials (rubber band) can withstand a great deal of elastic deformation. Brittle materials do not undergo plastic deformation when force is applied, and often require little force to reach failure. As we will see later, this principle and the amount of plastic deformation become important when assessing whether an insult was ballistic or blunt trauma.

Reaction to Tension

When equal loads are applied in a direction outward from the bone surface, tension is created. Maximum tensile stress occurs in a direction perpendicular from the applied force

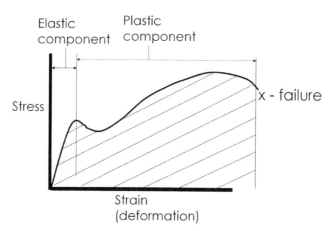

FIGURE 8.1   Stress–strain curve illustrating the stages of elastic and plastic deformation that bone undergoes before failure.

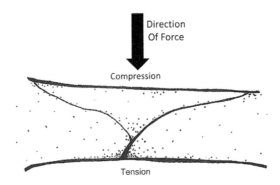

FIGURE 8.2   Butterfly fracture illustrating the direction of force.

(Nordin and Frankel, 1989). This force causes the material to narrow and lengthen. In bones, failure occurs at a microscopic level by the pulling apart of the osteons at the cement lines (areas of joining osteons) (Nordin and Frankel, 1989). Understanding that the bone will fail initially in the area of tension is also a key concept in fracture pattern interpretation. For example, a specific type of fracture commonly referred to as a **butterfly** or a wedge fracture is a great example of using fracture biomechanics for fracture pattern analysis. As the bone is loaded in a perpendicular direction, areas of both compression and tension are formed. The bone will fail first in the area of the tension, since bone is commonly weaker in tension than in compression, as discussed earlier. The fracture will then radiate back towards the area of compression, constantly changing due to the changing biomechanics of the bone as the fracture advances. While the moment-by-moment progression of this type of fracture is complex, a simple understanding of where the areas of tension and compression in the bone are can give an anthropologist the knowledge needed to correctly identify the direction of force (Figure 8.2).

TYPES OF TRAUMA IN THE HUMAN SKELETON

Historically, bone fractures have always been "classified" into the three separate categories of blunt, ballistic, and sharp trauma. These classifications serve to aid both pathologists and anthropologists in understanding the mechanism of injury; however, a proper understanding of the biomechanics behind the classification system is necessary to avoid confusion and incorrect interpretation of the fracture patterns.

Blunt Trauma

Blunt trauma is commonly thought of in terms of a slower loading force applied to tissue, such as is seen in cases of assault, battery, or even motor vehicle accidents. When examining bone that has been fractured by a blunt force type of mechanism, there are clues that the pathologist or anthropologist can identify. First, there is usually a clear sign of impact, which is the area where the fractures first originate from (Kroman et al., 2011). Two types of fractures are usually clearly identifiable, where long linear **radiating fractures** travel away from the area of impact, and are followed, given enough energy, by more circular **concentric fractures** (see Figure 8.3). Since the injury inflicted with blunt trauma is a relatively slow loading force (remember blunt force trauma is considered as occurring in miles per hour), the bone takes a longer time to reach the failure or fracture point, and will display a greater amount of **plastic deformation**. Also, if any areas of the skull are affected, there may be areas of **delamination**, in which the inner and the outer table of bone have become separated.

Ballistic Trauma

Ballistic trauma is also referred to as projectile trauma, and involves a much higher rate of acceleration (rate of change of velocity over time) than blunt trauma. Ballistic trauma is trauma sustained from any type of firearms or munitions. The speed of the impact as well as the surface area of the projectile are the critical components that create the difference between blunt and ballistic trauma fracture patterns. The most common types of ballistic trauma involve projectiles fired from firearms, but explosions fit into this category as well. The impact of the ballistic projectile into the bone often creates characteristic fracture patterns of an **entrance wound** and **exit wound**. These defects represent the entry and exit of the

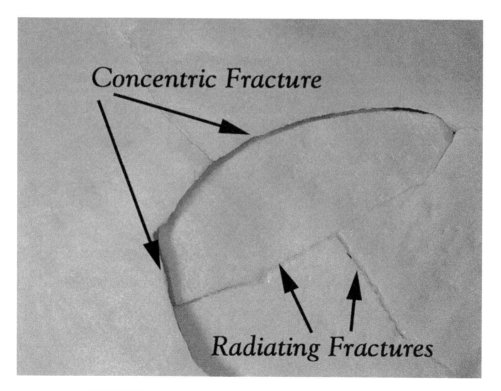

FIGURE 8.3 Concentric and radiating fractures in a cranial vault.

ballistic projectile into and out of the bone, and can be differentiated from one another based on the location of the bevel (angled edge of the fracture surface) surrounding the defect (for a more detailed explanation, please refer to Berryman and Symes, 1998).

Injuries from ballistic weapons also can have fracture patterns that are similar to those described in blunt trauma. Radiating and concentric fractures are often seen around the entrance and exit wound, and like blunt trauma simply represent the normal biomechanical response of the bone to the large amount of force being imparted on it. However, a lesser degree of plastic deformation is seen in ballistic trauma than in blunt trauma. A simple way to remember this is that ballistic trauma often results in pieces of bone that can be easily fit back together like a puzzle (elastic deformation) while blunt trauma often results in warped pieces of bone that cannot be fit back together (plastic deformation). To reiterate, this goes back to the high rate of speed of the applied force and the bone's response via reaching the fracture threshold more quickly.

Sharp Trauma

Sharp trauma is best conceptualized as a subcategory of blunt trauma. Like blunt trauma, sharp trauma is considered as occurring at a slower rate of loading. However, the major difference between blunt and sharp trauma is the surface area of the impacting weapon that interacts with soft tissue and bone. This then affects the resultant injury pattern. As we learned earlier, stress is calculated as force divided by area. This is a critical concept for understanding sharp trauma.

For example, imagine holding a 12-pound bowling ball in the palm of your hand. With the 12 pounds of force spread out over the 9 square inches of the palm, the amount of pounds per square inch (or psi) would be 1.33. While the bowling ball may be very heavy, with a psi of 1.33 you could easily hold this object in your hand. Now consider holding the same 12-pound bowling ball, however this time with a knifepoint in between the ball and your hand. Suddenly, the entire 12 pounds is focused in the 0.0001 square inches of the knifepoint, and the psi climbs to 120,000. Now you could not hold the bowling bowl in your hand without injury, as 120,000 psi exceeds the tissue threshold for injury (Kroman, 2007). It is this reduction in surface area that leads to the incised type of wound commonly seen with sharp trauma. However, it is important to note that since sharp trauma is a subcategory of blunt trauma the same type of fracture patterns can still result, with both radiating and concentric fractures being common.

Thermal Trauma

Fractures and damage to bone can also be caused by a variety of outside forces acting on the body. One of the most common forces that complicates trauma analysis is fire. Since fire is often used as a method by perpetrators to hide the true manner of death, it is important to understand how fire or thermal exposure damages bone in order to analyze the difference between fractures created by the fire as opposed to those that may have been created by events before the fire.

The study of thermal damage to bone is exceedingly complex and takes into consideration variables such as the heat of the fire, duration of the fire, and the amount of soft tissue present on the remains at the time of burning. All of these variables will influence the type of fractures and damage that the fire creates. For a comprehensive overview and great starting place for the study of thermal trauma to bone, please see the text by Schmidt and Symes (2008).

Understanding the Timing of Skeletal Trauma

Trauma research often revolves in part around questions regarding distinguishing between **perimortem** and **postmortem** trauma. Perimortem trauma is normally referred to as trauma at or around the time of death. However, as anthropologists define it based on the bony signature, perimortem trauma occurs when the bone is still wet, i.e., has collagen in it. This is because trauma occurring to a wet bone will have a different signature than trauma occurring to a dry bone. The bone can be wet for weeks or more following death. Postmortem trauma is trauma occurring after death, distinguishable from perimortem trauma by signs that the bone was dry when the trauma occurred. **Antemortem** trauma refers to trauma that occurred while the individual was alive and is distinguished by signs of healing. These definitions may seem simple but in practice it is challenging to distinguish perimortem from postmortem trauma and in some cases the prudent course is to state "undetermined." For more information on the timing of trauma, see Marden et al. (Chapter 9), this volume.

NEW THINKING: SKELETAL TRAUMA AS A CONTINUUM

While the standard classifications of trauma as described above have been the tried and true way of conceptualizing fractures, this way of thinking may still be problematic. In fact, trauma classification as defined above should be used as a loose guideline for classification, rather than as strict criteria that must be met. As discussed earlier, there are many areas of overlap between blunt and sharp trauma that are only discernible with a good knowledge of biomechanics. For example, some of the fracture characteristics of delamination, concentric fractures, and plastic deformation are often discussed when referring to blunt trauma, as was the case above. These are all typical osseous responses to a blunt trauma impact. However, this can mislead some anthropologists into thinking that those indicators are the absolute "signs" of blunt trauma alone, and their presence either confirms or denies an interpretation of blunt trauma.

The problem then deepens when the general categories (i.e., blunt, ballistic, and sharp) are viewed as exclusive weapons-based categories; for example, perceptions that *all* bullets create ballistic trauma, *all* hammers create blunt trauma, and *all* knives create sharp trauma, and they can all be neatly separated based on their own individual fracture characteristics. However, these neat classifications are not always accurate, as the force and velocity of impacting objects are essential factors. For example, Byers' (2002) interpretations encounter problems when he classifies any projectile (i.e., anything that flies through the air) as ballistic and therefore as ballistic trauma. Confusion further arises when there are mixed signs and the trauma cannot be easily classified based on the criteria being used. This type of viewpoint has led to the bizarre creation of new categories of trauma, such as "sharp-blunt trauma" or "blunt-ballistic trauma." By focusing on the biomechanics behind the trauma, the need for the creation of new trauma categories is eliminated.

Instead, skeletal trauma is best viewed biomechanically and conceptualized as a continuum, rather than as a series of discrete categories. This continuum is governed by a series of variables relating to the intrinsic properties of bone and the extrinsic characteristics of the force applied. The key extrinsic factors are (1) force of the impact, (2) surface area of the impacting interface, and (3) the acceleration/deceleration rate. The goal of research into skeletal trauma in biological anthropology should be in part to tease out the different interactions between these variables, as well as insight into the intrinsic properties of bone to understand how the injuries truly occur.

SKELETAL TRAUMA AS A COMPONENT OF ANTHROPOLOGICAL RESEARCH

As mentioned earlier, there are numerous avenues and modalities of research into skeletal trauma in biological anthropology. The two most widely used methods are clinical or case-based analysis research and experimental research. As with all areas of research there are both pros and cons to each research modality, and each modality is best utilized for examining certain types of questions. When selecting the best modality, it is critical to (1) clearly define the question being asked, (2) assess which variables need to be addressed to appropriately answer the research question, and (3) honestly evaluate the available resources. For example, if the research question demands a high level of experimental impact testing, but there are no resources or funding available, it is better to try to redesign the hypothesis to accommodate a different research modality than to try to conduct suboptimal research on the original question. Both the areas of case-based research and experimental research will be explored and described in the following, and descriptive case studies will be explored.

CASE-BASED ANALYSIS

Research involving case-based analysis is an important aspect of skeletal trauma research as a whole. In fact, it is often the case that this type of research serves to function as the "seed" research for further experimental testing down the road. For example, if a forensic anthropologist notices a trend in the fracture patterns observed in gunshot wounds to the head, it may spur them to do first a case-based review of their past cases (as well as cases from other colleagues) to elaborate on the observed trend, then secondly to expand and refine the research hypothesis to include an experimental-based design to test out the original idea.

Case-based trauma research is best suited for either investigating trends among a group or population or looking at characteristics of known injuries. It is a given constraint that case-based research is always a retrospective approach, meaning that you will always be looking at the fracture pattern as the result of an injury that has already occurred.

Case-based research is also the type of research most appropriately suited to looking at examples of violence and trauma in a historic or even prehistoric setting. This type of research provides unique challenges as well as unique sets of goals. In the evaluation of prehistoric cases of trauma and violence, the research is often focused on a broad spectrum of issues that encompasses more than just the mechanism of the injury. For example, in these cases anthropologists are concerned with types of violence, warfare, intergroup relations, social structure, and population dynamics. In these types of research questions, trauma is a key component that can help provide a window into the **population history** of past populations. For this type of research, anthropologists have to incorporate both a good understanding of trauma analysis from skeletal remains and a solid background in bioarchaeology. Several great sources to begin to dig deeper into this area of trauma research are Frayer and Martin (1998), Benson and Cook (2001), Murphy et al. (2010), Martin et al. (2012), and Tung (2012).

Positive Aspects of Case-Based Research

There are numerous positive aspects to case-based research, especially in the context of forensics. As mentioned above, clinical case evaluation often provides the initial start of a research idea. These great ideas often spring from forensic cases that prove to be difficult for trauma analysis, seem "different," or are unique. One of the greatest benefits of case-based research is that it affords the chance to see the real, uncontrolled results of injury biomechanics and provide an unadulterated glimpse into the material properties of bone and how they respond to force. These cases can often bring up new variables and new questions that may have not been considered in a strict experimental design, but are most certainly worth exploring.

Negative Aspects of Case-Based Research

Case-based research is always a retrospective approach to trauma. The injury that is being studied has already happened, and the research is constrained by the quality of information about the injury. A certain amount of basic information can be gained by analysis of the fracture pattern; however, if very specific biomechanical questions are being investigated, such as speed of the impact, force of the impact, or exact positioning of the victim, case-based research often lacks the required level of biomechanical detail and such questions are therefore better answered with experimental research.

What Questions Are You Trying to Ask?

With all types of research, the most critical step is clearly defining and outlining the main question that you want to tackle. In the area of trauma, this question can lead you down the path closer to either case-based analysis or experimental design (discussed in the next section). Examples of research questions best suited for case-based analysis would include the following: What types of fractures occurred most often in population X and why? In known motor vehicle accidents, what types of fractures are most commonly seen? In known cases of child abuse, are there any characteristic fracture patterns?

What Sample or Collection Will You Use?

The next important step after outlining your research question and deciding to conduct case-based research is to identify the sample that you will use. There are several key factors to keep in mind. First, you must have adequate access to a sample. You want to ensure that you have clearly outlined your hypothesis, research methodology, and research timeline to the curator of the collection and that everyone is in agreement. Also, be sure to be both realistic and generous with your timeline since more often than not research tends to take a little longer than planned. Nothing is more frustrating than trying to cram two months of research into a two-week time frame.

Second, make sure that the collection has an adequate sample size for your specific research project. For example, a skeletal collection may contain 800 individuals. However, if you are looking at skeletal trauma and only four individuals of the 800 exhibit trauma, this would not be an adequate sample size. The curator of the collection should be able to guide you here in advance. (Refer to DiGangi and Moore [Chapter 2], this volume for more information on project logistics).

Third, ensure that adequate records of the sample are available. Especially in the forensic area where you are trying to conduct research using known examples of trauma, make sure that the mechanism of injury is indeed "known" and more importantly, documented. For example, if you are conducting research on the sizes and shapes of entrance wounds and fracture patterns from different calibers of weapons, ensure that you have access to the official medical record that includes this information. It is best to adopt the standards of documentation used in medicine or forensic pathology in which documentation includes a medical record number or case number and an official document, not simply a self-stick note on the box.

I Have My Hypothesis and My Sample Set Up, Now What?

You are ready to start your research! Before you begin, however, there are some key factors to consider. First, decide how you will chart or document your observations. Having a clear and concise plan will guarantee that no detail is overlooked as well as ensure that the research is conducted more efficiently. Second, decide what type of imaging will be used as further documentation. As the saying goes, "a picture is worth a thousand words." Make sure that all examples of trauma are clearly photographed from all angles and that specimens are labeled in the photographs. (Refer to DiGangi and Moore [Chapter 2] and Smith [Chapter 7], this volume, for more information on taking photographs).

Third, ensure that you are protecting the individuals' privacy, especially relevant for studies of forensic cases. The United States Government Health Insurance Portability and Accountability Act (HIPAA) mandates that **no** identifiable information be associated with medical specimens or remains.[3] Be sure that you do not record the individual's name or date of birth on any of your records, or have this information visible in any photographs. If photographing radiographs or other images generated from sources such as **computed tomography (CT)** scans or **magnetic resonance imaging (MRI)** equipment, be sure the

---

[3]For more information about HIPPA please see www.hhs.gov.

individuals' names and dates of birth are obscured. Even though the "patients" are deceased, forensic records are medical records, and any violation of HIPAA, even in the context of forensic research, is a federal offense punishable by a fine or jail term. If doing your research in a country other than the United States, similar laws or standards may exist. Following the advice above will prevent any potential problems.

Other Considerations

Utilizing radiographs, other medical images, and national databases is another avenue for conducting trauma research using a case-based approach. While not traditionally used in forensics, these resources can contain a wealth of information. The best places to investigate these types of research projects are often in conjunction with the medical community. While in these cases, the benefit of actually examining the bone specimen does not exist, plain film radiographs as well as CT scans of patients with known injuries can provide a wealth of data into fracture pattern characteristics. See Moore [Chapter 14], this volume, for more on medical imaging technologies.

CASE STUDY: INVESTIGATION OF FRACTURE PATTERNS IN CHILD ABUSE USING A CASE-BASED APPROACH

Investigations in alleged child abuse are often a very delicate and sensitive subject for forensic pathologists, anthropologists, and law enforcement. To aid in the correct assessment of injuries in a child to make a determination of suspected abuse, the pathologist or anthropologist often relies on a suite of evidence, including multiple fractures showing different chronological episodes of abuse and fracture patterns (a pattern of abuse over time) indicative of assault type(s) of injury (Symes et al., 2002).

Mandibular fractures in children, especially young children who are not yet walking, are often very indicative of child abuse (Hobbs, 1984). These fractures commonly occur when an abuser strikes a child in the face, and due to the developing shape and structure of the mandible the most common location for fracture will be in the area below the mandibular condyle. To look at the occurrence of these types of fractures in known cases of abuse, a case analysis approach was used. Kroman and colleagues (2002) used a large forensic sample that they queried for cases of known abuse in children under two years of age. Out of the sample, four cases meeting the criteria were identified. Of these four cases, two had fractures of the mandibular condyle. In one case the fracture was acute, and associated with fractures of the frontal bone and rib fractures. In the other case, there were numerous acute fractures as well as fractures in various stages of healing. The mandibular condyle fracture and several rib fractures showed healing, which also helped to demonstrate a pattern of abuse (Kroman et al., 2002).

In this example, the research question best lent itself to a case-based analysis approach rather than an experimental design. While the sample size was small, this was expected when dealing with known and established cases of child abuse, as the aim was more in line with making descriptive conclusions rather than conclusions backed up by statistical analysis. For more information on child abuse and skeletal analysis, see the volumes by Love et al. (2011) and Ross and Abel (2011).

EXPERIMENTAL SKELETAL TRAUMA RESEARCH

As mentioned above, while case-based research can often provide interesting initial questions for research, experimental research is often the most appropriate methodology to refine your understanding of the variables involved. Experimental research affords the chance to investigate a very specific problem in a controlled environment. Resulting data can be very precise, and the experiment can be repeated on multiple specimens to help increase the accuracy of the results. This section will illustrate the important questions to ask when considering experimental research, critical steps that need to be addressed, and the basic methods used.

Positive Aspects of Experimental Trauma Research

Experimental trauma research affords a unique opportunity to investigate the very specific variables that were outlined in the brief overview of biomechanics at the beginning of this chapter. Only in an experimental setting can you really get down to the nitty-gritty aspects of bone and injury biomechanics. As mentioned above, this research design offers the chance to actually create trauma and get replicable results with extensive data.

Negative Aspects of Experimental Trauma Research

Experimental research in injury biomechanics necessitates extensive experience with physics, material science, biomechanics, and engineering; or ready access to an engineering department willing to help. Successful research in this area is both costly and complicated. There are numerous research designs with engineered impact devices to fit any variety of situations. If you can dream it, it can be designed, instrumented, and built. However, when addressing your initial research plan make sure that you either have access to equipment that you might need, or have the resources necessary to construct it.

What Question Are You Trying to Address?

Just as we saw with case-based analysis in skeletal trauma, there are research questions that are better suited to an experimental design. The best basic questions that are answered using experimental design are ones that investigate a specific variable or set of variables. For example, good questions conducive to experimental testing are, among others: At what force does the temporal bone fracture? How do fractures travel through bone? What type of impact is needed to create a cranial base fracture? How does the temperature of a fire influence thermal fracture patterns? How does axial load affect the creation of butterfly fractures?

What Are The Key Elements You Will Need?

Unfortunately, there is no concise list to make for all the equipment and resources needed to conduct experimental trauma. The necessary materials for the project will be dictated by the question that you are trying to ask. For example, a project involving the trauma caused by different types of large motor boat propeller blades dictated the use of a large torroidal pool and an outrigging set to hold and run the motor and propeller at a controlled speed (Kroman et al., 2007). On the opposite end of the spectrum, testing the fracture tolerance of human phalanges requires only a small drop tower set-up and force gauge, or a similar device used to monitor the force of the impact (Kroman, 2007). Drop tower constructs are commonly used in experimental biomechanics and can range from several stories high to small and portable.

The principle behind all of the constructs is the same—to deliver a reproducible impact with a set speed and force. They often involve a "tower" constructed of a linear rail system, and then an "impactor" that can often be changed depending on the size and shape needed. On a triggered release, the impactor travels down the rail at a set speed and impacts the object, which is stabilized at the bottom of the tower. To ensure that you have the correct equipment for the project, the best place to start is with your university's engineering department. Not only can they provide information on the best impact delivery device, they can assist with the best design for data collection as well. Since each project in this type of trauma research is unique, most of the testing equipment also has to be manufactured from scratch.

High-speed film is also a key component in experimental testing as it can provide critical data for the study. With high-speed film, it is possible to visualize the fracture patterns as they occur, offering anthropologists a unique opportunity to witness the injury as it is being created, rather than work backwards (Kroman et al., 2011). While the high-speed film set-up is very costly, most locations set up for impact already have a system in place that can be used. Again, collaboration with a facility familiar with experimental and impact testing is a key component to this type of research design.

Human Cadavers

The other critical component of experimental testing that needs to be addressed is the use of human cadaveric tissue. Human tissue is by far the gold standard for testing, and the preferred state of the tissue is what is described as a "fresh frozen" state; in other words, tissue that has not undergone a process of decomposition or embalming. The data may be influenced by changes in bone quality caused by decomposition, embalming, or drying (Reilly and Burnstein, 1974; Galloway, 1999). Bone quality can also be compromised by the chronological age of the individual (as bone density decreases with age), so it is also critical to outline your stipulations for the demographics of the cadavers that you are willing to accept (Bonfield et al., 1985; Oxnard, 1993). The preparation of the tissue is also very important, since soft tissue presence and/or condition influences the biomechanics, especially in the cranium (McElhaney et al., 1976). Removal of soft tissue from the impact site alters the elastic and biomechanical properties; however, in some cases it will be necessary in order to adequately collect the data or visualize the injury site.

Experimental testing is also restricted by the availability of human cadaveric material. Sample sizes may be small and limited in age, ancestry, and sex representation. The most common sources of cadaveric material are often from biomechanical research facilities or medical school donation programs. For anthropology students, the first source to check would be with your local medical school due to the fact that extra cadavers donated to the school are often used for research projects. It is important to keep in mind that costs may include administrative expenses and those for cadaver preparation. You should be prepared for returning all elements of the cadaver to the medical school for cremation at the end of the project. If your local medical school is not an option, other sources of cadaveric material include services that provide cadavers for surgical or medical research. However, these often come with a very hefty price tag in addition to tight restrictions on use. See DiGangi and Moore (Chapter 2), this volume, for information on the ethics inherent with studying human remains.

What About Animal Models?

With the paucity of available cadaveric material, and the ethical issues that accompany their use, it may seem very tempting to use an animal substitute in place of human cadavers. However, while easier to find and easier on the budget, there are also potential problems with the use of nonhuman models for studying trauma and fracture biomechanics. The main concern when dealing with the study of fracture biomechanics is the difference in the strength and structure of human bone compared to animal bone. When comparing nonhuman to human bone, the pig has the greatest similarity in bone structure to humans, and for that reason is often used in a variety of *in vivo* orthopedic implant research (Pearce et al., 2007). However, with that stated, pig models have consistently produced varying degree of experimental results. Additionally, many researchers use "butcher grade" animals due to easy availability. These animals are not fully skeletally mature, and their subadult status adds yet another confounding variable to the mix. Animal models can provide a helpful alternative in research design, but biomechanical studies utilizing human cadavers are still considered the gold standard in the field.

CASE STUDY: EXPERIMENTAL IMPACT BIOMECHANICS RESEARCH INTO CRANIAL BASE FRACTURES

As discussed, experimental testing is a research method that is well suited for application to questions regarding the specifics of fracture biomechanics. There are many areas of dispute in the literature regarding the etiology of fracture patterns, and one such area of dispute has focused on cranial base fractures. Cranial base fractures have been attributed to a wide range of injuries as their causation, including falls, blows to the top of the skull, and blows to the lateral or temporal area of the skull (Berryman and Symes, 1998). To address the questions of (1) how cranial base fractures are created and (2) how they travel or propagate through the skull, a cadaveric testing model was set up (Kroman et al., 2005). Fifteen fully fleshed, unembalmed human cadaver heads were used for this test, since an animal model was not biomechanically appropriate. A portion of the cranial vault was resected, along with the brain and dura, to allow for direct visualization of the cranial base and the capture of the fracture event by high-speed film. A drop tower system was utilized to ensure that a calibrated and fully monitored blow was delivered to the specimen each time.

The specimens were impacted in different areas, which included near the vertex (top of the vault), midway on the parietal, and from a lateral aspect. Five data acquisition load cells (small devices used to record force) monitored the response of the bone and calculated the compressive and shear stress during the impact in millisecond intervals. After testing, each specimen was dissected, photographed, charted, and analyzed. Each cranium was then processed down to clean bone to allow reconstruction and further visualization of the fracture pattern. The data from the high-speed camera were also reviewed.

The results from this experimental study showed that cranial base fractures are consistently created by blows to the lateral aspect of the skull, and the fracture radiates from the location of impact along the areas of least resistance within the base (Kroman et al., 2005). In this study, the question involved the biomechanics of how cranial base fractures are created, and was best answered by an experimental design. By using experimental research, not only was the general question answered ("How are cranial base fractures created?"), but information was also collected on other relevant topics such as "How much force does it take to create a cranial base fracture?" and "How do cranial base fractures propagate through the skull?"

FUTURE DIRECTIONS IN SKELETAL TRAUMA RESEARCH

Research into skeletal trauma has grown by leaps and bounds over the last two decades and will most likely grow exponentially in future years. As technology improves at an increasing rate, these advances will be applied to the field of experimental biomechanics and forensics. The field of trauma research will undoubtedly see changes and refinement in how fracture data are acquired during experimental research, how the experimental research is filmed, and how the research is analyzed. Another area that will likely become a mainstay of trauma analysis in the future is *finite element analysis*. Finite element analysis involves computational models of structures (from bridges to bones), which can be used to simulate force, such as an impact, and predict the response of the material or tissue. It is conceivable that in the near future cadaveric studies will be a thing of the past, and instead replaced by very complex finite element models.

For students who are interested in pursuing research or learning more about skeletal trauma, it would be wise to start with an immersion into the science behind the biomechanics of bone trauma. There are excellent texts on the basic principles of biomechanics, including Nordin and Frankel (1989) and Low and Reed (1996). An understanding of physics and biomechanics will serve as the foundation for your study and research into skeletal trauma. Once you have the basic foundation mastered, a good starting point is to read some of the applications of trauma analysis to biological anthropology, as seen in Galloway (1999) and Schmidt and Symes (2008). Once you have a question or a research project in mind, the final step would be a consultation with the anthropology and engineering departments, as well as your advisor and committee, to finalize the elements of the research design.

All of the recent changes and growth in the field are what make research into skeletal trauma one of the most exciting areas of skeletal biology and biological anthropology. For students, this is an extremely exciting and rewarding area of skeletal biology, and it will be the research by today's students that helps to truly drive this exciting field forward!

ACKNOWLEDGMENTS

Great thanks are due to the editors of this volume, Drs. Elizabeth A. DiGangi and Megan K. Moore for the chance to contribute and participate. Thanks are also due to Lucas B. Meadors for support and comments.

REFERENCES

Alms, M., 1961. Fracture mechanics. Journal of Bone and Joint Surgery 438, 162–166.

Antich, P., 1993. Ultrasound study of bone in vitro. Calcified Tissue International 53, S157–S161.

Ashman, R., Cowin, S., VanBuskirk, W., Rice, J., 1984. A continuous wave technique for the measurement of the elastic properties of cortical bone. Journal of Biomechanics 17, 349–361.

Benson, E.P., Cook, A.G. (Eds.), 2001. Ritual Sacrifice in Ancient Peru: New Discoveries and Interpretations. University of Texas Press, Austin.

Berryman, H., Symes, S., 1998. Recognizing gunshot and blunt cranial trauma through fracture interpretation. In: Reichs, K. (Ed.), Forensic Osteology: Advances in the Identification of Human Remains. Charles C. Thomas, Springfield, IL, pp. 333–352.

Bonfield, W., Behiri, J.C., Charalambides, C., 1985. Orientation and age related dependence of the fracture toughness of cortical bone. In: Perren, S.M., Schneider, E. (Eds.), Biomechanics: Current Interdisciplinary Research. Martinum Nijhoff Publishers, Dordrecht, pp. 185–188.

Bouvier, M., 1989. The biology and composition of bone. In: Cowin, S. (Ed.), Bone Mechanics. CRC Press, Boca Raton, FL, pp. 1–14.

Brinckmann, P., Forbine, W., Leivseth, G., 2002. Musculoskeletal Biomechanics. Thieme, New York.

Byers, S., 2002. Introduction to Forensic Anthropology. Allyn & Bacon, Boston.

Cowin, S., 1989. Mechanics of materials. In: Cowin, S. (Ed.), Bone Mechanics. CRC Press, Boca Raton, FL, pp. 15–42.

Crowder, C., Stout, S., 2012. Bone Histology: An Anthropological Perspective. CRC Press, Boca Raton, FL.

DiGangi, E.A., Moore, M.K., 2013. Application of the scientific method to skeletal biology. In: DiGangi, E.A., Moore, M.K. (Eds.), Research Methods in Human Skeletal Biology. Academic Press, San Diego.

Evans, F., 1970. Biomechanical implications of anatomy. In: Cooper, J. (Ed.), Selected Topics of Biomechanics: Proceedings of the C.I.C. Symposium on Biomechanics, Indiana University, pp. 3–30.

Evans, F., 1973. Mechanical Properties of Bone. Charles C. Thomas, Springfield, IL.

Frayer, D.W., & Martin, D.L. (Eds.). 1998. Troubled Times: Violence and Warfare in the Past. War and Society, vol. 3. Amsterdam: Overseas Publishers Association.

Frost, H., 1967. An Introduction to Biomechanics. Charles C. Thomas, Springfield, IL.

Galloway, A., 1999. Broken Bones: Anthropological Analysis of Blunt Force Trauma. Charles C. Thomas, Springfield, IL.

Gonza, E., 1982. Biomechanics of long bone injury. Biomechanics of Trauma. Williams and Wilkins, Baltimore, pp. 1–24.

Harkess, J., Ramsey, W., Ahmadi, B., 1984. Principles of fractures and dislocations. In: Rockwood, C., Green, D. (Eds.), Fractures in Adults. Vol. 1. Lippincott-Raven, Philadelphia, pp. 1–18.

Hobbs, C., 1984. Skull fractures and the diagnosis of abuse. Archives of Disease in Childhood 59 (3), 246–252.

Johnson, E., 1985. Current developments in bone technology. In: Schiffer, M. (Ed.), Advances in Archaeological Method and Theory. Academic Press, Orlando, FL.

Keaveny, T., Hayes, W., 1993. Mechanical properties of of cortical and trabecular bone. In: Hall, B. (Ed.), Bone. CRC Press, Boca Raton, FL, pp. 285–344.

Kennedy, K., 1989. Skeletal markers of occupational stress. In: Iscan, M., Kennedy, K. (Eds.), Reconstruction of Life from the Skeleton. Alan R. Liss, New York, pp. 129–160.

Kroman, A., 2007. Fracture Biomechanics of the Human Skeleton. Unpublished PhD dissertation, Department of Anthropology. The University of Tennessee, Knoxville, TN.

Kroman, A.M., Symes, S.A., Smith, O.C., Love, J.C., 2002. The hidden truth: mandibular condyle fracture in child abuse. Proceedings of the American Academy of Forensic Sciences 8, 250.

Kroman, A., Kress, T., Symes, S., 2005. Mandible and cranial base fractures in adults: Experimental testing. Proceedings of the American Academy of Forensic Sciences 11, 289.

Kroman, A., Kress, T., Porta, D., 2007. Propeller impacts: Injury mechanics and bone trauma. Proceedings of the American Academy of Forensic Sciences 13, 335–336.

Kroman, A., Kress, T., Porta, D., 2011. Fracture propagation in the human cranium: a re-testing of popular theories. Clinical Anatomy 24 (3), 309–318.

Love, J.C., Derrick, S.M., Weirsema, J.M., 2011. Skeletal Atlas of Child Abuse. Humana Press, New York.

Low, J., Reed, A., 1996. Basic Biomechanics Explained. Butterworth-Heinemann, Oxford.

Marden, K., Sorg, M., Haglund, W., 2013. Taphonomy. In: DiGangi, E.A., Moore, M.K. (Eds.), Research Methods in Human Skeletal Biology. Academic Press, San Diego.

Martin, D.L., Harrod, R.P., Perez, V.R., 2012. The Bioarchaeology of Violence. University Press of Florida, Gainesville.

McElhaney, J.E., Reynolds, V.L., Hilyard, J.F., 1976. Handbook of Human Tolerance. Japanese Automobile Research Institute, Tokyo.

Murphy, M.S., Gaither, C., Goyochea, E., Verano, J.W., Cock, G., 2010. Violence and weapon related trauma at Puruchuco-Huaquerones, Peru. American Journal of Physical Anthropology 142 (4), 636–649.

Nordin, M., Frankel, V. (Eds.), 1989. Basic Biomechanics of the Musculoskeletal System. Lea and Febiger, Philadelphia.

Oxnard, C.E., 1993. Bone and bones: architecture and stress, fossils and osteoporosis. Journal of Biomechanics 26 (1), 63–79.

Pearce, A.I., Richards, R.G., Milz, S., Schneider, E., Pearce, S.G., 2007. Animal models for implant biomaterial research in bone: a review. European Cell and Materials 13, 1–10.

Piekarski, K., 1970. Fracture of bone. Journal of Applied Physics 41 (1), 215–223.

Reilly, D.T., Burnstein, A.H., 1974. The mechanical properties of cortical bone. Journal of Bone and Joint Surgery 56 (5), 1001–1002.

Roark, R., Young, W., 1975. Formulas for Stress and Strain. McGraw Hill, New York.

Ross, A.H., Abel, S.M., 2011. The Juvenile Skeleton in Forensic Abuse Investigations. Humana Press, New York.

Schmidt, C.W., Symes, S.A., 2008. The Analysis of Burned Human Remains. Academic Press, San Diego.

Smith, M.O., 2013. Paleopathology. In: DiGangi, E.A., Moore, M.K. (Eds.), Research Methods in Human Skeletal Biology. Academic Press, San Diego.

Symes, S., Berryman, H., Smith, O., 1989. The changing role of the forensic anthropologist: pattern and mechanism of fracture propagation. Mountain, Swamp, and Beach Forensic Anthropology Meetings Gatlinburg, Tennessee.

Symes, S., Ferraro, C., Patton, S., Smith, O., Kroman, A., 2002. From Caffey (1946) to Kempe (1962): Historical perspectives on the recognition of child abuse. Proceedings of the American Academy of Forensic Sciences 8, 246–247.

Symes, S., L'Abbe, E., Champman, E., Wolff, I., Dirkmaat, D., 2012. Interpreting traumatic injury to bone in medicolegal investigations. In: Dirkmaat, D.C. (Ed.), A Companion to Forensic Anthropology. Wiley-Blackwell, New York, pp. 340–389.

Trammell, L., Kroman, A.M., 2013. Histology. In: DiGangi, E.A., Moore, M.K. (Eds.), Research Methods in Human Skeletal Biology. Academic Press, San Diego.

Tung, T.A., 2012. Violence, Ritual, and the Wari Empire: A Social Bioarchaeology of Imperialism in the Ancient Andes. University Press of Florida, Gainesville.

Turner, C., Burr, D., 1993. Basic biomechanical measurements of bone: a tutorial. Bone 14 (4), 595–608.

Weiss, E., 2004. Understanding muscle markers: lower limbs. American Journal of Physical Anthropology 125 (3), 232–238.

Wolff, J., 1892. Das Gesetz der Transformation der Knochen. A. Hirschwald, Berlin.

Woo, S., Kuei, S., Amiel, D., Gomez, M., Hayes, W.C., White, F., et al., 1981. The effect of prolonged biological training on the properties of long bone: a study of Wolff's law. Journal of Joint and Bone Surgery 63 (5), 780–786.

Zimmerman, L.J., Emerson, T., Willey, P., Swegle, T., Gregg, J.B., Gregg, P., White, E., Smith, C., Haberman, T., Bumstead, M.P., 1981. The Crow Creek Site (39BF11) Massacre: A Preliminary Report. US Army Corps of Engineers, Omaha District, Omaha.

9

Taphonomy

Kerriann Marden, Marcella H. Sorg, William D. Haglund

INTRODUCTION

We start with the premise that research about death and its resulting skeletal changes, i.e., taphonomy, is a relevant focus of study within human skeletal biology. **Taphonomy**[1] is the study of the postmortem processes (Efremov, 1940), encompassing all phases beginning at the moment of death, potentially extending even to fossilization. It is a field that was created when paleontologists realized that in order to correctly interpret the fossilized remains they were studying, they would have to mentally "strip away" the changes that had occurred to the bones since death, in order to reveal the biology of the organism. Therefore, taphonomy (from the Greek words for burial, "*taphos*," and law, "*nomos*") was originally envisioned as the study of death assemblages, involving postmortem phenomena. One had to understand—and essentially remove or ignore these phenomena—in order to reconstruct the characteristics of the (previously) living organism in its environment.

Efremov described taphonomy as "the study of the transition (in all its details) of animal remains from the biosphere into the lithosphere" (1940:85). However, with wider application in archaeology and forensic anthropology, use of the term has broadened to describe the study of all human and nonhuman processes that act upon an organism from the time of death through the moment of skeletal examination. Such increased scope is necessary for two reasons. First, human action—such as **perimortem** violence, corpse desecration, mortuary treatment, burial disturbance, and looting—can have an enormous impact on skeletal remains. Second, human action ranging from pre-depositional to post-collection effects on bone must be observed and understood in order to distinguish these effects from natural processes. Most archaeologists now recognize the importance of understanding taphonomic changes in "the reconstruction of perimortem and **postmortem** processes and the discrimination of natural from human-induced trauma" (Ubelaker, 1997a:77). Numerous studies have demonstrated the importance of rigorous standards in discerning the etiology of taphonomic modifications to bone (Brain, 1981; Potts and Shipman, 1981; Behrensmeyer et al., 1986; Blumenschine, 1988; Olsen, 1988; Bunn, 1989; Fiorillo, 1989;

---

[1]All bolded terms are defined in the glossary at the end of this volume.

Marshall, 1989; Cruz-Uribe and Klein, 1994; Ubelaker, 1997a; Sauer, 1998; Shipman and Rose, 1988; Saul and Saul, 2002).

The study of taphonomy thus extends beyond the natural processes of **diagenesis** (chemical changes to bone *in situ*, such as fossilization) to also include the effects of discovery, recovery, handling, and storage. This is the only means by which these latter effects can be discriminated from natural processes, trauma, or pathological conditions. Although many researchers do not like to admit it, "scratches, nicks and cuts from trowels frequently occur and can later be mistaken for perimortem trauma … The impacts of excavation and curation cannot be underestimated and both must be treated as important taphonomic variables" (Nawrocki, 1995:55). Therefore, the usage of the term "taphonomy" has shifted over time to encompass the full range of "natural and the cultural events, processes, and agents that modify human remains from the time of death until the time of analysis" (Stodder, 2008:72). **Mortuary treatment** of the corpse is also considered a taphonomic variable, as the way a body is prepared after death will affect its preservation and the impact of subsequent taphonomic forces (Ubelaker, 2000:55).

Taphonomic effects are sequential and cumulative, and they may affect each other. Human osteological remains "are a surviving sample of a dynamic system involving processes that added, modified and subtracted items of evidence" (Bunn, 1981:576). Myriad factors can influence the composition and condition of human bone assemblages recovered from forensic or archaeological contexts. It is critical to observe all of the layers of information in order to discriminate among them, and to perform research that encompasses disease processes that occurred during life as well as skeletal evidence of perimortem trauma (damage occurring at or around the time of death), and postmortem treatment of the body (Marden, 2011b; Sauer, 1998; Hackett, 1976; Wells, 1964). A comprehensive approach is necessary to consider the sum total of factors that might affect an assemblage—both human and nonhuman. See Table 9.1.

It seems straightforward that one would want to differentiate changes to bones that occur after death from skeletal features characteristic of the once-living individual, but it is not always easy to do so. Processes that change bone after death can mimic **antemortem** (before death) processes, generating "**pseudopathology**." The term for such mimicry is "**equifinality**," when the etiology (cause) is different, but the result is the same. In addition, postmortem processes (those occurring after death) can hide or distort biological characteristics. For example, scavengers can alter or completely remove signs of perimortem trauma. At the same time, pathological changes in life can weaken bone, making it more susceptible to destructive taphonomic agents and effectors. Therefore, it is essential that we study and understand the postmortem processes that might otherwise confound us, and to design research that adequately controls or accounts for these factors.

Although the field of taphonomy is over 70 years old, research advances continue to illuminate these complex issues. Human skeletal biologists have contributed a great deal to the field, building a substantial body of research, particularly in bioarchaeology, paleoanthropology, paleopathology, and forensic anthropology. But there is much that remains to be done. This chapter reviews the types of taphonomic research that have been conducted, focusing on methodological themes, and highlights some of the resulting implications for research design.

TABLE 9.1 Potential Taphonomic Processes Expressed in Stages from Living Animal to Collected Assemblage, Including Potential Preferential and Nonpreferential Alterations, Based upon Microdamage to the Makapansgat Limeworks Bone Breccia Material.

Stages	Related Processes	Potential Taphonomic Changes	
		Preferential Alterations[a]	Nonpreferential Alterations[a]
LIVING ANIMAL Transition to death ("perimortem" interval)	Senility, dehydration, starvation, disease, accident, human perimortem violence	Pathological conditions, blunt force trauma, projectile wounds, cutting or chopping (sharp force trauma), carnivore toothmarks	Pathological conditions, blunt force trauma, projectile wounds, cutting or chopping (sharp force trauma), carnivore toothmarks
DEAD ANIMAL Destruction of carcass	Defleshing, disarticulation, tool use, consumption, scavenging by carnivores, scavenging by other fauna (including avian species), chemical decomposition, insect scavenging, biological decay	Dismemberment cutmarks, hammerstone impact scars, carnivore toothmarks, bird talon and beak marks, cut and chop marks, abrasion, polish, wear, microchipping	Carnivore toothmarks, trampling scratches, soft part removal, abrasion, polish, wear
SKELETAL REMAINS Breakdown of skeletal remains	Weathering, trampling, insect boring, biological decay, rodent action, root etching	Gnawing marks	Borings, tunnels, abrasion, etching, soft part removal, gnawing marks
SKELETAL REMAINS AVAILABLE FOR BURIAL Burial	Sediment coverage, sediment infiltration, compression, trampling, depression, decay	Depression and compression features related to soil pressure	Abrasion, polish, root grooves, insect borings
BURIED REMAINS Fossilization	Impregnation, mineralization, leaching, cracking, shearing		
Transportation	Hill wash, water, wind, predators, faunal exploitation	Abrading of extruding parts	Abrasion, erosion, stomach acid etching, attrition, pitting
FOSSILIZED REMAINS Recovery	Erosion, excavation, blasting, drilling, wedging, levering		Abrasion, "fresh" scratches
RECOVERED REMAINS Preparation and conservation	Selection, mechanical preparation, acid preparation, surface coating		Excavation damage, preparator marks, applied coatings, etching, smoothing, obliteration of surface
STORED/DISPLAYED REMAINS Study	Handling, breakage, destruction, measuring, disappearance	Surface patina from handling	Labeling, repair, mounting (of remains that were curated in historical period)

[a]"Preferential alterations" are effects that occur at a preferred site on bone surface, whereas "nonpreferential alterations" are randomly distributed. The categories are not mutually exclusive.

Adapted from Schrenk, F. and J. Maguire 1988:287, 290, Tables 1 and 2.

THE TAPHONOMIC RESEARCH PERSPECTIVE

There are three key characteristics of the taphonomic research perspective, which in turn shape the field's research methods (Sorg and Haglund, 2002). First, postmortem changes cannot be understood outside their environmental context. Second, death is best understood as an ecological phenomenon: the corpse changes its immediate environment, the environment changes the corpse, and the entire process involves a complex relationship between communities of plants and animals, climate and weather, and soils and geology. The ecological perspective leads to the third characteristic of taphonomic research as an interdisciplinary research endeavor.

By interpreting human skeletal remains as a product of the context in which they were discovered, taphonomy adopts an ecological perspective, which focuses on human remains as the "centerpiece of a newly emerging **microenvironment**" (Sorg and Haglund, 2002:5). This perspective integrates information about ecological processes of decomposition, consumption by scavengers, dispersal, and assimilation involving plants, animals, and microorganisms that become associated with the decomposing body. All of these changes create a new microenvironment immediately surrounding the body that continues to change through time.

Ultimately, as a result of these natural processes, once-living organisms are reduced to their constituent molecules after death. The term for this process is **decomposition**, which quite literally refers to the breaking down of the organic composition of a once-living organism. Decomposition includes both (1) the self-destruction of cells by their own enzymatic action (**autolysis**) and (2) breakdown by other living organisms in the surrounding ecological community (**putrefaction** by microorganisms, consumption and assimilation by animal scavengers including insects, and chemical or physical breakdown caused by plants). In addition, nonbiological processes such as erosion, temperature, and moisture can speed, delay, or otherwise influence chemical reactions. It is important to note that these processes occur on land as well as in water environments.

Due to the wide-ranging effects of biological, chemical, and physical agents, taphonomy is interdisciplinary, potentially requiring a broad range of expertise spanning the natural sciences. The importance of context and the significance of ecological factors require the expertise of many disciplines in order to fully understand the various life forms involved, and their potential impact on the condition of the remains. Current taphonomic research is conducted cooperatively by zoologists, botanists, pedologists (soil scientists), and geologists, as well as archaeologists and biological anthropologists. For example, entomologists contribute knowledge about the identification of insects associated with the body and the timing of their developmental states, which allows them to estimate how much time has passed since the death. Botanists identify plants associated with the remains, which may reveal when a body was moved from one location to another.

In all forensic applications, the taphonomic approach views the human remains within the context of discovery. This means that collecting details about the location and environmental characteristics of the site where the remains were found is often just as important as information regarding the condition of the remains themselves. For example, bodies decompose more slowly in cooler temperatures, so knowing the temperature of the area where the body was found would contribute to understanding its taphonomic condition. Careful and comprehensive taphonomic documentation of the scene should include a wide range of ecological information about the microenvironment. Particularly important are those factors that either concentrate or limit the body's access to heat, moisture, and scavenging.

Perhaps the most important outcome of taphonomic research is the unequivocal demonstration that postmortem processes are context specific. Again, this seems straightforward, but may be inadequately appreciated by inexperienced skeletal biologists. As scientists, we look for patterns; we want to identify processes so that we can recognize and predict their results across many settings. But the lesson learned from 70 years of taphonomic research is that we must expand our models to address a wider range of specific environmental and contextual factors. Weathering processes, for example, will differ in the rate, the sequence, and the appearance of resulting changes to bone dependent upon relative moisture, solar radiation, and temperature. More holistic research is needed that can encompass and model variation that is microenvironmentally, regionally, and temporally specific (Marden and Sorg, 2011; Sorg, 2011, Sorg et al., 2012). To the extent that these perspectives are incorporated into taphonomic research, the result can yield much more accurate information about skeletal biology, when that taphonomic "overprint" is "stripped away" or "controlled" methodologically. Done properly, taphonomic research can also tell us more about the death event and about past environments, factors that contribute to understanding the organism's biological makeup and the events related to its death and deposition.

METHODOLOGY IN TAPHONOMIC RESEARCH

Focus: Taphonomic Interpretation of Bone Damage and Marks on Bone

A wealth of information can be gleaned from taphonomic analysis of osteological materials, the basis of which lies in the correct interpretation of bone modification (Bonnichsen and Sorg, 1989). For example, a vital function of forensic anthropology is "to properly interpret taphonomical factors (postmortem changes in the tissues) and distinguish them from evidence of foul play" (Ubelaker, 1997b:109). However, the reconstruction of past human behavior based upon marks on bone[2] depends heavily upon the accurate assessment of marks that are often grossly similar. Precise distinction between one type of mark and another is imperative for osteological analysis to be of any interpretative value, yet the reliable identification of human and nonhuman bone modifications has proven much more complex than originally presumed, and the body of knowledge remains dynamic.

Like archaeology, taphonomy is essentially a historical science, in that it requires reconstructing past events from currently observable evidence (Shipman, 1988). This "retrodiction" of unobservable actions and agents results in a somewhat inverted methodology wherein one

---

[2]"Marks" on bone refer to any observable change in bone color, texture, or surface contiguity relative to unmodified skeletal material. Note that virtually all skeletal material has "marks," even pristine medical specimens, which are often "marked" or modified by fixative or bleaching.

tries to accurately deduce a cause by observing the result—through examination of the product of a process, we attempt to replicate the process itself[3] (Shipman, 1988; Houck, 1998).

The process of determining the cause of marks of unknown origin relies upon what Lewis Binford referred to as an "argument of elimination," a deductive process that assumes that all possible causes have been recognized and considered, and that all but one of those possibilities can be satisfactorily rejected (Binford, 1981:83). Such disciplined reasoning is imperative in the study of processes related to the cause and manner of death and the disposition of human remains in a medicolegal context. Since the reproduction of past events is critical to forensic anthropology and other forms of skeletal biology research, an empirical paradigm based on actualistic experiments, explained below, can provide analogues to help interpret past processes.

Accurate interpretation of marks on bone requires the precise identification of not only the *actor* (e.g., human, carnivore, rodent, wind), but also the *effector* (e.g., hammerstone, tooth, abrasion). This procedure is potentially confounded by the fact that one actor may produce numerous and varied effects, and further, the same effect may be the result of very different processes (Schrenk and McGuire, 1988; Ubelaker and Adams, 1995). The potential for mimicry of human activity by nonhuman agents is great, posing tremendous challenges in interpreting skeletal material. Furthermore, bones in a naturally occurring deposition are likely to be altered by numerous taphonomic agents. The "taphonomic signatures" of various agents may intermingle, overlap, and obscure interpretation. Therefore, it is possible—indeed, probable—that the effects of multiple taphonomic agents will be superimposed upon one another over time, concealing or even obliterating the taphonomic signature of other processes (Andrews and Cook, 1985; Behrensmeyer et al., 1986; Schrenk and McGuire, 1988).

Weathering, trampling, abrasion, erosion, rodent and carnivore gnawing, or excavation and laboratory procedures—even simple washing—can eradicate diagnostic evidence of previous actors and effectors (Behrensmeyer et al., 1986). In one actualistic study, three minutes of trampling by humans in soft-soled shoes on a damp sand-and-gravel substrate was sufficient to obscure the distinguishing characteristics of intentional cutmarks on bone (Behrensmeyer et al., 1986). In a separate study, bones broken by humans to extract marrow proved attractive to carnivores, creating an overlap in different classes of marks (Blumenschine, 1988). In any naturally occurring skeletal assemblage, then, the distinction between various types of marks on bone can be dubious, and reference samples resulting from unobserved natural experiments are particularly problematic, because their ambiguous etiology does not permit their use as reliable control collections.

To accurately and reliably identify marks on bone, researchers must gain experience with reference collections produced by just one known actor and effector (Blumenschine, 1988; Pickering, 1989). Such investigation of past actions via examination of present systems can be termed **"actualism"** (Micozzi, 1991; Gifford, 1992). Actualistic research methodology can involve a range of approaches, including (1) ethnographic study of active practitioners of specific behaviors, such as butchering, providing direct observation of cause and effect relationships; (2) historical reconstruction, which can demonstrate cause and effect through comparison of archival documentation and physical collections; (3) natural experiment, in

---

[3]See Kroman and Symes (Chapter 8), this volume, for a discussion of how skeletal biologists also do this with analysis of trauma.

which results of natural processes are observed; and (4) experimental research design, in which a causal event is replicated in order to reproduce an observed effect. The ethnographic approach is beyond the scope of this chapter, but the other three approaches will be discussed in more depth below.

ACTUALISTIC METHODOLOGY: NATURAL AND EXPERIMENTAL

Natural Experiments

Perhaps the most effective research approach to determine the diagnostic characteristics of taphonomic bone modification is through comparison with marks on bone of known origin. Often this is accomplished through what is termed a "**natural experiment**," involving observation of bone changes produced by real events. One source for comparative collections from "natural experiments" is from archaeological contexts, wherein the etiology of marks is inferred from the depositional context and morphological features of the marks themselves. The drawback to this method is that the causative agent was not directly observed, and the interpretation is therefore limited to the judgment of the researcher, which may not actually be correct. A classic example of this method is the "taphonomic signature of cannibalism" in the pre-Columbian Southwest, in which the authors attribute a set of marks on bone to human cannibalism in early Puebloan communities (Turner and Turner, 1999:478), a conclusion that has recently been challenged on taphonomic grounds (Marden, 2011a).

Forensic cases can also offer comparative data for marks on bone, similarly functioning as "natural experiments." However, as in archaeological assemblages, these marks cannot always be reliably attributed to a specific actor and/or effector. Even in cases in which a confession describes the events surrounding the death event, it is not always possible to directly attribute a mark to a specific cause. For example, if a suspect admits to having stabbed the victim in the chest, it still cannot be assumed that linear marks observed on the thoracic skeleton are directly attributable to the acts related to the manner of death, to the exclusion of other explanations. Root etching, excavation trowels, autopsy scalpels, and other agents must also be considered.

Therefore, despite their tremendous value from having resulted from actual events, the precise etiology of marks on bone resulting from natural experiments is usually unknown, having been inferred or assumed rather than directly observed. Therefore, any errors in interpretation of the control collection will unwittingly be transferred to the analysis of the data in question. "Control collections can only be considered adequate if the actor and effector were actually observed to be the agent inflicting the surface modification .... For example, modern hyaena dens cannot be considered control collections" (Blumenschine, 1988:505).

There is a demonstrated need for caution when inferring evidence of human action on skeletal remains that have been affected by multiple agents, some of which may not even enter the imagination of the researcher (Andrews and Cook, 1985:688). For example, recent research in the Northeastern region of the United States has indicated the involvement of multiple faunal species, some never previously considered as an important part of the taphonomic sequence, such as bobcats and pine martens (Sorg, 2011; Sorg et al., 2012). The potential confusion of the signatures of numerous and varied processes necessitates a rigorous methodological approach to bone modification.

Controlled Actualistic Experiments

The most controlled form of actualistic methodology is **experimental research design**, which actively seeks to replicate the effect under study by reproducing the hypothetical causal event in a controlled setting (Binford, 1981; Micozzi, 1991). The importance of actualistic experiments in archaeological and taphonomic reconstruction cannot be overestimated, as they develop taphonomic profiles that can be used for reference in the identification of marks observed on skeletal remains in archaeological or medicolegal contexts.

The **uniformitarian principle** is implicit in such empirical studies of osteological material, in that researchers may assume that although species, environments, and behaviors may differ, the physical, mechanical, and chemical principles that control the alteration of bones will remain the same (Shipman, 1981; also see DiGangi and Moore [Chapter 2], this volume). Therefore, given adequate environmental controls, the researcher can assume that experimental agents and effectors will produce results on bone similar to those produced under natural conditions. Empirical actualistic studies provide a basic framework for the interpretation of taphonomic changes to skeletal remains (Saul and Saul, 2002).

Forensic Anthropology Research Facilities for Experimental Research

There are several forensic research facilities where controlled, actualistic anthropological experiments are carried out regularly, many related to taphonomic research questions. Best known among these is the Anthropological Research Facility at the University of Tennessee in Knoxville, initiated by Dr. William M. Bass in 1971, known informally as the "Body Farm."[4] Here, donated bodies are studied under experimental conditions within a secure outdoor setting, inaccessible to large scavengers. This facility allows monitoring of environmental variables such as temperature, moisture, and scavengers, and documentation of taphonomic changes through direct observation or camera imaging.

In the decades since the inception of this foundational approach, other facilities for the study of taphonomic processes have been developed at various locations around the country and abroad. These include the Forensic Osteology Research Station, or FOREST, at Western Carolina University in Cullowhee, North Carolina; the Outdoor Research Facility and Anatomical Sciences Laboratory at the Boston University School of Medicine; the Forensic Anthropology Research Facility at Texas State University, San Marcos; and the Taphonomic Research in Anthropology — Centre for Experimental Study (TRACES) at the University of Central Lancashire, UK, among others. Human bodies are used at some facilities, requiring adherence to both state and federal policies about donation, transport, and treatment of human remains. Nonhuman surrogates, such as pigs or rabbits, are used at other facilities; these are also subject to legal and procedural oversight. Laws and regulations differ from jurisdiction to jurisdiction, and community sensitivity may also influence facility policies. There are legal issues related to biological hazards, public health, and public safety. Development of such facilities requires a great deal of preparation, administrative care, and financial support.

Research from each of these facilities continues to contribute to the body of knowledge about the ways in which human and natural actions affect the processes of decomposition.

---

[4]Refer to Bass and Jefferson (2004) for more information.

Many other academic programs in anthropology also encourage actualistic research, although they may not have facilities dedicated specifically to taphonomic research on human remains. Individual actualistic studies involving human or nonhuman remains may be conducted in temporary research settings, without a fully developed facility; however, similar legal, health, and safety considerations still must be addressed by the institution authorizing the research. Experienced advisors can be invaluable.

Pseudopathology and Pseudotrauma

Actualistic research has provided tremendous insight on certain processes, such as when postmortem changes mimic traumatic or pathological defects and can lead to a misinterpretation of the causative agent. When taphonomic features mimic the effects of traumatic insult, this is termed **pseudotrauma**; when taphonomic changes are confused with pathological conditions, it is called **pseudopathology**. It is critical to consider taphonomic processes in the analysis of any defect on osseous material, and to be able to discern taphonomic damage from traumatic defects or pathological lesions when making a **differential diagnosis** (e.g., see Smith [Chapter 7], this volume).

Taphonomic analysis is important in the interpretation of the overall condition of the remains, yet some marks and features are ambiguous and difficult to classify. One highly experienced researcher has claimed that, of seven major classes of bone modification by tooth and tool, she is able to consistently identify only gnawing marks based on gross morphology of the marks alone (Shipman, 1981). The effects of sandy or rocky substrates on bone have been demonstrated to closely resemble the morphology of cutmarks (Shipman, 1981; Andrews and Cook, 1985; Behrensmeyer et al., 1986), and naturally occurring vascular grooves can easily be mistaken for intentional cutmarks (D'Errico and Villa, 1997). "Weathering cracks can resemble those produced by blunt force trauma. Trampling and carnivore chewing can cause spiral fractures similar to those caused by foul play-associated trauma. Fungus can cause a blackening of bones that simulates burning. Carnivore tooth-marks can appear very similar to sharp force trauma" (Ubelaker, 1997a:82). Water transport, sediment abrasion, avian activity, rodent or ungulate gnawing, insect activity, and root growth can all resemble human modification of bone (Potts and Shipman, 1981; Schrenk and Maguire, 1988; Raemsch, 1993; D'Errico and Villa, 1997; Sutcliffe, 1971 in Ubelaker, 1997a).

Layered analytic methods ranging from gross macroscopic examination to high-resolution microscopy can provide valuable information that cannot be obtained from one method alone. Despite the microscopic similarities between trampled bone and bone scored with stone tools (Shipman, 1988; Oliver, 1989), macroscopic characteristics such as distribution and patterning at the level of the organism or the assemblage can help to discern between various actors/effectors. For example, archaeological assemblages of butchered bone contain an average of 20–25% of bones bearing cutmarks, with most marked bones exhibiting between one and six cutmarks, whereas trampled assemblages commonly feature a much greater prevalence of markings and a far greater number of marks per bone[5] (Schrenk and Maguire, 1988). To understand an assemblage, not only must bones be examined at the microscopic level, mark by mark, but also for the frequency and distribution of cuts as they

---

[5]A notable exception to this trend is bones that have been processed to remove the periosteum, or to remove meat from areas of extensive muscle attachment (Andrews and Cook, 1985; Shipman, 1988).

represent the surface damage to each bone, and for the pattern of representation and damage to the bones at the assemblage level, must be investigated (Schrenk and Maguire, 1988).

Recognizing and Interpreting Marks on Bone

The first step toward the accurate interpretation of marks on bone is to observe their presence, analyze their morphology, and record their distribution pattern. Human skeletal remains must be interpreted as the result of a complex interaction of factors, which can add, modify, and remove evidence (Bunn, 1981). The potential confusion of the signatures of numerous and varied processes necessitates a rigorous methodological approach to bone modification, as previously stated. For example, the fact that cutmarks are rare even in assemblages generated by known butchering events highlights how radically the incorrect classification of marks on bone can skew the taphonomic analysis. The misidentification of even a few marks on human bone may result in a gross misinterpretation of taphonomic events (Behrensmeyer et al., 1986), and in the worst case scenario, can lead to a gross miscarriage of justice when applied in a forensic context. The most appropriate methods of analysis of marks on bone must be applied, allowing accurate comparison with experimental reference collections.

It has been well demonstrated that macroscopic similarities between markings of radically divergent origins can result in the misinterpretation of marks (Andrews and Cook, 1985; Shipman, 1988; Bunn, 1989; Bromage et al., 1991). The recognition of the potential for such macro-level similarities between bone modifications resulted in the development of research protocols involving microscopy, sometimes including high-resolution microscopic technology, to discern between the different taphonomic causes of marks on bone (Brothwell, 1969). It is argued that inspection with scanning electron microscopy (SEM) "reveals features that are unclear or invisible under the light microscope even when the magnifications are the same" (Shipman, 1981:360). Researchers have performed numerous actualistic experiments to produce a reference collection of "micromorphological profiles" to discern between various classes of marks on bone (Potts and Shipman, 1981; Shipman, 1981; Bromage, 1984; Bromage and Boyd, 1984; Behrensmeyer et al., 1986; Bromage et al., 1991).

However, it has also been shown that even at such a high level of resolution, the morphology of marks could bear striking similarities across classes. For example, abrasion marks could manifest the internal striae previously deemed the hallmark of stone tool cutmarks, and the shape of a mark in basal cross-section is not as diagnostic as once believed, as cutmarks, tooth scores, and abrasion scratches could all present as either V-shaped or U-shaped in cross-section (Behrensmeyer et al., 1986). Prevalent standards for analysis of bone markings are continually being tested, and some widely accepted diagnostic microscopic criteria have, over time, been discarded as overly simplistic (Shipman, 1988). Thus, although minute examination of markings on bone is indeed useful for identifying the taphonomic agent that produced the marks, such analysis can, in itself, prove misleading (Bunn, 1989).

Therefore, gross investigation using low magnification by hand lens or optic light microscopy remains not only the primary, but also the preferred technology used by microtaphonomists in the classification of marks on bone (Bromage et al., 1991). In comparison with other, "high-tech" methods like SEM, low magnification is less expensive, less labor intensive, and easier to accomplish in the field. Further, blind tests of interobserver reliability have demonstrated that even novice examiners can be trained to a near-perfect accuracy for identification of marks on bone using just a hand lens and angled light (White, 1992; Blumenschine et al., 1996).

The identification of human action on bone depends upon the recognition of patterns of modification that are characteristic of, if not unique to, human behavior, including such assemblage-level indicators as preferential selection and distribution of bones, and specific patterns of marking and breakage (Andrews and Cook, 1985). Micromorphology of individual marks, taken in combination with the macroscopic characteristics of modifications, is essential in taphonomic analysis. The anatomical location, distribution, and morphology are all equally significant in determining both the cause and the purpose of bone modification (Raemsch, 1993; Blumenschine et al., 1996). Even when microscopically indistinguishable, patterns of preferential alteration of particular bones or particular areas on bone can help to discern between disparate causative taphonomic processes (Schrenk and Maguire, 1988). "Diagnostically valuable contextual clues include the orientation of the mark with respect to a specimen's long axis, the number of marks present on a specimen, and the mark's location on a specimen in relation to anatomical landmarks, fracture features, and other marks" (Blumenschine et al., 1996:494).

Certain taphonomic signatures can only be distinguished by a macro-level analysis of their patterning and distribution (Behrensmeyer et al., 1986; Schrenk and Maguire, 1988). For example, despite the striking microscopic similarities between trampled bone and bone scored with stone tools, the placement of marks on the architecture of the bones and the frequency of marks within the assemblage are reliable indicators of the origins of the markings. Trampled bones classically show a tendency toward multiple, shallow, parallel striations oriented transversely or obliquely to the long axis (Behrensmeyer et al., 1986), so that when more than 70% of marks on long bones are oriented oblique to the long axis, it is likely that the marks are due to trampling (Shipman, 1988:267).

To accurately interpret the taphonomy of an osteological assemblage, analysis must occur on three levels, taken together: the individual morphology of each mark; the frequency and distribution of marks as they represent the surface damage to each bone; and the pattern of elemental representation and distribution of damage to the bones at the assemblage level (Schrenk and Maguire, 1988). Similarly, the importance of distribution within a single skeleton has been amply demonstrated in the accurate diagnosis of pathological lesions (Ortner, 2008). The pattern of distribution of marks across the skeleton is no less important in taphonomic analysis, and therefore, among the first tasks that must be performed is the careful reassociation of each set of skeletal remains. Not only the patterning of damage, but also the presence and absence of elements, can provide a wealth of information regarding perimortem action and postmortem treatment of remains.

TAPHONOMY AND SKELETAL BIOLOGY: TWO CASE STUDIES

Bones in either forensic or archaeological contexts are likely to be altered by numerous taphonomic agents. The signatures of various human and natural agents may intermingle, overlap, and obscure interpretation. These modifications can either confuse or illuminate the picture for the skeletal biology researcher. Therefore, skeletal biologists should consider the potential impacts of taphonomic change as they embark on their research.

The following two case studies illustrate the broad range and interconnectedness of research involving taphonomy and skeletal biology. In the first instance, a medicolegal homicide case, details that are discovered about the death enhance the understanding of the case as a natural experiment in bone modification and the identification of "perimortem" injuries. In the second case, known taphonomic signatures and investigation procedures assist in the interpretation of an archaeological mystery.

CASE STUDY: FORENSIC TAPHONOMY

Introduction

In one case that was certified as a homicide by the medical examiner in a northern New England state, the authors were brought in to provide forensic anthropology consultation, including an evaluation of skeletal damage. This case illustrates the potential overlap in the interpretation of trauma along with natural and human taphonomic processes. These modification agents were considered in helping to reconstruct the death event.

Documenting the Depositional Context

The death occurred about 8 weeks prior to the late November discovery of the body. The remains were left in a streambed, with a few large logs lying longitudinally over the body. The position of the logs suggested that they had been placed there intentionally, possibly in an effort to conceal the remains. The body was nude. An article of clothing that appeared to be a shirt was wrapped several times around the neck of the body, and then apparently knotted. Despite the log cover, much of the body was accessible to carnivores. Tri-colored fur from a carnivore was also found adhering to some of the exposed viscera.

Documenting the Condition of the Remains, Including Bone Modification

The soft tissue was still relatively fresh and the exposed bone was still well collagenated. Some bones of the torso and abdomen were chewed, the upper arm bones were dispersed, and the bones of the lower arm and hand were missing. The body exhibited some possible skeletal indications of perimortem trauma, but required confirmation. Specifically, there was bilateral breakage of the nasal bones and nasal margins, and one central incisor had been avulsed (forcibly removed).

Interpreting the Bone Damage with Multiple Taphonomic Indicators

The cause of the damage to the nasals was equivocal. Such breakage could indicate a blow to the face, which could help to reconstruct the events surrounding the death of this young woman. The broken nasal margins, especially that of the left maxilla, exhibited a slightly scalloped edge (see Figure 9.1) which is not characteristic of traumatic fracture. Also, the

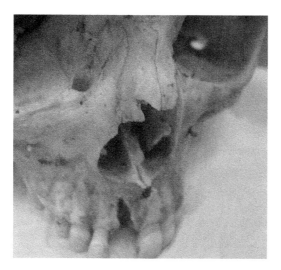

FIGURE 9.1   Close-up of mid-face of cranium, anterior-oblique view, illustrating irregular fracture margin of both nasal bones and the smoother fracture margin of the maxilla at the left lateral nasal aperture.

breakage of nasal bones, particularly the right nasal, appeared to have a punctate quality that is not generally characteristic of blunt force trauma to the nose and could be interpreted as more consistent with the damage caused by carnivore tooth puncture. Although this breakage is not typical of the "classic" facial damage resulting from interpersonal violence, neither is it typical of carnivore gnawing. Carnviores will preferentially scavenge the facial region (Haglund, 1997), but the utter absence of tooth scoring, tooth punctures, or other signs of gnawing on the facial skeleton or elsewhere on the cranium is not diagnostic of carnivore scavenging.

The anterior maxillary dentition also exhibited damage. The right central incisor was absent, and the bone of the anterior jaw was broken around the margin of the tooth root. See Figure 9.2. The left central incisor showed similar bone breakage along the outline of the tooth root, although this tooth was still in place. This type of breakage is consistent with tooth avulsion resulting from a blow to the mouth, in which the anterior teeth are levered out at the roots by force applied to the tooth crowns. However, the anterior alveolar bone on this individual was exceedingly thin and fragile, so that we could not rule out the possibility that this breakage resulted from weathering and drying during the period of post-mortem exposure. Furthermore, this type of dental damage could also result from rough postmortem handling of the body, which was found under heavy logs.

The damage to the nasal region is consistent with either perimortem trauma or carnivore modification, although the pattern is not highly typical of either. The damage to the anterior alveolar bone indicates blunt force applied to the front teeth resulting in avulsion, which could be related either to traumatic insult to the victim's face at or near the time of death, or to postmortem damage from transporting and attempting to conceal the body. The co-occurrence of these two forms of damage increases the likelihood that these are both skeletal indicators of traumatic insult to the face of the victim at or near the time of death. Taken in conjunction with the clothing bound about the neck and the apparent attempts at

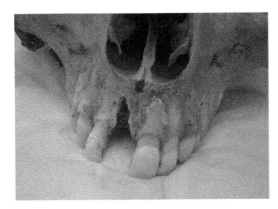

FIGURE 9.2   Close-up of maxillary anterior alveolus, showing breakage of right first incisor indicating tooth avulsion, but also depicting drying and cracking of thin bone at left first incisor.

concealment of the body, the evidence suggests but does not unequivocally demonstrate that the skeletal damage may be due to perimortem blunt force trauma.

Discussion

This case highlights the drawbacks of natural experiments, and demonstrates that even with meticulous analysis and strong reference collections from which to draw comparative samples, not all taphonomic damage can be reliably attributed to a specific actor and/or effector. It is possible that the damage to the victim's facial skeleton was caused by human action, resulting from intentional, violent assault. It is also possible that the breakage was caused by human action but inadvertently, as a result of reckless treatment of the corpse as the body was transported through the woods and covered with logs. However, it remains possible that this damage was caused by natural agents, including carnivores and weathering processes. Lastly, it is possible that human and natural agents had a **synergistic** effect, and that assault or rough damage by humans damaged the soft tissue of the nose, exposing blood and flesh and thus making it more attractive to carnivore scavengers.

It is critical to accept this ambiguity and resist overinterpreting the evidence, especially in a medicolegal context where anthropological conclusions have real-world consequences. Taphonomy is a critical component of any forensic anthropological analysis, but it cannot always provide definitive answers. Alexandre Lacassagne, a French physician who was among the earliest to apply anthropology in a medicolegal context in the late seventeenth century, is also credited with the quote, "One must know how to doubt" (Starr, 2010:105). Even now, almost a century after Lacassagne's death, these words must be heeded.

Yet each case that presents ambiguous evidence can also be seen as an opportunity for future research, perhaps by a graduate student at one of the facilities mentioned previously in this chapter. Students looking for ideas for research projects would be well served by speaking to their local board-certified forensic anthropologist or medical examiner regarding cases that have raised new questions. These gaps in the extant knowledge offer new directions for students to explore, eventually helping to answer the questions that remain elusive.

CASE STUDY: ARCHAEOLOGICAL TAPHONOMY

Introduction

In a case from Chaco Canyon, located in the San Juan River Basin of northwestern present-day New Mexico, a combination of taphonomic analysis and careful archival research has provided new insights on the treatment of human burials at the enigmatic pre-Columbian site of Pueblo Bonito, site 29SJ387 (Marden, 2011a, b). Taphonomic analysis has helped to demonstrate that these bones are indeed haphazardly distributed, probably by scavengers, rather than by elaborate ritual behavior to which their arrangement was previously attributed.

Documenting the Environmental and Recovery Context

The sealed outer doorway of a burial chamber in Pueblo Bonito referred to as Room 32 was breached by Harvard archaeologist George Pepper during his first field season in 1896. The room was filled with sand, suggesting that the doorway had remained open for a period of time after it had stopped being used regularly (Pepper, 1909:197). The first human remains encountered comprised a partial skeleton consisting of 13 vertebrae, a complete pelvic girdle, a femur, several ribs, a clavicle, and a scapula. Pepper also reported finding a human tooth, a "broken vertebra," "several vertebrae," and a "phalange" in this room (1896-47 Accession file), although descriptions of the numbers and locations of these last elements are extremely vague. Pepper described the discovery of these remains as follows:

> The human backbone and pelvis which were found in the southwest corner (p. 134) were the next objects to receive attention. They were intact and were lying northwest by southeast, the pelvis being toward the northern point and 6 inches above the level of the western doorway. The vertebrae were lying in an almost horizontal position, ten of them were intact and in position, as were also the sacrum and the pelvic bones. Three vertebrae fell in removing the surface dirt, but they had probably been in place when the body was found. [...] Wrapped around the bones and extending into the western doorway, there is a mass of burnt cloth, the greater part of which was simply woven textiles of finely spun yucca cord. **(Pepper, 1920:138)**

Pepper's field notes contain a sketch of these remains depicting the vertebrae and pelves in partial anatomical order *in situ*, consistent with his published description. The field notes also list the specific bones that were found in anatomical order:

> The back bone and pelvis were intact and were lying NW by SE, the pelvis being toward the former point. The pelvis was 6" above the level of the W doorway and the vertebrae were almost on a longitudinal plane. Ten of the vertebrae were intact and in position as were also the sacrum and the pelvic bones. The other vertebrae (3) fell when the man was removing the surface dirt and these too were probably in place. The vertebrae that were in place are numbered and run from 1 to 10, being numbered consecutively according to position. There were seven sticks that had been burnt off at one end, they were in a slanting position and rested against the lower part of the

vertebrae. They were on the western side. Under the vertebrae and extending into the western doorway was a mass of burnt cloth. (1896-47 Accession file).

Reassociating Remains with Morphological and Taphonomic Clues

A search of the records of the American Museum of Natural History (AMNH) in New York revealed that no skeletal elements in the collections were recorded as originating in Room 32, and previous researchers had reported that the remains could not be located (Akins, 1986:115). However, combined osteological analysis and archival research permitted the identification of the remains from Room 32. A large, commingled skeletal assemblage (curated at the AMNH) from the fill of the adjacent burial chamber, Room 33, contained the remains of 14 individuals: 12 adults and 2 infants.

Examination of the assemblage from Room 33 (Catalog Number H/3658) revealed that the skeletal elements from Room 32 were at some point incorporated into the Room 33 lot. Catalog Number H/3658 contains one set of ten vertebrae that—unlike any other bones—is marked with the numbers 1–10 in a careful hand. See Figure 9.3. This corresponds with Pepper's description of ten of the vertebrae found in Room 32 found "intact and in position" (1920:133), which he described in his notes as "numbered and run from 1 to 10, being

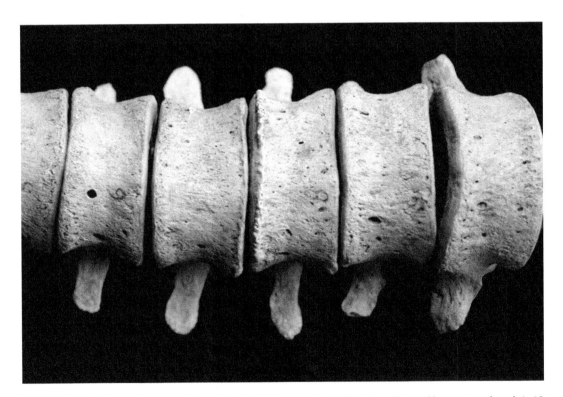

FIGURE 9.3 Ten contiguous vertebrae found in the commingled lot from Room 33 were numbered 1–10, consistent with Pepper's description of the vertebrae found in Room 32.

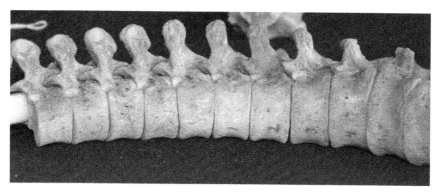

FIGURE 9.4 Three unmarked upper thoracic vertebrae are morphologically and taphonomically compatible with the numbered vertebrae, matching the description in the field notes of three vertebrae falling away from the block of ten that were numbered.

numbered consecutively according to position" (1896-47 Accession file). These ten numbered vertebrae were housed in a separate plastic bag in the drawer with all of the other vertebrae, along with three more thoracic vertebrae that reassociate perfectly to the ten numbered vertebrae to form a contiguous column. See Figure 9.4. This further supports the contention that these numbered vertebrae are the ten that Pepper found with the pelvis in Room 32, from which "other vertebrae (3) fell when the man was removing the surface dirt and these too were probably in place" (*ibid.*).

Unfortunately, none of the pelvic bones or sacra in this skeletal assemblage seem to bear any markings to indicate that they were from Room 32, but in the process of reassociation, a sacrum and pelvis in Catalog Number H/3658 were found to reassociate to the numbered vertebrae with perfect morphological integrity. The lumbosacral joint is highly specific, so a good fit between these elements is a very strong indication that these bones represent a single individual. The sacroiliac joint is also a highly specific joint for reassociation, and this joint is likewise strongly indicative that these bones represent a single individual. In this case, the surfaces of both pelves and the sacrum are also coated in adhesive, unlike any other bones in the assemblage, further confirming that these bones belong together. These bones are also consistent in their relative lack of arthritic changes and the excellent overall cortical quality.

Condition of Remains: Documenting Scavenger Modification, Leading to Additional Reassociation of Remains

These pelvic bones revealed a small amount of surface damage consistent with carnivore chewing. A pair of femora and tibiae that are consistent with the overall age, rugosity, robusticity, and cortical condition of this vertebral column and pelvis were also found among the commingled remains of H/3658. Like the pelvic bones, these lower limb bones exhibit damage consistent with having been chewed extensively by carnivores, including puncture marks, tooth furrowing, and tooth scoring (White, 1992; Haglund, 1997). No other femora of

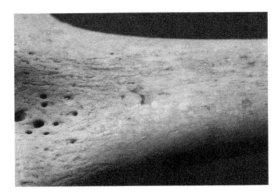

FIGURE 9.5 Oval-shaped black marking on anterior distal left femur that is consistent with Pepper's designation of the femur in Room 32 ("Left O" in his plan view sketches).

compatible age, sex, and cortical characteristics exhibited similar damage. Moreover, a distinctive ovoid mark drawn in black ink on the distal anterior left femoral shaft was noticed after these bones were reassociated to this individual. This mark appears to be the letter "O" consistent with the words "Left O" with which Pepper labelled the femur in Room 32 in his field sketch of these remains. See Figure 9.5. No other long bone in the assemblage was marked in ink in this way. This femur is an excellent morphological **antimere** for the right, leaving little doubt that the two bones are from the same individual.

Documenting the Condition of Remains: Taphonomic Signatures of Scavenger Modification and Mummification

Taken together, the skeletal and archival evidence indicates that part of this individual was recovered from Room 32, while the remainder was found in Room 33. The partial set of remains found in Room 32 consists of precisely the parts that are missing from the partial individual from Room 33 with which they have been reassociated; and the two partial skeletons are consistent in age, sex, and overall condition. The preponderance of evidence supports the interpretation that the remains in Room 32 and partial Skeleton #10 in Room 33 are the same individual.

Since partial Skeleton #10 and the partial remains from Room 32 almost certainly represent a single individual, it seems most likely that the body was first entombed in Room 33. The remains in Room 32 were found with a mass of cloth wrapped about them that Pepper concluded was their burial wrappings. This mass of cloth trailed into the doorway leading to Room 33, suggesting that it may have been dragged from that room with the bones. Actualistic evidence gleaned from forensic contexts has demonstrated the importance of understanding the potential of scavenging to destroy or scatter body parts, to alter or destroy evidence of the original context of the body's placement, and to create diagnostic damage to the remains (Haglund, 1997:367). All of these effects seem to have taken place in the case of the partial remains in Room 32. The sacrum, os coxa (pelvic bones), and femora of this individual show marks consistent with chewing, although this analysis did not attempt to identify the ribs among the large commingled lot. The most parsimonious explanation for the location of part of this body in Room 32 is that this thorax and pelvis were dragged there from their original burial location in Room 33 by scavengers, which would have held together relatively well due to its mummified condition (the leg and foot of Skeleton #10 in Room 33 were described as "desiccated" by Pepper). Vertebral elements can retain their anatomical association quite well due to their relatively strong ligamentous structures (Brain, 1981), especially when mummified. Furthermore, no other remains were buried above Skeleton #10 to impede scavenger access, and according to recent radiocarbon dating of these remains, the legs associated with this individual were among the last to be buried in this room (Plog and Heitman, 2010:19623, Table 1), suggesting that they would have been most accessible to scavengers.

Discussion: Contributions of Taphonomy to Archaeological Interpretation

The issue of whether these remains were originally entombed in Room 32 is important to the interpretation of this burial assemblage, because much has been made of the apparent ritual significance of a solitary, headless body found alone in this room. The configuration of the skeletal elements in Room 32 has been described previously as a "highly patterned association of the vertebrae and pelvis with burial goods, the preservation of the ceremonial sticks, arrows, and cloth, [with a]... patterned stratigraphic sequence" (Plog and Heitman, 2010:19622). However, taphonomic analysis and archival research instead indicate that the arrangement of the partial remains in this room was the result of carnivore scavenging, rather than a highly patterned association. The final location of this vertebral column has been invested with an archaeological significance that appears to be inconsistent with the taphonomic evidence resulting from direct analysis of the morphological characteristics of marks on the bones and their distribution in the skeletal assemblage.

CONCLUSION

Taphonomy is a critical component of the discipline of skeletal biology—a necessary first step in the analysis of skeletal material, whether it is archaeological or forensic in origin. Understanding the context in which a body became skeletonized, as well as the processes that may have acted on it *in situ*, during recovery, and since recovery should be the preliminary phase for all research on skeletal material. Taphonomic analysis should routinely include the following seven steps: (1) document context of skeletonization, recovery, and post-recovery; (2) document potential modifications resulting from exposure, recovery, and curation; (3) inventory and document all elements and fragments in the collection; (4) document the condition of the remains as a whole and for each element; (5) conjoin fractured fragments; (6) reassociate articulating elements; and (7) match antimeres (left/right paired elements) to the greatest extent possible. In addition, the following should be done: (1) assess potential for commingling; (2) assess potential for scavenging or other nonhuman animal modifications; and (3) assess the potential for postmortem modifications due to chemical, geological, climatological, or biological processes (e.g., burial, scavenging, water transport, geologic transport, and extreme temperatures, moisture, or dryness).

Empirical studies of taphonomic processes are of critical importance to skeletal biology, yet research about the postmortem processes that affect human remains is in many ways in its infancy. As the field grows, it is moving away from assumed taphonomic universals to incorporate an understanding of the broad ranges of variation across microenvironments, and to encompass input from interdisciplinary collaboration. Recent advances in biomolecular taphonomy and **DNA, mass spectrographic analysis** of the products of decomposition, and the taphonomic analysis of soil and water environments are all areas that potentially enrich skeletal biology research (Sorg et al., 2012). In addition, continued research about taphonomic signatures expands our ability to interpret remains with undocumented provenience or undocumented postmortem histories. Whether taphonomic research designs are naturalistic or experimental, they must incorporate an understanding of the skeletal remains within their environmental context, which frequently calls for interdisciplinary input and an ecological perspective. This three-part taphonomic perspective can inform the development of a new era of research that adds clarity and depth to our understanding of skeletal biology.

REFERENCES

1896-47 Accession file, Manuscript on file, Anthropology Department, American Museum of Natural History, New York.

Akins, N.J., 1986. A Biocultural Approach to Human Burials from Chaco, Canyon, New Mexico. Reports of the Chaco Center, No. 9. U.S. Department of the Interior. National Park Service, Santa Fe, New Mexico.

Andrews, P., Cook, J., 1985. Natural modifications to bones in a temperate setting. Man 20 (4), 675–691.

Bass, W., Jefferson, J., 2004. Death's Acre: Inside the Legendary Forensic Lab the Body Farm Where the Dead Do Tell Tales. Berkley Trade, New York.

Behrensmeyer, A.K., Gordon, K.D., Yanagi, G.T., 1986. Trampling as a cause of bone surface damage and pseudo-cutmarks. Nature 319 (6056), 768–771.

Binford, L.R., 1981. Bones: Ancient Men and Modern Myths. Academic Press, New York.

Blumenschine, R.J., 1988. An experimental model of the timing of hominid and carnivore influence on archaeological bone assemblages. Journal of Archaeological Science 15 (5), 483–502.

Blumenschine, R.J., Marean, C.W., Capaldo, S.D., 1996. Blind tests of inter-analyst correspondence and accuracy in the identification of cut marks, percussion marks, and carnivore tooth marks on bone surfaces. Journal of Archaeological Science 23 (4), 493–507.

Bonnichsen, R., Sorg, M.H., 1989. Bone Modification. Center for the Study of the First Americans, University of Maine, Orono, ME.

Brain, C.K., 1981. The Hunters or the Hunted? An Introduction to African Cave Taphonomy. University of Chicago Press, Chicago.

Bromage, T.G., 1984. Interpretation of scanning electron microscopic images of abraded forming bone surfaces. American Journal of Physical Anthropology 64 (2), 161–178.

Bromage, T.G., Boyde, A., 1984. Microscopic criteria for the determination of directionality of cutmarks on bone. American Journal of Physical Anthropology 65 (4), 359–366.

Bromage, T.G., Bermudez de Castro, J.M., Jalvo, Y.F., 1991. The SEM in taphonomic research and its application to studies of cutmarks generally and the determination of handedness specifically. Anthropologie 29 (3), 163–169.

Brothwell, D.R., 1969. The study of archaeological materials by means of the Scanning Electron Microscope: an important new field. In: Brothwell, D., D.R., Higgs, E. (Eds.), Science in Archaeology: A Survey of Progress and Research. Praeger, New York, pp. 564–566.

Bunn, H.T., 1981. Archaeological evidence for meat-eating by Plio-Pleistocene hominids from Koobi Fora & Olduvai Gorge. Nature 291 (5816), 574–577.

Bunn, H.T., 1989. Diagnosing Plio-Pleistocene hominid activity with bone fracture evidence. In: Bonnichsen, R., Sorg, M.H. (Eds.), Bone Modification. Center for the Study of the First Americans, Orono, Maine, pp. 299–315.

Cruz-Uribe, K., Klein, R.G., 1994. Chew marks and cut marks on animal bones from the Kasteelberg B and Dune Field Midden Later Stone Age sites Western Cape Province, South Africa. Journal of Archaeological Science 21 (1), 35−49.

D'errico, F., Villa, P., 1997. Holes and grooves: the contribution of microscopy and taphonomy to the problem of art origins. Journal of Human Evolution 33 (1), 1−31.

DiGangi, E.A., Moore, M.K., 2013. Application of the scientific method to skeletal biology. In: DiGangi, E.A., Moore, M.K. (Eds.), Research Methods in Human Skeletal Biology. Academic Press, San Diego.

Efremov, I.A., 1940. Taphonomy: a new branch of paleontology. Pan American Geologist 74, 81−93.

Fiorillo, A.R., 1989. Experimental study of trampling: implications for the fossil record. In: Bonnichsen, R., Sorg, M.H. (Eds.), Bone Modification. Center for the Study of the First Americans, Orono, ME, pp. 61−71.

Gifford, D.P., 1992. Taphonomy and paleoecology: a critical review of Archaeology's sister disciplines. In: Schiffer, M. (Ed.), Advances in Archaeological Method and Theory, Vol. 4. Academic Press, New York, pp. 365−438.

Hackett, C.J., 1976. Diagnostic Criteria of Syphilis, Yaws, and Treponarid (Treponematoses) and of Some Other Diseases in Dry Bones. Springer-Verlag, Berlin.

Haglund, W.D., 1997. Dogs and coyotes: postmortem involvement with human remains. In: Haglund, W.D., Sorg, M.H. (Eds.), Forensic Taphonomy: The Postmortem Fate of Human Remains. CRC Press, Boca Raton, pp. 367−381.

Houck, M.M., 1998. Skeletal trauma and the individualization of knife marks in bones. In: Reichs, K. (Ed.), Forensic Osteology: Advances in the Identification of Human Remains, 2nd ed. Charles C. Thomas, Springfield, IL, pp. 410−424.

Kroman, A.M., Symes, S.A., 2013. Skeletal trauma. In: DiGangi, E.A., Moore, M.K. (Eds.), Research Methods in Human Skeletal Biology. Academic Press, San Diego.

Marden, K., 2011a. Violence, taphonomy and cannibalism in Chaco Canyon: Discerning taphonomic changes from human action in the archaeological record. Abstracts of the Society for American Archaeology 76th Annual Meeting 206 (abstract).

Marden, K. 2011b. Taphonomy, Paleopathology and Mortuary Variability in Chaco Canyon: Using Bioarchaeological and Forensic Methods to Understand Ancient Cultural Practices. Unpublished doctoral dissertation, Department of Anthropology, Tulane University.

Marden, K., Sorg, M.H., 2011. Potential impacts of regional ecologies on the estimation of postmortem interval: Case comparisons from northern New England. Proceedings of the American Academy of Forensic Sciences 17, 388−389.

Marshall, L.G., 1989. Bone modification and the laws of burial. In: Bonnichsen, R., Sorg, M.H. (Eds.), Bone Modification. Center for the Study of the First Americans, Orono, ME, pp. 7−24.

Micozzi, M.S., 1991. Postmortem Change in Human and Animal Remains: A Systematic Approach. Charles C. Thomas, Springfield, IL.

Nawrocki, S.P., 1995. Taphonomic processes in historic cemeteries. In: Grauer, A. (Ed.), Bodies of Evidence: Reconstructing History through Skeletal Analysis. Wiley-Liss, New York, pp. 49−66.

Oliver, J.S., 1989. Analogues and site context: Bone damages from Shield Trap Cave (24CB91), Carbon County, Montana, U.S.A. In: Bonnichsen, R., Sorg, M.H. (Eds.), Bone Modification. Center for the Study of the First Americans, Orono, ME, pp. 73−98.

Olsen, S.L., 1988. Identification of stone and metal tools marks on bone artifacts. In: Olsen, S. (Ed.), Scanning Electron Microscopy in Archaeology Vol. 452, BAR International Series, Oxford, pp. 337−360.

Ortner, D.J., 2008. Differential diagnosis of skeletal lesions in infectious disease. In: Pinhasi, R., Mays, S. (Eds.), Advances in Human Palaeopathology. John Wiley & Sons, Chichester, pp. 191−215.

Pepper, G.H., 1909. The exploration of a burial room in Pueblo Bonito, New Mexico. In: Boaz, F. (Ed.), Putnam Anniversary Volume: Anthropological Essays, Presented to Frederic Ward Putnam in Honor of his Seventieth Birthday, April 16, 1909, by his Friends and Associates. G. E. Steckhert & Co., New York, pp. 196−252.

Pepper, G.H., 1920. Pueblo Bonito. University of New Mexico Press, Albuquerque.

Pickering, M.P., 1989. Food for thought: An alternative to cannibalism in the Neolithic. Australian Archaeology 28, 35−39.

Plog, S., Heitman, C., 2010. Hierarchy and social inequality in the American Southwest, A.D. 800−1200. Proceedings of the National Academy of Sciences 107, 19619−19626.

Potts, R., Shipman, P., 1981. Cutmarks made by stone tools on bones from Olduvai Gorge, Tanzania. Nature 291 (5816), 577−580.

Raemsch, C.A., 1993. Mechanical procedures involved in bone dismemberment and defleshing in prehistoric Michigan. Midcontinental Journal of Archaeology 18 (2), 217–239.

Sauer, N.J., 1998. The timing of injuries and manner of death: Distinguishing among antemortem, perimortem and postmortem trauma. In: Reichs, K. (Ed.), Forensic Osteology: Advances in the Identification of Human Remains, 2nd ed. Charles C. Thomas, Springfield, IL, pp. 321–332.

Saul, J.M., Saul, F.P., 2002. Forensics, archaeology, and taphonomy: The symbiotic relationship. In: Haglund, W.D., Sorg, M.H. (Eds.), Advances in Forensic Taphonomy: Method, Theory, and Archaeological Perspectives. CRC Press, Boca Raton, pp. 71–97.

Schrenk, F., Maguire, J.M., 1988. Actualistic SEM studies on the Makapansgat Limeworks grey breccia bone assemblage, Transvaal, South Africa. In: Olsen, S. (Ed.), Scanning Electron Microscopy in Archaeology. Vol. 452. BAR International Series, Oxford, pp. 287–301.

Shipman, P., 1981. Applications of scanning electron microscopy to taphonomic problems. In: Cantwell, A.M., Griffin, J.B., Rothschild, N.A. (Eds.), Research Potential of Anthropological Museum Collections. Annals of the New York Academy of Sciences, Vol. 376. New York Academy of Sciences, New York, pp. 357–385.

Shipman, P., 1988. Actualistic studies of animal resources and hominid activities. In: Olsen, S. (Ed.), Scanning Electron Microscopy in Archaeology. Vol. 452, BAR International Series, Oxford, pp. 261–285.

Shipman, P., Rose, J.J., 1988. Bone tools: an experimental approach. In: Olsen, S. (Ed.), Scanning Electron Microscopy in Archaeology. Vol. 452, BAR International Series, Oxford, England, pp. 303–335.

Smith, M.O., 2013. Paleopathology. In: DiGangi, E.A., Moore, M.K. (Eds.), Research Methods in Human Skeletal Biology. Academic Press, San Diego.

Sorg, M.H., 2011. Scavenging impacts on progression of decomposition in Northern New England. Proceedings of the American Academy of Forensic Sciences 17, 384–385.

Sorg, M.H., Haglund, W.D., 2002. Advances in forensic taphonomy: purpose, theory, and process. In: Haglund, W.D., Sorg, M.H. (Eds.), Advancing Forensic Taphonomy: Method, Theory, and Archaeological Perspective. CRC Press, Boca Raton, FL, pp. 3–29.

Sorg, M.H., Haglund, W.D., Wren, J.A., 2012. Taphonomic impacts of small and medium-sized scavengers in Northern New England. Proceedings of the American Academy of Forensic Sciences 18, 400.

Sorg, M.H., Haglund, W.D., & Wren, J.A., 2012. Research in forensic taphonomy. In: Dirkmaat, D.C. (Ed.), A Companion to Forensic Anthropology. Blackwell Publishing, Boston.

Starr, D., 2010. The Killer of Little Shepherds: A True Crime Story and the Birth of Forensic Science. Alfred A. Knopf, New York.

Stodder, A.L.W., 2008. Taphonomy and the nature of archaeological assemblages. In: Katzenberg, M.A., Saunders, S.R. (Eds.), Biological Anthropology of the Human Skeleton, 1st ed. John Wiley and Sons, New York, pp. 71–114.

Turner, C.G., Turner, J.A., 1999. Man Corn: Cannibalism and Violence in the Prehistoric American Southwest. University of Utah Press, Salt Lake City.

Ubelaker, D.H., 1997a. Taphonomic applications in forensic anthropology. In: Haglund, W.D., Sorg, M.H. (Eds.), Forensic Taphonomy: The Postmortem Fate of Human Remains. CRC Press, Boca Raton, pp. 77–90.

Ubelaker, D.H., 1997b. Latest developments in skeletal biology and forensic anthropology. In: Boaz, N.T., Wolfe, L.D. (Eds.), Biological Anthropology: The State of the Science. International Institute for Human Evolutionary Research, Bend, OR, pp. 101–115.

Ubelaker, D.H., 2000. Methodological considerations in the forensic applications of human skeletal biology. In: Katzenberg, M.A., Saunders, S.R. (Eds.), Biological Anthropology of the Human Skeleton, 1st ed. John Wiley and Sons, New York, pp. 41–67.

Ubelaker, D.H., Adams, B.J., 1995. Differentiation of perimortem and postmortem trauma using taphonomic indicators. Journal of Forensic Sciences 40 (3), 509–512.

Wells, C., 1964. Bones, Bodies and Disease: Evidence of Disease and Abnormality in Early Man. Thames and Hudson, London.

White, T.D., 1992. Prehistoric Cannibalism at Mancos 5MTUMR-2346. Princeton University Press, Princeton, NJ.

Dental Anthropology

Emily Hammerl

INTRODUCTION

With the wealth of information contained in the human skeleton, one might ask the question, "Why study teeth?" The answer is multifaceted as teeth can elucidate many interesting questions about living and past human populations. As teeth are the initial mechanism through which we obtain nourishment, they are under strict genetic constraints governing their development. After all, if you cannot eat, you cannot survive. Because of this, teeth are also less susceptible to environmental stressors such as poor nutrition and prolonged illness, both of which are well known to affect the completed length and form of the long bones.

Given the relative developmental stability of teeth in comparison to bone (Kieser, 1990; Bogin, 1999), it may seem that this would result in levels of variation too low to provide the researcher with much valuable information. Fortunately, this is not the case. As we will see, variation in tooth growth (e.g. Demirjian et al., 1973), form (e.g. Turner et al., 1991), size (e.g. Kieser, 1990), and wear (e.g. Gordon, 1988 or Unger et al., 2008) does exist at the species, population, and individual levels that can provide researchers with a wealth of data.

So what can teeth tell us? In short, different aspects of tooth growth and shape allow for the investigation of the basic age, sex, and ancestry aspects of the biological profile. As such, they can be good indicators of an individual's unique **life history**.[1] They are also excellent proxies for overall body growth and development. In this way, they are useful when attempting to interpret the life patterns of extinct species. Teeth can also provide insight into the behavior of both extinct and extant species through analysis of sexual dimorphism (which is strongly associated with the type of social organization in primates and other species), size and shape differences between species, and both macro- and microwear analysis. Additionally, the hard outer enamel surface is the strongest material produced by the body. This means that teeth (along with their associated "bony homes"—the maxilla and mandible), are the single most commonly found elements in the mammalian fossil record. For the same reasons, teeth and jaws are also more likely to be well preserved in various archaeological

---

[1] All bolded terms are defined in the glossary at the end of this volume.

and forensic contexts and consequently represent an excellent repository of information on the individuals from which they come.

At the species level, the shape and size of teeth as well as dental microwear can be useful in reconstructing broad dietary categories of different species. Due to the highly heritable nature of tooth form, the presence or absence of discrete traits and cusp patterns allows researchers to explore questions of **phylogeny** (the relatedness of different species) and **biological distance** (the evolutionary relationships between **populations** within humans, for example). Furthermore, the pace and pattern of tooth development can provide the information necessary to assess important species-level developmental and life history traits such as age at reproductive maturity, interbirth interval, and age at weaning.

At the population level, both distribution of tooth decay as well as micro- and macrowear can be used to learn more about the diet or activities of a group. Analysis of isotopes that become incorporated into teeth during their development can provide researchers with information about movement and location during life and potentially environmental conditions as well. Metric and nonmetric assessments of tooth crown morphology can help to distinguish between populations. Population health is often assessed through the study of dental pathologies including caries, periodontal disease, and enamel hypoplasia.

At the level of the individual, a variety of investigative methods exist that allow us to focus on the unique life history of a person. Age-at-death estimates can be informed by dental growth and tooth crown wear. Cementum annulations hold promise as yet another way to calculate age-at-death in adults (Obertová and Francken, 2009). Questions of ancestry and sex assessment can be explored through metric and nonmetric methods that describe tooth shape and size. Dental treatments (e.g., crowns, fillings, and other restorations) and **DNA** analysis may be helpful in establishing an individual identification. Tooth development errors such as **enamel hypoplasia** can illustrate periods of nutritional or dietary stress in an individual's early life when the teeth were still forming.

This chapter begins with an overview of dental anatomy including a description of metric and nonmetric methods for studying tooth size and shape. Next, a discussion of dental growth and development follows with a focus on the differences between available imaging techniques. Atypical dental growth and dental disease are then covered. This is followed by information on the relevance of molecular and isotopic studies to teeth. Finally, microwear analysis and its ability to provide insight into diet is presented. This chapter closes with an account of my own journey from initiation to implementation of a dental anthropology research project.

TEETH: A BRIEF INTRODUCTION

The following is a short overview of basic dental growth and anatomy. Those interested in a more in-depth understanding of the topic should consult *Dental Anthropology* by Simon Hillson (1996), which remains the most clear and concise text available for students of dental anthropology. Here, the fundamentals of tooth anatomy as it applies to humans will be reviewed along with a brief description of tooth developmental processes.

Like other primates, humans are **diphyodont,** meaning that we all have two sets of teeth during our lifetimes. First, the deciduous or primary teeth carry an individual through much of their childhood. The permanent teeth follow and are designed to fulfill masticatory requirements through the remainder of life. Humans are also **heterodonts**, which means that we have different types of teeth. Moving from the front to the back of the oral cavity, the four different types of teeth that we have include incisors, canines, premolars (or bicuspids), and molars (Figure 10.1).

Within the oral cavity, four quadrants are drawn from a line that runs anterioposteriorly along the sagittal plane between the central incisors. The tooth row runs posteriorly in a curved manner. Tooth surfaces closest to the midline, or facing more towards the front of the mouth within the curve of the dental arch are *mesial* while the more posterior surfaces facing away from the midline are *distal*. The surface facing the tongue is the *lingual* surface and the cheek side is the *buccal* surface (or *labial* when referring to the incisors). The chewing surface of the tooth crown is referred to as the *occlusal* surface (or *incisal* when referring to the incisors). The *cervical region* is where the crown meets the root, near what is called the *cementoenamel junction* (or CEJ), and the *apical region* is that nearest the bottom or apex of the root tip.

The four main components of a tooth as shown in Figure 10.2 are *enamel, dentin, cementum,* and *pulp*. Enamel is the outermost surface of the tooth crown. Dentin is the next layer, and in addition to forming the inner portion of the tooth crown, it makes up a large portion of the root of each tooth. The innermost layer of each tooth is the pulp chamber. Once the tooth is nearing full eruption, a layer of **cementum** begins to develop on the outside of the root. The portion of the jaws that the teeth sit in is called the *alveolus*. Teeth are held in place by periodontal ligaments that adhere to the cementum and the alveolus. The joint formed by this connection between the tooth and the alveolus is called a *gomphosis* and is relatively immovable.

In humans, the premolars and molars have separate cusps on their occlusal surfaces. The cusps on these teeth are separated by fissures or grooves that run between them. Premolars have a buccal cusp and a lingual cusp in keeping with the directional terminology presented above. Cusps in the molars are identified by their position on the tooth (i.e., mesiolingual, mesiobuccal, etc.), by numbers, and also by a naming system that derives from the ancestral tooth form (Figure 10.3).

Maxillary molars normally have four cusps, the three largest of which (mesiobuccal, mesiolingual, and distobuccal) form a somewhat raised triangle while the distolingual cusp (the hypocone) is often considerably smaller. In addition, the groove running between the distobuccal and mesiolingual cusps of the maxillary molars is known as the *crista obliqua*.

The first mandibular molars normally present with five cusps. In modern humans, the size of permanent molars tends to decrease from M1 (1st permanent molar) to M3 (3rd permanent

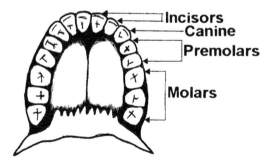

FIGURE 10.1 Tooth classes. From mesial to distal: incisors, canine, premolars, molars. Drawing by Lon Hunt.

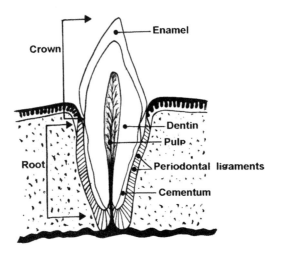

FIGURE 10.2　Cross-section of an incisor showing enamel, dentin, pulp, cementum, alveolus, and periodontal ligaments. Drawing by Lon Hunt.

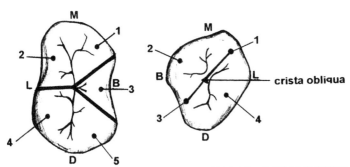

FIGURE 10.3　Molar morphology of the first mandibular molar (on left) and first maxillary molar (on right). M = mesial, D = distal, B = buccal, L = lingual. Cusps are labeled according to the standard numerical numbering system. Additional cusp naming systems include positional and ancestral terms. In this figure, the Y5 pattern and crista obliqua are also identified. Drawing by Lon Hunt.

Cusp #	Positional Term	Cusp Name	Cusp #	Positional Term	Cusp Name
1	Mesiobuccal	Protoconid	1	Mesiolingual	Protocone
2	Mesiolingual	Metaconid	2	Mesiobuccal	Paracone
3	Centrobuccal	Hypoconid	3	Distobuccal	Metacone
4	Distolingual	Entoconid	4	Distolingual	Hypocone
5	Distobuccal	Hypoconulid			

molar), and so frequently M2 (2nd permanent molar) and M3 display fewer cusps. The pattern of grooves between the M1 molar cusps approximates a shape in the form of the letter "Y" that opens to the distobuccal cusp and is known as the **Y5 pattern**, which is shared by all hominoids (apes and humans) (Figure 10.3). Variations of this characteristic pattern include both the +5 and X5 pattern where the slight shifting of cusps leads to a slightly different alignment of the grooves between them. Although less frequent, addition or subtraction of M1 cusps can lead to variants such as the +4 or Y6 pattern.

Among living primates, many different *dental formulae* exist. The dental formula is a notation for the number of different types of teeth in each quadrant in the mouth. Different taxa (i.e., taxonomic categories) within the order Primates have different numbers of teeth in the maxilla and mandible and these numbers also differ between the primary and permanent dentitions within species. Therefore, the notation appears as three or four numbers over three or four numbers, for the primary (deciduous) and permanent dentitions of the maxilla and mandible, respectively. The living primates have descended from a distant mammalian ancestor that had a permanent dental formula of $\frac{3143}{3143}$. This means that this ancestor had 3 incisors, 1 canine, 4 premolars, and 3 molars per quadrant in their permanent dentition.

In order to compare "apples to apples" when discussing dental evolution, it is important to make sure that like teeth are being compared with like teeth even if your study only involves modern human dental material. Through the general trend of dental reduction in the primate fossil record, it is clear to see that the third incisor and the first two premolars have been lost over the course of primate evolution in the catarrhines (the taxon consisting of Old World monkeys, apes, humans, and their ancestors). Thus, in the catarrhine primates, the teeth are numbered as I1 (central incisor), I2 (lateral incisor), C (canine), P3 (first premolar), P4 (second premolar), M1 (first molar), M2 (second molar), M3 (third molar) to reflect the loss of the first two premolars from a distant primate ancestor.

The human primary dental formula is $\frac{212}{212}$ while the human permanent dental formula is $\frac{2123}{2123}$. This means that humans have 2 incisors, 1 canine, and 2 molars per quadrant in their primary dentition, and 2 incisors, 1 canine, 2 premolars, and 3 molars in their permanent dentition.

TOOTH SIZE AND SHAPE

Descriptions of tooth form involve both measurements of the size and shape of the tooth and its features as well as the appearance or absence of various traits. Because the tooth roots are embedded in the maxilla and mandible during life, population and individual variation in tooth crowns is the most well-documented aspect of tooth form although there is certainly valuable variation to be studied in the tooth roots as well. For detailed descriptions of tooth crown and root traits and their variation see Scott and Turner's *The Anthropology of Modern Human Teeth: Dental Morphology and its Variation in Recent Human Populations* (1997).

Odontometrics

Measurements of the crown are frequently used to characterize size but can also be used to construct indices that describe the shape of the tooth. The most commonly reported tooth measurements are the mesiodistal and buccolingual distances of the tooth crown, which represent the maximum length and breadth of the tooth crown, respectively (Table 10.1). In humans, incisors are longer mesiodistally than buccolingually, canines tend to have nearly equal values, and premolars and maxillary molars are larger in the buccolingual dimension. Human mandibular molars are longer mesiodistally than they are wide buccolingually. The conventional practice is to record and report measurements to the nearest 0.1 mm using sliding dental calipers.

These basic measurements can then be used to calculate indices that are useful in describing the overall shape and proportions of a given tooth (Table 10.1). For example,

TABLE 10.1 Standard Dental Metric Measurements and Crown Indices after Hillson (1996) and Kieser (1990)

Metric/Index	Measurement
Mesiodistal (*length*)	Maximum crown diameter in the M-D direction. To be taken parallel to the buccal/labial surfaces.
Buccolingual (*breadth*)	Maximum crown diameter in the B-L direction. To be taken parallel to the mesial/distal surfaces.
Crown module	(mesiodistal diameter + buccolingual diameter)/2
Robustness index	mesiodistal diameter × buccolingual diameter
Summary tooth size	(summed robustness indices for all tooth classes)/(# of tooth classes)

the crown index is the buccolingual length divided by the mesiodistal length, multiplied by 100. Teeth that are wider than they are long have a value above 100 whereas teeth that are longer than they are wide have an index below 100. Other commonly used indices are the **crown module,** which gives an average of the size of a crown within a given tooth class; the **robustness index,** which is essentially the area of the crown; and the **summary tooth size,** which calculates the overall size of the dentition given the tooth classes included. A thorough reference on dental metrics that includes data to explore is *Human Adult Odontometrics* (Kieser, 1990). Within this volume, Kieser has compiled published mean and standard deviation data for mesiodistal and buccolingual measurements on populations worldwide.

As mentioned above, humans have characteristic tooth shapes that are useful in separating them from other species. Indeed, these same basic measurements are useful in discriminating into broad populations as well. Populations across the globe show differences in crown sizes, with Aboriginal Australians having the largest teeth overall and Western Eurasians having some of the smallest. Tooth shape, as measured by the crown index, also differs among human populations, with Polynesian and Western Eurasian groups having teeth with narrower mesiodistal widths than their Native American and Northeast Asian counterparts (Hanihara and Ishida, 2005).

Biological sex assessment from the teeth relies on the general trend of males having larger teeth than females (within populations). As with other primates, the canine remains the most dimorphic tooth in the human dentition. Just as adult bones are more sexually dimorphic than juvenile bones, permanent teeth are more dimorphic than are the primary teeth and so it follows that sex assessment from permanent teeth is more reliable than that from their primary predecessors. DeVito and Saunders (1990) achieved sex estimation accuracy rates of 75–90% from the deciduous tooth size, whereas Hassett (2011) achieved rates of 94% for sex discrimination from the adult canine dimensions.

It is important to note that standards for sexual differences in tooth size are subject to the same issues of overlapping distribution between the sexes as skeletal measurements. There is no clear cutoff for identifying male versus female dentition. While the trend exists for male teeth to be larger than female teeth, there are always exceptions to the rule as a part of the normal range of human variation. Therefore, dental measures should be considered in addition to as many other characteristics as possible in order to ensure the highest accuracy in sex estimation. Finally, population differences in the degree of tooth size dimorphism also exist, making it important to find a suitable reference sample for comparison and evaluation (Kieser, 1990; Hanihara and Ishida, 2005). See Moore [Chapter 4], this volume, for a more detailed investigation of sex estimation from the dentition.

Nonmetric Dental Traits

Nonmetric dental traits are features of dental morphology that show variation in their expression both within and between populations. One of the earliest published nonmetric traits was the shovel-shaped incisor described by Hrdlička (1920), who suggested a three-grade system for describing expression of the trait. This trait presents as an incisor with accessory ridges on both the mesiolingual and distolingual edges of the tooth, so that it looks similar to a shovel. As Hillson (1996) mentions, just as metric traits present along a continuum, so do nonmetric traits. However, due to difficulties in obtaining consistent measurements, the continuum of nonmetric traits is often best assessed on a graded basis.

The most widely used set of trait assessment standards to document such traits was developed by the Arizona State University Dental Anthropology Laboratory. The Arizona State University Dental Anthropology System (ASUDAS) consists of a series of plaques displaying the various grades of each defined trait made from dental casts as well as a manuscript that describes the interpretation and grading of such traits. The system describes the form of some 27 dental traits (Turner et al., 1991).

One such trait is the famous **Carabelli's trait**. First described in 1842 by Georg Carabelli, the trait ranges from a small groove or pit to a fully developed additional cusp. It appears on the mesiolingual surface of the first maxillary molar and occasionally on the second maxillary molar. As with other nonmetric dental traits, Carabelli's trait occurs on a continuum from slight to marked expression. This is an excellent example of the need for an additional scoring system to metric analysis as the form and nature of traits change with the degree of expression. This transformation in the form of a trait due to degree of expression eschews more traditional measuring techniques and therefore its classification is more amenable to the stage-based scoring technique used in the ASUDAS.

Certain nonmetric traits have gained a solid foothold within biological anthropology as characteristic of certain populations. For instance, the shovel-shaped incisor is commonly associated with Asian and Native American populations and Carabelli's trait is often used as evidence of European ancestry, and examples of these generalizations will be found in most introductory biological anthropology textbooks. While these are rather accurate characterizations due to the high prevalence of the individual traits in the given populations, as a student of skeletal biology it is wise to keep in mind that no single trait defines a population. In addition to seeking out further evidence for any assessment of the biological profile in the dentition through metric analysis, it is also best to consider the spectrum of nonmetric traits. Population affinity can be more confidently assessed using a suite of characteristics as different populations express different combinations of traits.[2] Finally, it is always best

---

[2]See DiGangi and Hefner (Chapter 5), this volume, for more information about population variation and the shovel-shaped incisor trait and Cabana et al. (Chapter 16), this volume, for a discussion of genetic trait distribution.

practice to combine information from the dentition with that available in the skeletal remains: use every element of the skeleton that is available to you.

TOOTH DEVELOPMENT AND WEAR

Studies of dental development include several different methods, each useful for different research questions. In order to describe the unique developmental patterns of primate species, researchers have studied dental emergence patterns, rate of growth of the first permanent molar, enamel secretion rates, and even the underlying dentinoenamel junction. To focus specifically on modern humans, development of the teeth is one of the most accurate ways to estimate age-at-death in subadults and dental wear is often useful in adult age assessment.

Emergence Patterns

The study of dental emergence patterns is perhaps of most interest to those studying primate and hominin dental evolution because the pattern differences between species indicate different paces of life, or life histories. However, the pattern of emergence of the teeth is also of use to those focused on modern human skeletal biology. It is useful to first point out the difference between *emergence* and *eruption*. Emergence is a single moment in the movement of the tooth when it breaks through either the gingiva or the alveolar bone. However, eruption is the entire process of tooth movement as it grows and moves through the jaw and soft tissues of the oral cavity.

The actual sequence of how teeth emerge into the oral cavity differs between species in a way that reflects their overall life history. Species that develop quickly tend to exhibit relatively early emergence of their permanent post-canine teeth while the emergence of the post-canine dentition tends to occur later in the overall sequence for longer lived species (such as humans) (Box 10.1). Because the order of emergence of the teeth is tied to both (1) *ecological independence* (Can the juvenile successfully ingest the food it needs to once it is weaned?) and (2) *longevity* (How long can these primary teeth hold up?) these sequences are under selection[3] for their ability to enable their carrier to process the food necessary to sustain life. Emergence sequences are also heritable, which preserves a genetic component to their expression; however, the selective effect mentioned above results in variation both within and between species.

In modern humans, the general sequence of emergence of the permanent teeth is M1 → I1 → I2 → P3 → C → P4 → M2 → M3. This reflects later emergence of the permanent molars due to an extended postnatal life. As a point of comparison, consider the relatively short-lived *Macaca nemestrina* (pigtailed macaque) where the sequence is generally M1 → I1 → I2 → M2 → P3 → P4 → C → M3. Due to the extreme sexual dimorphism in the canine of the pigtailed macaque, there is a distinct difference in the emergence sequence between males and females because of later canine placement in the sequence in males (Smith, 1994).

---

[3]See definition and explanation of **natural selection** in Cabana et al. (Chapter 16), this volume.

BOX 10.1

EMERGENCE PATTERNS OF A FAST GROWING
MAMMAL (TREE SHREW) AND A SLOW GROWING
MAMMAL (HUMAN)

In both tree shrews and humans, the deciduous teeth (iimm) emerge prior to the permanent teeth (I1, I2, M1, M2, M3). However, in the tree shrew all of the permanent molars emerge before the permanent incisors. In humans, the incisors emerge much earlier in the overall sequence. After Smith (1994).

Rapidly growing animal: **Tree shrew**

wave 1:	iimm	M1 M2 M3
wave 2:		I1 I2

Slowly growing animal: **Human**

wave 1:	iimm	M1 M2 M3
wave 2:		← I1 I2

Sequence Polymorphisms

Given the general sequence of emergence of human teeth presented above, there are characteristic differences in the emergence sequences between human populations, which were described early on by Schultz (1940) and Garn and colleagues (Garn et al., 1962; Garn and Lewis, 1963). The differences in emergence sequences are called **sequence polymorphisms** and are typically recognized in the written sequence by brackets surrounding the teeth that change order in ≥15% of individuals examined within a species. The modern human sequence is best described as [M1 I1] I2 [P3 C P4 M2] M3, indicating the tendency for M1 and I1 to reverse their emergence sequence and for the canine to alter the posterior emergence sequence (it may appear before P3 or after P4 and in extreme cases, after M2).

Smith and Garn (1987) demonstrated that there are differences in specific sequence polymorphisms between modern human groups. Utilizing data obtained from the Ten-State Nutrition Survey[4] they were able to discern significant differences between the emergence sequence polymorphisms present in female and male, and Black and White North Americans (as defined by the categories used in the study) (Smith and Garn, 1987). This sample represents one of the few large enough for the establishment of population standards of emergence sequence polymorphisms, none of which has been studied in this manner. We do not know, for example, what the common sequence polymorphisms are for the majority of human populations. Just as having specific population standards is necessary for accurate analysis of skeletal remains, the study of dental samples that include a large number of subadults

---

[4]The Ten-State Nutrition Survey was a federally funded study in the United States conducted between 1968 and 1970. Researchers collected anthropometric and dental growth data as well as clinical and nutritional status of low-income children in ten states from various regions of the United States. (Ten-State Nutrition Survey 1968–1970, 1972).

from different populations is crucial to expanding our knowledge and accuracy of interpretation of sequence polymorphisms. In addition to the benefits that this information would provide to the study of modern human populations, it would give us greater insight into the differences observed in fossil hominins.

VISUALIZING TOOTH GROWTH

Radiographic Methods

The study of radiographs is the most common method used for the development of population standards of dental growth. Images are relatively inexpensive and less time consuming to obtain in comparison with **computed tomographic (CT)** images, and histological and gross methods. It follows that inclusion of a higher number of individuals is usually possible. The cost of high-resolution digital radiographs is lower than that of CT scans and a number of truly portable machines are available commercially.

In addition to portable radiographs, there are table-style veterinary X-ray units with stationary beams (which are actually quite large and cumbersome when considering a project that involves collecting images at several sites). Additionally, handheld dental X-ray systems are available that are small enough to fit into a case the size of a carry-on style suitcase. The handheld models are perfectly suited for one who is interested in obtaining dental X-rays on skeletal specimens. This method is nondestructive, thus making it suitable for use in studies of museum collections, delicate specimens, and fossils. However, embedded matrix or sediment in fossil or archaeological specimens can sometimes prevent full visualization of the desired features. In these cases, other methods that can better distinguish between these materials must be sought out as discussed below (Conroy and Vannier, 1987).

One drawback is that radiographic analysis consistently underestimates the degree of **calcification** of teeth when compared with gross or histological methods (Simpson and Kunos, 1998). Calcification is the deposition of hydroxyapatite mineral that makes up a large portion of enamel and dentin. We look at the degree of calcification to determine the state of development of the root and crown. However, it is still a practical method because it allows for a relatively inexpensive and less time-consuming way to obtain greater amounts of data than would be possible through other analytical methods. Furthermore, available population standards are almost entirely based on the radiographic appearance of calcification and they present a clear and functional account of the calcification that can be useful in intra- and inter-population comparisons. As such, it remains the standard for producing population standards of dental development.

Analysis of Dental Development

Generally speaking, two different methods exist for the analysis of dental development via X-ray imaging: the **atlas approach** and the **dental age approach**. First, the atlas approach utilizes a set of developmental markers with associated ages as a basis for comparison with the individual. The individual is assigned a developmental age depending on where it fits most appropriately based on the markers in the predetermined model. Perhaps the most widely recognized atlas of human dental development is that of Schour and Massler

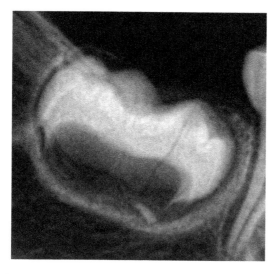

FIGURE 10.4 Radiograph of a chimpanzee permanent first mandibular molar at stage 4—crown completion to the cementoenamel junction. Small spicules of root growth are visible.

(1941). Reproduced in various forms in countless publications, this was one of the earlier examples of an illustrated publication depicting the appearance of the developing teeth for reference by dental clinicians. This reference chronicles the development of the human dentition from the early fetal stage through maturity and includes both the primary and permanent teeth. Although the population studied is not mentioned in the paper, AlQahtani and colleagues (2010) point out that Smith (1991) mentions the population as potentially being the same that appears in the earlier work of Logan and Kronfeld (1933).[5]

The second method, the dental age approach, assigns numbers to arbitrary stages of tooth development, indicating the degree of completion of the crown and root. With this method, the development of each tooth is ranked on a scale with each category representing a certain fraction of the crown or root growth. Teeth that are not visible radiographically are given a score of zero. Frequently, the stages represent roughly one-third of crown or root growth or refer to the proportion of the crown and root (e.g., "Root growth is less than crown height").

As an illustration, Figure 10.4 shows a digital X-ray of a developing mandibular molar in a chimpanzee at a stage of 4—crown completion—with small spicules of root formation present. The total amount of calcification that has taken place for each individual is then represented by the total of the numbers assigned to all teeth. This method was first proposed by Demirjian and colleagues (1973), and has been utilized in various forms by several authors (e.g., Sirianni and Swindler, 1985; Dean, 1987; Conroy and Mahoney, 1991; Simpson et al., 1991; Kuykendall, 1996; Simpson and Kunos, 1998).

[5]Interestingly, the population involved in the Schour and Massler atlas is somewhat of a mystery. It is not revealed in the original publication and so at this time, the primary reference for the population used is Smith's (1991) historical account.

Although they are useful for obtaining developmental standards in extant populations, assessments based on the "dental age" method are less useful on fragmentary specimens, as they require information on the entire dentition in order to make comparisons. A combination of the atlas method and the dental age approach is necessary for analyses of remains where more than one tooth is present and the teeth are in different stages of eruption. Analysis of individual teeth must rely largely on histological methods as described below.

An important contribution was recently made by AlQahtani and colleagues, who provided an updated atlas based on the study of over 500 individuals from a mixed sample including historic and modern Europeans as well as Bangladeshi immigrants to Great Britain. In addition to an atlas, they include useful information on alveolar emergence of both the primary and permanent teeth (AlQahtani et al., 2010).

Histology

Histological techniques are extremely informative in terms of tooth growth and development. Similar to the way that the growth rings of a tree record information about the tree's age and environmental conditions, teeth preserve a record of their development. Although they are not always reflected in the overall shape of the tooth, stresses affecting the individual during development of the teeth can be recorded in the microscopic structure of a tooth. Furthermore, if the tooth was still growing at the time of death, age assessment of the individual is possible. Other "stressful" occurrences in an individual's life such as birth or illness also produce disruptions in the developing enamel that are visible micro- or macroscopically.

It has long been assumed that the fine **cross striations** (or discontinuities in the enamel structure), visible in histological sections of teeth, are indicative of the daily amount of enamel secretion by **ameloblast** cells as they appear to divide **enamel prisms** (the "rod" of enamel that the ameloblast has formed). These fine striations are in turn separated into groups by brown **striae of Retzius**, which manifest on the surface of the tooth as **perikymata** (wave-like ridges) of the tooth crown. These features are all visible in Figure 10.5. In the dentin, similar lines are formed called Andresen lines that can be viewed internally. Like the perikymata in the enamel, these manifest on the root surface as **periradicular bands.**

The number of cross striae (representing daily incremental lines) between striae of Retzius (representing longer period features) varies among the primates, both within and between species from counts as few as 4−5 cross striations to as many as 10−12 (Hillson, 1996). In humans, the cross striae count ranges between 8 and 10. This means that if you were to count up the number of perikymata and periradicular bands on the outside of a *growing* tooth and then multiply that number by an average of the daily cross striation count (average of 9 in humans), you would arrive at a reasonably accurate estimate of the age-at-death of a subadult individual. Note that this method would not work in older subadults and adults with fully formed teeth.

When a stressful event such as illness or a period of malnutrition occurs during development, the event manifests as an **accentuated line.** This is because at the time of an insult, although the tooth continues to form, ameloblasts reduce their enamel secretion due to the stress on the individual. This leads to a defect. A classic example of an accentuated line is the "neonatal line" that indicates the time surrounding birth. Prolonged insults can manifest on the surface of the tooth as enamel hypoplasia. Analysis of these types of defects can have

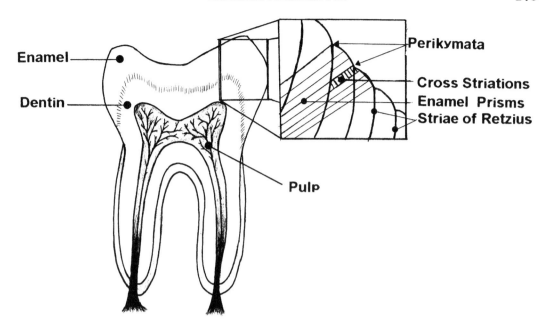

FIGURE 10.5 Cross-section of a molar with histologically visible structures of the enamel identified. Drawing by Lon Hunt.

relevance to understanding environmental pressures on individuals and populations at the time that teeth were forming.

Cross striae and striae of Retzius have a **circadian periodicity** (they occur at regular intervals) and the extension of this is that surface perikymata could be used to calculate the age of individuals. Bromage (1991) examined histological sections of maxillary first molars taken from known-age neonatal pigtailed macaques (*Macaca nemestrina*), to test this periodicity.

Prenatally, the macaques had been administered three different fluorescent bone labeling substances at two-week intervals both through their mother's bloodstream and directly into their hard tissues. These bone-labeling substances were taken up into the hard tissues and provided researchers with a clear way to measure bone and tooth growth within the specific time frame. Following sacrifice,[6] the teeth were removed, processed, and sectioned. As the absolute time between administrations of the dyes was known, disruption of the enamel formation could be compared with the appearance of the dyes (Bromage, 1991).

The assumption of circadian periodicity was confirmed by matching up the number of prisms between the labeled sections with the time of dye administration. In a series of papers including a greater number of observations, Smith and colleagues extended the implications of Bromage's paper by revealing additional features that seem to share a circadian periodicity with the striae (Smith, 2006, 2008; Smith et al., 2006).

Due to the record of growth and life history in the developing tooth, histological analysis of teeth can provide a remarkable longitudinal record of an individual's growth over the

[6]See DiGangi and Moore (Chapter 2), this volume, for a discussion of ethical concerns when doing research on humans or animals.

course of development. This has important implications for both paleoanthropology and forensic applications (Dean et al., 1993). See Trammell and Kroman (Chapter 13), this volume, for more information about dental and bone histology.

Cementum Annulation

Dental cementum is a living tissue that continues to grow throughout life. It is the calcified material that covers the outside of the tooth root, and provides the attachment site for the periodontal ligaments which hold the tooth to the alveolar bone within the socket. When looking at a horizontal slice through a tooth root, one can observe the layer of cementum covering the root. Under a microscope, alternating light and dark bands are visible. Because of the assumed annual periodicity of cementum annulations, counts of the naturally alternating light and dark bands that are characteristic of dental cementum formation have been used for estimating age-at-death in various animals, though the etiology is unclear (Charles et al., 1986; Hillson, 1996).

As discussed previously in this chapter and elsewhere in this volume, available skeletal and dental aging techniques are much more accurate on subadults as the processes that govern development are under rather strict genetic control (more so for teeth than the skeleton). The degenerative changes that are used to estimate age in adult skeletal and dental remains are inherently more variable due to environmental, individual lifestyle, and genetic differences that affect the various degenerative processes. Once tooth growth is completed, age estimations using the teeth must be based on dental wear. However, cementum annulation is a process that continues throughout life and thus holds great promise as a way to obtain age-at-death estimates in adults.

Age estimates using cementum annulation are made by adding the average age of emergence of the tooth to the number of dark and light line pairs counted because (1) cementum growth begins once the tooth is nearing functional occlusion and (2) it is assumed that each count of a light and dark band roughly equals one year of growth. Although the exact mechanism for formation of cementum annulations is still unclear, it appears that seasonal variation plays a large part in the degree of expression (Charles et al., 1986).

A primary challenge in the use of cementum annulations is the replicability of line counts, i.e., intraobserver and interobserver error. Part of the methodological complexity is in the difficulty inherent in reliably obtaining quality, readable slices for analysis in addition to the added step of having to slice the tooth (and thus damage it). Some authors report considerable difficulty in obtaining readable slices (Jankauskas et al., 2001; Renz and Radlanski, 2006). Furthermore, sections taken from different areas of a single tooth and sections taken from different teeth within the same individual can produce different counts. There is also no clear consensus on which tooth or portion of the root should be used to obtain the most accurate count (Renz and Radlanski, 2006). As pointed out by Renz and Radlanski (2006), if different teeth or even different portions of teeth display incongruous counts then the method would be less than desirable as a reliable indicator of age.

Once a readable slice is obtained, the thickness of a slice can also impede the ability of researchers to take reliable counts due to the superimposition of lower layers. Both Charles and colleagues (1986) and Condon and colleagues (1986) suggest demineralization of the tooth in order to obtain thinner slices to avoid this issue. They report obtaining significantly more reliable count results with 7 μm slices than with nondemineralized 80 μm slices (Charles et al., 1986; Condon et al., 1986). Despite these findings, many researchers opt instead for nondemineralized slices with a thickness between 50 and 100 μm (Wittwer-Backofen et al., 2004; Maat et al., 2006; Meinl et al., 2008). This is likely due at least in part to the increased time and cost involved in preparing the demineralized slices.

One further consideration is that similar to other aging techniques available for the skeleton, the accuracy of age estimations based on cementum annulation decreases as chronological age increases (Stein and Corcoran, 1994). Obertová and Francken (2009) tested this method on a sample of 116 teeth from 65 individuals. The method worked relatively well for individuals under the age of 40, but underestimated the ages of those individuals over 40 years. Again, as the processes governing the development of the annulations are poorly understood, it is hard to determine exactly what factors contribute to this age-related decline in accuracy. Does it have to do with diet? Perhaps age-related loss of other teeth and subsequent changes in jaw architecture and biomechanics? Both of these research questions need to be addressed. Understanding the exact nature of the alternating dark and light bands, the periodicity of the bands, and the age-related change in their expression will enable the use of cementum annulations with greater confidence. This is an interesting area of research with many questions awaiting answers.

Computed Tomography

The high-resolution images obtainable by computed tomography (CT) provide promise for the study of dental tissues. There is a discrepancy between appearance of calcification in X-rays and CT scans, making it potentially difficult to reconcile the population standards of extant primates obtained via radiographic analysis with the stunning CT images of fossilized, mummified, or otherwise preserved remains. All the same, both CT and microtomography (μCT) present researchers with exciting ways to analyze dental growth and tooth form.

Conroy and Vannier (1987) performed a series of scans on the Taung child (a juvenile *Australopithecus africanus* discovered in South Africa, dated to ~ 2.5 million years ago) in order to more clearly visualize the developing dentition and sinuses and more accurately characterize its development. This imaging technique enabled researchers to distinguish between the teeth and embedded matrix to show that the dental development evidenced in this specimen was not nearly as human-like has had been previously put forth by others (Dart, 1925; Conroy and Vannier, 1987).

Less than a year later, Conroy used CT analysis to examine the developing dentition of another hominin specimen, SK61, a juvenile *Paranthropus robustus*, whose dentition had been central to the discussion of whether robust australopithecines presented with a more human or more ape-like developmental pace (Conroy, 1988). Because the developing teeth still embedded in the jaws were not clearly visible in previous radiographic analyses, previous assessments of the specimen had either incorrectly identified the incisors in occlusion as the permanent incisors, or underestimated the stage of development of the I1 (Broom and Robinson, 1951; Dean, 1985).

This created an interesting situation that would indicate that *P. robustus* had a more human-like developmental schedule involving more advanced incisor development for the M1 stage relative to the condition in both apes and gracile australopithecines. In humans,

M1 and I1 emerge in a very short time frame, while in the apes and australopithecines I1 emerges roughly 2—2.5 years after M1 (Dean and Wood, 1981). The increased clarity of the CT images obtained in Conroy's study made it possible to confirm that in this specimen, the permanent central incisors were still developing and had just begun root growth, which is a lesser stage of development than would be expected if the specimen in question was on a modern human developmental trajectory.

It has been demonstrated that scoring standards developed for scoring traditional X-rays can be adapted for use with CT images of the developing dentition (Coquerelle et al., 2010). However, CT scanning remains a costly method that is often used for analysis of single specimens rather than the creation of population standards. For example, CT has been used to study dental wear and pathology in mummies (Melcher et al., 1997; Cesarani et al., 2003) although standardization of interpretive methods is yet to be done (Chhem, 2006). Still, others working with mummies have continued to use traditional dental or cephalometric X-ray imaging for the interpretation of dental growth and wear even when using CT to study the rest of the body (Previgliano et al., 2003; Kieser et al., 2004). In a forensic context, CT has been shown to be useful in aging fetuses and neonates by both dental and skeletal development (Sakurai et al., 2012).

In addition to the benefit of being able to distinguish between different materials that may be lodged in the dental and facial area, the smaller pixels of three-dimensional (3-D) microtomographic scans are able to distinguish between different portions of the tooth (enamel, dentin, pulp chamber) and to present, store, and analyze images in three dimensions. In this manner, the study of the topography of crown and root morphology and the enamel—dentin junction can progress beyond two-dimensional analyses at different sections along the tooth crown. Discrete metric analysis is also aided by the digital environment in which modern CT images are processed and viewed with the availability of 3-D landmark and volume analysis (Olejniczak et al., 2007). For more information on the applications of CT imaging, see Moore (Chapter 14), this volume.

Micro-CT

More recently, a special type of microtomography called *phase-contrast X-ray synchrotron* has been employed by dental anthropologists. This method is unique in that it allows the study of incremental tooth growth with exceptional clarity, enabling researchers to view and analyze tooth microstructure. Previously, determining such important developmental markers such as Retzius line periodicity would have required traditional, destructive histological techniques, as discussed earlier. Recent developments and research at the European Synchrotron Radiation Facility in Grenoble, France have provided researchers with a new way to assess such structures in precious fossil material without the need for sectioning. See Tafforeau and Smith (2008) for a thorough summary of the recent developments in this area.

Imaging Methods as Research Tools

In terms of studying dental development and teeth in general, consider the differences between traditional dental X-ray, dental histology, and CT. Understanding the benefits and limitations of different methods of analysis such as this is important when designing a study, particularly when it involves large numbers of specimens (Table 10.2).

TABLE 10.2 Basic Considerations When Choosing an Imaging Technique for Research in Dental Anthropology

Imaging Technique	Advantages	Disadvantages	Possible Uses
Dental X-ray	Low cost; rapid results; population standards available for comparison; nondestructive	Lower resolution than other methods, cannot see incremental development	Creation of population growth standards; individual ID; age-at-death estimation of individuals
CT and μCT	Possibility of 3-D model; with μCT, observation of enamel and dentin formation times; nondestructive	Relatively high cost; transport of specimens usually necessary	Study of individuals or small samples; morphology and dental development; with μCT—chronology of incremental development
Histology	Detailed study of enamel and dentin formation; most precise age-at-death estimation if teeth are still growing	Relatively high financial and time investment; destructive	Study of individuals or small samples; assessment of crown formation times, age-at- death, tooth mineralization rates

Dental X-ray is a cost-effective, portable, rapid method that allows for the inclusion of a large sample. In contrast, histological techniques, in addition to being destructive, require a much longer time investment, which translates into increased costs and smaller sample sizes. However, histological study can provide a level of detail that is unobtainable with traditional X-ray by actually examining the daily deposition of enamel and dentin and describing the timing of certain events in the development of the tooth. Likewise, CT analysis is cost prohibitive, which by extension limits the total possible sample size, but it allows for the study of teeth and adjacent structures in three dimensions.

DENTAL PATHOLOGY

Caries

Dental caries (a.k.a. "cavities") is caused by bacteria and their interaction with dietary carbohydrates. The bacteria produce acids that progressively demineralize the enamel and/or dentin, resulting in pits and decay in the teeth (Hillson, 1996). Initially, caries manifests as a microscopic white or brown speck on the surface of the tooth that grows as infection progresses. Once the infection grows, the white or brown area can be observed macroscopically and may also be observed in dental X-rays (X-ray visualization is possible most often only after the caries is detectable on the tooth surface).

Because of the link between consumption of carbohydrates and appearance of caries, it stands to reason that populations that consume increased levels of carbohydrates would present with more caries. Indeed, both historical (Silverstone et al., 1981) and prehistoric populations (Larsen et al., 1991) show this pattern. In particular, a dramatic increase in population levels of dental caries appears to have accompanied the transition to agriculture worldwide (e.g., see papers in Cohen and Armelagos, 1984). For a thorough review of the study of dental caries in archaeological material, see Larsen and colleagues (1991).

Hillson (2000) notes the differences in caries rates evident between populations that follow a low-carbohydrate diet (i.e., hunter-gatherer populations such as the !Kung Bushmen) and those that ingest greater amounts of carbohydrates. In the first group, caries are limited mainly to older adults with chipped or greatly worn teeth and are sparse in younger individuals. By extension, these distribution patterns can be applied to archaeological populations. Population differences in age distribution, missing teeth (which may be evidence of previous caries that necessitated extraction), and diagnostic error along with a host of other methodological issues accompany the recording of caries in a population. As such, Hillson (2001) recommends comparisons that are specific to tooth type, sex, age, and caries expression in order to accurately characterize caries rate in a given population.

Periodontitis

Dental plaque is a substance that consists of bacteria enmeshed in a biofilm that covers the surface of the teeth. Accumulation of dental plaque can lead to gingivitis (inflammation of the gums and soft tissues in the oral cavity) and also periodontitis. Early stages of infection of this sort are limited to inflammation of the oral soft tissues (gingivitis) and do not leave traces in the bone. With advanced cases that progress to periodontitis, the periodontal ligaments and alveolus become involved and it is at this point that the disease can be observed in skeletal remains.

Generally, the infection progresses into the gomphosis of the tooth and affects the periodontal ligaments holding the tooth in place. The resulting inflammation, accumulation of plaque, and loss of periodontal attachment result in alveolar bone resorption and loss (Hillson, 2000). This loss is most often found in the molars and ultimately presents as a recession of the alveolus and exposure of the root. The surface of the alveolus may present as porotic and may extend beyond a single tooth. Affected teeth may be loose in their sockets due to the bone resorption and loss of periodontal ligaments. Standards for the recording of periodontal disease can be found in Hildebolt and Molnar (1991).

Unlike caries, there appears to be a significant genetic component to the susceptibility to periodontal disease (Corey et al., 1993; Michalowicz et al., 2000). Michalowicz and colleagues (2000) estimate a heritability rate of 50% based on their study of twins. This indicates that earlier studies that had reported variation in prevalence between populations attributed to hygiene differences (Loe et al., 1992) may have overlooked the underlying genetic predisposition to periodontal disease.

Enamel Hypoplasia

Although the development of teeth is under tight genetic constraints and they are generally less susceptible to environmental insults than other elements of the skeleton, episodes of illness or malnutrition during the development of teeth can leave their mark. These episodes manifest in the enamel of the tooth as enamel defects or hypoplasias and result from stress-induced cessation of ameloblast activity (Duray, 1996). Enamel hypoplasias consist of deficiencies in enamel thickness, and this ranges from a single pit to entirely missing enamel (Goodman and Rose, 1991). These defects are easily detected in teeth, with linear enamel hypoplasia (LEH), represented by one or more transverse lines or grooves in the enamel surface, being the most common type seen.

While LEH is **nonspecific**[7] (meaning that the actual source of stress is unknown), it is recognized that it represents a serious and prolonged stress episode usually due to metabolic stress of some sort (Rose et al., 1985). For example, animal research has shown that anything disrupting growth such as disease or hormonal imbalance could lead to defects (Goodman and Rose, 1991). Further, the actual location of defects on the crown reflects how complete the crown was at the time of the stress episode (Lukacs, 1989). Therefore this allows the estimation of the age at which the insult occurred, given knowledge of dental development.

There also appears to be a general trend towards an increase in the development of defects around the time of weaning[8] according to studies of both contemporary and prehistoric populations (e.g., Cassidy, 1980; Schultz et al., 1998). In addition, it is clear that enamel hypoplasia frequency increased with the advent of agriculture, suggesting that stress episodes were not uncommon for these populations (e.g., see papers in Cohen and Armelagos, 1984).

Because of the relationship with metabolic stress episodes, enamel hypoplasia is an especially useful tool when examining population histories. Combining this indicator with other nonspecific indicators of stress (see Smith [Chapter 7], this volume) has the potential to reveal information specific to individual and population health in the past. Further, LEH (as well as caries) may be a clue in modern contexts with identifying skeletal remains in terms of indicating a possible population for the decedent, given that LEH would not be expected in individuals who had sufficient access to resources as children (good nutrition, medical care, etc.) (e.g., see Birkby et al., 2008).

TEETH AND GENETIC MATERIAL

DNA analysis involving the teeth is most often associated with forensic investigations to identify human remains. As with other parts of the body, genetic material is present in teeth. Fortunately, due to the strength of enamel and dentin capsule, and the location of the teeth within the oral cavity in a relatively protected space, DNA sampling from teeth has the potential to produce results when other areas of the skeleton cannot. As with other skeletal elements, degradation of the DNA in teeth can be accelerated due to exposure to high temperatures, extreme pH, water, and radiation. Fortunately, teeth are less susceptible to these elements than is the rest of the skeleton and therefore represent a great place to look for reliable DNA samples.

[7]See Smith (Chapter 7), this volume, for discussion of other nonspecific stress markers affecting the skeleton.

[8]See Smith (Chapter 7), this volume, for a discussion of the risks to health associated with weaning.

When preparing to extract DNA from teeth or to present materials to a lab for analysis (refer to Cabana et al. [Chapter 16], this volume, for information on sampling techniques), the molars are the best teeth to begin with due to their size (more material to sample) and relatively protected location within the oral cavity. Standard practice holds that harvesting DNA from the teeth is most fruitful from the dentin and dental pulp within the pulp chamber (Herschaft et al., 2007). As this area is the most protected from the outside world, contamination is less likely and the material is most often undisturbed. Barring the presence of dental pulp, the next best places to harvest from are the dentin and cementum (Herschaft et al., 2007). However, a recent study by Adler and colleagues (2011) found that the **mtDNA** content in dental cementum was up to five times higher than that present in the dentin, indicating that extraction from the root might also be a productive strategy.

ISOTOPE ANALYSIS

Isotope analysis is useful in forensic, bioarchaeological, and paleontological contexts. Teeth are the single most abundant element in the fossil record due to the relative durability of enamel. Tooth enamel is less susceptible to **diagenesis**, the process of chemical change and decay in organic remains following death, so isotopic evidence from teeth has the potential to produce more reliable results than can be obtained from bone. Because the mineralized portions of teeth are 20–25% higher than that of bone, they may very well provide a more faithful representation of the acquisition and integration of isotopes into body tissues during life. As with other elements of the skeleton, the most frequently studied isotopes in teeth include carbon, nitrogen, and strontium, which reveal information about diet (carbon, nitrogen) and geographic location (strontium).

The permanent teeth begin development while *in utero* and generally complete development in the late teenage years (with the exception of the variable third molar). Also, unlike bone, teeth do not remodel during life. Therefore, there is a somewhat truncated window for the uptake of isotopes into the teeth in relation to the rest of the skeleton. For a discussion of how this occurs, refer to Bethard (Chapter 15), this volume. As a result, analysis of isotope ratios in dental material is likely to reveal very good information about the early life of an individual, even providing information about diet surrounding the timing of weaning (Wright and Schwarcz, 1998). But although isotopic information from the teeth is particularly useful in regard to the area where individuals were born and spent their early years, it will not reflect changes in diet and environment that may have taken place later in life. However, isotope ratios in bone can reflect changes in diet and location as ratios turn over in bone roughly every ten years. For more detailed information on isotopic analysis, see Bethard (Chapter 15), this volume.

As an example, Sealey and colleagues (1995) studied the remains of five individuals from different temporal contexts and life situations from South Africa including two prehistoric Khoisan hunter–gatherers, two likely European soldiers, and a female in her fifties buried beneath the floor of a lodge where enslaved persons lived. Sealey and colleagues analyzed the isotopic ratios present in an earlier forming tooth (the first permanent molar or an incisor), the third permanent molar (which is the last tooth to form), and a sample from the skeleton, which as discussed above would have turned over within the ten years or so before death. This method of sampling from the remains ensured that they had samples from three points during each individual's life. In this way, a sort of personal life history could be reconstructed for the individuals.

Results indicated that the hunter—gatherers had maintained a nearly consistent diet and residence during their lives, whereas the possible soldiers had distinct differences between the earlier and later isotopic signatures between their bones and teeth, as would be expected for one traveling and dying quite a distance from their birthplace. The possible enslaved woman also demonstrated a marked change in isotope ratios during her life, particularly following the development of her third molar in her twenties and the subsequent uptake in her bones in the later years of her life that indicated a sharp shift from a more arid environment to one where seafood made up a larger portion of her diet (Sealey et al., 1995).

MICROWEAR

Since the surface of the tooth is subject to contact with the food eaten during life, teeth bear evidence of the diet of the individual in the form of tiny, microscopic scratches and pits referred to as **microwear**. Studies of microwear enable researchers to place individual specimens into broad dietary categories. Although specific records of foods eaten are not possible as microwear in an individual changes nearly weekly, assignment to broad dietary categories (e.g., frugivore vs. folivore) is possible. Studies analyzing microwear in archaeological populations have also noted differences in the *macrowear* patterns (grossly visible wear) between pre- and post-agricultural and industrial populations. Macrowear is often associated with agricultural diets or those diets that involve ingestion of plant materials containing high levels of silicates. Macrowear also includes *occupational wear* (e.g., using the teeth as tools) and *bruxism* (teeth grinding).

The chewing cycle places different amounts of wear and tear on different cusps and tooth surfaces, so an understanding of the basic chewing cycle mechanism and wear facets is crucial in order to compare wear on like facets in order to have an accurate basis for comparison. The chewing cycle begins with the closing stroke where the teeth of the upper and lower jaws first come into contact. This is followed by two power stroke phases, where in phase I, the lingual and buccal cusps of the maxillary molars come into contact and shear against the cusps of the mandibular molars. In phase II of the power stroke, the grinding action is continued with the lingual swing of the mandibular molars relative to the maxillary molars resulting in the inward facing mandibular buccal cusps grinding against the outward surface of the maxillary lingual cusps (Hillson, 1996). Given the different stresses being applied to the respective cuspal surfaces, wear facets involved in phase I and phase II are considered separately in microwear studies.

Initial studies of dental microwear examined the surfaces of teeth using optical light microscopy. Scanning electron microscopy (SEM) was then used due to the increased clarity and depth of field, with the most commonly used standards being those developed by Gordon (1988) and Walker and Teaford (Teaford and Walker, 1984; Walker and Teaford, 1989). Data collection using SEM is a costly and time-intensive endeavor. Some investigators have begun to return to low-level magnification analyses to make good use of the low cost and low time investment inherent in the technique. As with other research methods, the time and money that certain techniques require can greatly affect the types of research questions that might be explored. Limitations on sample sizes and the time and resources necessary to collect and analyze comparative samples should also be considered.

Pits and *scratches* are the two main features usually evaluated in microwear studies. Pits are somewhat circular indentations in the enamel surface and scratches are more linear features that are most often defined as having a length to width ratio of 4:1. Some researchers have used ratios of 2:1 or 10:1 to distinguish the more linear scratch from the "spot" of the pit (Ungar et al., 2008). However arbitrary these definitions may be, they are designed to distinguish between two different features that appear to be representative of different types of dietary abrasives.

One methodological issue that warrants consideration with both types of microscopy commonly used in microwear analysis (both SEM and low-level magnification) is the documentation, both qualitatively and quantitatively, of a three-dimensional surface and associated features with two-dimensional imaging techniques. That is to say that although we can recognize different features and count and group them in order to come up with profiles, we have a difficult time measuring depth of pits and scratches or the surface relief of a tooth.

In this vein, Ungar and colleagues (2008) have developed an automated method that tracks "surface complexity" rather than relying on manually collected data. They report that the method is fully automated, which reduces costs and time, and virtually eliminates the previously mentioned high rates of interobserver error. By examining measures that describe overall surface topography, their method records a three-dimensional account of the appearance of microwear on the tooth surface. Comparing like surfaces, this method found fewer surface complexities in folivores (leaf eaters) than in other primates. Significant differences also existed within species, indicating differential exploitation of available dietary resources.

To place this in a human context, we can consider the things that humans do with their teeth that might contribute to differences in their microwear patterns. In addition to diet, use of the teeth as a "tool" contributes to microwear variation between populations. For an extensive review on the occupational use of the dentition as a tool and appropriate recording methodologies, see Molnar (2011).

CASE STUDY: THE DEVIL IS IN THE DETAILS

My area of interest is dental development, and more specifically, how it relates to the evolution of life history in fossil hominins. As discussed earlier, in this area of research tooth growth is used to interpret the overall pace of life in our ancestors. To do this, we rely on our understanding of the complex interconnectedness of the body's systems. My work engages the interactions of these systems by using the teeth as a proxy for the chronology of important life history events such as age at weaning, menarche, and first reproduction.

My dissertation topic grew out of my Master's thesis, which studied the prenatal development of the teeth in *Macaca nemestrina* (the pigtailed macaque). I was lucky enough to be in a program where my advisor had an extensive collection of lateral X-rays from a collection of

M. nemestrina fetuses. Using these X-rays, I collected the data on tooth growth, analyzed them, and wrote up the results.

During that time, I was enrolled in several paleoanthropology courses that piqued my curiosity in life history evolution and I was searching for a way to connect these two interests. My advisors helped to guide me through independent reading lists for the topics and with tailoring my final projects for the other courses I was taking through the next two years. With this guidance I was able to begin exploration of the connections between life history and dental development.

During the literature review aspect for my dissertation, it stood out to me that currently we only use information about permanent tooth growth in primates to assess life histories for fossil hominin species. Moreover, the potential information that the deciduous teeth might give us is generally disregarded. It became apparent that the reason for this was a general lack of information on the growth and development of the deciduous teeth in living primates (even for humans). Even studies that meticulously detailed the growth of the permanent teeth rarely mentioned the deciduous teeth that were present in the very specimens that were being studied. The consequence of the dearth of knowledge in this area was that when an incredible specimen like the Dikika baby (DIK-1; a juvenile *Australopithecus afarensis*) was found, despite having a mouth full of deciduous teeth, only the permanent teeth received any attention in the analysis (Alemseged et al., 2006).

I brought this observation to the attention of my advisor and suggested a project that would examine the development of the deciduous teeth in chimpanzees. Because chimpanzees and humans are so closely related, studying the similarities and differences in their dental development could help with interpreting the teeth of our ancestors. Several considerations would have to be made: How would this project be more than a "filling in the gaps" style of study that simply reported on dental growth in chimpanzees? Although such studies are useful for expanding our knowledge base, a study of this type would not actively engage the question of hominin dental development that I was interested in exploring. Where would this study be best situated—in primate growth and development or paleoanthropology? Is the topic relevant—are there enough juvenile fossil hominids with deciduous teeth to make this study necessary and useful? These questions resulted in several more literature searches and reviews, further refinement of the study parameters and aim, and after a final consultation with my advisor I received permission to proceed with the project.

Part of the advanced exam protocol at my university involved constructing a grant proposal for an appropriate funding agency that would also serve as a template for my dissertation proposal. Knowing this in advance (and that regardless, I would need outside funding to complete the project) I began mapping out the logistics of the project. First and foremost, I would have to locate appropriate specimens. For my project, I would need over 100 fetal, neonatal, and juvenile chimpanzees in order to accurately characterize variation within the species for the subsequent statistical analyses.

After a couple of months of e-mails (returned and unreturned), follow-up phone calls (significantly more successful than e-mail in most cases), and out-of-pocket trips to several museums (which led on two occasions to getting shoulder deep in large vats filled with preserved specimens only to come up empty), I had located a grand total of *two* fetal chimpanzees. That's right, two.

Thankfully I had begun planning well in advance and had ample time to adjust and reframe my research questions. I was looking for information from the deciduous teeth of living primates that might enhance interpretation of the hominin fossil record. At this point, I am not aware of any fetal fossil hominins; please contact me if you have information to the contrary! However, there are quite a few juvenile fossil hominins that have a mixed set of deciduous and permanent teeth in place. Therefore, the question became whether or not museum collections had an ample number of chimpanzee specimens fitting this developmental stage. When I discovered that the answer was "yes," I changed my research questions. Studying the mixed primary and permanent dentition in living primates would also likely result in great insight into the mixed dentition present in dozens of fossil hominins.

As most often presented, the scientific method is a neat, orderly path from observation through to hypothesis testing, analysis, and presentation of findings. In reality, logistics often create unforeseen obstacles for completion of the ideal project. In my case, revision of my research question was necessary due to sample availability. Finding out what materials are available and what museums will actually let you do with their collections (e.g., in the case of destructive analyses or transporting specimens off-site for analysis) well in advance of your presumed start date is essential to getting the project completed on time. Refer to DiGangi and Moore (Chapter 2), this volume, for more advice on managing logistics.

While I was working on locating collections with specimens appropriate for my study, I was also considering equipment. I would be taking X-rays of the teeth of museum specimens to analyze for the project. It was necessary to ensure that all of the images were as clean, reliable, and as easy to read as possible. For my Master's project I had worked with traditional X-rays and knew that it was difficult to ensure that every exposure turned out well. Furthermore, small details like proper alignment of the film, tube, and specimen as well as exposure time could greatly affect the quality of the resulting image. Another consideration was that processing traditional X-rays takes a considerable amount of time. Using traditional methods, review of images would be delayed until after they were developed, leaving less time to retake images if necessary.

Fortunately, I had two colleagues who were working on their own projects using a portable X-ray source coupled with a digital film system. This technology makes the process much faster, with exposed film being scanned and directly uploaded to a computer. With this system, the film is then erased and reused. Watching the rapidity with which my colleagues imaged individual specimens intrigued me, so I set to work investigating the available options. Since their work dealt with full skeletons, they needed larger sensor plates and a much more powerful X-ray source. My project would be investigating teeth, so I could get the images I needed using bite-wing film (just like what is used in a dentist's office) and a handheld X-ray source. After several searches, I ended up locating separate dealers for the X-ray source and the sensor plates. Even better, I had found digital bite-wing sensor plates that connected via a USB port directly to my computer. This would considerably speed up image acquisition and review as images would open immediately on my laptop after exposure.

Since this system is expensive, I decided to rent rather than purchase it. Prior to rental, I had to arrange for training in the use of the equipment. The dealer of the sensor plates was kind enough to put me in touch with a veterinary dentist in my area who graciously agreed to show me how the sensor plates and associated computer software worked together. I took a couple of chimpanzee skulls with me to his office where he and I worked to find appropriate imaging angles so that I could ensure the best possible images of the teeth in the specimens I would be encountering "in the field."

Further, I also had to be certified by my home institution's office of radiation safety. They approved my use of the device and set me up with both a badge and ring dosimeter to measure my exposure to radiation during the study. This is a very important step, as many states have strict regulations regarding the operation of radiation-producing equipment. Although the radiation safety department was helpful with the regulations in my home state, I spent several hours on the phone and in e-mail contact with the state health departments in other states where I would be conducting research. It so happened that three of them had different regulations. Make sure that any similar logistics for your own projects are all sorted out well in advance to avoid problems while in the field. Especially in the busy summer months, many institutions book access to their collections on an extremely tight schedule. It is unlikely that you will have extra time for addressing any major issues once you arrive.

Now that arrangements for the equipment and collections to be used were established, I sent revised research requests to the four institutions I planned to visit. In these requests I explained in detail the protocol for my study including the use of the X-ray. This was an important consideration as it required that I have a room all to myself for the duration of my visit, with an outside wall at which I could aim the X-ray beam. All of the institutions had their own X-ray system available for use to other researchers, so I also had to explain why my handheld X-ray source was a better fit for my project than their stationary sources (which do not work well for bite-wing imaging). In the end, I was able to secure access to all collections that I had set out to include in my research. With their approval letters in hand, I was ready to apply for the funding necessary to cover expenses.

It is important to mention is that none of the steps proceeded in exactly the order outlined above. Indeed, it was much more complicated. Basically, the proposal had to come together before I could submit it to my committee, but then modifications were necessary once I realized that the samples did not exist. Whenever possible, I arranged to visit a museum to assess sample sizes. This was of course paid for out of my own pocket because I had not yet secured funding, and funding agencies love to know your sample sizes before they will give you any money! (Even though many museums have online databases of their collections, there is still no substitute for going in and checking them out in advance personally if at all possible.) This was also happening while I was contacting vendors regarding X-ray equipment rentals.

The closest thing I can liken this to is kitchen remodeling. All of the steps have to happen at a certain time and yet all at the same time (the sink cannot be installed until the countertops are in, but first the plumber has to come, then what about the electrician for the garbage disposal?). You cannot apply for funding until you have the project proposal in place, but receiving permission to work on a collection possibly years in advance seems strange. It is a juggling act extraordinaire to say the least, and certainly the first time around. The satisfaction of finally receiving funding for the project and the excitement of working with the collections of a world-famous museum for the first time are really life-changing experiences. Focus and perseverance will serve you well in the preparation and execution of a research project. Be prepared for the unexpected, because it is likely that something *will* go wrong. Be prepared for it all to take twice as long as you think it will, just in case it does. Finally, be prepared to be excited—you are finally a working anthropologist, congratulations!

MOVING FORWARD ...

This chapter has introduced the primary research foci of dental anthropology; however, the material presented here just scratches the surface. Although outside of the scope of this volume, which focuses on anatomically modern *Homo sapiens*, applications of the described methods can be taken in myriad directions involving not only modern humans, but also living and extinct primates as well as fossil humans. Indeed, most of the prominent texts on dental anthropology include research on these very topics. For further reading, the following are a few edited volumes that present an array of valuable scholarship in the field: Bailey, S.E., Hublin, J.-J. (Eds.), 2007. *Dental Perspectives on Human Evolution: State of the Art Research in Dental Paleoanthropology.* Dordrecht: Springer.

Irish, J.D., Nelson, G.C. (Eds.), 2008. *Technique and Application in Dental Anthropology.* Cambridge: Cambridge University Press.

Kelley, M.A., Larsen, C.S., 1991. *Advances in Dental Anthropology.* New York: Wiley Liss.

Scott G.R., Turner II, C.G. (Eds.), 1997. *The Anthropology of Modern Human Teeth: Dental Morphology and Its Variation in Recent Human Populations.* Cambridge: Cambridge University Press.

I strongly recommend that you consult these references and the others cited in this chapter for further exploration of the topics raised. Teeth are fascinating in that they are essentially time capsules. All one has to do is know how to break open the capsule and it will reveal a plethora of information about individuals and populations: modern, historic, and prehistoric.

ACKNOWLEDGMENTS

I thank the editors, Drs. Elizabeth DiGangi and Megan Moore, for the invitation to contribute to this unique volume and for their helpful comments during the writing of the chapter. Thanks are also extended to Lon Hunt for his thoughtful work on the illustrations.

REFERENCES

Adler, C.J., Haak, W., Donlon, D., Cooper, A., 2011. Survival and recovery of DNA from ancient teeth and bones. Journal of Archaeological Science 38 (5), 956–964.

Alemseged, Z., Spoor, F., Kimbel, W.H., Bobe, R., Geraads, D., Reed, D., Wynn, J.G., 2006. A juvenile early hominin skeleton from Dikika, Ethiopia. Nature 443 (7109), 296–301.

AlQahtani, S.J., Hector, M.P., Liversidge, H.M., 2010. Brief communication: The London atlas of human tooth development and eruption. American Journal of Physical Anthropology 142 (3), 481–490.

Birkby, W.H., Fenton, T.W., Anderson, B.E., 2008. Identifying Southwest Hispanics using nonmetric traits and the cultural profile. Journal of Forensic Sciences 53 (1), 29–33.

Bogin, B., 1999. Patterns of Human Growth 2nd Ed., Cambridge University Press, New York.

Bromage, T., 1991. Enamel incremental periodicity in the pig-tailed macaque: a polychrome fluorescent labeling study of dental hard tissues. American Journal of Physical Anthropology 86 (2), 205–214.

Broom, R., Robinson, J.T., 1951. Eruption of the permanent teeth in the South African fossil Ape-men. Nature 167 (4246) 443–443.

Cabana, G.S., Hulsey, B.I., Pack, F.L., 2013. Molecular methods. In: DiGangi, E.A., Moore, M.K. (Eds.), Research Methods in Human Skeletal Biology. Academic Press, San Diego.

Cassidy, C., 1980. Nutrition and health in agriculturalists and huntergatherers: a case study of two prehistoric populations. In: Jerome, N., Kendel, R., Pelto, G. (Eds.), Nutritional Anthropology: Contemporary Approaches to Diet and Culture. Redgrave, Pleasantville, NY, pp. 117–145.

Cesarani, F., Martina, M.C., Ferraris, A., Grilletto, R., Boano, R., Marochetti, E.F., et al., 2003. Whole-body three-dimensional multidetector CT of 13 Egyptian human mummies. American Journal of Roentgenology 180 (3), 597–606.

Charles, D.K., Condon, K., Cheverud, J.M., Buikstra, J.E., 1986. Cementum annulation and age determination in *Homo sapiens*. I. Tooth variability and observer error. American Journal of Physical Anthropology 71 (3), 311–320.

Chhem, R., 2006. Paleoradiology: imaging disease in mummies and ancient skeletons. Skeletal Radiology 35 (11), 803–804.

Cohen, M., Armelagos, G. (Eds.), 1984. Paleopathology at the Origins of Agriculture. Academic Press, New York.

Condon, K., Charles, D.K., Cheverud, J.M., Buikstra, J.E., 1986. Cementum annulation and age determination in *Homo sapiens*. II. Estimates and accuracy. American Journal of Physical Anthropology 71 (3), 321–330.

Conroy, G., 1988. Alleged synapomorphy of the M1/I1 eruption pattern in robust australopithecines and *Homo*: evidence from high-resolution computed tomography. American Journal of Physical Anthropology 75 (4), 487–492.

Conroy, G., Mahoney, C., 1991. Mixed longitudinal study of dental emergence in the chimpanzee, *Pan troglodytes* (primates, Pongidae). American Journal of Physical Anthropology 86 (2), 243–254.

Conroy, G.C., Vannier, M.W., 1987. Dental development of the Taung skull from computerized tomography. Nature 329 (6140), 625–627.

Coquerelle, M., Bayle, P., Bookstein, F., Braga, J., Halazonetis, D., Katina, S., et al., 2010. The association between dental mineralization and mandibular form: a study combining additive conjoint measurement and geometric morphometrics. Journal of Anthropological Sciences 88, 129–150.

Corey, L.A., Nance, W.E., Hofstede, P., Schenkein, H.A., 1993. Self-reported periodontal disease in a Virginia twin population. Journal of Periodontology 64 (12), 1205–1208.

Dart, R., 1925. *Australopithecus africanus*: the man-ape of South Africa. Nature 115, 195–199.

De Vito, C., Saunders, S.A., 1990. A discriminant function analysis of deciduous teeth to determine sex. Journal of Forensic Sciences 35 (4), 845–848.

Dean, M., Wood, B., 1981. Developing pongid dentition and its use for ageing individual crania in comparative cross-sectional growth studies. Folia Primatologica 36, 111–127.

Dean, M.C., 1985. The eruption pattern of the permanent incisors and first permanent molars in *Australopithecus (Paranthropus) robustus*. American Journal of Physical Anthropology 67 (3), 251–257.

Dean, M.C., 1987. The dental developmental status of six East African juvenile fossil hominids. Journal of Human Evolution 16 (2), 197–213.

Dean, M., Beynon, A., Reid, D., Whittaker, D., 1993. A longitudinal study of tooth growth in a single individual based on long- and short-period incremental markings in dentine and enamel. International Journal of Osteoarchaeology 3 (4), 249–264.

Demirjian, A., Goldstein, H., Tanner, J., 1973. A new system of dental age assessment. Human Biology 45, 211–277.

DiGangi, E.A., Hefner, J.T., 2013. Ancestry estimation. In: DiGangi, E.A., Moore, M.K. (Eds.), Research Methods in Human Skeletal Biology. Academic Press, San Diego.

DiGangi, E.A., Moore, M.K., 2013. Application of the scientific method to skeletal biology. In: DiGangi, E.A., Moore, M.K. (Eds.), Research Methods in Human Skeletal Biology. Academic Press, San Diego.

Duray, S.M., 1996. Dental indicators of stress and reduced age at death in prehistoric Native Americans. American Journal of Physical Anthropology 99 (2), 275–287.

Garn, S.M., Lewis, A.B., 1963. Phylogenetic and intraspecific variations in tooth sequence polymorphisms. In: Brothwell, D. (Ed.), Dental Anthropology. Pergamon, Oxford, pp. 53–73.

Garn, S.M., Lewis, A.B., Vicinus, J.H., 1962. Third molar polymorphism and its significance to dental genetics. Journal of Dental Research 42, 257–276.

Goodman, A.H., Rose, J.C., 1991. Dental enamel hypoplasias as indicators of nutritional status. In: Kelley, M., Larsen, C.S. (Eds.), Advances in Dental Anthropology. Wiley-Liss, New York.

Gordon, K., 1988. A review of methodology and quantification in dental microwear analysis. Scanning Microscopy 2, 1139–1147.

Hanihara, T., Ishida, H., 2005. Metric dental variation of major human populations. American Journal of Physical Anthropology 128 (2), 287–298.

Hassett, B., 2011. Technical note: estimating sex using cervical canine odontometrics: a test using a known sex sample. American Journal of Physical Anthropology 146 (3), 486–489.

Herschaft, E., Alder, M., Ord, D., Rawson, R., Smith, E. (Eds.), 2007. Manual of Forensic Odontology. American Society of Forensic Odontology. Impress Printing and Graphics, Albany.

Hildebolt, C., Molnar, S., 1991. Measurement and description of periodontal disease in anthropological studies. In: Kelley, M., Larsen, C. (Eds.), Advances in Dental Anthropology. Wiley-Liss, New York, pp. 225–240.

Hillson, S., 1996. Dental Anthropology. Cambridge University Press, Cambridge.

Hillson, S., 2000. Dental pathology. In: Katzenberg, M., Saunders, S. (Eds.), Biological Anthropology of the Human Skeleton. Wiley-Liss, New York, pp. 249–286.

Hillson, S., 2001. Recording dental caries in archaeological human remains. International Journal of Osteoarchaeology 11 (4), 249–289.

Hrdlička, A., 1920. Shovel-shaped teeth. American Journal of Physical Anthropology 3 (4), 429–465.

Jankauskas, R., Barakauskas, S., Bojarun, R., 2001. Incremental lines of dental cementum in biological age estimation. Homo—Journal of Comparative Human Biology 52 (1), 59–71.

Kieser, J., 1990. Human Adult Odontometrics. Cambridge University Press, Cambridge.

Kieser, J., Dennison, J., Anson, D., Doyle, T., Laing, R., 2004. Spiral computed tomographic study of a pre-Ptolemaic Egyptian mummy. Anthropological Science 112, 91–96.

Kuykendall, K.L., 1996. Dental development in chimpanzees (Pan troglodytes): the timing of tooth calcification stages. American Journal of Physical Anthropology 99 (1), 135–157.

Larsen, C., Shavit, R., Griffin, M., 1991. Dental caries evidence for dietary change: An archaeological context. In: Larsen, C.S., Kelley, M.A. (Eds.), Advances in Dental Anthropology. Wiley-Liss, New York, pp. 179–202.

Loe, H., Anerud, A., Boysen, H., 1992. The natural history of periodontal disease in man: prevalence, severity, and extent of gingival recession. Journal of Periodontology 63 (6), 489–495.

Logan, W., Kronfeld, R., 1933. Development of the human jaws and surrounding structures from birth to age fifteen. Journal of the American Dental Association 22, 3–30.

Lukacs, J.R., 1989. Dental paleopathology: Methods for reconstructing dietary patterns. In: İscan, M.Y., Kennedy, K.A.R. (Eds.). Alan R. Liss, New York, pp. 261–288.

Maat, G.J.R., Gerretsen, R.R.R., Aarents, M.J., 2006. Improving the visibility of tooth cementum annulations by adjustment of the cutting angle of microscopic sections. Forensic Science International 159, Supplement, S95–S99.

Meinl, A., Huber, C.D., Tangl, S., Gruber, G.M., Teschler-Nicola, M., Watzek, G., 2008. Comparison of the validity of three dental methods for the estimation of age at death. Forensic Science International 178 (2–3), 96–105.

Melcher, A., Holowka, S., Pharoah, M., Lewin, P., 1997. Non-invasive computed tomography and three-dimensional reconstruction of the dentition of a 2,800-year-old Egyptian mummy exhibiting extensive dental disease. American Journal of Physical Anthropology 103 (3), 329–340.

Michalowicz, B.S., Diehl, S.R., Gunsolley, J.C., Sparks, B.S., Brooks, C.N., Koertge, T.E., et al., 2000. Evidence of a substantial genetic basis for risk of adult periodontitis. Journal of Periodontology 71 (11), 1699–1707.

Molnar, P., 2011. Extramasticatory dental wear reflecting habitual behavior and health in past populations. Clinical Oral Investigations 15 (5), 681–689.

Moore, M.K., 2013. Functional morphology and medical imaging. In: DiGangi, E.A., Moore, M.K. (Eds.), Research Methods in Human Skeletal Biology. Academic Press, San Diego.

Moore, M.K., 2013. Sex estimation and assessment. In: DiGangi, E.A., Moore, M.K. (Eds.), Research Methods in Human Skeletal Biology. Academic Press, San Diego.

Obertová, Z., Francken, M., 2009. Tooth cementum annulation method: accuracy and applicability. Frontiers of Oral Biology 13, 184–189.

Olejniczak, A., Tafforeau, P., Smith, T., Temming, H., Hublin, J.-J., 2007. Technical note: Compatibility of microtomographic imaging systems for dental measurements. American Journal of Physical Anthropology 134 (1), 130–134.

Previgliano, C.H., Ceruti, C., Reinhard, J., Araoz, F.A., Diez, J.G., 2003. Radiologic evaluation of the Llullaillaco mummies. American Journal of Roentgenology 181 (6), 1473–1479.

Renz, H., Radlanski, R.J., 2006. Incremental lines in root cementum of human teeth—A reliable age marker? Homo—Journal of Comparative Human Biology 57 (1), 29–50.

Rose, J.C., Condon, K., Goodman, A.H., 1985. Diet and dentition: Developmental disturbances. In: Gilbert, R.I., Mielke, J.H. (Eds.), The Analysis of Prehistoric Diets. Academic Press, New York, pp. 281–306.

Sakurai, T., Michiue, T., Ishikawa, T., Yoshida, C., Sakoda, S., Kano, T., Oritani, S., Maeda, H., 2012. Postmortem CT investigation of skeletal and dental maturation of the fetuses and newborn infants: a serial case study. Forensic Science, Medicine, and Pathology [Epub ahead of print].

Schour, I., Massler, M., 1941. The development of the human dentition. Journal of the American Dental Association 28, 1153−1160.

Schultz, A., 1940. Growth and development of the chimpanzee. Contributions to Embryology 28, 1−63.

Schultz, M., Carli-Thiele, P., Schmidt-Schultz, T.H., Kierdorf, U., Kierdorf, H., 1998. Enamel hypoplasia in archaeological skeletal remains. In: Alt, K., Rosing, F., Teschler-Nicola, M. (Eds.), Dental Anthropology: Fundamentals, Limits, and Prospects. Springer-Verlag, New York.

Scott, G., Turner II, C., 1997. The Anthropology of Modern Human Teeth; Dental Morphology and its Variation in Recent Human Populations. Cambridge University Press, Cambridge.

Sealy, J., Armstrong, R., Schrire, C., 1995. Beyond lifetime averages: Tracing lifetime histories through isotopic analyses of different calcified tissues from archaeological human skeletons. Antiquity 69 (263), 290−300.

Silverstone, L., Johnson, N., Hardie, J., Williams, R., 1981. Dental caries. Aetiology, Pathology and Prevention. Macmillan, London.

Simpson, S.W., Kunos, C.A., 1998. A radiographic study of the development of the human mandibular dentition. Journal of Human Evolution 35 (4−5), 479−505.

Simpson, S.W., Lovejoy, C.O., Meindl, R.S., 1991. Relative dental development in hominoids and its failure to predict somatic growth velocity. American Journal of Physical Anthropology 86 (2), 113−120.

Sirianni, J., Swindler, D., 1985. Growth and Development of the Pigtailed Macaque. CRC Press, Boca Raton.

Smith, B., 1994. Sequence of emergence of the permanent teeth in *Macaca, Pan, Homo*, and *Australopithecus*: Its evolutionary significance. American Journal of Human Biology 6 (1), 61−76.

Smith, B., Garn, S., 1987. Polymorphisms in eruption sequence of permanent teeth in American children. American Journal of Physical Anthropology 74 (3), 289−303.

Smith, B.H., 1991. Standards of human tooth formation and dental age assessment. In: Larsen, C.S., Kelley, M.A. (Eds.), Advances in Dental Anthropology. Wiley-Liss, New York, pp. 143−168.

Smith, T., 2006. Experimental determination of the periodicity of incremental features in enamel. Journal of Anatomy 208 (1), 99−113.

Smith, T., 2008. Incremental dental development: methods and applications in hominoid evolutionary studies. Journal of Human Evolution 54 (2), 205−224.

Smith, T., Reid, D., Sirianni, J., 2006. The accuracy of histological assessments of dental development and age at death. Journal of Anatomy 208 (1), 125−138.

Stein, T.J., Corcoran, J.F., 1994. Pararadicular cementum deposition as a criterion for age estimation in human beings. Oral Surgery, Oral Medicine, Oral Pathology 77 (3), 266−270.

Tafforeau, P., Smith, T.M., 2008. Nondestructive imaging of hominoid dental microstructure using phase contrast X-ray synchrotron microtomography. Journal of Human Evolution 54, 272−278.

Teaford, M.F., Walker, A., 1984. Quantitative differences in dental microwear between primate species with different diets and a comment on the presumed diet of *Sivapithecus*. American Journal of Physical Anthropology 64 (2), 191−200.

Ten-State Nutrition Survey 1968−1970, 1972. U.S. Department of Health, Education, and Welfare, Centers for Disease Control, Atlanta, GA.

Turner, C., Nichol, C., Scott, G., 1991. Scoring procedures for key morphological traits of the permanent dentition: The Arizona State University Dental Anthropology System. In: Larsen, C.S., Kelley, M.A. (Eds.), Advances in Dental Anthropology. Wiley-Liss, New York, pp. 13−31.

Ungar, P., Scott, R., Scott, J., Teaford, M., 2008. Dental microwear analysis: Historical perspectives and new approaches. In: Irish, J.D., Nelson, G.C. (Eds.), Technique and Application in Dental Anthropology. Cambridge University Press, Cambridge, pp. 389−425.

Walker, A., Teaford, M.F., 1989. Inferences from quantitative analysis of dental microwear. Folia Primatologica 53, 177−189.

Wittwer-Backofen, U., Gampe, J., Vaupel, J.W., 2004. Tooth cementum annulation for age estimation: results from a large known-age validation study. American Journal of Physical Anthropology 123 (2), 119−129.

Wright, L.E., Schwarcz, H.P., 1998. Stable carbon and oxygen isotopes in human tooth enamel: identifying breast-feeding and weaning in prehistory. American Journal of Physical Anthropology 106 (1), 1−18.

11

Demography

Lyle W. Konigsberg, Susan R. Frankenberg

INTRODUCTION

In the past, the term "demography" as applied in skeletal biology was synonymous with the production of *life tables* (Jackes, 1992). A life table is simply a tabulation of the number of deaths within various age intervals, which is then used to calculate such related measures as the life expectancy for individuals who enter an age interval, the probability that someone who enters the age interval will die within that interval, or the living age distribution (population pyramid) implied by the distribution of deaths across age intervals. This life table approach allowed a division of labor where an osteologist could produce the counts of the number of deaths within age intervals after determining the age-at-death for each skeleton and a demographer could construct the life table. Oftentimes the osteologist or skeletal biologist would do it all, but even in this case there was a very clear order of operations where estimation of ages preceded the demographic analysis. The chapter structure of this book follows such an order, with the chapter on age estimation among the first in the "Research on Aspects of the Biological Profile" part, and this chapter on demography being the last.

We use the term "**demography**"[1] as a more specific version of its literal meaning derived from the Greek words "demos" (meaning "people") and "graphia" (meaning "description of"). So to us, the term "demography" means a description of people, and more specifically a description of their ages and sexes. To be meaningful, this description must move beyond the level of individual people. As we are often working with prehistoric populations, the description also must generally encompass far broader periods of time than would be typical in demographic studies of extant populations.

By the end of the previous millennium, the methods for demographic analyses of skeletal samples and the understanding of **paleodemography** had begun to shift substantially. This shift was triggered by Bocquet-Appel's and Masset's *Farewell to Paleodemography* (1982), and their work together with that of other researchers (Konigsberg and Frankenberg, 1992,

---

[1] All bolded terms are defined in the glossary at the end of this volume.

1994; Bocquet-Appel, 1994; Bocquet-Appel and Bacro, 1997, 2008; Aykroyd et al., 1999; Wood et al., 2002; Hoppa and Vaupel, 2002b; Boldsen et al., 2002; Frankenberg and Konigsberg, 2006; DeWitte and Wood, 2008; Redfern and DeWitte, 2011) is transforming the field. In its current configuration, demographic analysis of skeletal samples cannot be separated from the processes of age estimation or sex estimation. In other words, <u>individual age or sex estimates cannot be produced until **after** the demographic analyses have been performed</u>. We demonstrate how and why one should conduct demographic analyses prior to generating individual age and sex estimates, starting with sex estimation and estimation of the sex ratio since this is a simpler problem than age estimation. We then turn our attention to age estimation, the estimation of the age-at-death distribution, and the role of **hazard models**, including their relationship to traditional life table analysis. Finally, we briefly discuss the uses to which the results of such analyses can be put. These goals are relatively modest, but as the one thing demographers tend to do is enumerate things, we would do well to list the "order of operations" for this chapter. They are as follows:

1. <u>Estimating the sex ratio</u>: in this section we examine how to estimate the sex ratio (or really, the proportion of one of the sexes) such that it makes the observed "sexing" data as likely as possible to have been observed.
2. <u>Estimating the sex of individuals</u>: in this section we examine how to estimate individual sexes (or really, the probability that individuals are one particular sex) following on having already estimated the sex ratio from Step 1.
3. <u>Presentation of hazard models as a summary of mortality</u>: in this section we present hazard models as a direct alternative to life tables for summarizing mortality data.
4. <u>Simulating long bone growth</u>: in this section we show how to simulate long bone growth as a preamble to analyzing simulated data.
5. <u>Estimating the age-at-death structure</u>: in this section we use simulated data on long bone lengths (see Step 4) in order to demonstrate how one can fit a hazard model using "age indicator" data rather than using age estimates.
6. <u>Estimating ages-at-death</u>: in this section we show how to estimate "point ages" and the variance of the estimates from **Bayes' theorem** using the information on long bone growth and the hazard model fit in Step 5. By "point ages" we mean specific decimal ages such as 7.34 years old. Clearly, such estimates will require a statement about the possible error around the stated age, which is why we calculate the variance of the estimate.

Two explanations are in order before we dive into demographic analysis. First, demography is inherently technical, and requires a certain level of mathematical/statistical analysis and computer savvy. There is no avoiding algebra or calculus in this chapter. For those unfamiliar or uncomfortable with calculus, the integrals in Equations 11.17, 11.19, 11.21, and 11.22 can be thought of as summations across large spans with very small intervals. While Hoppa and Vaupel (2002b) have pointed out that "Pencil and paper or a computer is required," we note that neither pencil and paper nor computer spreadsheets or canned statistical packages are sufficient for the analyses presented here. Instead, we use an open source graphics, mathematical, and statistical package known as "R" (R Development Core Team, 2011), which "has become a de-facto standard among statisticians for the development of statistical software" (http://openwetware.org/wiki/R_Statistics). While the learning curve is a bit steep, there are a number of introductions and tutorials freely available (see the wiki cited above), and all of the code used for this chapter is available online[2].

Second, we make extensive use of simulated datasets rather than actual osteological data in this chapter. The advantage of using simulated data is that it is essentially known-age and known-sex because we created it, and we consequently can check that the demographic analyses are producing the correct answers. While we might accomplish the same thing with osteological data from known-age, known-sex collections, such collections are rare and often do not represent natural population profiles. Within our datasets, the osteological variables used to estimate sex or age are simulated to follow what is known about the statistical dependency of these traits on the demographic variables (actual sex and age) as realistically as possible. The simulations of the sex or age-at-death distributions that generate the dependent osteological traits also are designed to demonstrate particular properties of the analytical methods. All of the simulated datasets, as well as the code that generated them[2]. We believe firmly in learning by doing, and hope you will take advantage of the online materials to work through and play with the examples.

STARTING DATA FOR DEMOGRAPHIC ANALYSIS OF SKELETAL SAMPLES

If individual age or sex estimates cannot be produced until **after** the demographic analyses have been performed (for reasons that will become clear in subsequent sections), then what information from the skeletal sample initiates the demographic analyses? Hoppa and Vaupel (2002b) state that when working with age and ordered categorical data (such as pubic symphyseal scores), "the information that osteologists have regarding age and stages pertains to the probability of being in a specific stage given age, $Pr(c|a)$." Generalizing this statement, an osteologist needs two things in order to conduct a demographic analysis: (1) recorded information on individual sex or age indicators from each skeleton, and (2) a way to evaluate how these indicators depend, or are conditional, on known sex and/or age. The skeletal sample with unknown ages and/or sexes for which we wish to estimate population-level demographic parameters and individual ages and/or sexes forms a **target sample** (Konigsberg and Frankenberg, 1992), and it is from this sample that we will need to have the recorded information on individual sex and/or age indicators. It is imperative in constructing the demographic analysis that we have this basic observational information from each skeleton, so for example we will need the "scores" for each indicator. A proper demographic analysis of the target sample cannot begin with age estimates for each skeleton; it must begin with the basic observations that (traditionally) an osteologist would consider in making an age estimate. In order to effectively use observations on indicators from the target sample we must understand how these indicators are dependent on individual demographic variables (age and/or sex).

Generalizing Hoppa and Vaupel's $Pr(c|a)$ probability, we want to find the probability of various indicator states or values dependent on known individual age and/or sex. This information must come from a known age and/or sex **reference sample** (Konigsberg and

[2]https://netfiles.uiuc.edu/lylek/www/KF-Chap11.htm.

Frankenberg, 1992), or its equivalent. The reference sample should be a sample with known demographic information that is appropriate for application to the target sample. Unfortunately, the acceptance of a reference sample as being "appropriate" is often more of a leap of faith than anything else. For example, Shackelford et al. (2012) have applied data on dental formation and eruption from known age twentieth century children to estimate ages-at-death for Neandertal and early modern human fossils. In an actual analysis it may not be necessary to have access to a reference sample, provided that summary statistics of the relationship between osteological traits and known age and/or sex have been published in a useable format (for example, the mean and standard deviation of each indicator for each known age and/or sex). It also may be possible to combine information from different sources such as combining summary statistics on fetal long bone growth from ultrasound examinations with summary statistics on postnatal long bone growth from radiographs.

What is absolutely critical is that we have information on the indicator states given known age and/or sex. Much of the literature (see for example Todd (1920), Stewart (1948), McKern and Stewart (1957), Thompson (1979), Meindl and Lovejoy (1985)), because it focuses on estimating age and/or sex for individual skeletons, does not provide such information in a useable format. This early literature has instead provided summaries of the distribution of age (such as mean ages, standard deviations of age, or age ranges) within stages. Similarly, when trying to estimate sex we need information on the distribution of an osteological "indicator" of sex within known sex, and not the distribution of sex against the indicator.

As a brief example, presume that we have assigned sexes based on mastoid process size in a sample of known sex individuals, and that we have done this assignment without reference to the known sexes. To simplify the example, we will say that we treat the mastoid process size as a binary variable, so that we only assign sexes of "F" or "M." Now we go back and look at the two-by-two table of known sex (male or female) against the sex assigned from the mastoid process. The useful information in this table is $P("M"|male)$ and $P("F"|female)$, where $P("M"|male)$ is read as "the probability of scoring a mastoid process as being male given that the individual is an actual male." Complementary values can be obtained by subtraction (for example, $P("F"|male) = 1 - P("M"|male)$). The information contained in the "transposed conditionals" $P(male|"M")$ and $P(female|"F")$ is much less useful. This subtle distinction will be easier to demonstrate in concrete examples such as we present below.

ESTIMATION OF SEX AND OF THE SEX RATIO

While it may seem odd to refer to "estimation" of sex, it should be clear from Moore (Chapter 4), this volume, that the sex of skeletons can be treated as known only under certain circumstances. Specifically, if **DNA** sexing (Hummel and Herrmann, 1991; Stone et al., 1996; Faerman et al., 1998; Mays and Faerman, 2001; Matheson and Loy, 2001; Schmidt et al., 2003; Arnay-de-la-Rosa et al., 2007; De La Cruz, 2008; Gibbon et al., 2009) has been applied, then the sex of individual skeletons can be treated as known. Additionally, if the Phenice (1969) pubic bone characteristics are observable and unambiguous, then sex can be treated as nearly known, with correct identification of sex ranging between 95% and 98.5% (Kelley, 1978; Sutherland and Suchey, 1991; Konigsberg et al., 2002). One study (Lovell, 1989) did give a lower percentage of the correct identification of sex from the Phenice characteristics, but this study only examined a small sample of 50 individuals and included multiple observers, some of whom were novices. If we have at least some "known" sex skeletons from a population based on either DNA or Phenice characteristics, then we can use these as a calibration or training sample (in other words, as the reference sample) in order to sex additional skeletons (from that population) for which DNA or the Phenice characteristics are unavailable. To illustrate how this can be done we use an example from Konigsberg and Hens (1998).

Estimating the Sex Ratio

To estimate the sex ratio within a skeletal sample, we can simply estimate the proportion of one sex (either male or female) within that sample. Konigsberg and Hens (1998) gave a tabulation of how 114 crania from the Averbuch Site (Mississippian period, Middle Tennessee) would have been sexed on the basis of brow ridge morphology (see Table 11.1). Sixty of these 114 crania had previously been sexed as being from males on the basis of the Phenice characteristics from the associated pubic bones, while the remaining 54 individuals had been sexed as females on the Phenice characteristics. Note that the sexing from the brow ridges was done without knowledge of the sex from the Phenice characteristics. Further, Konigsberg and Hens originally selected the 114 individuals so that the identification of sex from their pubic bones was unambiguous. Consequently, these 114 individuals can be treated as a known sex reference sample. From the 60 males Konigsberg and Hens found that on the basis of the brow ridges they would have sexed 51 as being male, 5 as female, and 4 as indeterminate. From the 54 females they would have sexed 32 as being female, 16 as being male, and 6 as indeterminate. Now imagine that we score the brows in a sample of 100 crania from the same population (but without the ability to observe the Phenice characteristics) as 35 "male," 11 "indeterminate," and 54 "female." The immediate demographic task is not to attempt to determine the sex for each cranium, but instead to estimate the proportion of the sample that is either male or female. Following on from this, we can return to the problem of estimating sex for each cranium. For this example, we will estimate the proportion of individuals that are male, which we will show as p_m. The proportion of individuals that are female is then $p_f = 1 - p_m$.

To estimate p_m we will use the method of **maximum likelihood estimation** (MLE). There is a relatively gentle introduction to MLE by Purcell[3] and Myung (2003) gives a nice tutorial using MATLAB. MATLAB is a proprietary program, so in its place we use "R," which has an

TABLE 11.1   Tabulation of Estimated Sex from the Brow Ridge against the Phenice (1969) Characteristics of Sex from the Pelvis. 114 Individuals from the Averbuch Site (Konigsberg and Hens, 1998)

Phenice Characteristics	Indication from Brow		
	"M"	"?"	"F"
Male	51	4	5
Female	16	6	32

[3]http://statgen.iop.kcl.ac.uk/bgim/mle/sslike_1.html.

extensive MLE package (maxLik, see http://www.maxlik.org/). To use MLE we must first write the log-likelihood function, an element of which is what the probabilities are that brows would have been scored as "M," "?," or "F" given known sex. For the current example we will simply use our data from the reference sample. Thus, for a male the probability of an "M" score is 51/60, the probability of a "?" score is 4/60, and the probability of an "F" score is 5/60. For a female the probabilities of the three scores are 16/54, 6/54, and 32/54, respectively. In matrix form the log-likelihood function is

$$\ln LK = \ln\left(\begin{bmatrix} p_M & 1-p_M \end{bmatrix}\begin{bmatrix} 51/60 & 4/60 & 5/60 \\ 16/54 & 6/54 & 32/54 \end{bmatrix}\right)\begin{bmatrix} 35 \\ 11 \\ 54 \end{bmatrix}, \tag{11.1}$$

which after the matrix multiplications is

$$\ln LK = 35 \times \ln\left(\frac{17 p_m}{20} + \frac{8(1-p_m)}{27}\right) + 11 \times \ln\left(\frac{p_m}{15} + \frac{1-p_m}{9}\right)$$
$$+ 54 \times \ln\left(\frac{p_m}{12} + \frac{16(1-p_m)}{27}\right). \tag{11.2}$$

Since we harbor no particular affection for or facility with algebra, we obtained Equation 11.2 from Equation 11.1 using wxMaxima (see http://andrejv.github.com/wxmaxima/), a freeware symbolic algebra and calculus package that can be downloaded for Windows, Mac OS X, or as source code. Equation 11.2 has a single parameter (p_m), so we can have the max.-Lik object in "R" search across the function to find the maximum likelihood, which occurs at a value of 0.0982. This means that we estimate that about 10% of our sample of 100 crania is male and 90% is female, based on our previous scores of 35 crania with a "male" brow, 11 "undetermined," and 54 with a "female" brow.

Having a sample that is only 10% male seems like a substantial deviation from the expected 50% (based on the human sex ratio of approximately 1:1), so it would be useful to have some indication of how well the parameter is estimated. While skeletal biology articles are replete with analyses and reported percentages that do not have standard errors, this should and can be avoided. We calculate the variance of the estimate by taking the reciprocal of the negative of the second derivative of the log-likelihood. The second derivative of the log-likelihood can be found using the maxLik function "hessian." From this we obtain a standard error (the square root of the variance of the estimate) equal to 0.0855. Assuming a normal distribution, we expect about 95% of the estimates to fall within 1.96 standard errors of the true population value for the proportion of males. Consequently, we have a 95% confidence interval of 0.0982 ± 1.96 × 0.0855, or from −0.06938 to 0.26578. In other words, 95% of the estimates place the percentage of males in our sample between −6.95% and 26.58%, which removes a 1:1 (50%) sex ratio from the realm of possibility. Note that the percentage of males cannot be below 0%, or conversely that the percentage of females cannot be above 100%. We obtained a negative percentage because the percentage of males is low in this example and our estimate has a large standard error. It would be more correct in this setting to give a "one-tailed" 95% confidence interval (0.0982 + 1.64 × 0.0855) of from 0 to 23.84%, which again does not include a 1:1 sex ratio.

In general, increasing the size of a sample will reduce the size of the standard error of the estimates, but does not necessarily alter the proportion estimated. We can illustrate this by generalizing the above example. Equation 11.2 has a maximum that we can find explicitly without having to resort to numerical maximization. Setting the first derivative equal to zero and solving for p_m, we have the surprisingly ugly

$$P_m = \frac{20672U + 120497M + 64625F - 3\sqrt{\begin{array}{c} 346853376U^2 + 214651801M^2 + 1107225625F^2 \\ +U(1239427200F - 545720448M) + 975024050FM \end{array}}}{65780N},$$

(11.3)

where M is the number of crania with "male" brows (35 in the above example), U is the number with "indeterminate" brows (11 in the above example), F is the number with "female" brows (54 in the above example), and N is the total sample size (100 in the above example). We can also explicitly find the "information" (the negative of the second derivative) of Equation 11.2 as

$$I = \frac{4U}{2025\left(\frac{p_m}{15} + \frac{1 - p_m}{9}\right)^2} + \frac{89401M}{291600\left(\frac{17p_m}{20} + \frac{8(1 - p_m)}{27}\right)^2} + \frac{3025F}{11664\left(\frac{p_m}{12} + \frac{16(1 - p_m)}{27}\right)^2},$$

(11.4)

where p_m is the maximum likelihood estimate from Equation 11.3. The reciprocal of the information is an estimate of the variance, so the square root of this reciprocal is the standard error. We can use Equations 11.3 and 11.4 for a new example where we have 10 times as many crania ($N = 1000$), but with brow indicators in the same proportions (350 "male," 110 "indeterminate," and 540 "female"). From Equation 11.3 we get an estimated proportion of males at 0.0982, identical with our previous example. The addition of 900 crania to the original 100 does, however, decrease the standard error (from Equation 11.4) to 0.0270, giving a 95% confidence interval of from 0.0453 to 0.1511, or 4.53% to 15.11% male. Having an estimate of the proportion of the target sample that is male is absolutely "mission critical" in obtaining individual estimates of sex, as we directly show in the next section.

Estimating the Sex of Individuals (or the Probability that Individuals were Male)

In demographic terms, estimating the sex of an individual in fact means estimating the probability that an individual was a male, or the probability that an individual was a female. This is a different way of thinking about estimating sex compared to traditional osteological analyses. The results of an osteological analysis might identify individuals as male, probably male, possibly male, possibly female, probably female, female, and unknown or indeterminate. These are largely unquantifiable statements, as we have no way of knowing how much more likely a "probable male" was to have been male than would be the case for a "possible male." Instead of producing such qualitative sex estimates, we want to quantitatively estimate the probability that an individual was male.

The probability that the individual was female is then one minus the probability that they were male.

To illustrate the importance of estimating the sex ratio (the demographic parameter)—what we just did above—before generating individual sex estimates, imagine that we had followed tradition and charged headlong into estimating sex individually for each cranium in our target sample first. One way to do this is to use numbers directly from our original data, so that for each additional cranium we score as having a "male" brow, we would say that there is a $51/(51+16) = 0.7612$ chance that the individual was actually a male. But this is a classic inverse probability problem in that we are calculating probabilities given known sex that the brow will be "sexed" as "male," "indeterminate," or "female," when what we really want is the *probability of sex given our observation on the brow*. We could consequently apply Bayes' theorem:

$$P(M|"M") = \frac{P("M"|M)P(M)}{P("M"|M)P(M) + P("M"|F)P(F)},$$
(11.5)

where we use quotation marks to represent "brow sex" and unquoted characters to represent actual sex. $P(F)$ and $P(M)$ are the prior probabilities of being female versus male. We might assume that $P(M) = P(F) = 0.5$, (because we might assume that there is a 50/50 chance of a skeleton being male versus female) in which case the prior probabilities cancel and we have

$$P(M|"M") = \frac{P("M"|M)}{P("M"|M) + P("M"|F)}$$

$$= \frac{51/(51 + 4 + 5)}{51/(51 + 4 + 5) + 16/(16 + 6 + 32)}.$$
(11.6)

From Equation 11.6, the probability that a cranium was from a male if we decide that the brow $\pm$ "male" is 0.7415, which is slightly different $\pm$ the probability we estimated earlier (0.7612). Our estimate of the proportion of individuals who are male (p_m), which is also the prior probability that someone was male from our sample of 100 crania ($P(M)$), was 0.0982, so we should instead have

$$P(M|"M") = \frac{51/(51 + 4 + 5) \times 0.0982}{51/(51 + 4 + 5) \times 0.0982 + 16/(16 + 6 + 32) \times (1 - 0.0982)},$$
(11.7)

or 0.2380. Thus, the probability that an individual with a "male brow" ridge in our example was actually a male is 0.2380 and the probability that the same individual was female is 0.7620 (1−0.2380). The highly skewed sex ratio in favor of females in our example (target sample) has decreased the probability that an individual we classified as a "male" based on brow morphology was actually male. This all happened because our naïve assumption of a 50/50 sex ratio that led to Equation 11.6 was far off the mark. In fact, now that we have an estimate of the percentage of males in the target sample which is significantly less than 50%, when we see a male-looking brow in the target sample the individual is less likely to be an actual male than if they had come from a target sample where males were more common.

Simulating Data for Sex Ratio Estimation and Extending MLE to Other Traits

The example of 100 crania scored on brow morphology as 35 "male," 11 "indeterminate," and 54 "female" used above is a simulated dataset based on an ordinal categorical trait with three categories. The trait is femaleness of the brow, with "male" as the least female, "indeterminate" as intermediate, and "female" as the most female (or alternatively we could say maleness of the brow with "female" as the least male, "indeterminate" as intermediate, and "male" as the most male). We deterministically simulated this dataset by assuming that out of a sample of 100 crania 10 were from males and 90 were from females, so that we had

$$
\begin{bmatrix} 10 \\ 90 \end{bmatrix}
\begin{bmatrix} 51/60 & 16/54 \\ 4/60 & 6/54 \\ 5/60 & 32/54 \end{bmatrix}
=
\begin{bmatrix} 35.1667 \\ 10.6667 \\ 54.1667 \end{bmatrix}
\approx
\begin{bmatrix} 35 \\ 11 \\ 54 \end{bmatrix}.
\tag{11.8}
$$

Note that our estimated proportion of males (0.0982) is very close to the actual proportion (0.1). Had we not insisted on using integer counts for the number of crania, we would have precisely recovered the proportion of males.

The types of demographic analysis exemplified so far (estimation of the sex ratio and the probability of being male or female) can be extended to other single ordinal categorical traits by simple substitution. Extending this type of demographic analysis to multiple ordinal categorical traits generally requires adoption of a *cumulative probit model*, as discussed by Konigsberg and Hens (1998). But what about using measurements on one or more skeletal traits that display sexual dimorphism to estimate the sex ratio or the probability of being male or female?

To illustrate this, next we provide an example of a univariate (single) metric trait application using Black's (1978) published summary statistics for circumference of the femur at the midshaft from 63 males and 51 females from the Libben Site, Ohio. Among these 114 individuals who had been sexed on the basis of Phenice characteristics, the male mean femoral circumference was 63 ($\pm$ 4.1) millimeters and the female mean was 51 ($\pm$ 4.2), where the parenthetical terms give the standard deviations. Figure 11.1 shows these parameters as normal distributions. To simulate an example dataset we use the random normal generator in "R" and simulate data from 100 males and from 900 females using Black's means and standard deviations, with the simulated values rounded to the nearest millimeter.

A simple, albeit incorrect, method to estimate the sex ratio from this example dataset is to use the measurement halfway between the female and male means (51 and 63 mm, respectively) as a sectioning point (see Figure 11.1). Thus, we sex individuals with measurements below 57 mm as female, those above 57 mm as male, and divide those at 57 mm equally between male and female. From our simulated dataset 820 of the females have values below 57 mm, 29 are at 57 mm, and 51 are above 57 mm. For males 7 are below 57 mm, 3 are at 57 mm, and 90 are above 57 mm. Our estimated proportion of males in the sample using this (incorrect) method is $(51+14.5+1.5+90)/1000 = 0.157$, which is higher than the actual proportion of 0.1. Why did we overestimate the proportion of males?

The calculation of 57 mm as the sectioning point rested on two assumptions, only one of which is supportable. The first assumption is that the male and female standard deviations are equal, which they are nearly so. The second assumption is that the sex ratio is 1:1, which it is not. If we knew *a priori* that there was only one male for every nine females then we could solve

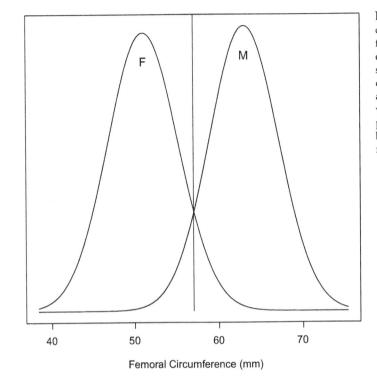

FIGURE 11.1 Normal densities for male and for female femoral circumferences (in millimeters). The summary statistics for drawing these two densities are from Black (1978), and the vertical line is the "sectioning point" (at 57 mm) that could be used to sex individuals as male versus female.

$$0.9 \times \phi(x, 51, 4.2) - 0.1 \times \phi(x, 63, 4.1) = 0, \qquad (11.9)$$

for the sectioning point x, in which case we find that the correct sectioning point should be 60.2, which we round down to 60 mm. Figure 11.2 shows a plot of this new situation. In Equation 11.9 the ϕ symbol is the normal density evaluated at point "x" with the specific mean and standard deviation. Using this new sectioning point, we find that 882 females have values less than 60 mm, 8 have a value of 60 mm, and 10 are above 60 mm. For males, 17 have values below 60 mm, 6 have a value of 60 mm, and 77 are above 60 mm. This gives our estimated proportion of males as $(4+10+3+77)/1000 = 0.094$, close to the correct value of 0.1. So we needed to have some form of information about the sex ratio *before* we ever began trying to sex individual femora. When we assumed a 50:50 sex ratio we got biased results in the application to a sample where the real ratio was 10:90.

Since we do not always have access to the correct proportion of males when conducting demographic analysis of actual skeletal data, MLE is a useful approach. The log-likelihood is

$$\ln LK = \sum_{i=1}^{N} \log(p_m \times \phi\{x_i, \ 63, 4.1\} + (1 - p_m) \times \phi\{x_i, \ 51, 4.2\}). \qquad (11.10)$$

Here, the proportion of males and proportion of females are each multiplied by a normal density based on the observed mean and standard deviation, instead of by a matrix of trait score probabilities as in the ordinal categorical case. Using "maxLik"

FIGURE 11.2 Normal densities for male and for female femoral circumferences (as in Figure 11.1), but with nine females to every one male. Note how this uneven sex ratio shifts the sectioning point up to 60.2 mm from the previous value of 57 mm.

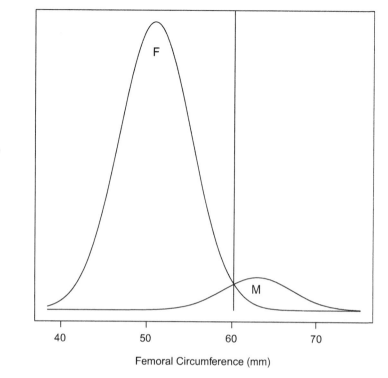

and "hessian" we find an estimated proportion of males of 0.1005 with a standard error of 0.0114. As with our previous example from the brow, we can now use Bayes' theorem to find the probability that an individual with a given measurement is male (or female):

$$P(M|x) = \frac{\phi\{x, 63, 4.1\} \times 0.1005}{\phi\{x, 63, 4.1\} \times 0.1005 \; + \; \phi\{x, 51, 4.2\} \times (1 - 0.1005)} \; . \tag{11.11}$$

For a measurement of 60.2 mm (which we saw was our correct sectioning point) the probability that the individual was a male is 0.4996, or essentially 0.5. This is the 50:50 that we would expect for someone at the proper sectioning point. In contrast, for a measurement of 57 mm (our original sectioning point) the probability that the individual was a male is 0.0981. Again, if this were the correct sectioning point the probability that an individual was male at this measurement should be 0.5.

ESTIMATION OF AGE AND OF THE AGE-AT-DEATH STRUCTURE

In the past, analysis of the age-at-death structure in skeletal samples rested on the construction of life tables from counts of individuals (or deaths) within particular age indicator states. Then in the 1980s and 1990s, scholars began cross-tabulating one or more age indicators in a target sample against age categories in a reference sample in order to esti- mate proportions of deaths by age category for the target, in what we (Konigsberg and Frankenberg, 2002) have called "contingency table paleodemography." Although there have been major new developments in these methods (Bocquet-Appel and Masset, 1996; Eshed et al., 2004; Bonneuil, 2005; Bocquet-Appel and Bacro, 2008; Caussinus and Cour- geau, 2010) the explicit use of hazard models (see section below) has increased (Boldsen et al., 2002; Hoppa and Vaupel, 2002b; Konisgberg and Herrmann, 2002; Müller et al., 2002; Wood et al., 2002; DeWitte and Wood, 2008; Gage, 2010; Redfern and DeWitte, 2011) and is starting to supplant life tables. We focus here on the estimation of age-at-death and of the parameters of hazard models, leaving coverage of life tables to a previous publi- cation (Frankenberg and Konigsberg, 2006).

Hazard Models

Hazard models are a class of statistical models that specify the time until particular events occur. In our case, the event of interest is the death of individuals, and so the times until the events (deaths) are the ages-at-death. Hazard models are simply a tool that can be used to represent a continuous age-at-death distribution using a relatively small number of param- eters, where the parameters are numbers that characterize the age-at-death distribution. We start with the simplest of possible models: an exponential hazard. In the exponential hazard model the survivorship to age t is

$$S(t|\lambda) \;=\; \exp(-\lambda t), \tag{11.12}$$

where λ is the instantaneous hazard of death (risk of dying), which is constant across age. This is a completely unreasonable model for most human mortality, but it serves as a good starting point. Note that at age zero we have the exponentiation of zero, which is one, so the survivorship at the initial age is 1.0. The distribution of ages-at-death will be

$$f(t|\lambda) \;=\; \lambda \exp(-\lambda t). \tag{11.13}$$

As the example in this section we will use a hazard of $\lambda = 0.34$. (There is no logic behind choosing this particular value except that 34 is LWK's favorite number.) In the exponential hazard model the mean age-at-death is $1/\lambda$ while the median age-at-death is $\ln(2)/\lambda$, so we have about three years for the mean age-at-death and about two years for the median age-at-death. Again, this is a completely unreasonable model for human mortality, but if you persevere we will get to more reasonable models.

Figure 11.3 shows a simulation of 10,000 deaths from the exponential hazard model, where the histogram represents the simulated ages-at-death and the dashed curve is the expected distribution given the hazard parameter of 0.34. The exponential hazard model represents a constant hazard of death, and as such the hazard does not change across age. This model is sometimes used to represent a constant "baseline" hazard in a five- parameter model known as the Siler model (Siler, 1979; Gage and Dyke, 1986). The Siler model has three components of mortality: (1) juvenile mortality represented by a negative **Gompertz model**, (2) senescent (old-age) mortality represented by a positive Gompertz model, and (3) a baseline age-independent hazard represented by the exponential model.

FIGURE 11.3 Simulation of 10,000 deaths from an exponential hazard model where the hazard is 0.34. The histogram shows the "binned" ages from the simulation, while the dashed line shows the **probability density function** for age-at-death when the hazard is equal to 0.34.

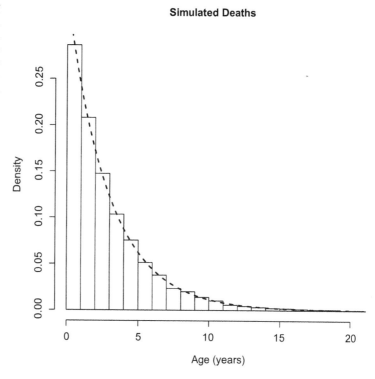

The five parameters in the Siler model consist of one parameter for the baseline hazard, two parameters (the magnitude and rate of decline) for juvenile mortality, and two parameters (the magnitude and rate of increase) for senescent mortality. Figure 11.4 shows the hazard for each of the three mortality components and for total mortality (the dashed line) for Coale and Demeny's (1983) Model West 1 life table for females plotted on a logarithmic scale. On a logarithmic scale each of the components of mortality will be a straight line, with the immature component decreasing with age, the senescent component increasing with age, and the baseline hazard staying constant with age. For a quick read of Figure 11.4, note where the immature and senescent component lines cross at about six years of age. At this point both components have small values so that the total hazard is only slightly above the baseline hazard. At young ages the total hazard is "driven" by the immature component of mortality, while at advanced ages the total mortality is "driven" by the senescent component of mortality.

Our first task in the estimation of age structure for target sample populations is to simulate individual ages-at-death based on the hazard model. Note that we are NOT yet estimating individual ages-at-death in the skeletal sample. Instead, we are creating (numerically generating) a test case against which we will ultimately compare the observed data. "R" has a few hazard models, such as the exponential and the Weibull (another model not discussed here) that can be directly simulated (using "rexp" and "rweibull," respectively), and that use the inversion method to simulate values. This inversion method can

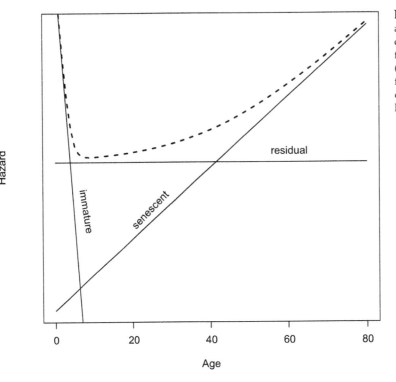

FIGURE 11.4 Log hazards for each of the three components in a Siler model fit to Coale and Demeney's (1983) Model West 1 for females. The unlabeled dashed line is the total log hazard.

also be used to simulate hazard models not available in "R." To use inversion, we simulate survivorship values and then "look these up" to see what ages they translate into. This "looking up" of ages forms the inversion step, since we are simulating survivorship and converting it to age, rather than following the actual process where one's survivorship depends on both age and random events. If U is a random uniform number (i.e., a random number that is uniformly distributed such that $0 < U \leq 1$), then we can solve Equation 11.12 for age to find that

$$t = -\frac{\ln(U)}{\lambda}.$$

(11.14)

Equation 11.14 was used to simulate the ages in Figure 11.3, although the function "rexp" in "R" could be used directly. For single component hazard models such as the Gompertz model, one can also solve the **survivorship function** for age in order to simulate ages. The Gompertz model has survivorship to age t of

$$S(t) = \exp(a_3/b_3 (1 - \exp(b_3 t))),$$

(11.15)

where we number the a and b parameters with a "3" to represent the third component of mortality in the Siler model. Equation 11.15 can be solved for age at a given survivorship, just as we did for the exponential hazard, so that ages at death can be simulated from

$$t = \ln(1 - b_3 \ln(U)/a_3)/b_3. \qquad (11.16)$$

Multiple component models do not generally have explicit solutions, but one can solve the survivorship numerically using "uniroot" in "R." Figure 11.5 shows the results of simulating 10,000 deaths from a combined negative and positive Gompertz model that Nagaoka et al. (2006) fit to a Medieval Japanese archaeological skeletal collection. For completeness, Figure 11.5 also shows the hazard function, the survivorship function, and the age-at-death distribution from the hazard model.

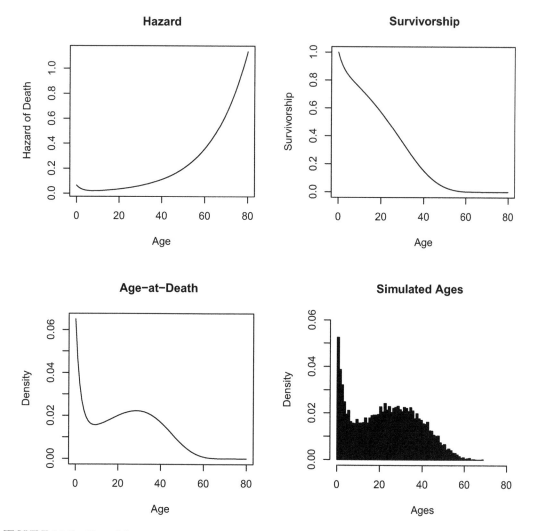

FIGURE 11.5 Hazard function, survivorship function, and probability density function (for age-at-death) from a negative and positive Gompertz model taken from Nagaoka et al.'s (2006) analysis of a Medieval Japanese archaeological skeletal collection. The final panel shows a simulation of 10,000 deaths from the modeled distribution.

This section on simulating ages-at-death may seem excessive, but the ability to simulate ages-at-death is a useful tool for demonstrating, and particularly for testing, demographic methods. While simulations can always be criticized for being unrealistic, they have the advantage that we can control various aspects of the data production so that in the end we can compare our analysis to the results we "should have gotten" given that we know the way that the data were simulated. In the next section we examine the simulation of "age indicators" in order to produce test cases for demographic analysis. To keep the example simple, we use only the exponential hazard model and limit it to immature individuals, specifically children ages 0 to 12 years. While age estimation at the younger ages is generally not problematic, the simulations and methods we present can be used in applications for older individuals.

Simulating Long Bone Growth

We use quotation marks around the term "age indicators," because we need to decouple the processes of growth and development and of progressive skeletal change in adults from the idea of "indicators," particularly when dealing with senescent processes. There is a long history of using skeletal markers or indicators as predictors for age-at-death, and a consequent tendency for researchers to use models that make age dependent on the markers or skeletal variables. Bocquet-Appel and Masset (1982) point out the error in this approach for ordered skeletal traits (such as Todd phases), and Aykroyd et al. (1999) and Konigsberg et al. (1997) point out the problem for continuous traits. The idea that age is the dependent variable (rather than the skeletal variables being the dependent variables depending on age) is logically inconsistent, and runs counter to studies of growth and development (McCammon, 1970; Roche et al., 1988; Cameron, 2002). For children it is very unusual to see age treated as the dependent variable, although a few publications do present regressions of fetal gestational ages in weeks on long bone lengths (Scheuer et al., 1980; Sherwood et al., 2000).

In order to simulate records for children between birth and 12 years of age, we chose length of the femur diaphysis as an "age indicator," and drew summary data from Maresh's (1970) radiographic longitudinal growth study. From his study we use the means and standard deviations of bone lengths for males observed at two months, four months, six months, and then at six month intervals up until age 12 years (these are given in Maresh's Table F-7). In order to simulate bone lengths at any given age on a continuum, we need to smooth Maresh's tabular interval data. We accomplish this using fractional polynomials, which do not require the powers in the polynomial to be integers and which can produce simpler equations (Royston and Altman, 1994; Sauerbrei et al., 2006). Polynomial regression is a commonly applied tool that can be used to fit long bone length to powers of age. As an example, Figure 11.6 shows a third-degree polynomial that regresses long bone length on age, the square of age, and the cube of age as a dashed line, and the fractional polynomial as a solid line, both fit to the means from Maresh. While the dashed line appears to fit reasonably well, the solid line also fits well.

In the case of the Maresh data, the best fitting fractional polynomial model is femur length $= 3.6 + 9.78\sqrt{age}$, so the power is 0.5. The best fitting fractional polynomial model for the standard deviations from Maresh is actually the linear model, resulting in

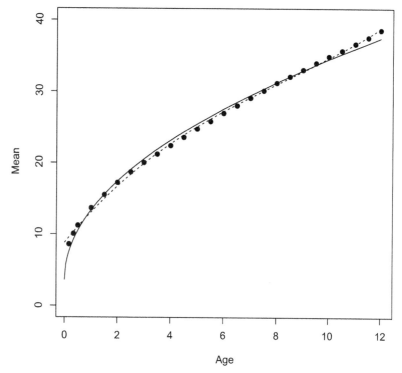

FIGURE 11.6 Plot of mean femoral length against age in boys. The filled points are from Maresh's (1970) radiographic study, the dashed line was fit as a third-degree polynomial, and the solid line was fit using fractional polynomials.

standard deviation $= 0.52 + 0.11 \times$ age. Figure 11.7 shows a plot of the mean femur length plus and minus two standard deviations as a continuous curve from birth to age 12 years. To simulate long bone lengths based on the hazard model age-at-death structure, we simulate 250 deaths from the exponential hazard model with the hazard parameter equal to 0.34. We then take the simulated age-at-death for each "individual" in this dataset and simulate a femur length using a draw from a normal distribution with the mean and standard deviation predicted for the given age.

Estimating the Age-at-Death Structure

To estimate the age-at-death structure of an actual skeletal sample we write the log-likelihood for obtaining the observed (or in our case, simulated) femur length data conditional on the exponential hazard parameter. For an individual femur length (FL) measurement the point probability of getting that measurement conditional on the exponential hazard parameter is

$$f(FL|\lambda) = \int_t \phi(FL|age)\, \lambda \exp(-\lambda age), \tag{11.17}$$

where the integration is across age, for which we use a lower limit of $\exp(-10)$, which is approximately 4.5×10^{-5} years and an upper limit of $\exp(3.4)$ or approximately 30 years.

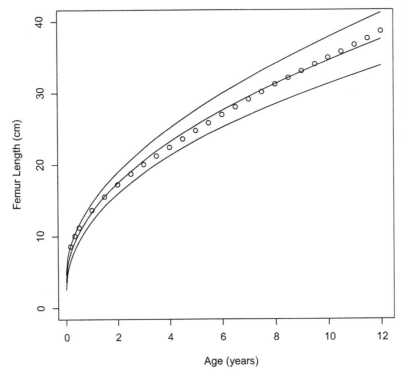

FIGURE 11.7 Plot of the predicted mean femoral length plus and minus two standard deviations across age. The open points are as in Figure 11.6, while the lines for the mean and plus and minus two standard deviations were drawn using fractional polynomials.

We treat age in the logarithmic scale and then exponentiate within the likelihood function itself to reduce numerical difficulties in calculating the likelihood. The integral across age is easily handled using the "integrate" function in "R."

From the individual likelihoods we can write the total log-likelihood as

$$\sum_{i=1}^{250} \ln(f(FL_i|\lambda)). \qquad (11.18)$$

We again use "maxLik" in "R" to find the maximum likelihood estimate (and its error) for the exponential hazard parameter. This results in an estimated exponential hazard parameter of 0.3451 with a standard error of 0.0220. Figure 11.8 shows a Kaplan–Meier plot (Kaplan and Meier, 1958) of the survivorship from the actual (albeit simulated) ages-at-death and the 95% confidence intervals for survivorship estimated from the simulated femur length data. The fit is good, which is to be expected given that we used the same models and assumptions to simulate and analyze the data. Specifically, we simulated the deaths under an exponential hazard and analyzed the simulated femoral length data assuming that the mortality could be modeled using an exponential hazard. We also simulated growth and then used the same underlying equations to model growth.

In an actual analysis of a skeletal sample we will not know the true underlying form of the hazard of death against age, we may run the risk of applying growth standards that are not appropriate for the given sample, and we certainly will not have access to the true ages. For

FIGURE 11.8 Kaplan–Meier plot (Kaplan and Meier, 1958) of the survivorship from 250 simulated ages-at-death (solid line step function) and the 95% confidence intervals for survivorship estimated from the simulated femur length data (dashed smooth curves).

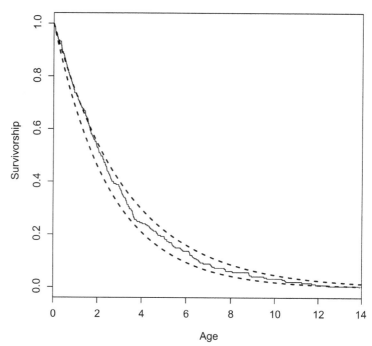

Simulation of 250 Immature Deaths

these reasons, it is important to assess the goodness of fit between functions empirically generated from observed skeletal data and those from the fitted model. As an example, consider the goodness of fit between the empirical cumulative density for the femur lengths (that we simulated) and the cumulative density that our estimated parameter(s) in the hazard model implies. The empirical cumulative density function is just a step function that rises by $1/n$ at each value of, in this case, sorted femoral length. From Equation 11.17 we can write the modeled cumulative density function (cdf) for femoral length as

$$cdf(FL) = \int_{x=0}^{FL} f(x|\lambda). \tag{11.19}$$

Figure 11.9 shows the empirical cumulative density function and the modeled one from Equation 11.19. The fit appears quite good in this example for the same reasons as in the preceding paragraph.

Estimating the Ages-at-Death

As with estimating the sex of individuals following estimation of the sex ratio, we often want to estimate individual ages-at-death after estimating the age-at-death structure. We first approach this as a problem in point age estimation, where we want to estimate the most likely

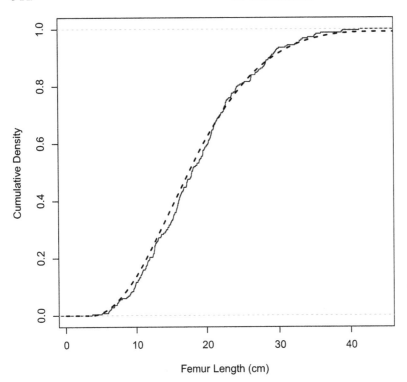

FIGURE 11.9 Comparison of the empirical cumulative density function for 250 simulated femoral lengths (shown as a solid line step function) and the modeled cumulative density shown as a dashed line.

age-at-death for each individual given the estimated age-at-death structure and the "age indicators." We do this using Bayes' theorem as follows:

$$f(age|FL, \lambda) \propto \phi(FL|age)f(age|\lambda), \tag{11.20}$$

where the symbol $\propto$ means proportional to rather than equal to. In Equation 11.20 the first term on the right-hand side is the normal density for femur length given age (see Figure 11.6) and the second term is from Equation 11.13. Given femur length, we then search across Equation 11.20 to find the maximum density, which gives the best estimate of age for the individual based on what we know about the age-at-death structure from the exponential hazard model.

In Figure 11.10 we have plotted these age estimates for femur lengths of $8 - 20$ cm in 1 cm increments and of $20 - 40$ cm in 1 mm increments. We again use fractional polynomials to fit a curve that allows us to quickly estimate age from any given femur length. The equation for this curve is $age = \exp(-3.542 - 13.464/FL + 1.748 \times \log(FL))$ and is shown as a solid line. This line runs entirely through the plotted points. Another possibility is to solve the regression of femur length on age from the Maresh data ($FL = 3.6 + 9.78\sqrt{age}$) for age, in which case we get $age = 0.1355 - 0.0753 \times FL + 0.0104 \times FL^2$, plotted as a second solid line in

FIGURE 11.10 Plot of age estimates against femur lengths. The individual points are shown at centimeter intervals of femoral lengths from 8 to 20 cm and at millimeter intervals from 20 to 40 cm. There is one solid line shown that passes entirely through the points and is from a fractional polynomial fit. The additional line that departs from the points at greater femur lengths is from solving the regression of femur length on age.

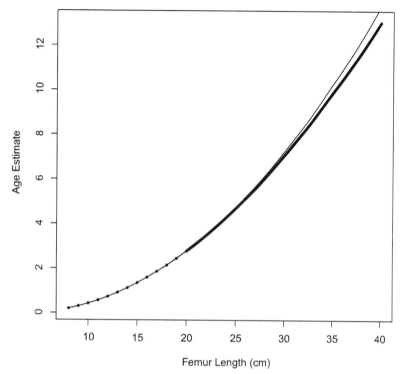

Figure 11.10. These two lines are very similar, because the majority of information on age is coming from the femur length. However, the line from inverting the Maresh equation departs at longer femoral lengths because the prior density $(f(t|\lambda))$ provides relatively little information at later ages.

Obtaining simple point estimates for individual ages-at-death ignores the fact that these ages are not precisely known, but are instead estimated with some uncertainty. We can, and should, recover the uncertainty in these age estimates. In place of Equation 11.20 we can write the density function for age-at-death as

$$f(age|FL, \lambda) = \frac{\phi(FL|age)f(age|\lambda)}{\int_{t=0}^{\omega} \phi(FL|t)f(t|\lambda)}, \tag{11.21}$$

where ω represents the maximum age we are willing to consider. The variance of age-at-death given a femur length (and the estimated exponential hazard parameter) can be found numerically as

$$\int_{t=0}^{\omega} f(t|FL, \lambda) \times (t - \mu)^2, \tag{11.22}$$

where μ is the best estimate of age from Equation 11.20. We have plotted the square roots of the variances from Equation 11.22 as individual points connected by a solid line in Figure 11.11, which looks very much like Figure 11.10. The fractional polynomial fit to these points, shown as a dashed line in Figure 11.11, gives us a standard error of the estimate of age as equal to $\exp(-7.647 + 2.145\sqrt{FL} - 0.238\sqrt{FL} \times \log(FL))$. We then use these standard errors to calculate 95% confidence intervals for ages-at-death, following the same procedure as with sex ratio confidence intervals.

Figure 11.12 plots the 95% confidence intervals for age-at-death given femur length. Although these intervals should include 95% of the data or about 238 out of 250 individuals, they actually include only 92% of the data, or 230 of 250 cases. Additionally, the 50% confidence interval, which should include 125 individuals, actually includes 51.6% of the data or 129 cases. This type of wobble is to be expected for relatively small sample sizes, and it is important in these cases to assess whether or not the calculated confidence intervals are themselves reliable. We do this by examining the coverage for the sample at all possible confidence limits. Figure 11.13 shows a plot of the actual coverage versus the stated coverage for the 250 individuals in the simulated sample. The stated coverage is simply the claimed confidence interval, formed from percentage values of 1/250, 2/250, 3/250 ... 249/225, 250/250 and shown in this graph as a diagonal line of identity. The actual coverage is the number of cases (counted up and converted into a percentage) that fall within the stated confidence

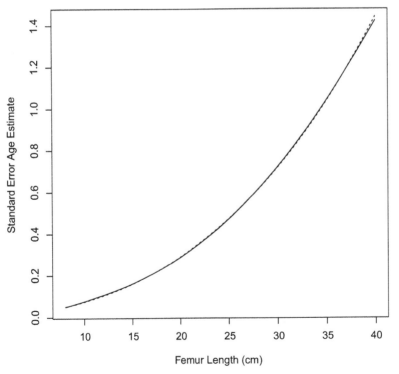

FIGURE 11.11 Plot of standard error of age estimates against femur length. The solid line is from the calculation, while the dashed line is a fractional polynomial fit to the calculated values.

FIGURE 11.12 Plot of 250 simulated ages against femoral lengths. The solid lines show the 95% confidence intervals for age estimates, which contain 230 of 250 cases (92% of the data).

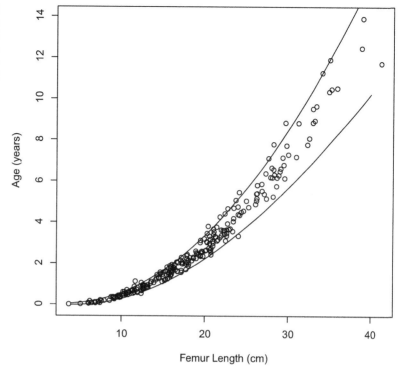

Femur Length (cm)

limits, plotted in Figure 11.13 as a step function. Based on the comparison of stated and actual coverage, the wobble in the calculated 95% confidence intervals is negligible.

WHAT SEX RATIOS AND AGE-AT-DEATH STRUCTURES CAN TELL US ABOUT PAST POPULATIONS

This chapter provides tools for estimating the sex ratio and age-at-death distribution for a skeletal sample using reference information and demographic models prior to estimating individual sex or age-at-death. Conducting the analyses in this order allows you to generate probabilities and reliability estimates for the skeletal data relative to what is known or expected for the relationship between osteological indicators and sex and/or age. The examples amply demonstrate that relying on individual sex estimates and "age indicators" from the skeletal sample to initially generate the demographic parameters (treating skeletal "sex estimates" or "age indicators" as known) will produce incorrect results. Following the course prescribed above also gives you the analytical basis on which to make a broad range of biologically and culturally based demographic comparisons as we outline below.

Skeletal biology has long contained elements of both a descriptive and an analytical science, although much of earlier skeletal biology was relegated to simple osteological descriptions in the appendices to various reports, as Buikstra (1991) notes. Current skeletal

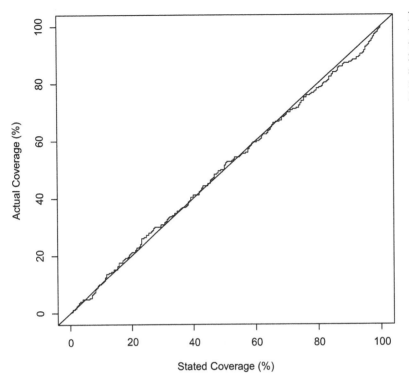

FIGURE 11.13 Plot of the actual coverage versus the stated coverage for the 250 individuals in the simulated sample (step function line). The diagonal line is the line of identity.

biology analyses that appear purely descriptive on the surface typically have some comparative basis, and are consequently analytically oriented. For example, attempting to estimate the sex ratio for neonatal skeletons using DNA methods may begin as a descriptive endeavor, but comparing the results to an expected sex ratio for perinatal deaths of near 1:1 and finding a large departure warrants some explanation and further analysis. Alternatively, researchers might begin with a hypothesis that a past population may have been practicing sex-biased infanticide or differential neglect, as for example in Faerman et al. (1998). Other studies with a stronger comparative and thus analytical bent include Andrushko et al.'s (2010) work on "trophy victims" (i.e., individuals who had body parts removed at or near death during warfare) from prehistoric central California. This study, which demonstrated that 50% of trophy victims were young adults (18–25 years old) whereas only 17.6% of individuals from the remainder of the skeletal sample died as young adults, would have had a much stronger inferential basis if the entire age-at-death structure for trophy victims and for the general skeletal sample had been estimated. Although it is beyond the level of this chapter, the method of maximum likelihood can be used in a fairly straightforward manner to develop tests of whether two or more age-at-death structures differ substantially, allowing inferences into why or why not.

Because the demographic structure for populations is fundamentally related to so many factors, estimation of sex ratios and/or age-at-death structure should be an integral part of a complete skeletal biological analysis. For example, DeWitte and Wood (2008) have attempted to relate aspects of the age-at-death structure to the presence of the Black Death (bubonic plague) while Redfern and DeWitte (2011) have examined the effect of "Romanization" on age-at-death structures. Although the analyses become increasingly more difficult as one pushes further back in time, there is now research and lively debate over the origins of modern human mortality based on data from Australopithecines through modern humans (Caspari and Lee, 2004, 2006; Hawkes and McConnell, 2005; Minichillo, 2005). Bocquet-Appel and Arsuaga (1999) have presented evidence that two important Neandertal skeletal samples represent mortality from catastrophes rather than from ordinary accretional deaths. Such findings are important, because they alter our views about the representational nature of skeletal assemblages. On a more recent scale, Bocquet-Appel (2002) and Bocquet-Appel and Naji (2006) have examined the demographic transition that occurred with the Neolithic transition. All these studies demonstrate the need for, and benefit of, integrating demographic analyses into skeletal biology research.

WHAT ROLE CAN SEX RATIOS AND AGE-AT-DEATH STRUCTURES PLAY IN FORENSIC ANTHROPOLOGY?

This chapter has primarily focused on paleodemography, and as such we have had nothing yet to say about the role of sex ratios and age-at-death structure in forensic anthropology. On the surface, it would not appear that demography plays any particular role in forensic anthropology. Why would we want to estimate the sex ratio and/or the age-at-death structure in a forensic setting? In fact, demographic analysis can be vitally important in the forensic setting. To look at the role that demography can play in forensic anthropology we need to consider two different settings. Konigsberg and colleagues (Konigsberg et al., 2006, 2008, 2009; Steadman et al., 2006) have referred to these two different settings as a problem in estimation versus a problem in building evidence for identification of an individual. We begin with a brief discussion of the estimation problem and then turn to a discussion of the evidentiary problem.

The estimation problem is the one that traditionally was handled by an osteologist who would build a biological description that might aid in the eventual identification of the individual from a missing persons list. Where the demographic analysis is concerned, the osteologist would estimate the age-at-death and sex from the remains. But here we need to be careful to separate the acts of observing, scoring, and possibly measuring the bones and teeth from the actual act of estimating the age-at-death and sex of the remains. Steadman and Konigsberg (2009) discuss "the problem of bias" that can arise if an osteologist enters into their analysis with prior knowledge about the case. If the osteologist has been told by law enforcement "we think these are the bones of a particular missing person who was 34 years old," then this can no doubt influence the osteologist. So the osteologist must make their basic observations blind to any possible identification. But once an osteologist has made their basic observations then the context of the case becomes very important. Note that the use of Bayes' theorem (such as in Equations 11.5, 11.11, and 11.20) required prior demographic information, and this prior information must come from the context of the case.

The evidentiary process also should proceed with the osteologist blind to any prior information when they do their basic data collection, but once again the contextual information becomes vitally important in completing the analysis. The evidentiary problem should always proceed by calculating what is referred to as a **likelihood ratio**. A likelihood ratio in this setting is just the probability of getting the observed data if a putative identification is correct divided by the probability of getting the observed data if the putative identification is incorrect. How one calculates the probabilities contained in the likelihood ratio is beyond the scope of this chapter, but Steadman and colleagues (2006) provide a worked example. Their example is for what could be referred to as an "open" population setting, in that if the identification was incorrect then they must consider the "population at large" to find the probability in the denominator. Defining the "population at large" is indeed problematic. In a "closed" population setting (see Hackman (2009) for a good description of "open" versus "closed" populations), as for example in a plane crash where the flight manifest enumerates everyone, the denominator probability is much less problematic. The first author of this chapter is currently producing a worked example of an application to such a "closed" population setting.

CONCLUSION: WRAPPING IT UP

The paleodemographic world is certainly much more complicated than when the first author of this chapter published his first journal article (Konigsberg, 1985) over half a lifetime ago. That paper on the paleodemography of a classic Ohio Hopewell site violated just about every proscription we have written here and even (shudder) included the use of life tables. The paper also included a "Table 1" that gave individual age estimates "ahead" of doing any demographic analysis, precisely what we have argued against doing in this chapter. But with the benefit of increasing age, and the possible accumulation of wisdom, how would we approach a paleodemographic analysis now and what would we recommend to others who undertake this endeavor?

The simple answer to this question, unfortunately, is not simple. Life tables can be conveniently calculated within computer spreadsheets and even hazard models can be fit to life table type data within such spreadsheets[4]. However, the vast majority of the methods we have described in this chapter cannot be easily handled either within spreadsheets or using standard statistical analysis packages. Dr. Darryl Holman at the University of Washington-Seattle has long provided his program "mle," which is a workhorse for fitting models to demographic data[5]. Dr. Jesper Boldsen's software for transition analysis (ADBOU), an advanced technique we have not described here, has recently been made available for downloading from the web from Dr. George Milner's website.[6] One of the common opinions voiced at a number of workshops on paleodemographic methods at the Max Planck Institute for Demographic Research in Rostock, Germany is that any methods under development

[4]See https://netfiles.uiuc.edu/lylek/www/LibbenHaz.xlsx for an example of both.

[5]The software and manuals are freely available from http://faculty.washington.edu/djholman/mle/index.html.

[6]http://www.anthro.psu.edu/projects_labs/bioarch/bioarch_lab.shtml.

would need to be supported by easily available and easy to use software. Unfortunately, a decade has now passed since the publication of the "Rostock volume" (Hoppa and Vaupel, 2002a) and with the exception of the ADBOU software, we are not substantially further along in terms of having the software tools necessary to do paleodemography. This is an area open for contribution.

Our discussion in this chapter has made clear the importance of the demographic approach for questions in skeletal biology, especially those pertaining to age and sex estimations. While it may seem overwhelming, with hard work, sweat of the brow, and learning some "R" and some math (especially calculus), any current or aspiring skeletal biologist can learn how to incorporate demographic methods into their research program.

REFERENCES

Andrushko, V.A., Schwitalla, A.W., Walker, P.L., 2010. Trophy taking and dismemberment as warfare strategies in prehistoric central California. American Journal of Physical Anthropology 141 (1), 83—96.

Arnay-de-la-Rosa, M., González-Reimers, E., Fregel, R., Velasco-Vázquez, J., Delgado-Darias, T., González, A.M., Larruga, J.M., 2007. Canary Islands aboriginal sex determination based on mandible parameters contrasted by amelogenin analysis. Journal of Archaeological science 34 (9), 1515—1522.

Aykroyd, R.G., Lucy, D., Pollard, A.M., Roberts, C.A., 1999. Nasty, brutish, but not necessarily short: a reconsideration of the statistical methods used to calculate age at death from adult Human skeletal and dental age indicators. American Antiquity 64 (1), 55—70.

Black III, T.K., 1978. A new method for assessing sex of fragmentary skeletal remains: femoral shaft circumference. American Journal of Physical Anthropology 48 (2), 227—232.

Bocquet-Appel, J.-P., 1994. Estimating the average for an unknown age distribution in anthropology. In: Borgognini-Tarli, S., Di Bacco, M., Pacciani, E. (Eds.), Statistical Tools in Human Biology. World Scientific, Singapore, pp. 197—202.

Bocquet-Appel, J.-P., 2002. Paleoanthropological traces of a Neolithic demographic transition. Current Anthropology 43 (4), 637—650.

Bocquet-Appel, J.-P., Arsuaga, J.L., 1999. Age distributions of hominid samples at Atapuerca (SH) and Krapina could indicate accumulation by catastrophe. Journal of Archaeological Science 26 (3), 327—338.

Bocquet-Appel, J.-P., Bacro, J.N., 1997. Brief communication: Estimates of some demographic parameters in a Neolithic rock-cut chamber (approximately 2000 BC) using iterative techniques for aging and demographic estimators. American Journal of Physical Anthropology 102 (4), 569—575.

Bocquet-Appel, J.-P., Bacro, J.N., 2008. Estimation of its confidence intervals using an iterative Bayesian procedure and a bootstrap sampling approach. In: Bocquet-Appel, J.-P. (Ed.), Recent Advances in Paleodemography. Springer, Dordrecht, pp. 63—82.

Bocquet-Appel, J.-P., Masset, C., 1982. Farewell to paleodemography. Journal of Human Evolution 11, 321—333.

Bocquet-Appel, J.-P., Masset, C., 1996. Paleodemography: expectancy and false hope. American Journal of Physical Anthropology 99, 571—583.

Bocquet-Appel, J.-P., Naji, S., 2006. Testing the hypothesis of a worldwide Neolithic demographic transition. Current Anthropology 47 (2), 341—365.

Boldsen, J.L., Milner, G.R., Konigsberg, L.W., Wood, J.M., 2002. Transition analysis: a new method for estimating age from skeletons. In: Hoppa, R.D., Vaupel, J.W. (Eds.), Paleodemography: Age Distributions from Skeletal Samples. Cambridge University Press, New York, pp. 73—106.

Bonneuil, N., 2005. Fitting to a distribution of deaths by age with application to paleodemography: the route closest to a stable population. Current Anthropology 46, 29—45.

Buikstra, J.E., 1991. Out of the appendix and into the dirt: comments on thirteen years of bioarchaeological research. In: Powell, M.L., Bridges, P.S., Mires, A.M.W. (Eds.), What Mean These Bones? University of Alabama Press, Tuscaloosa, AL, pp. 172—188.

Cameron, N. (Ed.), 2002. Human Growth and Development. Academic Press, San Diego, CA.

Caspari, R., Lee, S.H., 2004. Older age becomes common late in human evolution. Proceedings of the National Academy of Sciences 101 (30), 10895−10900.

Caspari, R., Lee, S.H., 2006. Is human longevity a consequence of cultural change or modern biology? American Journal of Physical Anthropology 129 (4), 512−517.

Caussinus, H., Courgeau, D., Mandelbaum, J., 2010. Estimating age without measuring it: a new method in paleodemography. Population-E 65 (1), 117−144.

Coale, A.J., Demeny, P., 1983. Regional Model Tables and Stable Populations, 2nd ed. Academic Press, New York.

De La Cruz, I., González-Oliver, A., Kemp, B.M., Román, J.A., Smith, D.G., Torre-Blanco, A., 2008. Sex identification of children sacrificed to the ancient Aztec rain gods in Tlatelolco. Current Anthropology 49 (3), 519−526.

DeWitte, S.N., Wood, J.W., 2008. Selectivity of Black Death mortality with respect to preexisting health. Proceedings of the National Academy of Sciences 105 (5), 1436−1441.

Eshed, V., Gopher, A., Gage, T.B., Hershkovitz, I., 2004. Has the transition to agriculture reshaped the demographic structure of prehistoric populations? New evidence from the Levant. American Journal of Physical Anthropology 124 (4), 315−329.

Faerman, M., Bar-Gal, G.K., Filon, D., Greenblatt, C.L., Stager, L., Oppenheim, A., Smith, P., 1998. Determining the sex of infanticide victims from the late Roman era through ancient DNA analysis. Journal of Archaeological Science 25 (9), 861−865.

Frankenberg, S.R., Konigsberg, L.W., 2006. A brief history of paleodemography from Hooton to hazards analysis. In: Buikstra, J.E., Beck, L.A. (Eds.), Bioarchaeology: The Contextual Analysis of Human Remains. Elsevier, New York, pp. 227−261.

Gage, T.B., 2010. Demographic estimation: indirect techniques for anthropological populations. In: Larsen, C.S. (Ed.), A Companion to Biological Anthropology. Wiley-Blackwell, New York, pp. 179−193.

Gage, T.B., Dyke, B., 1986. Parameterizing abridged mortality tables tables: The Siler three-component hazard model. Human Biology 58 (2), 275−291.

Gibbon, V., Paximadis, M., Strkalj, G., Ruff, P., Penny, C., 2009. Novel methods of molecular sex identification from skeletal tissue using the amelogenin gene. Forensic Science International: Genetics 3 (2), 74−79.

Hackman, L., 2009. DVI and anatomy. Axis: The Online Journal of CAHId 1 (2), 26−40.

Hawkes, K., O'Connell, J.F., 2005. How old is human longevity? Journal of Human Evolution 49 (5), 650−653

Hoppa, R.D., Vaupel, J.W., 2002a. Paleodemography: Age Distribution from Skeletal Samples. Cambridge University Press, New York.

Hoppa, R.D., Vaupel, J.W., 2002b. The Rostock manifesto for paleodemography: the way from stage to age. In: Hoppa, R.D., Vaupel, J.W. (Eds.), Paleodemography: Age Distributions from Skeletal Samples. Cambridge University Press, New York, pp. 1−8.

Hummel, S., Herrmann, B., 1991. Y-chromosome-specific DNA amplified in ancient human bone. Naturwissenschaften 78 (6), 266−267.

Jackes, M., 1992. Paleodemography: Problems and techniques. In: Saunders, S.R., Katzenberg, M.A. (Eds.), Skeletal Biology of Past Peoples: Research Methods. Wiley-Liss, New York, pp. 189−224.

Kaplan, E.L., Meier, P., 1958. Nonparametric estimation from incomplete observations. Journal of the American Statistical Association 53, 457−481.

Kelley, M.A., 1978. Phenice's visual sexing technique for the os pubis: a critique. American Journal of Physical Anthropology 48 (1), 121−122.

Konigsberg, L.W., 1985. Demography and mortuary practice at Seip Mound One. Midcontinental Journal of Archaeology 10 (1), 123−148.

Konigsberg, L.W., Frankenberg, S.R., 1992. Estimation of age structure in anthropological demography. American Journal of Physical Anthropology 89 (2), 235−256.

Konigsberg, L.W., Frankenberg, S.R., 1994. Paleodemography: not quite dead. Evolutionary Anthropology 3 (3), 92−105.

Konigsberg, L.W., Frankenberg, S.R., 2002. Deconstructing death in paleodemography. American Journal of Physical Anthropology 117 (4), 297−309.

Konigsberg, L.W., Hens, S.M., 1998. Use of ordinal categorical variables in skeletal assessment of sex from the cranium. American Journal of Physical Anthropology 107 (1), 97−112.

Konigsberg, L.W., Herrmann, N.P., 2002. Markov chain Monte Carlo estimation of hazard model parameters in paleodemography. In: Hoppa, R.D., Vaupel, J.W. (Eds.), Paleodemography: Age Distributions from Skeletal Samples. Cambridge University Press, New York, pp. 222–242.

Konigsberg, L.W., Frankenberg, S.R., Walker, R.B., 1997. Regress what on what? Paleodemographic age estimation as a calibration problem. In: Paine, R.R. (Ed.), Integrating Archaeological Demography: Multidisciplinary Approaches to Prehistoric Population. SIU Press, Carbondale, IL, pp. 64–88.

Konigsberg, L.W., Herrmann, N.P., Wescott, D.J., 2002. Commentary on: McBride DG, Dietz MJ, Vennemeyer MT, Meadors SA, Benfer RA, Furbee NL. Bootstrap methods for sex determination from the os coxae using the ID3 algorithm. Journal of Forensic Sciences 47 (2), 424–426.

Konigsberg, L.W., Ross, A.H., Jungers, W.L., 2006. Estimation and evidence in forensic anthropology: determining stature. In: Schmitt, A., Cunha, E., Pinheiro, J. (Eds.), Forensic Anthropology and Medicine: Complementary Sciences from Recovery to Cause of Death. Humana Press, Totowa, NJ, pp. 317–331.

Konigsberg, L.W., Herrmann, N.P., Wescott, D.J., Kimmerle, E.H., 2008. Estimation and evidence in forensic anthropology: Age-at-death. Journal of Forensic Sciences 53 (12), 541–557.

Konigsberg, L.W., Algee-Hewitt, B.F., Steadman, D.W., 2009. Estimation and evidence in forensic anthropology: sex and race. American Journal of Physical Anthropology 139 (1), 77–90.

Lovell, N.C., 1989. Test of Phenice's technique for determining sex from the os pubis. American Journal of Physical Anthropology 79 (1), 117–120.

Maresh, M.M., 1970. Measurements from roentgenograms, heart size, long bone lengths, bone, muscles and fat widths, skeletal maturation. In: McCammon, R.W. (Ed.), Human Growth and Development. Charles C. Thomas, Springfield, IL, pp. 155–200.

Matheson, C.D., Loy, T.H., 2001. Genetic sex identification of 9400-year-old human skull samples from Çayönü Tepesi, Turkey. Journal of Archaeological Science 28 (6), 569–575.

Mays, S., Faerman, M., 2001. Sex identification in some putative infanticide victims from Roman Britain using ancient DNA. Journal of Archaeological Science 28 (5), 555–559.

McCammon, R.W., 1970. Human Growth and Development. Charles C. Thomas, Springfield, IL.

McKern, T.W., Stewart, T.D., 1957. Skeletal Age Changes in Young American Males. US Army, Quartermaster Research and Development Command.

Meindl, R.S., Lovejoy, C.O., 1985. Ectocranial suture closure: a revised method for the determination of skeletal age at death based on the lateral-anterior sutures. American Journal of Physical Anthropology 68 (1), 57–66.

Minichillo, T., 2005. Paleodemography, grandmothering, and modern human evolution: a comment on Caspari and Lee (2004). Journal of Human Evolution 49 (5), 643–645.

Moore, M.K., 2013. Sex estimation and assessment. In: DiGangi, E.A., Moore, M.K. (Eds.), Research Methods in Human Skeletal Biology. Academic Press, San Diego.

Müller, H.G., Love, B., Hoppa, R.D., 2002. Semiparametric method for estimating paleodemographic profiles from age indicator data. American Journal of Physical Anthropology 117 (1), 1–14.

Myung, I.J., 2003. Tutorial on maximum likelihood estimation. Journal of Mathematical Psychology 47 (1), 90–100.

Nagaoka, T., Hirata, K., Yokota, E., Matsu'ura, S., 2006. Paleodemography of a medieval population in Japan: Analysis of human skeletal remains from the Yuigahama-minami site. American Journal of Physical Anthropology 131 (1), 1–14.

Phenice, T.W., 1969. A newly developed visual method of sexing the os pubis. American Journal of Physical Anthropology 30 (2), 297–302.

R Development Core Team, 2011. R: A Language and Environment for Statistical Computing. R Foundation for Statistical Computing, Vienna.

Redfern, R.C., DeWitte, S.N., 2011. A new approach to the study of Romanization in Britain: A regional perspective of cultural change in late Iron Age and Roman Dorset using the Siler and Gompertz–Makeham models of mortality. American Journal of Physical Anthropology 144 (2), 269–285.

Roche, A.F., Chumlea, W.C., Thissen, D., 1988. Assessing the Skeletal Maturity of the Hand–Wrist: Fels Method. Charles C. Thomas, Springfield, IL.

Royston, P., Altman, D.G., 1994. Regression using fractional polynomials of continuous covariates: parsimonious parametric modelling. Journal of the Royal Statistical Society. Series C (Applied Statistics) 43 (3), 429–467.

Sauerbrei, W., Meier-Hirmer, C., Benner, A., Royston, P., 2006. Multivariable regression model building by using fractional polynomials: description of SAS, STATA and R programs. Computational Statistics & Data Analysis 50 (12), 3464—3485.

Scheuer, J.L., Musgrave, J.H., Evans, S.P., 1980. The estimation of late fetal and perinatal age from limb bone length by linear and logarithmic regression. Annals of Human Biology 7 (3), 57—265.

Schmidt, D., Hummel, S., Herrmann, B., 2003. Brief communication: Multiplex X/Y PCR improves sex identification in aDNA analysis. American Journal of Physical Anthropology 121 (4), 337—341.

Shackelford, L.L., Harris, A.E.S., Konigsberg, L.W., 2012. Estimating the distribution of probable age-at-death from dental remains of immature human fossils. American Journal of Physical Anthropology 147 (2), 227—253.

Sherwood, R.J., Meindl, R.S., Robinson, H.B., May, R.L., 2000. Fetal age: methods of estimation and effects of pathology. American Journal of Physical Anthropology 113 (3), 305—315.

Siler, W., 1979. A competing-risk model for animal mortality. Ecology 60 (4), 750—757.

Steadman, D.W., Konigsberg, L.W., 2009. Multiple points of similarity (revised). In: Steadman, D.W. (Ed.), Hard Evidence: Case Studies in Forensic Anthropology, 2nd ed. Prentice Hall, Upper Saddle River, NJ, pp. 68—79.

Steadman, D.W., Adams, B.J., Konigsberg, L.W., 2006. Statistical basis for positive identification in forensic anthropology. American Journal of Physical Anthropology 131 (1), 15—26.

Stewart, T.D., 1948. Medico-legal aspects of the skeleton: I. Age, sex, race and stature. American Journal of Physical Anthropology 6 (3), 315—321.

Stone, A.C., Milner, G.R., Pääbo, S., Stoneking, M., 1996. Sex determination of ancient human skeletons using DNA. American Journal of Physical Anthropology 99 (2), 231—238.

Sutherland, L.D., Suchey, J.M., 1991. Use of the ventral arc in pubic sex determination. Journal of Forensic Sciences 36 (2), 501—511.

Thompson, D.D., 1979. The core technique in the determination of age at death in skeletons. Journal of Forensic Sciences 24 (4), 902—915.

Todd, T.W., 1920. Age changes in the pubic bone. I: The male white pubis. American Journal of Physical Anthropology 3, 285—334.

Wood, J.W., Holman, D.J., O'Connor, K.A., Ferrell, R.J., 2002. Mortality models for paleodemography. In: Hoppa, R.D., Vaupel, J.W. (Eds.), Paleodemography: Age Distributions from Skeletal Samples. Cambridge University Press, New York, pp. 129—168.

PART III

TECHNOLOGICAL ADVANCES

12

Geometric Morphometrics

Ashley H. McKeown, Ryan W. Schmidt

INTRODUCTION

Geometric morphometrics is a suite of methods for powerful analysis of shape variation. Geometric morphometrics provides the tools to capture the geometry of a form, retain those geometric properties throughout analysis, and visualize shape variation among specimens or groups. The focus in geometric morphometrics is analyzing and visualizing shape variation in the absence of size differences among specimens. By using *Cartesian* (x, y, and z) coordinates to record morphological structures, the form of a specimen is captured as a two- or three-dimensional configuration. The coordinates that define the configuration simultaneously contain information about landmark location in multiple planes (anterior—posterior (A-P), superior—inferior (S-I), and medial—lateral (M-L)). The configuration can be plotted as a two- or three-dimensional object. When geometric morphometric approaches are used for analysis, this multidimensional information is utilized.

The most popular geometric morphometric approaches offer efficient scaling methods enabling the analysis of shape variation independent of size. In studies of morphological variation, size can be an informative parameter or it can be a confounding factor. For example, there is size and shape variation in craniofacial morphology across human populations. When trying to estimate sex, size differences between males and females can be informative. However, when trying to assess variation in morphology across many populations, size differences can obscure similarities in shape. Geometric morphometrics provides methods for working solely with shape variation or for integrating size back into the analysis. This flexibility makes these approaches highly suitable for research in human skeletal biology.

Further benefits include graphical depictions of morphological variation that can be used to explain statistical results. Identifying specific differences in landmark location between groups can provide more in-depth answers about how the variation is patterned, which can ultimately lead to better interpretations of variability within an evolutionary framework.

This chapter provides an overview of geometric morphometrics as it is currently applied to research in human skeletal biology. It is designed to introduce the topic and associated resources to the reader. Anyone interested in employing geometric morphometrics in their

325

research should have a background in **multivariate statistics**[1] and conduct a thorough review of the original publications concerning the mathematical and theoretical aspects of the methods. The availability of free statistical packages that conduct geometric morphometric analyses may make it seem that little background knowledge is necessary; however, this cannot be farther from the truth. In order to use geometric morphometrics, one must have an in-depth understanding of the theoretical foundations for the suite of methods including the assumptions and caveats associated with a particular method being employed. As you utilize a geometric morphometric program, you will be asked to make choices that require comprehensive knowledge about the analyses being conducted by the program. Making theoretically and statistically sound choices require greater understanding than can be acquired from a review chapter. Further, we will refer to several statistical concepts herein that will not necessarily be fully explained. Many terms and concepts are included in the glossary at the end of the book, but some basic knowledge of statistics will be needed, or you can refer to one of the statistical texts cited in the chapter.

For those interested in geometric morphometrics, we strongly encourage you to explore well beyond the boundaries of this chapter and immerse yourself in the original literature. You can also look for workshops offered periodically that provide intensive training in these methods (see the "Conclusion and Additional Resources" section at the end of the chapter for websites where such workshops are advertised). Finally, as this is a rapidly developing area, one should conduct an exhaustive literature search to appreciate the current state of the field and the way methods are being applied to various research questions.

TRADITIONAL MORPHOMETRICS

Any discussion of geometric morphometrics must start with at least a brief review of traditional morphometrics, defined by Marcus (1990) as the use of measurements or linear distance data to quantify phenotypic variation analyzed with an array of exploratory and confirmatory multivariate statistical methods. In biological anthropology, measurements of lengths, breadths, and heights of anatomical structures or units were utilized for investigating morphological variation among and within human groups and have dominated quantitative research for decades. In particular, multivariate morphometrics became popular in studies of human skeletal biology as the objectively observed measurements were evaluated with statistical methods that enabled the investigation of patterns of variation and the testing of proposed hypotheses as well as evaluating the validity of those results (i.e., statistical significance testing). Thus, morphometrics held great appeal to skeletal biologists who desired to apply the rigor of the scientific method and to pursue research grounded in the developing body of evolutionary theory as applied to phenotypic variation. Additionally, the observation of osteological measurements is technologically simple and extensive datasets could be easily amassed for large series of human skeletal remains. The nondestructive nature of linear measurements ensured the continuation of traditional morphometric approaches after the passage of the *Native American Graves Protection and Repatriation Act* in

---

[1]All bolded terms are defined in the glossary at the end of this volume.

the United States in 1990[2] and the dawn of the genomic era. For a discussion of the value of traditional morphometrics in an age of geometric morphometrics and ancient **DNA** analyses, see Pietrusewsky (2008).

Morphometric research within biological anthropology has been particularly fruitful. Studies using cranial measurements, such as Howells' (1973) analysis of samples from around the world and Jantz's (1973) analyses of regionally defined samples, clearly demonstrated the capacity of these approaches for exploring morphological variation and integrating evolutionary models. While measurements of postcranial elements were employed to estimate sex and stature, explore **secular changes** (phenotypic differences in a population through time), and evaluate health status among other things, the primary focus of morphometric research in skeletal biology was the study of **biological distance** (biodistance), the evolutionary relationships of groups based on **phenotypic** similarity or dissimilarity (Buikstra et al., 1990; Stojanowski and Schillaci, 2006).

Initial applications of morphometrics to studies of biodistance primarily focused on two areas. One was explanations of change in craniofacial morphology as a product of migration versus *in situ* change due to evolutionary forces or secular change. The other was ancestry estimation for application in modern forensic casework (i.e., Giles and Elliot, 1962). Many of these studies employed **canonical variates analysis (CVA)** to explore variation among groups and in some cases construct possible temporal sequences. This analysis is quite appealing as it generates **Mahalanobis distance (D^2)** among groups and the **canonical scores** can be plotted in two or three dimensions for visual interpretation of the degree of phenotypic similarity or dissimilarity present. In many cases Mahalanobis distances (D^2) were used as biological distances between populations using the assumption that smaller Mahalanobis distances reflect greater phenotypic similarity and more closely related groups (Buikstra et al., 1990; Stojanowski and Schillaci, 2006). Others used **discriminant function analysis (DFA)** to classify an unknown specimen based on multivariate distance to reference group **centroids** or a DFA score (e.g., Giles and Elliot, 1962, 1963). While these studies were informative, the inability to account for environmental influences on the phenotype limited interpretations and permitted criticism by those who saw craniofacial morphology as containing minimal genetic information.

In 1982, Relethford and Lees outlined the application of population genetic analyses to quantitative traits (i.e., morphometrics) and began the integration of quantitative genetic models into morphometric research designs. Relethford and Blangero (1990) developed an extension of the model from Harpending and Ward (1982) for calculating genetic variation based on multivariate quantitative traits such as morphometrics. The theoretical framework for the model holds that expected levels of heterozygosity are proportional to total phenotypic variation in the population, and, as such, **parameter** estimates such as **gene flow** and **genetic drift** can be made. The model also permits heritability to be less than 1. This means that the amount of phenotypic variance in a trait within a population can be explained by partitioning environmental and genetic transmission. For example, many studies have used an average heritability for craniometric traits of 0.55 (after Devor, 1987), which means that, overall, the additive genetic transmission to the total phenotypic variance for craniometric traits is on

---

[2]Public Law 101-601; 25 U.S.C. § 3001 et seq. Also see DiGangi and Moore (Chapter 1), this volume, for a discussion.

average 55%. That is, **shape** and size components of craniofacial traits are moderately heritable from generation to generation. This approach has been successfully applied to numerous studies employing craniometric data; perhaps the most notable are studies by Relethford (1994, 2001, 2002, 2004, 2009, 2010) demonstrating that patterns of within- and between-group variation based on craniofacial morphology are congruent with genetic studies. The Relethford–Blangero model, as it is now known, has now been successfully applied to numerous studies in skeletal biology for identifying population structure and inferring population histories in evolutionary terms.

The 1990s also saw an explosion in the growth of forensic anthropology and an increasing need for reliable methods for assessing biological characteristics for unknown individuals. *Social race* can be an important identifier for searching missing persons reports and methods for estimating genetic ancestry (which can approximate social race) were clearly needed. Jantz and Ousley (1996–2005) developed the program FORDISC for use with craniometrics and postcranial metrics. The program generates custom discriminant functions for classifying unknown individuals based on comparison with a series of reference samples. It also provides plots of canonical scores so that the distance between the unknown and any comparison group **centroid** can be visually evaluated. While the program is user friendly, it still requires understanding of the basic statistical procedures and underlying assumptions associated with DFA and CVA to properly interpret results. The use of craniometrics for classifying unknown individuals has demonstrated a fairly high rate of accuracy (Ousley et al., 2009). For more information on this topic and approach, see DiGangi and Hefner (Chapter 5), this volume.

Traditional Morphometric Data

For the biological anthropologist, all measurements of skeletal elements fall under the rubric of **osteometrics**. Measurements of the cranium and mandible are typically referred to as **craniometrics**. **Postcranial metrics** include measurements of the rest of the skeleton. Measurements of dental dimensions are **odontometrics**. The typical tool kit for observing skeletal and dental dimensions includes spreading and sliding calipers, a radiometer, a coordinate caliper, an osteometric board, and a measuring tape. The craniometric canon was established by Howells (1973). Buikstra and Ubelaker (1994) provide a list of recommended cranial, postcranial, and dental measurements to standardize measurements of human skeletal remains for the purposes of documentation and analysis. Definitions for these measurements are provided in the aforementioned volumes. Anyone interested in morphometric research should *carefully read the definitions and practice observing the measurements* before proceeding with data collection. The measurements chosen and the accuracy of observation can have a significant effect on the validity of the research results.

Raw linear distances contain both size and shape information. For example, males typically have larger crania than females and on average have a greater maximum cranial length (glabella-occipital length). This difference is due to both the larger overall size of the male cranium (on average) and shape differences in the glabellar and occipital regions between the sexes. Thus, a major source of variation in samples composed of both males and females is size related to sexual dimorphism. Therefore, without standardizing data transformations such as **Z-scores** or applying a size correction such as scaling variables by the **geometric**

mean after Darroch and Mosimann (1985) to the data, males and females must be analyzed separately. Without a size correction, both within- and between-group shape variation can be obscured by size differences and many morphometric researchers are more interested in shape variation alone. While traditional morphometric variables can be scaled or size corrected through the approaches mentioned above, there is no consensus on which method works best and different techniques for size removal may mean that the results of studies are not comparable.

Traditional Multivariate Statistics

The range of statistical methods available for answering anthropological questions adds to the allure of traditional morphometrics with techniques for investigating patterns of morphological variation as well as procedures that assess the validity of a statistical hypothesis. While Marcus (1990) includes a wide range of multivariate statistical methods employed in morphometric studies in many different disciplines, only a subset of these are regularly used in human skeletal biology. Methods such as principal component analysis, canonical variates analysis, discriminant function analysis, regression, multivariate analysis of variance, and the related multivariate analysis of covariance provide statistical tools for exploring variation and accepting (or not accepting) hypotheses.

Principal components analysis (PCA) allows the exploration of the range of variation and interrelationships present in the entire dataset. PCA transforms intercorrelated variables into uncorrelated variables known as **principal components** (PC). Each PC is a linear combination of the original variables that maximize the variance (think variation) represented (Rencher, 1995; Afifi and Clark, 1996). The principal components are organized such that the first component contains the greatest variance with the remaining components ordered by decreasing variance. Since most of the sample variation is usually explained by the first few components, individual specimen PC scores or group mean scores can be plotted in two or three dimensions to explore the variation present between groups or individuals. PCA can also be used to reduce the dimensionality of a dataset for further analysis. This can be useful in anthropological morphometrics, as sometimes sample sizes are smaller than the number of variables available (which results in a singular covariance matrix making certain analyses, such as canonical variates analysis and discriminant function analysis, impossible).

Further, PCA resolves *multicollinearity* (correlation among multiple variables) by generating uncorrelated variables. In morphometrics, principal components can sometimes be interpreted in terms of morphology based on the correlation between the principal component coefficients and the original variables. These properties make PCA an attractive exploratory method for assessing the distribution of overall sample variation and the intercorrelation of variables as well as a useful tool for reducing the dimensionality of the original dataset without losing significant information.

An exploratory method for grouped data, *canonical variates analysis* (CVA), generates *Mahalanobis distances* between groups based on sample centroids. It also produces canonical variates (CV) from rotation and scaling of the centroids (Marcus 1990). In morphometrics, Mahalanobis distances (D^2) can be interpreted in terms of similarity or dissimilarity between groups. The canonical variates are linear combinations of the original variables that maximally separate groups. Similar to PCA, individual or group mean scores can be plotted to interpret patterns of variation across the groups being analyzed. It should be noted that the canonical axes are not truly *orthogonal*, so distances in canonical plots may be slightly skewed; nevertheless, canonical variates plots can provide visual representation of the biological distances among groups.

Discriminant function analysis (DFA) calculates the multivariate distance from an unknown specimen to the centroids for reference groups (Marcus, 1990) for the purpose of classification. The DFA will classify the individual based on the smallest distance (indicating that the specimen is most similar to that group mean). Discriminant analysis also generates a linear (classification) function consisting of coefficients and a constant. For each individual specimen, a discriminant score can be calculated by multiplying the original variables by the DF coefficient and adding the constant. Canonical and discriminant analysis are often used together to assess patterns of intergroup variation and identify the biological affinity of individual specimens.

Regression analysis can test the relationship between independent and dependent variables (Afifi and Clark, 1996). Descriptive regression analysis evaluates the type and strength of the relationship between the independent and dependent variables based on the correlation coefficient. If a strong relationship exists, then regression analysis can also be used to generate an equation that predicts the dependent value given the independent variables. In skeletal biology, regression analysis is used for both purposes.

Multivariate analysis of variance (MANOVA) is the multivariate extension of the analysis of variance (ANOVA) and tests for differences between group centroids (Marcus, 1990). The **multivariate analysis of covariance** (MANCOVA) also tests for differences between group means while allowing for a covariate, such as age. The MANCOVA assesses the effect of the covariate on the multivariate model permitting the testing of hypotheses about patterns of biological variation.

The use of the Relethford and Blangero (1990) R matrix analysis has seen widespread application, particularly after John Relethford's program RMET became available. The R matrix method employs quantitative phenotypic data in a population genetics-based analysis. This is particularly appealing as it provides greater insight into the evolutionary forces that may be acting on phenotypic traits in populations. Recent studies of craniometric variation suggest that most craniofacial morphology is relatively neutral and carries a strong genetic signal useful for tracing population histories.

GEOMETRIC MORPHOMETRICS

At one time known as the "New Morphometry," (Marcus and Corti, 1996) geometric morphometrics have become widespread in studies of shape variation within anthropology and numerous other fields. Indeed, we have gone from the "revolution in morphometrics" of the early 1990s (Rohlf and Marcus, 1993) to the regular application of these techniques in the various subareas of biological anthropology, including modern human skeletal biology, paleoanthropology, and primatology. Human skeletal biology has seen great benefit from the integration of geometric morphometrics into the array of methods employed to quantify morphology and analyze it within an evolutionary framework.

Current methods in geometric morphometrics rely on the theoretical foundation of shape space as defined by Kendall (1984). Now known as **"Kendall's shape space,"** it is non-Euclidean (curved, nonlinear) multidimensional space where configurations of two or more dimensions can be plotted as a single point. For the simplest shape, a triangle, Kendall's shape space takes the form of a sphere. For shapes with more than three landmarks, the shape space is a more complex, manifold surface in hyperspace that cannot be depicted. This means that coordinate-based configurations do not exist in Euclidean space, which may confound linear statistical methods commonly used in traditional morphometrics.

Slice (2001) demonstrates that the coordinates for configurations fitted via a **generalized Procrustes analysis** (the most popular method for more than two configurations) do not actually exist in Kendall's shape space, but are instead associated with a hemisphere that has properties very similar to Kendall's space. Fortunately for both Kendall's shape space and the Procrustes hemisphere, the point corresponding to the average configuration for a group is approximately tangent to a linear vector plane. This creates a link to Euclidean space, where the coordinates for configurations can be projected for use in linear statistical analyses. In order to analyze Procrustes coordinates with standard, linear statistical procedures, the tangent space can be constructed for projection of coordinates into a Euclidean plane. Alternatively, some linear statistical methods such as principal components analysis approximate the curved shape space and are often used to bypass the more statistically complex projection into tangent space. This brief overview of "Kendall's shape space" and the Procrustes hemisphere attributes and implications for geometric morphometrics should be augmented by reading Kendall (1984) and Slice (2001) as well as reviews found in Slice (2005) and Mitteroecker and Gunz (2009).

Types of Data

Currently there are two primary data types common in geometric morphometric research in biological anthropology. Since the type of data employed in a study depends on the research question being investigated, it is useful to consider the benefits of each data type. Modes of data acquisition for each of the data types are also presented.

Landmark Coordinates

The most common type of coordinate data employed in biological anthropology is from anatomical landmarks, many of which are endpoints of standard craniometrics or other linear distances on the skeleton. Typically, landmark coordinates are collected relative to arbitrary axes that are specific to each specimen, meaning that they are not comparable until differences due to orientation and location have been eliminated. Not all landmarks are created equal, as the quality of anatomical information contained in landmarks varies based on location. It is desirable for landmarks to be **homologous**; in other words, they are discrete structures or features that occur in approximately the same location on all specimens.

Recognizing that not all landmarks have the same degree of homology, Bookstein (1991:63–66) defined three types of landmarks. *Type I landmarks* are defined as locations based on distinct structures that intersect or are juxtaposed. The cranial landmark, bregma, is a Type I landmark, as it is the intersection of the sagittal and coronal sutures in the midsagittal plane. This landmark occurs in the same anatomical location on each cranium. *Type II landmarks* are located at points of sharpest curvature along tissue boundaries. Jugale, the deepest incurvature along the posterior edge of the zygomatic between the frontal and temporal processes (Howells, 1973:175), is an example of a Type II landmark. *Type III landmarks* are relational points whose placement is dependent on the location of another landmark. These are often endpoints of measurements like maximum cranial breadth (euryon) and maximum cranial length (opisthocranion). Problems with Type III landmarks include a lack of biological meaning independent of the other landmark/endpoint and the high degree of variability in the landmark location from individual to individual.

Type I and II landmarks are fairly common on the cranium and provide relatively complete coverage of the craniofacial form. The same cannot be said of the postcranial elements where most landmarks tend to be Types II and III. The emphasis of the cranium in the application of geometric morphometrics is not surprising, given the ease of identifying biologically meaningful landmarks on the cranium and that craniofacial morphology has already been the focus of traditional morphometric research in skeletal biology for several decades.

Figure 12.1 depicts common cranial landmarks employed in geometric morphometric research. For definitions of these landmarks, refer to Howells (1973), Moore-Jansen et al. (1994), and Buikstra and Ubelaker (1994). It is strongly suggested that you *carefully read the landmark definitions found in the original sources* listed above before trying to locate them on a cranium, as you cannot always fully appreciate the intended location of a landmark from two-dimensional images such as Figure 12.1. The definitions are detailed and standardized to decrease the likelihood of observer error in landmark placement. It is critical that you be well-versed in the anatomical features that define a particular landmark and understand how to handle exceptions from expected morphology.

RECORDING LANDMARKS

Landmark coordinates can be recorded from a photograph or radiograph of a specimen with a two-dimensional digitizing tablet or from a three-dimensional digitizer, such as a Microscribe (http://www.3d-microscribe.com/) or Polhemus (http://polhemus.com/). Three-dimensional digitizers can also be used to observe coordinates directly on a dry bone specimen (see Figure 12.2). While these types of digitizers will transmit coordinates to programs such as Excel, Notepad, or AutoCad, there are also specialized software programs to facilitate data collection. Landmark data can also be acquired from laser surface scans and volumetric (**computed tomography (CT)** or **magnetic resonance imaging (MRI)**) scans. For more on these technologies, see Moore (Chapter 14), this volume.

A popular Windows-based program for acquiring landmark coordinates and craniometrics from the cranium and mandible is **3Skull** written by Stephen Ousley. An early version of this program is described in Ousley and McKeown (2001), and it is designed to work with a three-dimensional digitizer such as the Microscribe or Polhemus. The program provides a straightforward interface page for recording catalog and/or identification information about the specimen, and then prompts the observer for each landmark to be digitized. The basic list of landmarks provided in Ousley and McKeown (2001) includes all the landmarks associated with the suite of Howells' (1973) craniometrics plus numerous other landmarks to provide comprehensive coverage of important anatomical features of the skull.

The program is also designed to record continuous coordinates along a series of arcs (frontal, parietal, occipital, and others). The arcs are used to calculate the location of some

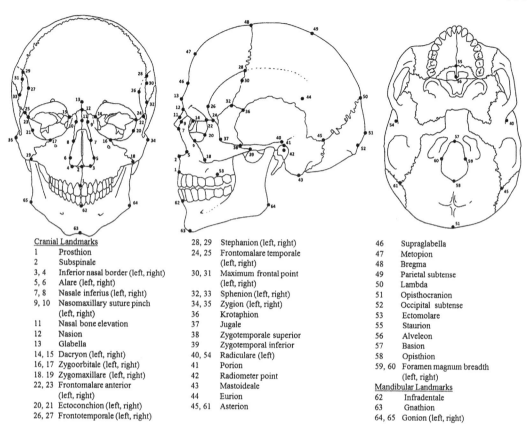

Cranial Landmarks

1	Prosthion
2	Subspinale
3, 4	Inferior nasal border (left, right)
5, 6	Alare (left, right)
7, 8	Nasale inferius (left, right)
9, 10	Nasomaxillary suture pinch (left, right)
11	Nasal bone elevation
12	Nasion
13	Glabella
14, 15	Dacryon (left, right)
16, 17	Zygoorbitale (left, right)
18, 19	Zygomaxillare (left, right)
22, 23	Frontomalare anterior (left, right)
20, 21	Ectoconchion (left, right)
26, 27	Frontotemporale (left, right)

28, 29	Stephanion (left, right)
24, 25	Frontomalare temporale (left, right)
30, 31	Maximum frontal point (left, right)
32, 33	Sphenion (left, right)
34, 35	Zygion (left, right)
36	Krotaphion
37	Jugale
38	Zygotemporale superior
39	Zygotemporal inferior
40, 54	Radiculare (left)
41	Porion
42	Radiometer point
43	Mastoideale
44	Eurion
45, 61	Asterion

46	Supraglabella
47	Metopion
48	Bregma
49	Parietal subtense
50	Lambda
51	Opisthocranion
52	Occipital subtense
53	Ectomolare
55	Staurion
56	Alveleon
57	Basion
58	Opisthion
59, 60	Foramen magnum breadth (left, right)

Mandibular Landmarks

62	Infradentale
63	Gnathion
64, 65	Gonion (left, right)

FIGURE 12.1 Landmarks of the human skull commonly used in geometric morphometrics. (Note: not all landmarks that can be used are identified in this figure, just the most common.) **Left**—anterior view that depicts facial and mandibular landmarks; **middle**—lateral view with lateral facial, vault, and mandible landmarks; **right**—inferior view showing landmarks of the basicranium and palate. Landmark names by number are provided. (Note: some bilateral landmarks are only visible from left lateral perspective; nevertheless, there is a right **antimere** that is not depicted).

Type II and III landmarks useful for both craniometrics and coordinate-based analyses (e.g. metopion, parietal subtense point, vertex radius point, opisthocranion, and occipital subtense point). Additionally, the coordinates associated with these arcs could be used as **semilandmarks** to analyze the profile outlines (see discussion of semilandmarks in the next section).

3Skull employs the coordinate data to calculate a complete set of Howells' (1973) measurements that are in turn utilized to error check many of the landmark coordinates. Both the three-dimensional coordinates and the craniometrics are saved in separate databases. Users can create a custom landmark list, although the current landmark database is fairly exhaustive. An accessory program can calculate the distance between any set of landmarks, allowing researchers to utilize unconventional measurements in traditional morphometric analyses. The program is distributed as freeware and researchers interested in this program

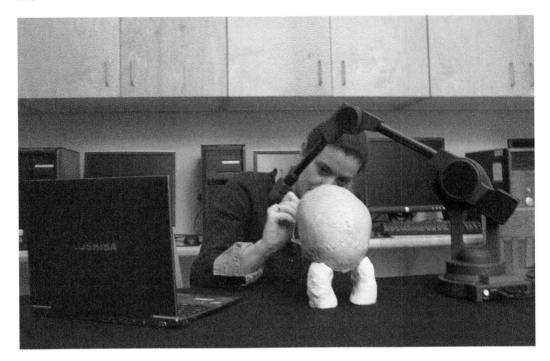

FIGURE 12.2   A researcher using a three-dimensional digitizer to observe landmark coordinates on a cranium. Photograph by Roselyn Campbell.

should contact Dr. Ousley directly (http://mai.mercyhurst.edu/personnel/stephen-d-ousley/). Other programs for recording landmark data are presented in Table 12.1 along with relevant attributes and procurement information.

When working with a three-dimensional digitizer with an internal origin (0, 0, 0 point), it is important to keep the digitizer and the skeletal structure, photograph, or radiograph

TABLE 12.1   Programs for Recording Landmark Coordinates[a]

Program Name	Mode of Data Acquisition	How to Access
3Skull (Stephen Ousley, 2011)	Landmarks—3D digitizer connected to computer	Contact Stephen Ousley http://mai.mercyhurst.edu/personnel/stephen-d-ousley/
DSDIGIT (Dennis Slice)	Landmarks—3D digitizer connected to computer	http://life.bio.sunysb.edu/morph/ Software page, Data Acquisition
Landmark Editor (IDAV/UC-Davis)	Landmarks and semilandmarks from laser surface scans	http://graphics.idav.ucdavis.edu/ research/EvoMorph
tpsDIG2 (F. James Rohlf)	Landmarks and outlines from image files, scans and video	http://life.bio.sunysb.edu/morph/ Software page, Data Acquisition

[a]*This is not a complete list of all available programs, more are available at http://life.bio.sunysb.edu/morph/, Software page, Data Acquisition.*

immobile during the digitizing process. This keeps the landmark coordinates for each specimen in the same coordinate system as a coherent configuration. The need for the specimen and digitizer to be stationary requires securing the cranium, skeletal element, or two-dimensional image such that all landmarks or structures to be traced are accessible. When working with dry bone specimens, they must be placed in a stable and secure configuration, as the safety of the skeletal material is a critical consideration. Figure 12.3 shows a cranium positioned for digitizing with a Microscribe or Polhemus. All landmarks can be reached with the stylus tip and the arcs can be traced without interruption. A mirror can be used to facilitate tracing the occipital arc.

Laser scanners do not have the same restrictions; here the specimen is typically placed on a platform that rotates and all observable surfaces are scanned. The specimen often needs to be repositioned and rescanned, so that all surfaces are captured. Computer software programs associated with the laser scanners then "stitch" the scans together to produce three-dimensional renderings of the entire specimen.

The observation of landmark coordinates is subject to error due to inaccurate identification of landmark location (lack of precision) and variation among observers (lack of repeatability). Several studies (Corner et al., 1992; Richtsmeier et al., 1995; Aldridge et al., 2005; Ross and

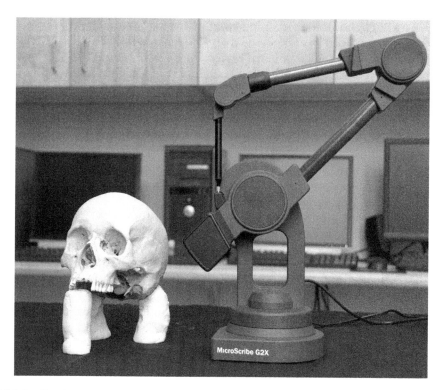

FIGURE 12.3 Cranium positioned for data collection with a three-dimensional digitizer. Photograph by Roselyn Campbell.

Williams, 2008; Sholts et al., 2011a) have evaluated the precision of various landmark types and error associated with different coordinate observation techniques. In summary, these studies find a fairly high degree of precision and repeatability for Type I and II landmarks across different observation modalities. Further, thorough knowledge of landmark definitions and locations and practice using a digitizer increase a researcher's precision when observing landmark coordinates (yes, practice, practice, practice, and then practice some more).

When conducting research that includes coordinate data, an assessment of measurement error should be part of the research design. Currently, there are several methods for evaluating the precision and repeatability of landmark coordinate data. The most popular approaches are critically reviewed by von Cramon-Taubadel and colleagues (2007) and the authors propose an alternate method for assessing measurement error. Anyone interested in using coordinate data should carefully read this article before choosing a method for their research.

Semilandmarks

Some of the original data types of interest in geometric morphometrics were as outlines or curves, such as the midsagittal profile of the frontal bone. In humans we know there are differences in the curvature of the frontal bone between the sexes, across human populations, and through time due to secular change. While the curve or outline may be anchored by Type I landmarks at either end, the intervening coordinates that define the curve or outline lack homology, necessitating different methods to enable meaningful analyses. This is an important endeavor as many of the anatomical regions of interest are not defined by Type I or II landmarks, yet these surfaces and curves contain important information for interpreting aspects of morphological variation. The ability to explore this variation by quantifying the curvature and testing differences with rigorous statistical analysis would be beneficial to studies of human variation.

Semilandmarks (also called **sliding landmarks**) can be acquired from curves and outlines by tracing with a three-dimensional digitizer set to collect coordinates spaced equidistant apart (e.g., every 0.05 mm) and downloaded to a custom program such as 3Skull (described earlier), which can record coordinates along an arc, or to a utility program such as Microsoft Excel. Semilandmarks can also be sampled from laser surface scans or from volumetric (CT or MRI) scans. The custom program, Landmark Editor (see Table 12.1), can be used to place semilandmarks across surfaces captured with laser scans.

Currently, most geometric morphometric research in biological anthropology employs landmark coordinates observed on the cranium. The long-standing interest in craniofacial variation, the ease of data collection, the numerous biologically meaningful landmarks on the cranium, and the suite of available sophisticated analytical packages make this method a natural inclination. Nevertheless, studies utilizing landmark coordinates characterizing the morphology of postcranial elements do exist (e.g., Stephens and Strand Viðarsdóttir, 2008; Bytheway and Ross, 2010; De Groote et al., 2010; De Groote, 2011a, 2011b). It is likely that similar studies will be more plentiful in the future. Although the methodological developments regarding the use of semilandmarks are relatively new, there are now several programs capable of analyzing semilandmarks, and it is expected that this approach will see significant growth in the coming years.

GEOMETRIC MORPHOMETRIC METHODS

Originally geometric morphometrics included several methods for analyzing shape information encoded in coordinate data that were widely used in biological anthropology. Analytical approaches such as **Euclidean distance matrix analysis** (EDMA) and **elliptical Fourier analysis** (EFA) were included in early discussions of the suite of geometric morphometric methods (e.g., Richstmeier et al., 2002). While EFA is useful for certain research designs (e.g., Christensen, 2005; Sholts et al., 2011b) and many geometric morphometrics programs are capable of performing this analysis, EDMA is no longer as common as once it was. Rohlf (2003) compared error and bias in estimation of mean shapes for several geometric morphometric methods including generalized Procrustes analysis (described below) and EDMA. This study demonstrated that generalized Procrustes analysis generated the least error and no bias when used to estimate mean shape. For this review of methods, only the most common methods currently in use are presented.

Procrustes Methods

Coordinate data, the basis for geometric morphometric methods, define a **form** under investigation by encoding its geometric properties. Each configuration is defined by a set of arbitrary axes where the coordinates are relative only to each other, meaning that multiple configurations are not comparable to one another. Configurations composed of raw coordinates also contain size information. The most popular approach to removing the differences in location, orientation, and size among configurations is the **Procrustes superimposition** (Adams et al., 2004; Slice, 2005, 2007; Mitteroecker and Gunz, 2009).

Procrustes superimposition uses a least-squares solution to bring multiple configurations into a common coordinate system and align homologous landmark coordinates through rotation (Rohlf and Slice, 1990). Typically, Procrustes superimposition is set to scale configurations to a common **Centroid Size** without the use of a least-squares estimate, known as a partial Procrustes fitting. Specifically, configurations are translated into a common coordinate system by aligning the centroid of the coordinates for each configuration. Often, this is accomplished by locating all centroids at the shared coordinate system's origin. Next, the configurations are scaled to a common Centroid Size, which is the measure of the distances (square root of the sum of the squared distances) from all landmark coordinates to the configuration centroid. For Procrustes superimposition, Centroid Size is typically set to equal one. This removes uniform size differences among configurations. Finally, the configurations are rotated so that sum of the squared distances is minimized between the **homologous** landmark coordinates. In the case of two configurations, this is fairly straightforward, but for more than two configurations, an iterative rotation process is needed.

The generalized Procrustes analysis (GPA) translates and scales the configuration as described above, and then rotates all configurations to a least-squares fit with one of the configurations from the sample. After this initial fitting process, the average of all coordinates is calculated to generate a first-round mean configuration. The process is then continued with each configuration again being fit to the estimated mean configuration leading to the arrival at a new mean configuration. This iterative process continues until the sum-of-the-squared deviations between the fitted configurations and the means meet some criterion (minimal deviation) or convergence (no significant change in mean configuration from one iteration to the next) occurs.

The details of the mathematical and algorithmic basis for Procrustes superimposition are beyond the scope of this chapter, and for a thorough understanding of the theoretical underpinnings of Procrustes methods, the reader is directed to literature documenting the development of these methods (Gower, 1975; Rohlf and Slice, 1990; Goodall, 1991; Dryden and Mardia, 1993) and to the review found in Slice (2005). The process of Procrustes superimposition is visually represented in Figure 12.4, and an example of cranial landmark configurations both before and after generalized Procrustes analysis is shown in Figure 12.5.

The purpose of the scaling step in Procrustes superimposition is to facilitate assessment of shape variation without the confounding factor of size differences. It also permits the aggregation of males and females from a group, which can be useful in biological anthropology both due to research designs and to remedy small sample sizes. When desired, size can be reincorporated in the statistical analysis by using Centroid Size or the natural logarithm of Centroid Size as a variable.

After a GPA, the fitted coordinates are **Procrustes shape coordinates**, which can be statistically manipulated for further analysis. Since the shape coordinates do not exist in Euclidean space and will not produce a variance–covariance matrix of full rank, either they need to be

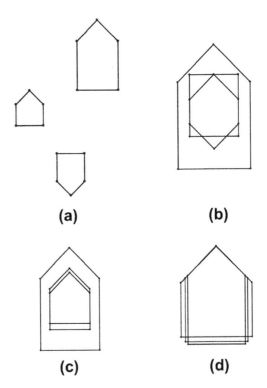

FIGURE 12.4   The steps of a Procrustes superimposition starting with (a) raw coordinate-based configurations that undergo (b) Step 1—translation, then (c) Step 2—rotation, and finally (d) Step 3—scaling.

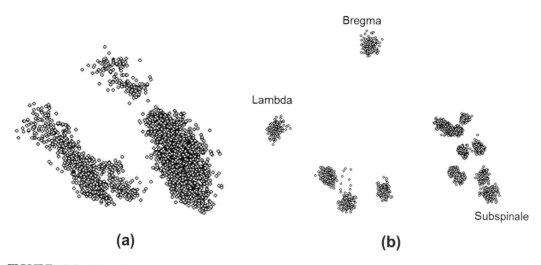

FIGURE 12.5 Three-dimensional coordinate date from 20 cranial landmarks from 164 individuals (lateral view with facial landmarks to the right and vault landmarks to the left): (a) before Procrustes superimposition and (b) after Procrustes superimposition.

projected into the linear space tangent to the Procrustes hemisphere or nonparametric statistical methods can be applied. Alternately, a linear statistical analysis, such as principal component analysis, that approximates the curved shape space and reduces the dimensionality of the shape coordinates can be used. In some cases, the principal component scores will illustrate differences among groups, both in scatter plots and in shape variation by visualizing shape change associated with scores along the principal component axes. The principal component scores based on the shape coordinates can also be used for standard morphometric analyses such as CVA, DFA, MANOVA or MANCOVA, regression, and R matrix analysis with a program such as RMET (by John Relethford).

Group means can be visually compared by graphically displaying the coordinate configurations together so that differences in the locations of landmarks can be seen. Difference-vector diagrams enhance this capacity by showing vectors extending from the location of a landmark on one configuration (usually the group mean) to the homologous landmarks of the other configuration (usually the other group mean) (Slice, 2007). The direction and magnitude of the differences can easily be appreciated from these graphical depictions of shape variation. Figure 12.6 illustrates the superimposition of group means from samples of Euro-American and African-American males from the **Robert J. Terry Anatomical Skeletal Collection** housed at the Smithsonian Institution's National Museum of Natural History in Washington, D.C. The figure clearly shows variation in the location of certain landmarks between the two group means.

The most obvious differences are in the vault, with the African-American mean having more posteriorly oriented landmarks, particularly bregma, mastoideale, basion and lambda. This suggests an overall elongated vault when compared to the more anterior position of these landmarks in the Euro-American male mean. Additionally, the more laterally positioned landmarks mastoideale and asterion indicate a broader vault for the Euro-American

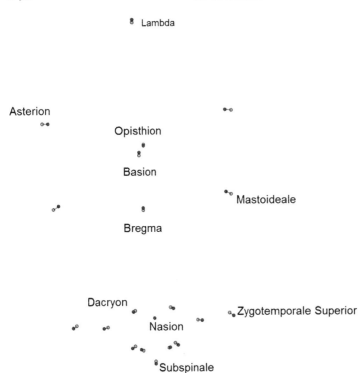

FIGURE 12.6 Group mean configuration (Euro-American and African-American male) overlays from superior view. Euro-American landmarks are represented by open circles and African-American landmarks are represented by solid circles.

male mean. In the face, the more anteriorly positioned subspinale and the more laterally positioned alares, dacryons, and other facial landmarks suggest a wider mid-face region and overall broader face in the African-American male mean.

The presence of shape variation in these landmarks of the face and vault for these two American populations contributes to the ability of statistical programs to distinguish between these groups based on craniofacial dimensions; however, we are just beginning to understand the reasons for this pattern of variation. Climatic adaptation has been considered as an explanation for these differences and may very well hold true for the nasal and mid-face region (see the review of Noback et al., 2011 later in this chapter). Nevertheless, research has also demonstrated secular change in craniofacial form for both Euro-Americans and African-Americans (see review of Wescott and Jantz, [2005] later in this chapter as well as Jantz and Meadows Jantz [2000] and Jantz [2001]). While these trends have been documented, the reasons (environment, gene flow, or some combination) have not been completely elucidated; therefore, assigning explanations to the variation depicted in this mean shape configuration overlay is premature, but an area ripe for further research.

Case Study: Biodistance Analysis Using Geometric Morphometrics

An example of using landmark coordinates from crania to investigate shape variation among groups for the purposes of biodistance analysis is drawn from the dataset collected for McKeown (2000). Here, three-dimensional coordinates from 22 facial landmarks for eight samples from sites associated with the Arikara of the Middle Missouri region of South Dakota are analyzed using geometric morphometrics and traditional statistical methods. The landmarks employed in this study are depicted in Figure 12.7. The samples are from sites along the Missouri River and vary temporally and geographically as shown in Figure 12.8. The temporal and cultural period assignments for the various components are drawn from Jantz (1997) and McKeown (2000).

In this example, three-dimensional coordinates observed on crania from each site component are analyzed in order to explore the pattern of morphological variation that exists among individuals from these sites. A three-dimensional digitizer and the program 3Skull were used to record the coordinate data. The coordinate-based configurations were subjected to a generalized Procrustes analysis (GPA) using MorphoJ (Klingenberg, 2011), which accounts for the effects of object symmetry, which means the structure is symmetric in itself and has an interior line or plane, so that its left and right halves are mirror images of each other, such as the vertebrate skull (Klingenberg et al., 2002).

Since crania have object symmetry and numerous bilateral landmarks are included in the dataset, it is useful to only analyze the symmetric component of the morphological variation (leaving out the intra-individual asymmetric component). MorphoJ partitions these two components, permitting the analysis of the symmetric component alone, making it

Landmarks
Prosthion
Subspinale
Alare (L, R)
Nasion
Bregma
Dacryon (L, R)
Zygoorbitale (L, R)
Zygomaxillare (L, R)
Ectoconchion (L, R)
Frontomalare anterior (L, R)
Frontomalare temporale (L, R)
Frontotemporal (L, R)
Zygomaticotemporale Superior (L, R)

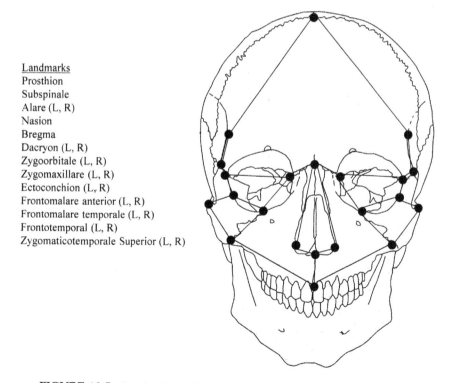

FIGURE 12.7 Landmarks used in the biological distance analysis case study.

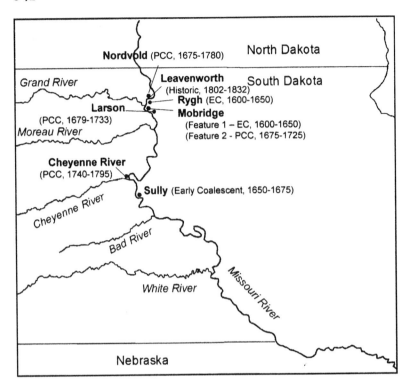

Nordvold (PCC, 1675-1780)　North Dakota

Grand River

Leavenworth South Dakota
(Historic, 1802-1832)
Rygh (EC, 1600-1650)
Larson　**Mobridge**
(PCC, 1679-1733)
Moreau River
(Feature 1 – EC, 1600-1650)
(Feature 2 - PCC, 1675-1725)

Cheyenne River
(PCC, 1740-1795)

Cheyenne River

Sully (Early Coalescent, 1650-1675)

Bad River

White River

Missouri River

Nebraska

FIGURE 12.8 Map of the sites used in the case study example with temporal information. EC is the Extended Coalescent and PCC is the Postcontact Coalescent. All site dates are approximate. North is to the top of the figure.

particularly suited for the analysis of crania. Post GPA, MorphoJ provides for further analysis of the fitted coordinates. One method projects the configurations into the tangent plane that has Euclidean properties allowing for standard statistical analysis of the coordinates. The other conducts principal components analysis (PCA) of the fitted coordinates and the PC scores can then be used in traditional statistical procedures. In this case, the projected coordinates are selected and a canonical variates analysis (CVA) is conducted to maximally separate the sites and generate plots that can be interpreted as biodistance maps.

Additionally, configurations depicting the morphological pattern associated with group averages are generated, facilitating interpretations of shape variation. The ability to graphically depict morphological patterns is one of the great benefits of geometric morphometrics, which is not possible using traditional morphometrics. Figure 12.9 is a plot of the mean canonical scores for each component along the first two canonical variates axes (CV1 and CV2) along with configurations illustrating the average morphological pattern associated with each group. The configurations have been scaled by a factor of 5 to facilitate visualization of shape difference. Table 12.2 provides the pairwise Mahalanobis distances among site components with those that are significant based on 10,000 permutations indicated; both the Mahalanobis distances and the significance testing were conducted in MorphoJ.

The canonical variate plot (Figure 12.9) depicts a clear separation along CV1 between the cluster of early northern site components (Rygh and Mobridge Feature 1) and all the other sites. The similar shape of the average face from Rygh and Mobridge Feature 1 is evident

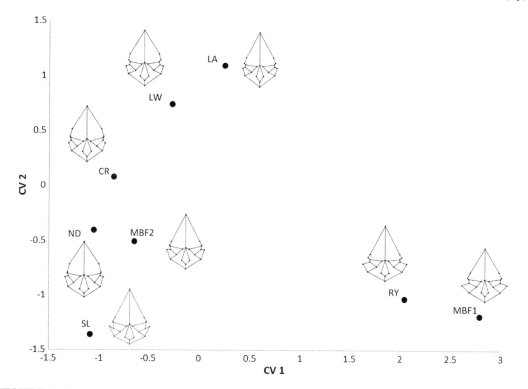

FIGURE 12.9 Graph of group means along canonical variates 1 and 2 for site components in case study with wireframe depictions of average group morphological variation. RY=Rygh; MBF1=Mobridge Feature 1; MBF2=Mobridge Feature 2; ND=Nordvold; CR=Cheyenne River; SL=Sully; LW=Leavenworth.

TABLE 12.2 Mahalanobis Distances among Site Components.

	CR	LA	LW	MBF1	MBF2	ND	RY
LA	2.2557*						
LW	2.2593*	1.7896*					
MBF1	4.0636*	3.5111*	3.9566*				
MBF2	1.8595	1.9918*	2.2224*	3.6554*			
ND	1.7408	2.7088*	2.5547*	4.242*	1.8266*		
RY	3.773*	3.06*	3.2383*	1.932	3.0451*	3.7109*	
SL	2.5177*	2.8952*	2.7429*	4.0668*	1.7342*	2.5516*	3.4804*

* Distances that are significant at $p < 0.01$ are marked with an asterisk (*).

from the wireframe configurations. The more laterally positioned superior zygomatic suture points and more inferiorly located bregmas distinguish them from the other groups in this analysis. CV2 provides separation among the other samples with Sully, Rygh, and Mobridge Feature 1 having the most negative mean canonical scores. Nordvold, Mobridge Feature 2, and Cheyenne River form a loose cluster that reflects geographic proximity, common temporal period, and similar facial shape. Interestingly, Leavenworth is positioned between Larson and Cheyenne River, which corresponds to hypotheses about Leavenworth being an aggregate village for both Bad River peoples similar to those who occupied Cheyenne River, and Le Beau peoples similar to those who occupied Larson after significant depopulation primarily due to infectious diseases. Morphologically Leavenworth is also intermediate between the patterns seen in Larson and Cheyenne River.

The Mahalanobis distances between site components indicate that based on facial morphology almost all the components are significantly different from one another. The few exceptions are the Cheyenne River, Mobridge Feature 2, and Nordvold, which formed a loose cluster on the CV plot. One can visually appreciate the similarities in average facial shape. The other exception is the lack of significant difference between Rygh and Mobridge Feature 2, which cluster together well away from all other sites in the CV plot and share a similar average facial shape.

Both McKeown (2000) and McKeown and Jantz (2005) present results for these sites using landmark coordinates for the face and vault. These studies used Mantel tests (Mantel, 1967; Manly, 1986; Smouse et al., 1986) to compute the correlation between the biological distance matrix (based on the Mahalanobis distances), the temporal distance matrix (calculated as differences in mean site dates), and the geographic distance matrix (calculated as linear distance between site locations). In both studies, the correlation between biological and geographic distance matrices was positive and statistically significant ($p < 0.01$). Conversely, the correlation between biological and temporal distance matrices was not statistically significant. This is consistent with a model of isolation by geographic distance where sites that are biologically more similar to each other are also geographically closer and vice versa (Konigsberg, 1990).

This short case study demonstrates that geometric morphometrics methods are well suited to biological distance studies as the coordinate data provide greater information about the range and pattern of morphological variation in an anatomical unit such as the face. By capturing three-dimensional variation in landmark location (i.e., the geometry of the form), it increases the level of morphological variation available for statistical analysis. Output from geometric morphometric techniques such as GPA can be analyzed by standard statistical procedures and employed in tests of models regarding reasons for certain patterns of morphological variation. The graphical depictions of morphological variation add considerably to our understanding of shape variation among groups as we can visually interpret the differences based on variation in landmark location. This takes us beyond interpreting variation simply as "faces becoming taller through time" and provides the tools for describing the exact change in morphology (e.g., nasion is more superiorly located or prosthion is more inferiorly located or both) that produces that overall difference in shape.

Thin-Plate Spline Methods

The **thin-plate spline** (TPS) (Bookstein, 1991) provides a sophisticated approach to visualizing differences between coordinate-based configurations. In particular, it can be used to depict the shape variation between two group mean configurations in terms of the shape deformation necessary for one mean configuration to be mapped directly onto the other mean configuration. This is accomplished with an algorithm to exactly map the homologous coordinates while smoothly interpolating the interlandmark space. The smoothness of the interpolation is maximized by minimizing the **bending energy** required to generate the deformation. Typically the TPS results are viewed as grid-based deformations, where the differences in interlandmark space are visible as deformations in the grid surface. Figure 12.10 shows an example of TPS visualization using mean configurations from samples of Euro-American and African-American males from the Terry Collection generated using the program PAST (Hammer, 2011). The two-dimensional thin-plate spline was produced by mapping the Euro-American male consensus configuration onto the African-American male consensus configuration. This figure shows the morphological differences between the two groups both in the face and in the vault shape viewed from a lateral perspective. The areas requiring the greatest degree of warp to map the corresponding landmark locations are indicated by the darker colors in the grayscale gradient across the grid. The minimal degree of interlandmark deformation in the spline grid indicates that the differences between these two mean shape configurations are limited and mainly confined to a few landmarks of the anterior face (alare and dacryon) and the inferior cranial vault (basion, mastoideale, and asterion).

Thin-plate spline analysis can also be used to generate relative warp scores by deforming each individual configuration onto the grand mean configuration. These scores can be used for subsequent statistical analysis.

Semilandmark Methods

Semilandmarks (defined earlier) can now be analyzed by allowing the semilandmarks to slide along vectors tangent to the curve or surface until some criterion is minimized. Initially

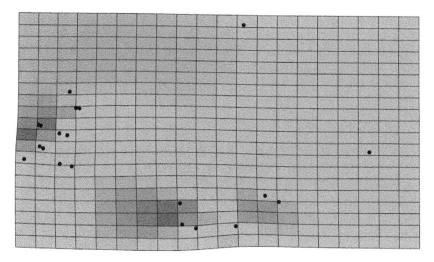

FIGURE 12.10 Thin-plate spline deformation grid showing that morphological variation between mean forms for samples of Euro-American and African-American males is largely confined to the anterior face and inferior cranial vault. The configurations are shown from a lateral view with landmarks for the face at the left of the image and vault landmarks to the right.

described by Bookstein (1991), semilandmarks can be "fitted" across the curve or surface by using one of two different algorithms. One algorithm uses the TPS to map each set of coordinates onto the sample mean such that the *bending energy* is minimized. The other algorithm seeks to minimize the Procrustes distance across the sets of coordinates. Both methods require iterations of sample mean computation, sliding of the landmarks along the tangent vectors so as to meet the optimization criterion, and sliding the semilandmarks back to the nearest point along the curve or surface (Gunz et al., 2005; Mitteroecker and Gunz, 2009). Once the semilandmarks have been "fitted" by one of the two possible algorithms, they can be treated as homologous landmarks and subjected to further statistical analyses. Williams and Slice (2010) demonstrate how semilandmarks can be effectively used to identify variation in facial structures that are not well defined by traditional landmarks. The curvature of the nasal aperture, the orbit, the zygomatic bone and arch, and the maxillary alveolar process were recorded as semilandmarks and then analyzed for age-related changes. This study found changes in the shape of these structures associated with age as well as population and sex-related variation.

Programs for Data Analysis

There exists a wide range of software packages that perform various geometric morphometric analyses. There are utility programs for post-collection data processing, programs that conduct specific analyses, and comprehensive programs for both geometric morphometric and standard statistical analyses. Table 12.3 includes some of the more popular geometric morphometric programs used in biological anthropology along with their capabilities and access information. The free statistical computation and graphical program R: A Language and Environment for Statistical Computing (R Development Core Team, 2011, http://www.r-project.org/) is also capable of performing many geometric morphometric analyses and code for various geometric morphometric procedures is freely available, both from R and from other sources on the Internet, including the SUNY-Stony Brook Morphometrics site (http://life.bio.sunysb.edu/morph/). For using R for both traditional and geometric morphometrics, the text *Morphometrics with R* (Claude, 2008) is a good place to start.

CURRENT APPLICATIONS OF GEOMETRIC MORPHOMETRICS IN SKELETAL BIOLOGY

Skeletal biologists have eagerly adopted the tools of geometric morphometrics and have applied them to a wide range of research questions. This process has integrated the approaches to data collection and analysis into biological anthropology, and at times, the needs of anthropological analyses have helped shape advances within geometric morphometrics (Slice, 2007). A survey of current applications of geometric morphometrics to human skeletal biology is presented below and organized by research area. Since the focus of this text is human skeletal biology, the review does not include studies involving nonhuman primates or paleoanthropology, although there is a considerable body of geometric morphometric

TABLE 12.3 Popular Programs for Geometric Morphometric Analysis in Biological Anthropology[a]

Program Name	Capabilities	How to Access
MorphoJ (Klingenberg, 2011)	Procrustes superimposition, partitions symmetric and asymmetric components, PCA, regression, CVA, DFA	http://www.flywings.org.uk/MorphoJ_page.htm
Morpheus et al. (Slice, 2000)	Data acquisition, Procrustes superimposition, TPS, visualization	http://www.morphometrics.org/
EVAN TOOLBOX (EVAN-society)	Data acquisition, Procrustes superimposition, PCA, TPS, visualization	http://evan-society.org/node/23 (access requires $100 yearly membership fee)
R Version 2.14.1 (R Foundation for Statistical Computing, 2011)	Procustes superimposition, PCA, TPS, visualization, standard statistical analyses	http://www.r-project.org/
tpsRegr (F. James Rohlf)	Multivariate multiple regression of partial warp scores from TPS and uniform shape onto independent variables	http://life.bio.sunysb.edu/morph/ Software page, Thin Plate Spline
tpsRelw (F. James Rohlf)	Relative warp analysis from TPS, visualizations, semilandmark fitting	http://life.bio.sunysb.edu/morph/ Software page, Thin Plate Spline
tpsSplin (F. James Rohlf)	Pairwise thin-plate spline deformations	http://life.bio.sunysb.edu/morph/ Software page, Thin Plate Spline
3d-id (Slice and Ross, 2009)	Classification of unknown specimen based on landmark coordinates	http://www.3d-id.org/

[a]*This is by no means a complete list of all available programs. Many more programs can be found on the Software page of http://life.bio.sunysb.edu/morph/.*

research in both of these areas. Because of the extreme volume of publications, this survey is not exhaustive, but hopefully provides the reader with a grasp of the current state of geometric morphometric research in our field.

For a single volume that contains critical theoretical and methodological content as well as a diverse series of applications of geometric morphometrics to anthropological questions, *Modern Morphometrics in Physical Anthropology* edited by Dennis Slice (2005) is recommended. Nevertheless, be aware that geometric morphometric methods have progressed rapidly, and one should conduct a thorough literature search to identify the most recent publications on a particular topic or method to ensure that research designs take advantage of the most current knowledge and innovations in the field.

Sexual Dimorphism

Patterns of sexual dimorphism in craniofacial morphology and postcranial elements have been investigated with geometric morphometrics. Since sexual dimorphism is a function of both shape and size, geometric morphometric methods provide significant insight into how each contributes to dimorphism and clarify the shape differences between males and females that exist independent of size.

Using a generalized Procrustes analysis (GPA) of three-dimensional coordinates from 16 craniofacial landmarks observed on Euro-American and African-American males and females of known sex, Kimmerle et al. (2008) investigated shape and size variation associated with sexual dimorphism. A MANCOVA procedure employing principal component scores derived from the Procrustes coordinates and Centroid Size indicated that sex had a significant effect on shape for both groups, but that size did not influence shape for either group (meaning that within each sex, shape was the same regardless of size). Based on this finding, they suggest that varying degrees of sexual dimorphism across human populations may be the result of size differences, rather than allometric variation.

Gonzalez et al. (2011) used crania from the Coimbra collection in Portugal to explore patterns of sexually dimorphic shape and size in the cranium. They used 12 landmarks and 25 semilandmarks to quantify the shape of the glabella and the malar, mastoid, and frontal processes. The PCA results indicated a low degree of dimorphism in shape and discriminant analysis produced poor classification results. When Centroid Size was included in the analysis, correct classification increased, reflecting the marked difference in size between the sexes.

Sexual dimorphism in subadults was investigated by Franklin et al. (2007) utilizing a sample of 96 known subadult mandibles using coordinates from 38 landmarks. Results indicated little sexual dimorphism in the subadult mandible for all populations and classification results were poor (only 59% correctly classified overall). However, the authors found some significant shape variables associated with different populations. The authors suggest that variation in mandibular shape may be attributed to morphology established early in ontogeny and the result of inherited genetic traits.

In an effort to quantify morphological traits typically assessed through visual observation for estimating sex, Pretorius et al. (2006) analyzed a sample of South Africans comparing three areas that may be sexually dimorphic: the shape of the greater sciatic notch, mandibular ramus flexure, and shape of the orbits. The coordinate data were analyzed using relative warp scores, thin-plate splines, and CVA. As expected, the greater sciatic notch provided the best separation of the sexes. Surprisingly, a greater degree of accuracy for estimating sex was obtained from the orbits as opposed to the ramus. Bigoni et al. (2010) also found a high degree of classification using landmarks of the orbits, suggesting that the orbits are a region of sexual dimorphism that previously was not identified using traditional methods.

In application of geometric morphometric methods to postcranial elements, Bytheway and Ross (2010) attempted to define landmarks on the os coxa that might be useful for quantifying the morphological variation employed in sex estimation. Three-dimensional coordinates for 36 landmarks were observed on adult os coxae from a sample composed of African-Americans and Euro-Americans. GPA was used to fit the coordinates, which were then subjected to PCA. The PC scores were utilized as data for a MANCOVA and discriminant analysis. Results indicated that both size and sex have a significant effect for both groups and that these landmarks produce highly accurate sex estimation. For more information on sexual dimorphism and sex estimation/assessment, see Moore (Chapter 4), this volume.

Population Structure and History

Geometric morphometric analyses have been applied to studies of biological distance, population structure, and history. Early applications of geometric morphometrics to biological distance analyses include McKeown (2000) and McKeown and Jantz (2005). The use of geometric morphometrics has been extended to larger, more geographically diverse samples and has also been applied to questions regarding the interplay of genetics and environment on the phenotype.

Building on previous geometric morphometric research into the peopling of the Americas (Perez et al., 2007; Gonzalez-Jose et al., 2008), Perez et al. (2009) tested the discrepancy between morphological variation and genetic data in explaining the number of founding populations into the Americas. The degree of biological diversity during the Holocene (which began about 12,000 years ago) as shown in craniofacial morphology among populations in North and South America has resulted in the proposal of two hypotheses regarding the peopling of the Americas. One states there were multiple migrations and the second proposes a single migration with local diversification. The two competing hypotheses are based on whether one is using craniometric data (multiple migrations) or genetic data (local diversification).

To test these hypotheses, Perez et al. (2009) sampled Holocene remains from Central Argentina and compared morphological and ancient genetic data. The authors used both two-dimensional landmarks and semilandmarks digitized in the Frankfurt plane from photographs taken on the facial and vault regions of the skull. **mtDNA** *haplogroup* data were obtained from previous studies using the same Holocene remains from Argentina. They found a lack of concordance between the molecular data and craniofacial morphology, similar to a previous study (Perez et al., 2007). Their results demonstrated that even for the early Holocene samples that show a distinct morphology from modern Native Americans, the mtDNA haplogroups are the same. These findings might imply a single migration from Northeast Asia or southern Siberia as detected in a recent study using whole-genome sequencing (Dulik et al., 2012). If the rapid peopling of the continent occurred coupled with extreme ecological diversity, a scenario of localized diversification is probable.

Smith et al. (2007) investigated variation in the temporal bone and the relative contributions of genetics and environment. Coordinates from 22 landmarks observed on temporal bones from 11 modern population samples were registered with GPA. PC scores based on the GPA output were used to assess variation across the groups sampled as well as to test for concordance among group distances based on the coordinate and genetic data. Differences in the shape of the temporal bone were found across all groups and discriminant analysis was able to correctly classify individual specimens with a relatively high degree of accuracy. The distance matrices based on coordinate and genetic data for the Old World samples were significantly correlated; however, this did not hold true when Native Americans were included in the matrix correlation analyses. While temporal bone size did show strong correlation with climate (temperature and latitude) suggestive of selective forces, shape was correlated with geography and conformed to a model of isolation by distance. This research indicates that temporal bone shape is selectively neutral and useful for distinguishing among groups.

In a follow-up to a previous study, Smith (2009) used coordinate data from 83 landmarks collected on skulls from 14 modern populations. The dataset was broken into seven subsets representing anatomical units, including the entire cranium, that were employed to calculate biological distances among the groups that were compared to molecular distances among the same or similar groups. The coordinate data were subjected to GPA and the projected coordinates were used to compute PC scores which were analyzed with the program RMET (R matrix analysis) for the purposes of generating biological distance matrices. The anatomical units with the highest correlations with the neutral molecular distances were the basicranium, temporal bone, upper face, and the entire cranium, suggesting these may be the best regions of the cranium for assessing population structure and relationships based on morphological data.

With a similar goal, von Cramon-Taubadel (2009) tested the shape of the temporal bone against other individual cranial bones to ascertain if other elements show a pattern of selective neutrality similar to the temporal bone. Employing coordinates observed on landmarks from 7 individual cranial bones as well as the entire cranium from 15 samples of modern humans, biological distance matrices were calculated in RMET based on PC scores from GPA registered coordinates. These matrices were compared to molecular distance matrices and results indicated that the temporal bone does show the strongest correlation with neutral genetic data; nevertheless, the shape of the sphenoid, frontal, and parietal bones also shows significant correlations with the molecular data.

In another study utilizing coordinate data from cranial landmarks, von Cramon-Taubadel (2011) tested the efficacy of functional and developmental cranial units for reconstructing human population history and delineating suitable cranial units related to congruence with neutral molecular data. She tested to see if the basicranial region is more reliable to reconstruct population history than other regions of the human cranium. The study also tested the hypothesis that cranial regions associated with a single sensory function are less reliable indicators of neutral genetic history. The results showed little support for the "basicranium hypothesis" as other regions of the cranium showed just as much genetic congruence. She also found less support for defining cranial regions on the basis of anatomical or functional complexity as this did not provide a consistent way to predict phylogenetic relationships or population history. Overall, she suggested future research should be focused on identifying areas that are particularly unreliable (such as the zygomatic and occipital bones) and removing these from analyses.

Martinez-Abadias et al. (2012) studied the question of morphological integration of the cranium by applying geometric morphometrics and quantitative genetic theory to the study of a sample from the Hallstatt, Austria ossuary that are individually identified. Results suggested that the face, cranial base, and cranial vault should not be seen as independent units, but rather are strongly integrated structures. Their methodology has an advantage over previous research that used phenotypic covariance structure as a proxy for genetic data (Smith et al., 2007; von Cramon-Taubadel, 2011). Instead, they estimated a genetic covariance matrix directly from the quantitative traits of the Hallstatt sample, since associated genealogical information is available for this sample. They found strong integration for cranial shape throughout the entire skull as genetic variation was concentrated in only a few dimensions, thus indicating a strong genetic component and integration to overall cranial shape change. This means that, overall, the skull behaves as a composite, and changes in one region will produce correlated phenotypic changes in other regions, similar to studies in mouse and newt skulls (Ivanovic and Kalezic, 2010), and previous studies of the human skull (Bookstein et al., 2003; Bastir et al., 2010).

In order to test the hypothesis that within extreme environments (cold, dry, hot, humid) nasal cavities will exhibit features that enhance turbulence and air-wall contact to improve conditioning of the air, Noback et al. (2011) sampled 10 modern human populations residing in extreme climates and analyzed the shape of the bony nasal cavity using 21 landmarks. This study demonstrated a high degree of correlation between nasal cavity morphology and climatic variables. The authors concluded that nasal cavity morphology appears mostly related to temperature, whereas morphology of the nasopharynx is associated with humidity. Similar to previous studies, they found that the shape of the nasal aperture is higher and narrower in cold climates compared to hot–humid climates. These shape changes in cold–dry climates appear to be functionally consistent with an increase in contact with air and mucosal tissue through greater turbulence during respiration and a higher surface-to-volume ratio in the upper nasal cavity.

Growth and Development

Several studies have used geometric morphometrics to detect ontogenetic scaling and allometric trajectories in human growth and development. As morphological variation develops during growth, the study of ontogenetic series could identify forces (genetic or environmental) responsible for the size and shape differences observed among adult crania.

Strand Viðarsdóttir et al. (2002) explored the ontogenetic basis for craniofacial variation in 10 groups of modern humans ranging in age from infancy to adulthood. GPA was performed on coordinates from 21 landmarks. PCA was used to assess shape differences and discriminant analysis was used to classify individual crania. Results indicate that human facial form from birth contains population-specific morphologies. These distinct trajectories lead to further developmental differences later in ontogeny and carry over to adult morphology.

In another growth and development study, Gonzalez et al. (2010) analyzed the ontogeny of facial robustness among prehistoric South American groups. Similar to Strand Viðarsdóttir et al. (2002), these authors found the pattern of interpopulation variation in shape and size of facial form is established by the age of five, indicating that processes acting on facial morphology during ontogeny contribute to the observed differences seen in adult variation. Whether the observed developmental differences for robusticity are the result of random changes, or more localized, adaptive processes, the authors could not conclude. This is an area for further research.

Secular Change

Significant trends have occurred during the last 200 years in a number of human populations, including the U.S., Europe, and Japan. Significant attention has been paid to secular changes in craniofacial morphology. These changes include increased cranial vault height and changes in cranial vault width and have been seen in numerous populations, including Euro-American and African American populations, and in both males and females. Wescott and Jantz (2005) calculated two-dimensional coordinate data for 13 landmarks from craniometric data and use the data to investigate secular trends in nineteenth and twentieth century Euro-American and African American cranial morphology. Individuals with birthdates in the nineteenth century were obtained from the **Hamann-Todd Human Osteological Collection**[3] and the Robert J. Terry Anatomical Skeletal Collection while twentieth century samples were obtained from the **Forensic Databank**. Given that these collections are composed of known individuals, sex, ancestry, and birth year were available for all individuals. Data were subjected to Procrustes superimposition and multivariate regression was performed on the partial warp scores based on TPS. They found the most prominent change is associated with the cranial base for both groups. The authors concluded that proximate causes for this change are associated with the rapid neural growth trajectory of the basicranium in early development or growth rate **allometry**. Ultimate causes for these changes, the authors posit, are associated with improved health and nutrition.

Kimmerle and Jantz (2005) studied secular trends in asymmetry by analyzing craniofacial traits in a large sample of Euro- and African-Americans born between the years 1820 and 1980. Building on previous research for cranial morphological secular trends within this dataset, these authors tested the possible relationship for increased asymmetry during periods of rapid morphological change. Seven bilateral landmarks were chosen for their analysis. Coordinate data were subjected to GPA and differences in asymmetry were assessed through a MANOVA. Centroid Size was used for analyses of size asymmetry. Two-way ANOVAs were performed to test for the main effects of side to test for *directional asymmetry* (the propensity for a particular side of a trait to develop more than the other), individual, and the interaction between side and individual on size and shape for both sex and ancestral groups. *Fluctuating asymmetry* (subtle deviations that exist between paired structures due to random perturbations of developmental processes) over time was assessed via regression analysis.

The only group to exhibit some degree of developmental instability was African American females. The interpretation of developmental instability is challenging given the various genetic and environmental components that might result in the observed asymmetry. Interestingly, not all American samples showed a significant degree of fluctuating asymmetry as might be expected from such vast environmental change during the period under study. Nineteenth century America saw many environmental changes for African Americans, including nutritional deficiencies, infectious disease, and parasitic load as well as detrimental social conditions (i.e., segregation and social discrimination). The authors conclude that perhaps a combination of the effects of slavery, the American Civil War, Reconstruction, and the Depression in the Southern United States had a significant effect on cranial asymmetry. This study not only illustrates the efficacy of geometric morphometrics for studying shape change through time, but it also reminds us that biological variation is the product of both genetics and environment acting on the phenotype and that social conditions and stress are components of environmental factors (e.g., see Gravlee, 2009).

Weisensee and Jantz (2011) examined secular change in cranial morphology in the New Lisbon collection, a documented skeletal collection from Lisbon, Portugal with birth years ranging from 1806 to 1954. This period represents significant changes in the population, including increased urbanization, population growth, and changes in mortality and fertility patterns. As this population is from a more geographically restricted space compared with

---

[3]This collection is curated by the Cleveland Museum of Natural History in Cleveland, Ohio.

the previous studies of Euro-American and African-American samples (Wescott and Jantz, 2005), the confounding variables were more easily controlled. The authors tested two hypotheses found in previous studies: (1) cranial morphology will change as a result of demographic transitions (population growth, urbanization, etc.) and (2) allometry will have a localized effect on cranial shape, specifically in areas of variation found to be important in growth and development.

They tested these hypotheses by using geometric morphometrics on 67 cranial landmarks, and dividing the series into an ontogenetic (subadult) series and an adult series. Multiple regression on the symmetric components of the Procrustes coordinates on year of birth and Centroid Size were used to examine shape change over time and examine patterns of allometry. The sample was further divided by sex into 25-year birth cohorts to assess the relative position of the birth cohorts in the multivariate analyses. A secular trend was indicated by the chronological ordering of birth cohorts in the data as detected in CVA. The multiple regression of shape on year of birth in the sample indicates a strong and statistically significant temporal change over the last 150 years. The changes that occurred during this time period in Portugal were mostly to the cranial base, a region of the skull that experiences an early growth curve. Weisensee and Jantz (2011) argued that this change was most likely associated with declines in childhood morbidity and mortality.

Forensic Anthropology

The use of geometric morphometrics within the field of forensic anthropology is varied, and includes methods for sex estimation and ancestry analyses. The following are just a few examples of the use of geometric morphometrics in the field over the last decade or so.

In an early attempt at using geometric morphometrics to differentiate groups based on craniofacial morphology, Ross et al. (1999) compared a sample of Euro-Americans and African Americans to test for differential morphological patterns. A total of 14 cranial landmarks was recorded. After Procrustes superimposition, the crania were subjected to discriminant analysis. This early study was successful in the classification of crania and demonstrated how these methods could be employed as a tool to locate specific regions of morphological variation important to distinguishing between groups.

Similar to the estimation of sex in subadult skeletal material, the estimation of ancestry is equally difficult. Buck and Strand Viðarsdóttir (2004) analyzed mandibular morphology for ancestral estimation as skeletal remains in forensic cases are often found incomplete. Their study sample represented five distinct morphological groups and included both adult and subadult mandibles. Seventeen unilateral landmarks were digitized on the mandibular ramus and corpus. Coordinate data were subjected to Procrustes superimposition. PCA of the fitted coordinates was used to account for the principal axes of variation within the sample and discriminant analysis was applied to the data in order to classify individuals. Their results show that significant classification is achieved for the complete mandible (> 70%), with slightly less accurate classification results for incomplete mandibular remains. The results suggest that mandibular shape might be useful in the estimation of ancestry in subadult skeletal material.

Using facial contours, Sholts et al. (2011b) examined the midfacial skeleton in modern human groups, as this region of the skull has been found to have higher predictive value for group classification. They analyzed the midfacial skeleton employing digital scans of crania from three groups (Norway, China, U.S.) to obtain cross-sectional contours defined by a geometric plane using three standard craniometric landmarks: nasion, and right and left zygomaxillare. The contours were then subjected to elliptic Fourier analysis and Fourier coefficients were extracted for statistical analysis, in this case discriminant analysis. The classification results are similar to other methods, with crania classifying correctly 86% of the time. This finding, although based on a small sample size, is promising considering the range of geographic provenience for remains found in places like the Western United States (see DiGangi and Hefner [Chapter 5], this volume).

CONCLUSION AND ADDITIONAL RESOURCES

This short review of current geometric research in human skeletal biology clearly illustrates the wide range of applications available with this approach to quantification and analysis of morphological variation. Research is expanding into the use of semilandmarks from curves and surfaces and the application of these methods to the morphology of postcranial elements. So the revolution continues as these new approaches expand the range of research questions that can be investigated with coordinate data and we expect to see rapid changes in the tool kit for geometric morphometrics.

There are some excellent resources online for anyone interested in geometric morphometrics. The most comprehensive of these is the SUNY Stony Brook Morphometrics site (http://life.bio.sunysb.edu/morph/) that contains a wide range of resources for both novice and experienced researchers. Arguably the most important components of this site include a Software page, which provides a compilation of analytical programs for geometric morphometrics that can be downloaded directly from the site and links to other sites where programs can be accessed, and the Glossary (Slice et al., 2009), which contains a wide-ranging list of terms, concepts, and methods with definitions. The site also provides information on workshops and conferences, hardware for data collection, available datasets, a list of researchers from around the world interested in geometric morphometrics with areas of specialization and contact information, and bibliographies with important publications in geometric morphometrics.

Another excellent resource is MORPHMET (http://morphometrics.org/morphmet.html), a morphometrics mailing list moderated by Dennis Slice. Subscribers can post questions about any aspect of morphometric research and the MORPHMET community provides answers to the best of their ability. Several senior geometric morphometric researchers and software designers subscribe to MORPHMET and often provide feedback to questions posed. Overall the list provides an opportunity to get answers to specific questions as well as learn from the questions asked by others. Workshops for learning about geometric morphometric are often advertised through this list so it is an excellent way to get exposed to the field.

Students interested in further exploration of geometric morphometrics should explore online resources such as Morphometrics at SUNY Stony Brook and Morphometrics.org. Then move into the literature (this chapter's bibliography is a great place to start) and explore the wide range of methods and research designs being implemented in studies that use geometric morphometrics. We urge you to remember that this is an area that has seen extraordinary growth in theory, method and application since the "revolution," and this is expected to continue at a furious pace as biological anthropologists find ever more innovative ways to apply geometric morphometrics to studies of human variation.

ACKNOWLEDGMENTS

The authors would like to thank the editors of the volume for their insightful comments and suggestions that assisted in the production of this chapter. We appreciate the contributions of Elizabeth Agosto to the case study presented and the programming assistance provided by Patrick McKeown. Thanks are due to Roselyn Campbell for the photographs used in this chapter and to Jonathan Bethard for his assistance with figure formatting. Funds for the purchase of the three-dimensional digitizer utilized to collect the data employed in the case study were provided by the William M. Bass III Endowment and the Office of Research at the University of Tennessee-Knoxville.

REFERENCES

Adams, D.C., Rohlf, F.J., Slice, D.E., 2004. Geometric morphometrics: ten years of progress following the "revolution". Italian Journal of Zoology 71, 5—16.

Afifi, A.A., Clark, V., 1996. Computer-aided Multivariate Analysis. Chapman & Hall, London.

Aldridge, K., Boyadjiev, S.A., Capone, G.T., DeLeon, V.B., Richtsmeier, J.T., 2005. Precision and error of three-dimensional phenotypic measures acquired from 3dMD photogrammetric images. American Journal of Medical Genetics 138A, 247—253.

Bastir, M., Rosas, A., Stringer, C.B., Cuetara, J.M., Kruszynski, R., Weber, G.W., Ross, C.F., Ravosa, M.J., 2010. Effects of brain and facial size on basicranial form in human and primate evolution. Journal of Human Evolution 58, 424—431.

Bigoni, L., Veleminská, J., Brůžek, J., 2010. Three-dimensional geometric morphometric analysis of cranio-facial sexual dimorphism in a Central European sample of known sex. Homo 61 (1), 16—32.

Bookstein, F.L., 1991. Morphometric Tools for Landmark Data. University of Cambridge Press, London.

Bookstein, F., Schafer, K., Prossinger, H., Seidler, H., Fieder, M., Stringer, C., Weber, G.W., Arsuaga, J.L., Slice, D.E., Rohlf, F.J., Recheis, W., Mariam, A.J., Marcus, L.F., 1999. Comparing frontal cranial profiles in archaic and modern Homo by morphometric analysis. Anatomical Record 257, 217—224.

Bookstein, F.L., Gunz, P., Mitteroecker, H., Prossinger, K., Schaefer, K., Seidler, H., 2003. Cranial integration in Homo: singular warps analysis of the midsagittal plane in ontogeny and evolution. Journal of Human Evolution 44 (2), 167—187.

Buck, T.J., Strand Viðarsdóttir, U., 2004. A proposed method for the identification of race in sub-adult skeletons: a geometric morphometric analysis of mandibular morphology. Journal of Forensic Sciences 49 (6), 1—6.

Buikstra, J.E., Ubelaker, D.H., 1994. Standards for data collection from human skeletal material: Proceedings of a seminar at the Field Museum of Natural History. Arkansas Archaeological Survey, Fayetteville, AR.

Buikstra, J.E., Frankenburg, S.R., Konigsberg, L.W., 1990. Skeletal biological distance studies in American physical anthropology: Recent trends. American Journal of Physical Anthropology 82 (1), 1—7.

Bytheway, J.A., Ross, A.H., 2010. A geometric morphometric approach to sex determination of the human adult os coxa. Journal of Forensic Sciences 55 (4), 859—864.

Claude, J. (2008). Morphometrics with R. Springer, New York.

Christensen, A.M., 2005. Assessing the variation in individual frontal sinus outlines. American Journal of Physical Anthropology 127 (3), 291—295.

Corner, B.D., Lele, S., Richtsmeier, J.T., 1992. Measuring precision of three-dimensional landmark data. American Journal of Physical Anthropology 3, 347—359.

Darroch, J.N., Mosimann, J.E., 1985. Canonical and principal components of shape. Biometrika 72 (2), 241–252.

De Groote, I., 2011a. Femoral curvature in Neanderthals and modern humans: a 3D geometric morphometric analysis. Journal of Human Evolution 60 (5), 540–548.

De Groote, I., 2011b. The Neanderthal lower arm. Journal of Human Evolution 61 (4), 396–410.

De Groote, I., Lockwood, C.A., Aiello, L.C., 2010. Technical note: A new method for measuring long bone curvature using 3D landmarks and semi-landmarks. American Journal of Physical Anthropology 141 (4), 658–664.

Devor, E.J., 1987. Transmission of human craniofacial dimensions. J. Craniofacial Genet. Dev. Biol. 7, 95–106.

DiGangi, E.A., Hefner, J.T., 2013. Ancestry estimation. In: DiGangi, E.A., Moore, M.K. (Eds.), Research Methods in Human Skeletal Biology. Academic Press, San Diego.

DiGangi, E.A., Moore, M.K., 2013. Introduction to skeletal biology. In: DiGangi, E.A., Moore, M.K. (Eds.), Research Methods in Human Skeletal Biology. Academic Press, San Diego.

Dryden, I.L., Mardia, K.V., 1993. Multivariate shape analysis. Indian Journal of Statistics 55A, 460–480.

Dulik, M.C., Zhadanov, S.I., Osipova, L.P., Askapuli, A., Gau, L., Gokumen, O., Rubinstein, S., Schurr, T.D., 2012. Mitochondrial DNA and Y chromosome variation provides evidence for a recent common ancestry between Native Americans and indigenous Altaians. American Journal of Human Genetics 90 (2), 229–246.

Franklin, D., Oxnard, C.E., O'Higgins, P., Dadour, I., 2007. Sexual dimorphism in the subadult mandible: quantification using geometric morphometrics. Journal of Forensic Sciences 52 (1), 6–10.

Giles, E., Elliot, O., 1962. Race identification from cranial measurements. Journal of Forensic Sciences 7, 147–157.

Giles, E., Elliot, O., 1963. Sex determination by discriminant function analysis of crania. American Journal of Physical Anthropology 21 (1), 53–68.

Gonzalez, P.N., Perez, S.I., Bernal, V., 2010. Ontogeny of robusticity of craniofacial traits in modern humans: a study of South American populations. American Journal of Physical Anthropology 142 (3), 367–379.

Gonzalez, P.N., Bernal, V., Perez, S.I., 2011. Analysis of sexual dimorphism of craniofacial traits using geometric morphometric techniques. International Journal of Osteoarchaeology 21 (1), 82–91.

Gonzalez-Jose, R., Bortolini, M.C., Santos, F.R., Bonatto, S.L., 2008. The peopling of America: craniofacial shape variation on a continental scale and its interpretation from an interdisciplinary view. American Journal of Physical Anthropology 137 (2), 175–187.

Goodall, C., 1991. Procustes methods in the statistical analysis of shape. Journal of the Royal Statistical Society 53 (2), 285–339.

Gower, J.C., 1975. Generalized procrustes analysis. Psychometrika 40, 33–51.

Gravlee, C.C., 2009. How race becomes biology: embodiment of social inequality. American Journal of Physical Anthropology 139 (1), 47–57.

Gunz, P., Mitteroecker, P., Bookstein, F.L., 2005. Semilandmarks in three dimensions. In: Slice, D.E. (Ed.), Modern Morphometrics in Physical Anthropology. Kluwer Academic, New York, pp. 73–98.

Hammer, Ø., Harper, D.A.T., Ryan, P.D., 2001. PAST: Paleontological statistics software package for education and data analysis. Palaeontologia Electronica 4, 9pp.

Harpending, H.C., Ward, R., 1982. Chemical systematics and human evolution. In: Nitecki, M. (Ed.), Biochemical Aspects of Evolutionary Biology. University of Chicago, Chicago, pp. 213–256.

Howells, W.W., 1973. Cranial variation in man: A study by multivariate analysis of patterns of differences among recent human populations. Peabody Museum, Harvard University, Cambridge, MA.

Ivanovic, A., Kalezic, M.L., 2010. Testing the hypothesis of morphological integration on a skull of a vertebrate with a biphasic life cycle: a case study of the alpine newt. Journal of Experimental Biology Part B: Molecular and Developmental Evolution 314 (7), 527–538.

Jantz, R.L., 1973. Microevolutionary change in Arikara crania: a multivariate analysis. American Journal of Physical Anthropology 38 (1), 15–26.

Jantz, R.L., 1997. Cranial, postcranial and discrete trait variation. In: Owsley, D.W., Rose, J. (Eds.), Bioarchaeology of the North Central United States. Arkansas Archaeological Survey, Fayetteville, AR, pp. 240–247.

Jantz, R.L., 2001. Cranial change in Americans: 1850–1975. Journal of Forensic Sciences 46, 784–787.

Jantz, R.L., Meadows Jantz, L., 2000. Secular change in craniofacial morphology. American Journal of Human Biology 12 (3), 327–338.

Jantz, R.L., Ousley, S.D., 1996–2005. FORDISC 3.0: Personal computer forensic discriminant functions. Department of Anthropology, The University of Tennessee, Knoxville, TN.

Kendall, D.G., 1984. Shape manifolds, procrustean metrics, and complex projective spaces. Bulletin of the London Mathematical Society 16 (2), 81–121.

Kimmerle, E.H., Jantz, R.L., 2005. Secular trends in craniofacial asymmetry studied by geometric morphometry and generalized Procrustes methods. In: Slice, D.E. (Ed.), Modern Morphometrics in Physical Anthropology. Kluwer Academic, New York, pp. 247–263.

Kimmerle, E.H., Ross, A.H., Slice, D.E., 2008. Sexual dimorphism in America: geometric morphometric analysis of the craniofacial region. Journal of Forensic Sciences 53 (1), 54–57.

Klingenberg, C.P., 2011. MorphoJ: an integrated software package for geometric morphometrics. Molecular Ecology Resources 11 (2), 353–357.

Klingenberg, C.P., Barluenga, M., Meyer, A., 2002. Shape analysis of symmetric structures: quantifying variation among individuals and asymmetry. Society for the Study of Evolution 56 (10), 1909–1920.

Konigsberg, L.W., 1990. Analysis of prehistoric biological variation under a model of isolation by geographic and temporal distance. Human Biology 62 (1), 49–70.

Lele, S., Richtsmeier, J.T., 1991. Euclidean distance matrix analysis: a coordinate free approach for comparing biological shapes using landmark data. American Journal of Physical Anthropology 86 (3), 415–428.

Manly, B.F.J., 1986. Randomization and regression methods for testing for associations with geographical, environmental, and biologial distances between populations. Researches on Population Ecology 28 (2), 201–218.

Mantel, N., 1967. The detection of disease clustering and generalized regression approach. Cancer Research 27, 209–220.

Marcus, L.F., 1990. Traditional morphometrics. In: Rohlf, F.J., Bookstein, F.L. (Eds.), Proceedings of the Michigan Morphometrics Workshop. The University of Michigan Museum of Zoology, Ann Arbor, MI, pp. 77–122.

Marcus, L.F., Corti, M., 1996. Overview of the new, or geometric morphometrics. In: Marcus, L.F. (Ed.), Advances in Morphometrics. Plenum Press, New York, pp. 1–13.

Martinez-Abadias, N., Esparza, M., Sjovold, T., Gonzalez-Jose, R., Santos, M., Hernandez, M., Klingenberg, C.P., 2012. Pervasive genetic integration directs the evolution of human skull shape. Evolution 66, 1010–1023.

McKeown, A.H., 2000. Investigating Variation among Arikara Crania using Geometric Morphometry. Unpublished PhD dissertation. Department of Anthropology, University of Tennessee, Knoxville.

McKeown, A.H., Jantz, R.L., 2005. Comparison of coordinate and craniometric data for biological distance studies. In: Slice, D.E. (Ed.), Modern Morphometrics in Physical Anthropology. Kluwer Academic, New York, pp. 215–230.

Mitteroecker, P., Gunz, P., 2009. Advances in geometric morphometrics. Evolutionary Biology 36, 235–247.

Moore, M.K., 2013. Functional morphology and medical imaging. In: DiGangi, E.A., Moore, M.K. (Eds.), Research Methods in Human Skeletal Biology. Academic Press, San Diego.

Moore, M.K., 2013. Sex estimation and assessment. In: DiGangi, E.A., Moore, M.K. (Eds.), Research Methods in Human Skeletal Biology. Academic Press, San Diego.

Moore-Jansen, P.M., Ousley, S.D., Jantz, R.L., 1994. Data collection procedures for forensic skeletal material. Report of Investigations no. 48, Department of Anthropology, The University of Tennessee, Knoxville, TN.

Noback, M.L., Harvati, K., Spoor, F., 2011. Climate related variation of the human nasal cavity. American Journal of Physical Anthropology 145 (4), 599–614.

Ousley, S.D., McKeown, A.H., 2001. Three dimensional digitizing of human skulls as an archival procedure. In: Williams, E. (Ed.), Human Remains: Conservation, Retrieval and Analysis. Archaeopress, Oxford, pp. 173–184.

Ousley, S.D., Jantz, R.L., Fried, D., 2009. Understanding race and human variation: why forensic anthropologists are good at identifying race. American Journal of Physical Anthropology 139 (1), 68–76.

Perez, S.I., Bernal, V., Gonzalez, P.N., 2007. Morphological differentiation of aboriginal human populations from Tierra del Fuego (Patagonia): implications for South American peopling. American Journal of Physical Anthropology 133 (4), 1067–1079.

Perez, S.I., Bernal, V., Gonzalez, P.N., Sardi, M., Politis, G.G., 2009. Discrepancy between cranial and DNA data of early Americans: implications for American peopling. PloS ONE 4 (5) e5746.

Pietrusewsky, M., 2008. Metric analysis of skeletal remains: methods and applications. In: Katzenberg, M.A., Saunders, S.R. (Eds.), Biological Anthropology of the Human Skeleton. John Wiley & Sons, Hoboken, NJ, pp. 487–532.

Pretorius, E., Steyn, M., Scholtz, Y., 2006. Investigation into the usability of geometric morphometric analysis in assessment of sexual dimorphism. American Journal of Physical Anthropology 129 (1), 64—70.

R Development Core Team, 2011. R: A Language and Environment for Statistical Computing. R Foundation for Statistical Computing.

Relethford, J.H., 1994. Craniometric variation among modern human populations. American Journal of Physical Anthropology 95, 53—62.

Relethford, J.H., 2001. Global analysis of regional differences in craniometric diversity and population substructure. Human Biology 73 (5), 629—636.

Relethford, J.H., 2002. Apportionment of global human genetic diversity based on craniometrics and skin color. American Journal of Physical Anthropology 118 (4), 393—398.

Relethford, J.H., 2004. Global patterns of isolation by distance based on genetic and morphological data. Human Biology 76 (4), 499—513.

Relethford, J.H., 2009. Race and global patterns of phenotypic variation. American Journal of Physical Anthropology 139 (1), 16—22.

Relethford, J.H., 2010. Population-specific deviations of global human craniometric variation from a neutral model. American Journal of Physical Anthropology 142 (1), 105—111.

Relethford, J.H., Blangero, J., 1990. Detection of differential gene flow from patterns of quantitative variation. Human Biology 62, 5—25.

Relethford, J.H., Lees, F.C., 1982. The use of quantitative traits in the study of human population structure. Yearbook of Physical Anthropology 25, 113—132.

Rencher, A.C., 1995. Methods of Multivariate Analysis. John Wiley & Sons, New York.

Richtsmeier, J.T., Paik, C.H., Elfert, P.C., Cole, T.M., Dahlman, H.R., 1995. Precision, repeatability, and validation of localization of cranial landmarks using computed tomography scans. Cleft Palate-Craniofacial Journal 32 (3), 217—227.

Richtsmeier, J.T., DeLeon, V.B., Lele, S.R., 2002. The promise of geometric morphometrics. Yearbook of Physical Anthropology 45, 63—91.

Rohlf, F.J., 2003. Bias and error in estimates of mean shape in geometric morphometrics. Journal of Human Evolution 44 (6), 665—683.

Rohlf, F.J., Marcus, L.F., 1993. A revolution in morphometrics. Tree 8 (4), 129—132.

Rohlf, F.J., Slice, D.E., 1990. Extensions of the Procrustes method for optimal superimposition of landmarks. Systematic Zoology 39 (1), 40—59.

Ross, A.H., Williams, S.E., 2008. Testing repeatability and error of coordinate landmark data acquired from crania. Journal of Forensic Sciences 53 (4), 782—785.

Ross, A.H., McKeown, A.H., Konigsberg, L.W., 1999. Allocation of crania to groups via the new morphometry. Journal of Forensic Sciences 44 (3), 584—587.

Sholts, S.B., Flores, L., Walker, P.L., Warmlander, S.K.T.S., 2011a. Comparison of coordinate measurement precision of different landmark types on human crania using a 3D laser scanner and a 3D digitiser: implications for applications of digital morphometrics. International Journal of Osteoarchaeology 21 (5), 535—543.

Sholts, S.B., Walker, P.L., Kuzminsky, S.C., Miller, K.W.P., Warmlander, S.K.T.S., 2011b. Identification of group affinity from cross-sectional contours of the human midfacial skeleton using digital morphometrics and 3D laser scanning technology. Journal of Forensic Sciences 56 (2), 333—338.

Slice, D.E., 2000. Morpheus et al: Software for morphometric research. Department of Ecology and Evolution, State University of New York, Stony Brook, NY.

Slice, D.E., 2001. Landmark coordinates aligned by Procrustes analysis do not lie in Kendall's shape space. Systematic Biology 50 (1), 141—149.

Slice, D.E., 2005. Modern morphometrics. In: Slice, D.E. (Ed.), Modern Morphometrics in Physical Anthropology. Kluwer Academic/Plenum Publishers, New York, pp. 1—24.

Slice, D.E. (Ed.), 2005. Modern Morphometrics in Physical Anthropology. Kluwer Academic, New York.

Slice, D.E., 2007. Geometric morphometrics. Annual Review of Anthropology 36, 261—281.

Slice, D.E., Ross, A., 2009. 3D-ID: geometric morphometric classification of crania for forensic scientists. http://www.3d-id.org.

Slice, D.E., Bookstein, F.L., Marcus, L.F., Rohlf, F.J., 2009. A glossary for geometric morphometrics. Morphometrics at SUNY Stony Brook. (http://life.bio.sunysb.edu/morph/index.html).

Smith, H.F., 2009. Which cranial regions reflect molecular distances reliably in humans? Evidence from three dimensional morphology. American Journal of Physical Anthropology 21, 36—47.

Smith, H.F., Terhune, C.E., Lockwood, C.A., 2007. Genetic, geographic, and environmental correlates of human temporal bone variation. American Journal of Physical Anthropology 134 (3), 312—322.

Smouse, P., Long, J., Sokal, R., 1986. Multiple regression and correlation extensions of the Mantel test of matrix correspondence. Systematic Zoology 35 (4), 627—632.

Stevens, S.D., Strand Viðarsdóttir, U., 2008. Morphological changes in the shape of the non-pathological bony knee joint with age: a morphometric analysis of the distal femur and proximal tibia in three populations of known age at death. International Journal of Osteoarchaeology 18 (4), 352—371.

Stojanowski, C.M., Schillaci, M.A., 2006. Phenotypic approaches for understanding patterns of intracemetery biological variation. Yearbook of Physical Anthropology 49, 49—88.

Strand Viðarsdóttir, U., O'Higgins, P., Stringer, C., 2002. A geometric morphometric study of regional differences in the ontogeny of the modern human facial skeleton. Journal of Anatomy 201 (3), 211—229.

von Cramon-Taubadel, N., 2009. Congruence of individual cranial bone morphology and neutral molecular affinity patterns in modern humans. American Journal of Physical Anthropology 140 (2), 205—215.

von Cramon-Taubadel, N., 2011. The relative efficacy of functional and developmental cranial modules for reconstructing global human population history. American Journal of Physical Anthropology 146 (1), 83—93.

von Cramon-Taubadel, N., Frazier, B.C., Lahr, M.M., 2007. The problem of assessing landmark error in geometric morphometrics: theory, methods, and modifications. American Journal of Physical Anthropology 134 (1), 24—35.

Weisensee, K.E., Jantz, R.L., 2011. Secular changes in craniofacial morphology of the Portuguese using geometric morphometrics. American Journal of Physical Anthropology 145 (4), 548—559.

Wescott, D.J., Jantz, R.L., 2005. Assessing craniofacial secular change in American blacks and whites using geometric morphometry. In: Slice, D.E. (Ed.), Modern Morphometrics in Physical Anthropology. Kluwer Academic, New York, pp. 231—245.

Williams, S.E., Slice, D.E., 2010. Regional shape change in adult facial bone curvature with age. American Journal of Physical Anthropology 143 (3), 437—447.

Bone and Dental Histology

Lindsay H. Trammell, Anne M. Kroman

INTRODUCTION

Biological anthropologists are constantly tasked with studying and identifying unknown human remains from modern, historic, and prehistoric contexts. In forensic circumstances, for example, the anthropologist is pivotal in the development of a biological profile from which a positive identification may be established. This profile includes age-at-death, sex, stature, and ancestry estimation from the remains, as discussed extensively in earlier chapters. Many of these estimations are based on gross morphological methods (refer to Uhl [Chapter 3]; Moore [Chapter 4]; DiGangi and Hefner [Chapter 5]; and Moore and Ross [Chapter 6], this volume). The presence of multiple individuals, along with confounding perimortem and postmortem circumstances, can make the analysis more difficult.

Successful application of the biological profile employs a variety of traditional methods. A key disadvantage is the necessity of near complete remains and proper preservation of target elements to make reliable estimations. Instances where traditional gross odontoskeletal features are not present force anthropologists to rely on bone or dental histology.

Bone histomorphology,[1] or the structure of bone tissue at the microscopic level, has potential utility for numerous anthropological disciplines. Histological studies have led to developments in ascertaining species identification, assessing age, analyzing trauma in peri- and postmortem environments, and understanding certain pathological conditions (Bell, 1990; Martin, 1991; Ericksen et al., 1994; Pfeiffer, 2000; Crowder and Stout, 2012). **Quantitative bone histology** is most commonly utilized in estimating age-at-death and has been employed by researchers since as early as 1911 when Balthazard and Lebrun produced the first written report in this area.

These applications will be discussed later in the chapter. To understand how to utilize bone histology as a research tool, it is first necessary to appreciate the basics of bone biology. We will provide a basic review below; however, the aspiring histologist should become intimately familiar with bone biology. Therefore, we recommend the following texts as a starting

[1]All bolded terms are defined in the glossary at the end of this volume.

point for further study: Enlow (1963), Martin and Burr (1989), Carter and Beaupre (2001), and Hall (2005).

Bone Biology

Bone is a very dynamic tissue (Enlow, 1963; Martin and Burr, 1989; Carter and Beaupre, 2001; Hall, 2005). It functions to provide mechanical support, protect vital structures, aid in **hematopoiesis** (generation of blood cells), and maintain mineral **homeostasis**. It is a composite material with both organic and inorganic components including a collagen matrix comprised of **hydroxyapatite** crystals.

To comprehend the structure and function of bone, it is necessary to grasp the types of cells involved in cortical bone **modeling** and **remodeling**. Bone modeling involves the sculpting of bone during growth and development. New bone, or primary bone, is produced or resorbed as individuals grow and there are shifts in areas of stress and strain being placed on the bone (Enlow, 1963). Modeling induces cortical bone changes in length and in width depending on the location and function of the type of bone.

Bone remodeling involves the removal and replacement of old bone with new bone. Enlow (1963) discusses this remodeling process of bone growth as a systematic coordination between bone building cells (**osteoblasts**) and bone resorbing cells (**osteoclasts**). Bone remodeling occurs throughout life at differing rates. This normal process is often affected by age and pathological, or inflammatory processes (Recker, 1983; Hall, 2005), and results in secondary bone. These terms and processes will be elaborated upon in subsequent sections in this chapter.

Bone Function

Bone is enveloped by two membranes. The **periosteum**, a double-layered protective covering on the outer bone surface, is comprised of a fibrous layer of dense cartilaginous tissue surrounding an inner **osteogenic** layer composed of osteoblasts and osteoclasts. This layer is rich in nerve fibers, blood, and lymphatic vessels and is secured to the bone via **Sharpey's fibers**. The **endosteum** is a membranous layer lining the internal surface of the medullary cavity. Bone modeling or remodeling can occur on either the periosteal or endosteal surfaces (Frost, 1963, 1964; Lacroix, 1971; Ortner, 1975; Recker, 1983; Martin and Burr, 1989; Martin et al., 1998).

There are two general types of human bone: compact or **cortical bone** and spongy or **trabecular bone**. The cortical bone is the outer layer and is harder and denser than the inner spongy bone (Recker, 1983; Martin and Burr, 1989; Carter and Beaupre, 2001; Hall, 2005). The cortical and trabecular bone lies between the periosteum and endosteum. Cortical bone is primarily found in varying thicknesses in the shafts, or diaphyses, of long bones, and surrounding the trabeculae. The organization of cortical and trabecular bone allows for maximum absorption of energy with minimal trauma to the bone structure itself (Martin and Burr, 1989).

Spongy bone is located within the medullary cavity as well as in the ends of long bones, inside the bodies of vertebrae, and between cortical bone layers in the flat bones of the cranium (Recker, 1983; Martin and Burr, 1989; Carter and Beaupre, 2001; Hall, 2005).

It consists of extensively connected bony trabeculae that are oriented along the lines of stress for osseous mechanical support. The presence of trabeculae increases the load-carrying capacity of a bone without increasing mass, thus improving structural efficiency (Robling et al., 2006).

Bone Cells

There are several important cells involved in bone formation, maintenance, and remodeling: **osteoprogenitor** cells, osteoclasts, osteoblasts, and **osteocytes**. Osteoprogenitor cells are derived from **mesenchymal** tissue during embryonic development. They have the ability to differentiate into a number of different cell types. They can modify their morphologic and physiologic characteristics in response to specific stimuli (Frost, 1964; Recker, 1983; Martin and Burr, 1989).

Osteoclasts are large, multinucleated cells that work to resorb or break down the established bone matrix. They are believed to affix themselves to a bony surface and break down the bone matrix in that area via enzymal and acidic chemical secretions. Osteoclastic cells resorb both cortical and trabecular bone. They lie within enzymatically etched resorptive bays in the bone matrix known as **Howship's lacunae.**

Osteoblasts are small, single-nucleated, cuboid cells that secret **osteoid** and build bone (Frost, 1964; Recker, 1983; Martin and Burr, 1989; Carter and Beaupre, 2001). Osteoid is an unmineralized organic tissue that eventually undergoes calcification and is deposited as lamellae or layers in the bone matrix. **Lamellar bone** is structured and uniform in organization and is present in both compact and spongy bone (Enlow, 1962b; Frost, 1964; Recker, 1983; Martin and Burr, 1989; Martin et al., 1998; Hall, 2005). Lamellae are layers of bone that differ in pattern of organization based on the type of bone in which it is present. Osteoblasts are thought to originate from mesenchymal stem cells and can be the product of osteoprogenitor cells or bone lining cells that can differentiate. They line the periosteal or endosteal surface of bone tissue to form new bone (Heersche, 1978; Baron et al., 1984).

Osteocytes are another type of bone cell that are actually former osteoblasts that have become surrounded and encased by their own secreted bone matrix. Osteocytes reside in **lacunae,** which permeate the lamellar bone and function by facilitating communication between bone cells and by maintaining bone integrity. These cells are linked by an extensive interconnecting network of tunnels or finger-like extensions called **canaliculi**; these aid in nutrient transmission and cell-to-cell communication (Martin et al., 1998; Carter and Beaupre, 2001). Also helping to maintain cell nourishment are **Volkmann's canals,** which traverse the bone matrix and connect Haversian canals (Figure 13.1). An **osteon** is the structural unit of compact bone. A central **Haversian canal** penetrates the osteon and serves as a passage for blood cells, lymph vessels, and nerves.

Bone Modeling

The formation and subsequent maintenance of bone occur during growth and development via bone modeling as previously introduced. Bone modeling refers to the initial bone mineralization in the embryonic stage. Large areas of bone structure need to be shaped so that the bone architecture is practical and functional. Modeling can build or remove bone

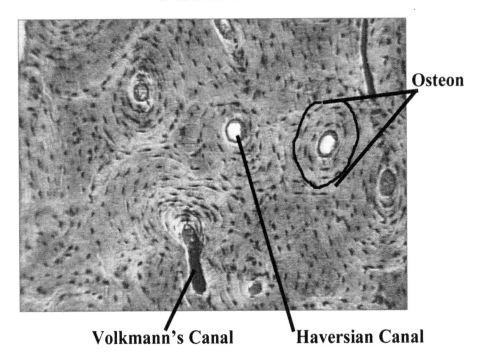

Osteon

Volkmann's Canal   **Haversian Canal**

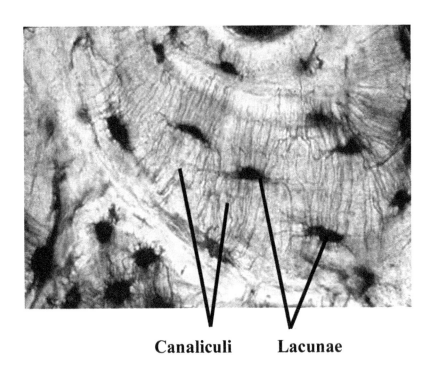

Canaliculi   Lacunae

FIGURE 13.1   Basic bone histological features.

at different rates by osteoblastic or osteoclastic activity on specific areas of bone. For example, for long bones, osteoblasts increase the diameter of the shaft by adding bone to the periosteal surface while osteoclasts remove bone from the endosteal surface (Frost, 1964; Lacroix, 1971; Sharpe, 1979; Martin and Burr, 1989).

Prior to bone modeling, bone tissue is comprised of loosely organized **woven bone**. Woven bone is immature bone with randomly oriented collagen fibers. It is temporary and eventually replaced by lamellar bone. It generally disappears when children are very young (Martin and Burr, 1989) and is usually not found in adults unless in response to pathology or trauma. Woven bone can be rapidly produced to provide temporary mechanical strength during skeletal repair. It is unique in that it is the only type that can be deposited *de novo,* or without any previous cartilaginous or tissue model in place (White et al., 1977; Martin and Burr, 1989).

There are three different types of primary bone that can be deposited during the modeling process (Martin and Burr, 1989). The first, *primary lamellar bone,* is organized in a circumferential pattern between the periosteal and endosteal layers of bone. The second, **plexiform bone**, is formed very rapidly. Since it is common for plexiform bone to develop in response to the need for increased biomechanical support, it is often seen in larger, faster growing mammals than humans, including cows, sheep, or deer (Currey, 2002). It is very rarely, if ever, seen in humans, and if present, it will be in extremely young individuals (Mulhern and Ubelaker, 2001). It is characterized by rectangular, brick-like shapes (Figure 13.2) and stems from mineral buds that grow first perpendicular and then parallel to the outer edge of bone surface (Jowsey, 1966; Martin and Burr, 1989).

The third type, *primary osteonal bone,* is comprised of circular or concentric layers of lamellae surrounding a vascular canal. These layers, the central vascular canal, and osteocytes make up a primary osteon (Jaffe, 1929; Currey, 1982; Martin and Burr, 1989). In primary bone, there is a shorter distance between osteocytes and the blood supply than in secondary bone allowing for easier access to nutrients for growth and development (Dempster and Enlow, 1959).

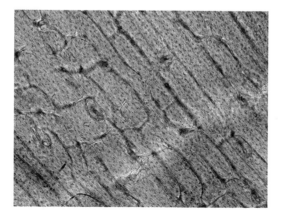

FIGURE 13.2 Plexiform bone.

Bone Remodeling

Bone is in a constant state of turnover. Bone remodeling involves the continuous process of resorption and deposition. Remodeling is the replacement of primary bone with secondary bone. **Basic multicellular units** (or BMUs) are complex arrangements of cells responsible for remodeling (Frost, 1964; Martin and Burr, 1989; Junqueira et al., 1998). Unlike bone modeling, bone remodeling occurs at a specific site and in a consecutive order—**activation**, **resorption**, and **formation** (**ARF**). During the processes of bone remodeling, the osteoclasts and osteoblasts work sequentially to resorb and deposit new bone in response to normal turnover, biomechanical factors, hormonal changes, increases or decreases in activity patterns, or from injury or trauma.

Bone remodeling can involve the removal or resorption of older bone and the deposition of newer bone to help alleviate biomechanical stress, damage, or increased strain. Martin and Burr (1989) describe "normal" bone remodeling occurring in six successive phases. The first, activation, involves the procurement of differentiated cells from available stem cell populations. In the second phase, bone resorption, the newly derived osteoclasts begin to break down bone. The third phase, reversal, is the transitional period between the resorptive and formative stages. Osteoclastic activity converts at varying rates to osteoblastic activity. During this time secondary osteons are formed and surrounded by **cement reversal lines** (Frost, 1964; Lacroix, 1971; Recker, 1983). These lines are mineral-deficient layers of the bone matrix that separate secondary osteons from the lamellar bone.

Bone formation is the fourth phase. Osteoblasts deposit osteoid and lay down concentric lamellae leaving a centralized Haversian canal to serve as a pathway for blood vessels and nerves. The fifth phase, mineralization, involves the calcification of the secreted osteoid. Over 60% of the osteoid becomes mineralized within the first 24 hours of its secretion (Martin and Burr, 1989). The final phase is quiescence. During this sixth step, osteoclasts have vanished and most of the osteoblasts have become osteocytes or have disappeared (Martin and Burr, 1989).

The total amount of time required to move through these six phases is called "**sigma**." Frost (1963) coined this term with "Sigma R" referring to resorption time and "Sigma F" referring to refilling time. Refilling time refers to bone formation. In cortical bone, it would take an estimated 120 days (30 days for resorption and 90 days for formation) to move from the initial phase and resorption cavity to a completed secondary osteon (Frost, 1963; Martin and Burr, 1989).

These six consecutive phases can occur in different locations in the bony matrix and at varying magnitudes and rates. An increase or decrease in the lag time between subsequent phases can affect bone structure and integrity.

Bone remodeling forms secondary bone and secondary osteons. The **secondary osteon** is characterized by lamellar bone surrounding a central Haversian canal with a clear cement or reversal line marking its boundary. Secondary osteons replacing primary bone are solely the result of remodeling. Mature compact bone is comprised of secondary osteons (Figure 13.3).

Being able to distinguish between primary and secondary osteons is vital to histological research. As mentioned, the primary osteon is initial bone tissue laid down on an existing bone surface (immature woven bone) and surrounded by concentric rings of lamellar bone. These concentric rings allow for the protection of the central blood vessel that passes through each osteon. If these primary osteons do not have concentric lamellae, they are called

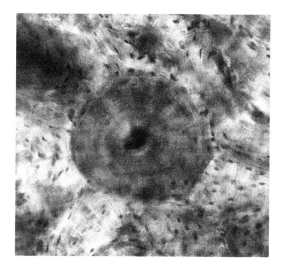

FIGURE 13.3   Secondary osteon surrounded by reversal line.

non-Haversian systems. Primary osteonal bone and non-Haversian bone are present in both human and nonhuman bone. The organization of these and the differentiation of secondary osteons from primary osteons can help separate human from nonhuman bone (Jowsey, 1966; Mulhern and Ubelaker, 2001; Horni, 2002).

Primary osteonal bone is different than secondary osteonal bone in its method of formation and in its level of structure. It is believed that primary osteons are formed via the mineralization of cartilage while secondary osteons are the result of a remodeling process that replaces existing bone (Frost, 1964; Sharpe, 1979).

Primary osteons are usually smaller than secondary osteons (Figure 13.4) and tend to have fewer concentric rings of lamellar bone. They do not have cement reversal lines separating them from lamellar bone as is definitive of secondary osteonal bone (Frost, 1964; Kerley, 1965; Lacroix, 1971; Recker, 1983; Martin and Burr, 1989; Hall, 2005).

Bone Formation

There are two models of bone growth. The first, **endochondral ossification**, meaning "within cartilage," creates bone by replacing hyaline cartilage-formed models. This is common in the long bones of the appendicular skeleton. The second model, **intramembranous ossification**, creates bone from a fibrous membrane. This is common in the bones of the neurocranium and other flat bones such as those of the face and pelvis. We review these processes below, but Scheuer and Black (2000) provide a detailed discussion to which you should refer to learn more.

Endochondral Ossification

As mentioned, growth of long bones occurs as a result of endochondral ossification. This model involves a specific sequence of events beginning in the second trimester of

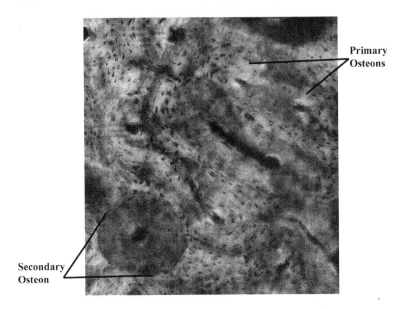

Primary
Osteons

Secondary
Osteon

FIGURE 13.4 Differences in primary and secondary osteons.

development and continuing into the first stages of adulthood (Martin and Burr, 1989; Carter and Beaupre, 2001). Initial endochondral osteogenesis takes place in hyaline cartilage starting with the development of the bone *collar*, or model. The bone collar is initially formed via intramembranous ossification. Once blood enters the mixture, with the surrounding peri-chondrium, the membrane of fibrous connective tissue covers the surface of cartilages except at the joints (Martin and Burr, 1989; Junqueira et al., 1998; Carter and Beaupre, 2001).

Following this process, a primary growth center appears at the rudimentary base of the diaphysis and secondary ossification centers form at the epiphyses (or ends) of the bone (Leeson and Leeson, 1981; Carter and Beaupre, 2001). Longitudinal growth occurs by *chondrocytes* (carti-lage-forming cells) in an area near the ends of bone called the *growth plate* or *physis*. The physis serves as a boundary between the bone epiphysis and *metaphysis* (zone between the epiphysis and diaphysis) (Martin et al., 1998). The growth plate is divided into several zones: resting, proliferative, hypertrophic, and provisional calcification. Chondrocytes progress through these above-mentioned subsequent phases during their life cycle ultimately resulting in a calcified cartilage matrix (Martin et al., 1998) followed by a zone of ossification (Leeson and Leeson, 1981). During this process, osteoblasts accumulate at these calcified areas to lay down bone.

Intramembranous Ossification

Intramembranous bone development occurs within the flat bones of the skeleton, including the neurocranium, the pelvis, and some bones of the face. It is also responsible for the thickening of long bones undergoing endochondral growth (Junqueira et al., 1998; Carter and Beaupre, 2001). This process is seen as early as the eighth week of gestation. During this time, undifferentiated mesenchymal cells directly differentiate into osteoblasts and begin to deposit osteoid. This unmineralized bone matrix eventually surrounds the oste-oblast and mineralizes. The encased osteoblasts are now known as osteocytes, which are housed in lacunae, as already discussed. During bone growth, osteoblasts develop on the periosteal surface of preexisting bone and deposit on these areas to increase bone thickness (Leeson and Leeson, 1981).

BONE HISTOLOGY AND ANTHROPOLOGY

This section of the chapter will briefly discuss the various ways that anthropologists can utilize bone histology. Each subsection includes useful references for additional sources should the reader wish to learn more about a specific topic.

Species Identification

Bone histological research generally focuses on mammalian bone, specifically the Haversian system including such variables as secondary osteon and Haversian canal size and osteon, osteocyte, and lacunae counts (Enlow and Brown, 1956, 1957, 1958; Enlow, 1962a; Jowsey, 1966; Frost, 1987; Burr et al., 1990; Harsanyi, 1990; Pfeiffer, 1998; Mulhern and Ubelaker, 2001). The size, shape, and density of the Haversian system and organization of bone differ between human and nonhuman remains as well as from one mammalian species to another (Jowsey, 1966; Mulhern and Ubelaker, 2001; Horni, 2002). These dissimilarities can help determine whether fragmentary remains discovered in a forensic or archaeological context are the result of a natural process. If not, and the remains are human, this may be cause for a medicolegal death investigation.

Biological Profile and Age-at-Death Estimations

Bone biologists and anthropologists have recognized that with increasing age, there are concurrent microstructural changes in bone (Enlow, 1963; Frost, 1963, 1964, 1987; Kerley 1965; Lacroix, 1971; Kerley and Ubelaker, 1978; Ubelaker, 1989; Stout, 1989; Martin and Burr, 1989; Curtis, 2003; Crowder and Stout, 2012). Monro (1776) was the first to acknowledge that as an individual gets older, loss of bone occurs through expansion of the medullary cavity and related cortical thinning as well as loss of bone within the cortex itself.

There is a large amount of research that discusses the potential relationship between changes in human bone microstructure and increasing age. Age-at-death estimates are based on the process of bone remodeling. They consider the correlation between increasing age and bone microstructure; this is often done with regression analyses. Regression analyses focus on the correlation between dependent and independent variables (in this case age and bone microstructure). This correlation is used in bone histology to predict age. As individuals get older and bone is remodeled, secondary osteons generally decrease in overall area and increase in overall density. Because of this, the secondary osteon is commonly quantified or measured. **Histomorphometrics** is the quantitative study of the microscopic organization and structure of a tissue (such as bone).

For example, Kerley (1965), Kerley and Ubelaker (1978), and Thompson (1979) have utilized secondary osteon counts to estimate age-at-death. Similarly, Ahlqvist and Damsten (1969), Thompson (1979), and Ericksen (1991) examined osteon population densities to estimate age-at-death. Stout and Stanley (1991) tested both secondary osteon counts and percent **osteonal bone** and found counts to be more accurate in predicting age estimates.

Secondary osteons are measured in several ways. Mean osteonal area, perimeter, and maximum and minimum diameters have been used to predict age-at-death estimates (Thompson, 1979; Watanabe et al., 1998; Pfeiffer et al., 2006). The Haversian canal of every secondary osteon is similarly quantified utilizing average canal area, perimeter, and diameters to estimate age (Thompson, 1979; Thompson and Gunness-Hey, 1981; Watanabe et al., 1998). Research suggests that during aging, these variable measurements decrease in response to increased bone remodeling and the addition of more secondary osteonal bone (Thompson, 1979; Thompson and Gunness-Hey, 1981; Watanabe et al., 1998; Pfeiffer et al., 2006). See Figure 13.5.

Additionally, researchers have looked at primary osteonal counts and **fractional volume** of primary osteons as well as percent lamellar bone (Kerley, 1965; Ahlqvist and Damsten, 1969). The fractional volume refers to the percentage or ratio of bone comprised of primary osteons versus secondary (or remodeled) osteonal bone. As age increases, the number of primary osteons as well as the percentage of lamellar bone decrease and are replaced by secondary osteons.

Other variables considered to estimate age-at-death include average cortical thicknesses (Thompson, 1979; Thompson and Gunness-Hey, 1989), secondary osteon circularity (Ortner, 1975; Britz et al., 2009), and number of secondary osteonal fragments (Kerley, 1965; Clarke, 1987; Ericksen, 1991; Cool et al., 1995).

The reliability of these age estimators is dependent upon the individual bone (as mentioned in the upcoming paragraph) and on methodology. Through decades of research, the technique developed by Kerley (1965) and later fine-tuned (Kerley and Ubelaker, 1978) has produced the most reliable age-at-death estimations. Kerley considered the following variables: number of whole osteons, number of fragmentary osteons, percentage circumferential lamellar bone, and number of non-Haversian canals. Stout and Stanley (1991) found

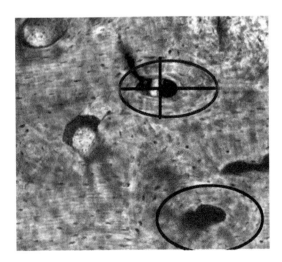

FIGURE 13.5   Example of measurements taken by imaging software.

that utilizing Kerley's osteon count method in the entire cross-section of the fibula produces the best results. Support for Kerley's methodology is echoed in more recent literature such as Robling and Stout (2008: 164), who stated, "Age estimates determined by averaging the estimates for all Kerley predicting formulas produced the greatest accuracy and reliability for all age classes."

Not only are a multitude of variables considered in current bone histological methods, multiple skeletal elements have also been of interest. These include the femur (Kerley, 1965; Ahlqvist and Damsten, 1969; Singh and Gunberg, 1970; Thompson, 1979; Ericksen, 1991), tibia (Kerley, 1965; Singh and Gunberg, 1970), fibula (Kerley, 1965), humerus (Thompson, 1979; Yoshino et al., 1994), ulna (Thompson, 1979), clavicle (Stout and Paine, 1992; Stout et al., 1996), mandible (Singh and Gunberg, 1970), ribs (Stout, 1986; Stout and Paine, 1992; Stout et al., 1996; Cho et al., 2002; Kim et al., 2007), and neurocranium (Clarke, 1987; Cool et al., 1995; Curtis, 2003; Trammell, 2012).

Biological Profile and Sex Estimation

It is important that the skeletal biologist consider both **intrinsic** and **extrinsic factors** that affect age and how these may subsequently affect histological aging methods. One key variable to consider is sex. Kerley (1965) and Stout and Paine (1992) indicate that differences in sex have very little to no effect on age-at-death estimation techniques. Other researchers, however, have noticed significant differences between male and female histomorphometrics (Thompson, 1980; Samson and Branigan, 1987; Ericksen, 1991).

Ericksen (1991) developed linear regression equations separately for males and females as well as for the sexes combined and found that the number of secondary osteons and secondary osteon fragments differs between males and females and, because of these findings, emphasized the importance of using sex-specific analyses (Ericksen, 1991). Thompson (1980) indicates that with increasing age, females experience a much more significant decline in cortical thickness and bone mineral density than do males. Females also experience more significant age-related changes in Haversian canal areas than males (Thompson, 1980).

Since some findings suggest that males and females undergo bone remodeling at different rates, this lends credibility to the potential utility of histomorphometrics to estimate sex. Though past histological analyses have not particularly focused on estimating sex as part of the biological profile, recent research (Trammell, 2012) indicates the promising potential of using the microstructure itself to classify individuals as males or females using a **discriminant function analysis**. When histomorphometric variables (such as secondary osteon and Haversian canal area and perimeters and minimum and maximum secondary osteon and Haversian canal diameters) from the frontal, parietal, and temporal are considered in a single analysis, the discriminant function is very accurate at classifying males and females—90% correct classification for males and 80% correct classification for females (Trammell, 2012).

Nutrition and Pathology

Microstructural analysis of bone can discern pathology as well as signs of nutritional and metabolic stress (Jowsey, 1977; Martin and Burr, 1989; Bell, 1990; Ericksen et al., 1994; Pfeiffer,

2000; Schultz, 2001). Junqueira and Carneiro (2003) describe histological indications of osteomalacia in bone. Osteomalacia is a nutritional deficiency of vitamin D causing inadequate calcification of new bone concurrent with partial resorption of existing bone (Junqueira and Carneiro, 2003). In addition, hyperparathyroidism is a hormonal imbalance described by Robling and Stout (2008) as a condition where an excess of the parathyroid hormone is released. Though it does not have a direct effect on bone remodeling, it does affect the activation frequency (Robling and Stout, 2008). They noted that individuals suffering from hyperparathyroidism have a greater number of osteons than healthy individuals.

Osteoporosis (a loss of bone density typically associated with aging) causes intracortical bone thinning and results in increased porosity within the bone. Jowsey (1977) discovered that bone depositional rates remained the same while resorption rates rapidly increased with osteoporosis. This is caused by an extended lag time between the resorption and formation stages of ARF remodeling (Frost, 1964; Recker, 1983; Martin and Burr, 1989).

Schultz (2001, 2003, 2012) states that paleohistopathology is valuable in disease diagnoses. Essentially, if a disorder initiates a bony response, these reactions are visible histologically. Inflammatory processes, lesions, bony tumors, and certain types of bone disease are manifested at the microscopic level and may even be visible before macroscopic indicators are observable (Schultz, 2003). Paleohistopathology can also enable the discernment between **lytic** removal versus deposition of bone (see Smith [Chapter 7], this volume). Also, refer to Schultz (2001) for comprehensive treatment of the different pathologies recognizable histologically.

Physical Activity and Biomechanics

Bone responds to both mechanical and nonmechanical factors. The bone remodeling process is constant and is partly regulated by the body's hormonal system, a process independent of mechanical adaptation. Aside from physiology, bone is also subject to forces and stress of varying magnitudes (Kroman and Symes [Chapter 8], this volume; Petrtyl et al., 1996; Hughes-Fulford, 2004). Once bone modeling is complete, biomechanical stressors and forces still affect the gross morphology of bone. Bone adapts to its mechanical environment and does so through ARF remodeling or damage repair. These effects will be visible at the microscopic level (Currey, 1959; Ascenzi and Bonucci, 1967, 1968).

Wolff's law (Wolff, 1892; Petrtyl et al., 1996; Hughes-Fulford, 2004) states that bone can adapt or remodel in response to forces or demands placed upon it from mechanical factors. Studies have additionally been conducted to research how habitual action (or inaction), obesity, loading, and other biomechanical factors affect the skeleton at the macroscopic level (Ribot et al., 1987; Frost, 1997; Beaupre et al., 2000; Moore and Schaefer, 2011). Research indicates that obese individuals exhibit an increase in overall bone mass and a reduction in bone loss with age (Wheatley, 2005; Miyabara, et al., 2007; Moore, 2008). Obesity in postmenopausal women provided for a higher bone mineral density than for women considered to be healthy or thin (Ribot et al., 1987). Frost (1997) suggests that because overweight individuals require stronger muscle forces to move, these forces cause extra strain and stress on bone, resulting in increased levels of bone remodeling and more secondary osteonal bone. This topic is discussed further in the chapter on medical imaging and functional morphology (Moore [Chapter 14], this volume).

Diagenesis

Diagenesis refers to physical and chemical degradation of organic materials, thus fitting under the auspices of taphonomy (see Marden et al., [Chapter 9], this volume). This can occur in bone and these taphonomic processes can be visible histologically. Histotaphonomy examines diagenesis at the microstructural scale (Bell, 2012; Crowder and Stout, 2012). Such changes can give indications about post-depositional environments. For example, taphonomic changes to human remains that have decomposed in marine environments (Bell et al., 1996, 2008) will differ in timing and manifestation than those found in a burial or arid setting. The time frame of different types of postmortem change to bone microstructure is not only useful to the forensic anthropologist but also of interest to the paleoanthropologist, skeletal biologist, and bioarchaeologist.

One of the earliest types of taphonomic change to affect bone microstructure is microbial, or bacterial, attack (Jans et al., 2004). For example, Bell and colleagues (1996) looked at how bones were taphonomically altered in terrestrial, intertidal, and lacustrine contexts. They found evidence of microbial attack in bone as soon as 3 months postmortem and as late as 83 years postmortem. The bone with a postmortem interval of 83 years was interred in a dry coffin and exhibited no macroscopic or histological evidence of alteration while the tibial fragment recovered after 3 months postmortem from carnivore scat in a wet environment had evidence of focal destruction (Bell et al., 1996). They also found microscopic destruction in a rib found 15 months postmortem on the surface of a waterlogged musket bog. Bell and colleagues demonstrated the vital importance of postmortem environment as it relates to destruction of bone.

Hackett (1981) has classified and described four categories of postmortem microstructural focal destructive changes that can be observed histologically. These are called *Wedl*, *linear longitudinal*, *budded*, and *lamellate* (Hackett, 1981; Bell, 2012). **Wedl** microbial attack causes tunneling while the additional three categories are assumed to be bacterial in nature and can be distinguished by size and shape histologically (Wedl, 1864; Hackett, 1981; Jans et al., 2004).

BASIC CONCEPTS IN DENTAL HISTOLOGY

Due to their unique physiology and anatomy, teeth bear the special distinction of being both the most durable part of the hard tissues and the only part directly exposed to the environment during the life of the individual. These two facts make dentition a gold mine for anthropologists to collect information regarding the biology, phylogeny, and health of human populations—both past and present (Scott and Turner, 1988). Teeth also have the unique distinction in the human body of recording their own growth during their creation. They provide tiny snapshots into the life and health of an individual during the period that the teeth were being formed.

In the field of human evolution and paleoanthropology, there are numerous areas of research analyzing dentition from both a morphological and a histological perspective (for complete reviews see Dean, 2006). Dental histology also contributes heavily to the field of forensic anthropology. Numerous studies have been conducted looking at a variety of histological methods used to estimate the age of an individual, as well as form conclusions regarding their overall state of health (Skinner and Anderson, 1991). As you can see, there is a wide spectrum of research opportunities in the field of dental anthropology, including but not limited to forensic anthropology, human evolution, morphology, and population health (Scott and Turner, 1988). However, the scope of this section will be limited to the aspect of dental research concerning histology. Refer to Hammerl (Chapter 10), this volume, for a complete overview of research in dental anthropology.

Definitions and Basic Principles of Dental Histology

The main components of dentition that are examined during histological analysis are enamel and dentin, and to a lesser degree cementum and the pulp chamber of the tooth. These structures develop from different embryological origins, have different functions during the life of the individual, and thus have different appearances in histological thin sections.

Enamel

Enamel is the heavily mineralized layer that covers the crowns of the dentition. Enamel is the hardest material in the human body, which is what makes it such a durable tissue, and therefore so important in the field of skeletal biology. Unlike all of the other tissues that make up the dentition, enamel has an embryonic ectodermal origin (Junqueira and Carneiro, 2003). Enamel is a noncellular structure that is formed by cells referred to as *ameloblasts*, which differentiate out of epithelial cells located in the internal enamel epithelium (Sadler, 2006). Enamel formation by the ameloblasts starts at the apex of the tooth and works downwards to form the crown of the tooth.

The enamel is secreted by ameloblast cells in two different stages. The first stage involves the secretion of a matrix that will be the framework for the structure of the enamel. This matrix has both an organic component and an inorganic component. The matrix is secreted out of the end of the ameloblast, from a protuberant area referred to as the *Tome's process*. Any disruption of the ameloblast, from either mechanical or metabolic causes, can lead to a constriction of the Tome's process (Hillson, 1996). This constriction of the Tome's process leaves a permanent line in the formation of the enamel matrix. This line is a permanent mark in the enamel, and is visible on histological section. These lines of discontinuity are commonly referred to **striae of Retzius**. These striae of Retzius have an implication in the anthropological world as well. For example, a case report by Skinner and Anderson (1991) investigates whether striae of Retzius can be used to correlate with specific times of stress in an individual's life in an attempt to provide a basis for presumptive identification of unknown remains. If the stress to which an individual is exposed continues for a prolonged period of time, these lines of discontinuity can become visible macroscopically as **linear enamel hypoplasias**.

The second stage of enamel formation is the mineralization or maturation stage. Once the matrix has been secreted by the ameloblasts, they undergo a transformation and start to break down the organic component of the matrix (Hillson, 1996). While the ameloblasts are taking away the organic component of the enamel, crystals are also forming in the nonorganic component. Once maturation is complete, only the nonorganic material remains. However, any incongruities left from the enamel formation, such as the striae of Retzius, are still present. See Hammerl (Chapter 10), this volume, for more information on episodes of stress recorded by enamel.

Dentin

The bulk of the tooth is made of dentin. Dentin, like bone and enamel, is also a calcified tissue. In fact, dentin is harder than bone but not as hard as enamel (Junqueira and Carneiro, 2003). Dentin is formed by specialized cells called *odontoblasts,* which are derivatives of embryologic neural crest cells. The odontoblasts are polarized cells that travel from the internal border of the enamel towards the area that will become the pulp cavity; they secrete an organic matrix called *predentin.* As the odontoblasts secrete predentin they leave their long apical extensions called *odontoblast processes* trailing behind them. These slender cellular extensions reside in hollow tubules located throughout the dentin, called *dentinal tubules.* These tubules contain the protoplasmic extension of the odontoblast cells lining the pulp chamber and provide a link between enamel and the pulp organ. The tubules may contain nerve, vascular and lymphoid tissues from the pulp organ.

Once secreted, the predentin begins the mineralization process, which is controlled by another part of the odontoblasts called the matrix vesicles, which cause the **hydroxyapatite** crystals to grow and harden. Unlike enamel, dentin is sensitive to outside factors such as temperature, trauma, and acidic pH (Junqueira and Carneiro, 2003). Any stimuli to the dentin are interpreted as the sensation of pain.

Cementum

Cementum covers the outside of the root, and is very similar to bone but without any blood or nerve innervations and without the Haversian systems seen in bone (Junqueira and Carneiro, 2003). The layer of cementum functions to attach the root of the tooth to the periodontal ligament, which helps to provide critical stabilization of the tooth in the bone of either the mandible or maxilla. The cementum primarily covers the root, with some portion overlapping the crown. The cementum is made by specialized mesenchymal cells located on the outside of the tooth root. Once these cells come into contact with the dentin that has just been made, some differentiate and turn into *cementoblasts* (Sadler, 2006). Once these cells become trapped within the matrix of the cementum, they live on as *cementocytes.* Like osteocytes in bone, cementocytes are reactive cells and can secrete cementum to help keep the tooth stable within the socket (Junqueira and Carneiro, 2003).

Pulp Cavity

The pulp cavity is a space on the interior of the tooth that is filled with cellular material and soft tissue. The pulp cavity has two areas, each defined by location. The *pulp chamber* is the area of the pulp cavity that is located within the crown portion of the tooth, and the *root canal* is the hollow portion located within the root of the tooth (Junqueira and Carneiro, 2003). The root canal extends all the way down the root of the tooth, where it exits the tooth through the *apical foramen.* The apical foramen allows for the entrance and exit of nerves, lymphatic tissues, and blood vessels to the living cells of the tooth.

The pulp inside the pulp cavity is a highly innervated and vascular tissue. The cells inside the pulp cavity are mainly loose connective tissue, fibroblasts, and odontoblasts, and ground substance. The nerve cells within the pulp only respond to the sensation of pain.

Age Estimation from Dental Histology

Gustafson Method and Derivatives

One of the most well-known methods for estimating age-at-death from histological thin sections of teeth is the Gustafson method. First developed in 1947, and later revised in 1950, the method is based on the scoring of six age-related factors identified in the histological sections of the teeth. The six factors that are studied are (1) dental attrition, (2) periodontosis, (3) secondary dentin deposition, (4) cement apposition, (5) root resorption, and (6) transparency of the root (Gustafson, 1950). The original method by Gustafson utilized a simple linear regression between the total score based on all six components and the age of the individual at death. There have been numerous revisions and recalculations based on the original Gustafson method. For review of the method and the revisions see Johanson (1971), Maples (1978), Rice and Maples (1979), and Lucy and Pollard (1995).

Cementum Annulations

In many large mammals, the age estimation technique of correlating the amount of cementum on the root of the tooth with age is commonly used (Morris, 1978; Stott et al., 1980; Lieberman, 1993; Hillson, 1996). The first study to attempt to apply the methodology to the human species was by Stott et al. (1982). The theory behind using cementum annulations for age-at-death estimation is similar to counting the rings on a tree trunk. The premise is that cementum is deposited on the root of the tooth at a constant rate during the life of the individual, and by measuring the thickness of the cementum, age-at-death can be calculated. However, as noted by several authors the biologic basis behind this theory has not been clearly demonstrated (Hillson, 1996).

Once a tooth has been sectioned, the cementum annulations are visible as alternating bands of light and dark, when using either microradiography or polarized light microscopy. There have been multiple studies on a variety of different methods utilizing this technique, but the results can be considered variable at best (for a review see Miller et al., 1988; Lipsinic et al., 1986; Charles et al., 1989; and Hillson, 1996). The greatest success in utilizing this technique involves teeth sectioned with a Microtome (see upcoming section on histological methods), which have been decalcified and stained with hemaotoxylin preparations. This preparation can be extremely destructive and is often problematic for archaeological samples. As studies have shown, teeth can have a highly variable distribution of cementum along the root, so the ideal situation involves multiple sections per tooth (Hillson, 1996).

CASE STUDY OF DENTAL HISTOLOGY IN FORENSIC ANTHROPOLOGY: THE PROBLEM OF PINK TEETH

The phenomenon of "pink teeth," which is described as a postmortem pink discoloration of the teeth, was first documented by Bell (1829) and others in the middle nineteenth century, and was always associated with "unnatural death" and "foul play." However, it was the pink teeth of the two buried victims of the high-profile Christie murders in the early 1950s that

[2]This research was conducted at the University of Tennessee and presented by Kroman and Marks (2003).

activated modern interest in this phenomenon by forensic odontology and pathology.[3] Histological sections made from multiple teeth of those victims revealed that the discoloration was confined to the dentin adjacent to the pulp chamber of the tooth. Miles and coworkers (1954) were the first to suggest that the pink discoloration of the teeth was simply an artifact of the **decomposition** process, and not just a byproduct of homicide. This hypothesis marked a turning point in the way that the forensic field viewed the pink teeth problem.

Over the years, pink teeth have been studied under a variety of case-based and experimental conditions. The appearance has been linked to three etiologies: (1) **perimortem** physical trauma from asphyxia (strangulation and hanging) and head trauma; (2) peri- and **postmortem** moisture exposure (drowning, wet grave); and (3) postmortem longevity between death and discovery (see Dye et al., 1995 for a research review).

In wet decomposition, Beeley and Harvey (1973) noted differential dentin staining and Van Wyk (1987) concluded that the roots of the anterior teeth are most vulnerable to coloration as a result of advanced decomposition. In a similar manner, Brondum and Simonsen (1987) noted a high correlation between putrefaction, adipocere formation, and the occurrence of pink teeth. Clark and Law (1984) examined the phenomenon in drowned bodies and discovered differential staining on the left arcade of one victim with the left side of the head in a dependent position. Besides Clark and Law (1984), Whittaker and McDonald (1989) also considered discoloration as "maybe analogous to postmortem lividity stains at the most dependent parts of the body."

Methods

The outdoor Anthropological Research Facility at the University of Tennessee in Knoxville, Tennessee affords an opportunity to study postmortem decomposition. To assess whether pink teeth form in relation to gravitational lividity, five cadavers were positioned in head-dependent, face-down posture from April to December. Once teeth exhibited pink discoloration, they were documented, extracted, and thin sectioned for histological examination using standard petrographic technique. Light micrographs were taken at $10\times$ and $60\times$ magnification followed by scanning electron microscopy analysis and photography.

Results

All cadavers demonstrated some degree of dentin discoloration. This was documented through gross and histological examination. Thin sections revealed blood infusion into the dentin (Figure 13.6), as did SEM (Figure 13.7). The appearance of pink teeth is not immediate in nontraumatized remains. It gradually appears similar to generalized decomposition and may persist long into the skeletal stage. Discoloration is a byproduct of the decomposition process whereby the vascular integrity in the pulp chamber becomes structurally compromised and leaks vessel contents. Simple gravity allows seepage of the red blood cells into the tubules. Subsequent discoloration may persist until the remains are righted (or their position is changed) and the appearance subsides when the pulp chamber once again becomes

[3]John Christie was a serial killer active in England during the 1940s and 1950s. He is known to be responsible for the deaths of at least eight women between 1943 and 1953.

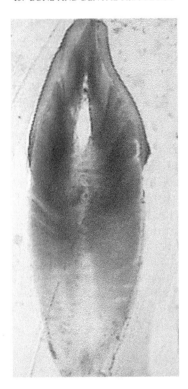

FIGURE 13.6   Thin section showing the red pigmentation from the red blood cells in the dentin. Color version of figure is available in the online version of this volume.

a gravity-dependent reservoir. There is a strong correlation between dependent positioning of the head and creation of pink teeth.

Conclusions

The findings of Kroman and Marks (2003) did not negate the relationship of pink teeth with a variety of peri- and postmortem situations. However, they did experimentally produce their occurrence as a byproduct of decomposition and gravity without trauma. These results confirm the earlier speculation of Clark and Law (1984) and Whittaker and MacDonald (1989). When pink teeth are discovered in decomposed or skeletal remains in the absence of tell-tale traumatized soft and osseous tissue (i.e., a broken hyoid bone), guess-timations about perimortem violence are unfounded. Similar to postmortem soft tissue lividity, pink teeth are an indicator of body position.

SO YOU'RE INTERESTED IN DENTAL HISTOLOGY

If you are interested in learning about and starting research in the area of dental histology, the first place to start is with a good foundation in oral biology as well as in dental

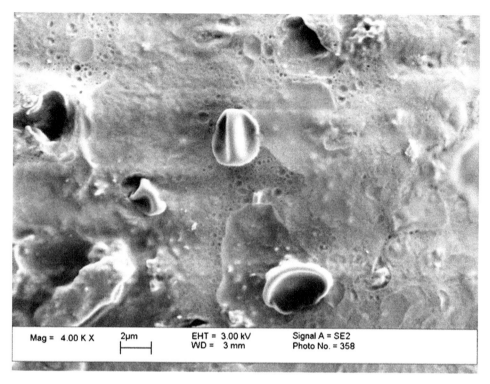

Mag = 4.00 K X   2μm   EHT = 3.00 kV   Signal A = SE2
                                      WD =   3 mm   Photo No. = 358

FIGURE 13.7   SEM photograph showing a red blood cell located in a dentin tubule. Color version of figure is available in the online version of this volume.

anthropology. To understand the anatomy of teeth on a microscopic, histological level, it is best to first understand them from a macroscopic, gross anatomical level. Once you have a good foundation in oral biology and dental anthropology, begin to learn about the basic methods and techniques for histology as introduced in this chapter.

HISTOLOGICAL METHODS

This section of the chapter demonstrates one simple methodology to make slides for microscopic analysis. As the methodology and technique are very similar for both dental tissue as well as bone, please refer to the methodology here for dental sections as well. This section will address common questions and research design concerns anthropologists face when conducting bone histological analyses. The anthropologist should keep in mind that human bone samples are very difficult to obtain for histological research due to the destructive nature of the procurement process (refer to DiGangi and Moore [Chapter 2], this volume, for a discussion of ethical concerns with destructive analyses); because of this, careful attention to detail is very important, as is the production of good quality **thin sections** (the slices of bones or teeth cut). Keep in mind that depending on the type of project or research, there are times that mandate different types of staining or etching techniques. As always, be sure to outline your research project and be sure of the type of thin sections and sample preparation needed before you start.

Sample Selection

Bone samples taken for histological analysis should be chosen carefully. It is extremely important that if a specific methodology is used as a template or guide for histomorphometric research, the procured samples should be selected from the same bone and location presented in that resource's methods. For example, research has demonstrated that histological structures are not uniform throughout the shaft of a long bone (Jowsey, 1966; Pfeiffer et al., 1995; Tersigni, 2005). Kerley's (1965) pioneering study utilized complete midshaft cross-sections. If an age estimate based on Kerley's methodology is made at the midshaft of a bone as well as at the distal and proximal ends, the three estimates will not produce the same results (Tersigni, 2005).

In addition to consistency in bone sample selection, researchers emphasize the need for **population-specific** methods (Thompson and Gunness-Hey, 1981; Aiello and Molleson, 1993; Cho et al., 2002). As mentioned earlier, sex-specific analyses are also recommended (Thompson, 1980; Samson and Branigan, 1987; Ericksen, 1991). Separate equations may be necessary for different ancestral groups as well due to **biological distance**, but this is yet to be investigated. As with gross morphological methods, histological aging methods are most reflective of the reference sample upon which they were developed (Thompson and Gunness-Hey, 1981; Aiello and Molleson, 1993; Cho et al., 2002).

Essentially, when conducting bone histomorphometric analyses, if the anthropologist is basing their methodology on a previous publication, then they should strictly adhere to that methodology including (1) the choice of population, (2) the choice of bone, and (3) the choice of specific location on the bone. If the anthropologist seeks to develop an innovative technique, controlling for specific variables is vital to the replicability and applicability of the research.

Sample Procurement

Just as important as sample selection and location is the means by which bone is procured for histological analysis. If you are adhering to standard methodologies presented in previous research, bone samples should be procured via a similar process to ensure comparability in results, as mentioned.

Options include the removal of complete bone cross-sections (Kerley, 1965; Ahlqvist and Damsten, 1969; Stout and Stanley, 1991), windows, or wedges (Ericksen, 1991). These types of samples can be taken with a *Stryker*®[4] saw or a *Dremel*®[5] rotary tool. Another option is to remove a bone core (Thompson, 1979; Curtis, 2003). Curtis (2003) utilized

[4]Stryker Corporation, Kalamazoo, Michigan.

[5]Robert Bosch Tool Corporation.

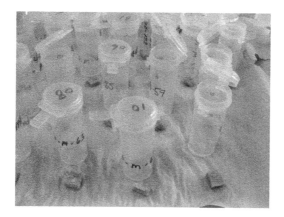

FIGURE 13.8   Bone samples drying prior to embedding.

a 3/8-inch plug-cutting bit and a standard electric hand drill. When removing bone samples for histological analyses, it is important to section areas not affected by pathology, trauma, or other skeletal abnormalities, unless, of course, the anomaly is the region of interest.

Embedding and Slide Preparation

The **embedding** and slide preparatory procedures discussed below are for unaltered cortical bone samples (following similar approaches utilized by Ubelaker, 1989; Stout, 1989a; and Anderson, 1982). The term "embedding" refers to the process of fixing small pieces of bone into a plastic resin. This helps the bone samples maintain integrity during the preparation of thin sections. Bones with more structural integrity, i.e., long bone shafts, do not always necessitate embedding. Samples that are not embedded are sectioned in a similar process as discussed below but then are affixed to glass slides with Permount™ mounting medium and cover slips. This methodology, however, makes it more difficult to produce a usable thin section of the ideal size and without air bubbles. Additionally, this method may be messy and not as durable in the long term as is embedding.

The technique presented here does not involve either the **decalcification** of the bone samples or tissue staining. These processes are not always necessary and depend on the detail of the variables to be observed and the overall goal of the histological analysis. Refer to Maat et al. (2001) and Schenk et al. (1984) for more information on these procedures.

See Box 13.1 for a detailed list of simple steps involved for the novice anthropologist conducting histological research. However, the reader should additionally be sure to consult the following references that detail methods in this area: An and Martin (2003), Paine (2007), and Cho (2012). Further, in line with the advice given elsewhere in this volume (Bethard [Chapter 15]; Cabana et al. [Chapter 16]), when undertaking the methods as outlined in Box 13.1, the

BOX 13.1

BASIC HISTOLOGICAL METHODS

Step Detail

1   Once bone samples have been removed, place them in a simple formalin solution until ready for embedding. Make sure to record the source of the sample as well as the anatomically correct orientation of each sample.

2   Assign each bone sample a designated label and record this in a lab notebook so that the demographics are available.

3   Record information such as bone sample and the ascribed designated numeric designation (from Step 2) on a small adhesive label to be placed inside each peel-away mold.

4   If samples are archaeological or devoid of soft tissue, lightly clean the samples with distilled water and allow them to dry for at least 48 hours (Figure 13.8).

5   If samples still have adherent tissue, a hot soapy water mixture followed by a drying period will help deflesh and degrease the bone samples. If samples are still greasy they can be soaked in solution mixture of 60% industrial grade alcohol and 40% xylene (following Nawrocki, 1997). Do not use bleach and/or hydrogen peroxide (Fenton et al., 2003) because these materials will degrade bone.

6   Mix five parts *Buehler® EPO-THIN®*[6] resin and two parts *Buehler® EPO-THIN®* hardener in a glass beaker. Make sure to stir the solution until the color fades to clear.

7   Fill square peel-away molds ¼ full and allow to set overnight. Make sure you prepare enough molds for your sample size.

8   Place each bone sample into the molds and superglue to the bottom. Make sure to note the orientation of the bone (anterior, posterior, etc.).

9   Again, mix five parts *Buehler® EPO-THIN®* resin and two parts *Buehler® EPO-THIN®* hardener in a glass beaker. Make sure to stir the solution until the color fades to clear.

10   Fill the peel-away molds to the top with the prepared solution, making sure to cover the entirety of each bone sample (Figure 13.9).

11   Vacuum-seal the samples to ensure there are no air bubbles in the mixture surrounding the bone (Figure 13.10). Allow the samples to sit for at least 24 hours prior to sectioning.

12   Peel the plastic molds from the embedded blocks.

13   With an etching pencil, mark the glass slides with labels corresponding to each bone sample.

14   Attach the embedded block to the chuck (Figure 13.11) of a *Buehler® Isomet® Low Speed Oil-cooled Diamond Saw. Buehler®* and *Leica®*[7] are two examples of companies that manufacture saws for thin-section preparation.

15   Pay careful attention to the orientation of the block to ensure that the cut is made in the proper direction (this is usually perpendicular to the diaphysis when sectioning a long bone).

16   Make an initial cut to bisect the block; then, prepare at least one thin section of approximately 80–100 μm. Multiple thin sections are recommended in case of error.

(Continued)

BOX 13.1 *(cont'd)*

17 Using forceps, gently place the bone section onto a thin layer of superglue and adhere to slide (Figure 13.12).

18 If necessary, grind samples down using grit paper. The slide can be placed in a grinding fixture to secure it during grinding (Figure 13.13). The ideal thin section is translucent against the light. An example of a grinder/polisher that can be used for slide preparation is a *Dual Wheel Mark V*[®][8] *Laboratory* grinder/polisher.

19 Polish the sample prior to examination of histomorphological features under the microscope. Polishing will remove or lessen any scratches on the slide from the grinding process.

20 Save the remaining portions of the blocks of embedded bone samples for future research (Figure 13.14).

[6]Buehler, Lake Bluff, Illinois.
[7]Leica Microsystems, Wetzlar, Germany.
[8]Mark V Laboratory, East Granby, Connecticut.

FIGURE 13.9 Bone samples in peel-away molds with embedding medium.

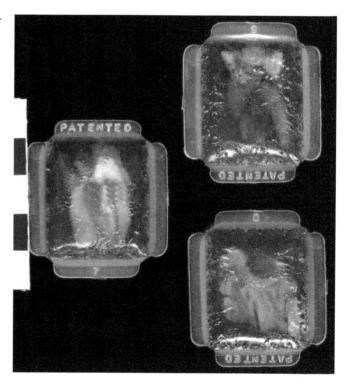

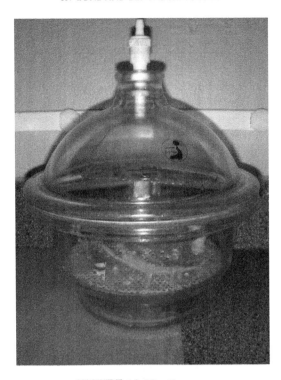

FIGURE 13.10   Vacuum.

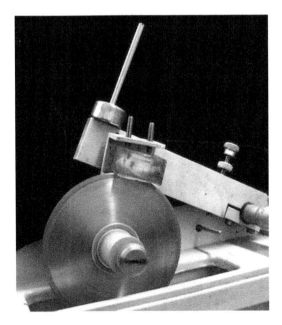

FIGURE 13.11   Embedded bone block attached to the chuck of a microtome.

III. TECHNOLOGICAL ADVANCES

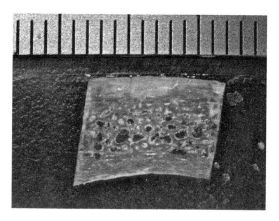

FIGURE 13.12   Prepared thin section.

reader should ensure that they have access to and help from a person who is experienced in this area.

HISTOLOGICAL ANALYSES

Microscopy

Light microscopy is ideal for histological research endeavors. If the prepared bone section is thin enough, the light penetrates the slide and allows the histological features to be visible with the microscope. An anthropologist interested in using bone histology to determine human from nonhuman remains, to estimate elements of the biological profile, to document or diagnose diseases and taphonomic processes, or to assess nutritional and biomechanical

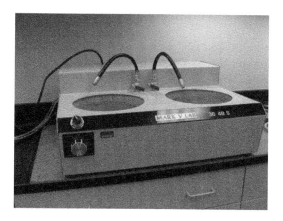

FIGURE 13.13   Grinder and polisher.

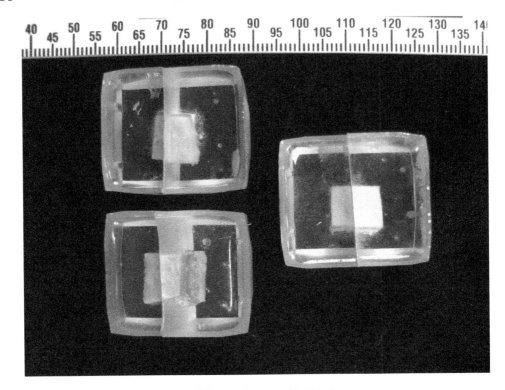

FIGURE 13.14   Embedded blocks.

status can do so with a simple light microscope (Figure 13.15). An example is the *Leica*®
DMRX light microscope. It has multiple magnification options, 1.6×/0.05, 40×, 100×, and
200×, allowing for all of the aforementioned types of analysis.

Also useful is image analysis software. Two very reputable and sophisticated options are
Bioquant®[9] and *Image-Pro*® *Express*.[10] These packages often include a digital camera attachment allowing for live imaging and easier analyses. They have the capability to take a variety
of quantitative measurements and can mark and number each measurement to ensure there
are no missing or duplicate data.

ImageJ[11] is a free and easy-to-use downloadable program that is also helpful in histological research. Take care to periodically ensure that the calibration between the microscope
and image analysis software is correct. Refer to the help guide supplied with the image analysis software program you choose to use.

[9]BIOQUANT Image Analysis Corporation, Nashville, Tennessee.

[10]Media Cybernetics, Inc., Bethesda, Maryland.

[11]http://rsbweb.nih.gov/ij/index.html.

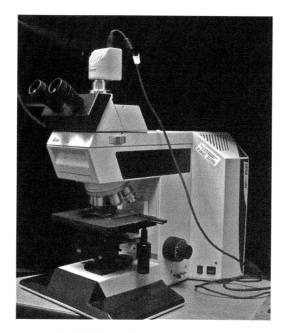

FIGURE 13.15 Light microscope.

CASE STUDIES: BONE HISTOLOGY

Case Study 1

I (LHT) did my Master's research on differentiating human and nonhuman bone microstructure. Therefore, when I first began in the doctoral program at the University of Tennessee in biological anthropology, I welcomed the opportunity to histologically examine fragmentary remains discovered under various circumstances.

A professor approached me one day with a question that led to the development of my dissertation. He handed me three small, flat bony fragments and asked: "Is this human?" Based on my background in osteology and zooarchaeology, I was able to confidently say yes and identify the remains as human cranial bone. However, his next question was "Well … what else can you tell me from this?" Because of my previous research and coursework in bone histology, I knew that at the microscopic level I could discern answers to questions concerning numerous interests of the skeletal biologist, namely, estimating aspects of the biological profile.

The majority of relevant histological research that discusses estimating age-at-death is focused on numerous bones, including the ribs, clavicles, and mandible, but the primary focus is the long bones. The discovery of fragmentary cranial remains made me consider the possibility of using the microstructure of these elements to estimate age-at-death. After an extensive literature review, I learned that the neurocranium has not often been employed in histological age research and only a few studies have attempted to quantify microscopic traits of the skull (Clarke, 1987; Cool et al., 1995; Curtis, 2003). Based on this, I decided a contribution examining this area would be valuable.

When considering my research design, I chose three neurocranial elements for analysis—the frontal, parietal, and temporal bones. Both the frontal and parietal have been previously discussed in relation to age estimations (Clarke, 1987; Curtis, 2003) so one purpose of my research was to compare findings. Additionally, there was no evidence in previous literature that the temporal bone had been examined so another goal was to attempt an entirely new approach.

Because of the paucity of neurocranial histological research, I decided to begin with basic questions about the microstructure of these elements before considering too many variables. I chose to use European American males and females based on the demographics of East Tennessee as well as the possibility of needing specific methodologies for different ancestral groups. The bone samples were procured from autopsied individuals at the University of Tennessee Medical Center in Knoxville. The existing literature was skewed towards older individuals so my research addressed this gap and focused on age groups below 50 years. I followed the embedding and sectioning procedures discussed earlier in this chapter and utilized variables similar to Curtis (2003) as her study also focused on the cranium.

I reached the following significant conclusions:

- There are no differences in the histomorphometrics (or *subvariables*) between the internal and external tables of the frontal, parietal, and temporal bones.
- There are significant differences in the subvariable mean values between males and females. Sex-specific analyses are necessary.
- There are significant differences in the subvariable mean values between bones when controlling for sex.
- The correlations of subvariable mean values and age are similar to the trends found in previous neurocranial studies.
- These correlation trends are additionally comparable to long bone histomorphometric research indicating similar processes of cortical remodeling.

As the conclusions indicated that sex-specific analyses were necessary for neurocranial histology, I created a discriminant function analysis based on the collected histomorphometrics to estimate sex. I used a combination of subvariables from the frontal, parietal, and temporal bones for this purpose and was successful, with 80% correct classification for females and 90% correct classification for males.

Finally, I was able to eventually return to that same professor and tell him that I could estimate age and sex from those small cranial bone fragments that he had initially approached me with.

Case Study 2

Bone histology proved to be pivotal in relation to a 1985 homicide investigation as presented by Owsley and colleagues (1985). A woman was shot and killed by two shotgun blasts; her humerus was fractured during the event leaving a portion of her diaphysis missing and never recovered. During the course of the investigation, fragmentary remains were discovered inside a pickup truck of a potential suspect. The man claimed to be an avid hunter and asserted that the small bony fragments were from deer he had recently killed during the hunting season.

Bone samples were procured from the extant portion of the victim's humerus as well as from the forearm of a recently killed deer. These samples were embedded, sectioned, and examined under a microscope for comparative histological analysis. Owsley et al. (1985) took measurements of cortical thicknesses and examined the sections for the presence and organization of osteonal bone.

The known deer bone was characterized by plexiform bone and primary osteons. The unidentified bony fragments, however, were comprised of remodeled secondary osteonal bone. The cortical thicknesses of these remains were consistent with the samples taken from the victim at autopsy. Also, there was no evidence of plexiform bone in the unknown sample from the pickup truck.

Therefore, the researchers were able to rule out deer as the source of the unidentified remains as well as demonstrate the likelihood that the bone fragments were from the victim. The suspect in question admitted to the murder before his trial.

If this homicide were a present-day investigation, the question may arise as to why histo-morphological analyses were preferred to DNA analyses. Under certain circumstances, bone histology can be a more expeditious, less expensive, and in some cases, perhaps a less destructive technique.

SO YOU'RE INTERESTED IN BONE HISTOLOGY

Bone and dental histological research is a tedious process. It can be painstaking and time consuming but it is fascinating and the future potential of the field is wide open. For the anthropologist interested in pursuing histology, a strong grasp of bone and tooth biology and bone biomechanics is essential. A solid understanding and awareness of the key histo-morphological innovators and their methodologies is strongly recommended. Many of these have been discussed within this chapter.

Keep in mind the importance of sample selection and adhering to the specificities of a technique as it is described. Useful bone histology references include the recent publication, Crowder and Stout (2012), as well as works by Kerley (1965), Kerley and Ubelaker (1978), Stout (1989, 1992), and Robling and Stout (2008), to name only a few. Becoming familiar with these sources as well as bone biology texts such as Enlow (1963), Martin and Burr (1989), Carter and Beaupre (2001), and Hall (2005) is strongly recommended for the aspiring bone histology researcher.

The microscopic analysis of hard tissues is very useful to anthropologists. As discussed, bone and dental histology contribute to partial estimation of the biological profile as well as providing insight into nutritional, pathological, biomechanical, and taphonomic research. These fields are ripe with unexplored and unanswered questions. A better understanding of how biomechanical stress and strain affect bone structure is necessary as is a need to further substantiate current histological aging techniques and potential sexing methodologies. An appreciation of this potential and a desire to pursue these avenues will greatly benefit the future of the field. With the recent advancements in imaging and microscopy technology, there exists a valuable opportunity for young researchers to jump in at an exciting time and leave their mark on the field.

ACKNOWLEDGMENTS

Thank you to the editors, Elizabeth A. DiGangi and Megan K. Moore, for the invitation to contribute to this useful text.

REFERENCES

Acsádi, G., Nemeskéri, J., 1970. History of Human Life Span and Mortality. Akademiai Kiado, Budapest.
Ahlqvist, J., Damsten, O., 1969. A modification of Kerley's method for the microscopic determination of age in bone. Journal of Forensic Sciences 14, 205–212.
Aiello, L.C., Molleson, T., 1993. Are microscopic ageing techniques more accurate than macroscopic ageing techniques? Journal of Archaeological Science 20 (6), 689–704.
An, Y.H., Martin, K.L., 2003. Handbook of Histology Methods for Bone and Cartilage. Humana Press, New Jersey.
Anderson, C., 1982. Manual for the Examination of Bone. CRC Press, Boca Raton, FL.
Ascenzi, A., Bonucci, E., 1967. The tensile properties of single osteons. Anatomical Record 158 (4), 375–386.
Ascenzi, A., Bonucci, E., 1968. The compressive properties of single osteons. Anatomical Record 161 (3), 377–391.
Baron, R., Vignery, A., Horowitz, M., 1984. Lymphocytes, macrophages and the regulation of bone remodeling. In: Peck, W.A. (Ed.), Bone and Mineral Research Annual. Elsevier, Amsterdam, pp. 175–225.
Beaupre, G.S., Stevens, S.S., Carter, D.R., 2000. Mechanobiology in the development, maintenance, and degeneration of articular cartilage. Journal of Rehabilitation Research and Development 37 (2), 145–151.
Beeley, J., Harvey, W., 1973. Pink teeth appearing as a post-mortem phenomenon. Journal of the Forensic Science Society 13 (4), 297–305.
Bell, L.S., 1990. Palaeopathology and diagenesis: an SEM evaluation of structural changes using backscattered electron imaging. Journal of Archaeological Science 17 (1), 85–102.
Bell, L.S., 2012. Histotaphonomy. In: Crowder, C.M., Stout, S.D. (Eds.), Bone Histology, An Anthropological Perspective. CRC Press, Boca Raton, pp. 241–251.
Bell, L.S., Elkeron, A., 2008. Human remains recovered from a sixteenth century mass fatality: unique marine taphonomy in human skeletal material from the medieval warship the Mary Rose. International Journal of Osteoarchaeology 18, 523–535.
Bell, L.S., Skinner, M.F., Jones, S.J., 1996. The speed of post mortem change to the human skeleton and its taphonomic significance. Forensic Science International 82 (2), 129–140.
Bell, T., 1829. Anatomy, Physiology, and Disease of Teeth. Highly, London.
Bethard, J.D., 2013. Isotopes. In: DiGangi, E.A., Moore, M.K. (Eds.), Research Methods in Human Skeletal Biology. Academic Press, San Diego.
Britz, H.M., Thomas, C.D., Clement, J.G., Cooper, D.M., 2009. The relation of femoral osteon geometry to age, sex, height and weight. Bone 45 (1), 77–83.
Brondum, N., Simonsen, J., 1987. Postmortem red coloration of teeth: a retrospective investigation of 26 cases. American Journal of Forensic Medical Pathology 8 (2), 127.
Buikstra, J.E., Ubelaker, D.H., 1994. Standards for Data Collection from Human Skeletal Remains. Arkansas Archaeological Survey, Fayetteville, AR.
Burr, D., Ruff, C.B., Thompson, D.D., 1990. Patterns of skeletal histological change through time: Comparison of an archaic Native American population with modern populations. Anatomical Record 226 (3), 307–313.
Cabana, G.S., Hulsey, B.I., Pack, F.P., 2013. Molecular methods. In: DiGangi, E.A., Moore, M.K. (Eds.), Research Methods in Human Skeletal Biology. Academic Press, San Diego.

Carter, D.R., Beaupre, G.S., 2001. Skeletal Form and Function. Mechanobiology of Skeletal Development, Aging, and Regeneration. Cambridge, New York, Melbourne: Cambridge University Press.

Charles, D., Condon, K., Cheverud, J., Buikstra, J., 1989. Estimating age at death from growth layer groups in cementum. In: Iscan, M.Y. (Ed.), Age Markers in the Human Skeleton. Charles C. Thomas, Springfield, IL, pp. 277–316.

Cho, H., 2012. The histology laboratory and principles of microscope instrumentation. In: Crowder, C.M., Stout, S.D. (Eds.), Bone Histology, An Anthropological Perspective. CRC Press, Boca Raton, pp. 341–359.

Cho, H., Stout, S.D., Madsen, R.W., Streeter, M.A., 2002. Population-specific histological age-estimating method: A model for known African-American and European-American skeletal remains. Journal of Forensic Sciences 47 (1), 12–18.

Clark, D., Law, M., 1984. Postmortem pink teeth. Medicine, Science, and the Law 24 (2), 130.

Clarke, D.F., 1987. Histological and Radiographic Variation in the Parietal Bone in a Cadaveric Population. Unpublished Master's thesis. University of Queensland, Australia.

Cool, S.M., Hendrikz, J.K., Wood, W.B., 1995. Microscopic age changes in the human occipital bone. Journal of Forensic Sciences 40 (5), 789–796.

Crowder, C.M., Stout, S.D., 2012. Bone Histology, An Anthropological Perspective. CRC Press, Boca Raton.

Currey, J.D., 1959. Differences in the tensile strength of bone of different histological types. Journal of Anatomy (London) 93 (1), 87–95.

Currey, J.D., 1964. Some effects of ageing in human Haversian systems. Journal of Anatomy 98 (1), 69–75.

Currey, J.D., 2002. Bones: Structure and Mechanics. Princeton University Press, New Jersey.

Curtis, J.M., 2003. Estimation of Age at Death from the Microscopic Appearance of the Frontal Bone. Unpublished Master's thesis. Graduate School of the University of Indianapolis.

Dean, M., 2006. Tooth microstructure tracks the pace of human life-history evolution. Proceedings of the Royal Society of Biology 273 (1603), 2799–2808.

Dempster, W.T., Enlow, D.H., 1959. Patterns of vascular channels in the cortex of the human mandible. Anatomical Record 135 (3), 189–205.

DiGangi, E.A., Hefner, J.T., 2013. Ancestry estimation. In: DiGangi, E.A., Moore, M.K. (Eds.), Research Methods in Human Skeletal Biology. Academic Press, San Diego.

DiGangi, E.A., Moore, M.K., 2013. Application of the scientific method to skeletal biology. In: DiGangi, E.A., Moore, M.K. (Eds.), Research Methods in Human Skeletal Biology. Academic Press, San Diego.

Dye, T., Lucy, D., Pollard, A., 1995. The occurrence and the implications of post-mortem pink teeth in forensic and archaeologic cases. International Journal of Osteoarchaeology 5 (4), 339.

Gustafson, G., 1950. Age determination on teeth. Journal of the American Dental Association 41, 45–54.

Enlow, D.H., 1962a. A study of the post-natal growth and remodeling of bone. American Journal of Anatomy 110 (2), 79–101.

Enlow, D.H., 1962b. Functions of the Haversian system. American Journal of Anatomy 110 (3), 269–305.

Enlow, D.H., 1963. Principles of bone remodeling. In: Enlow, Donald H. (Ed.), American Lecture Series. Charles C. Thomas, Springfield, IL.

Enlow, D.H., Brown, S.O., 1956–58. A comparative histological study of fossil and recent bone tissues: Parts I, II and III. Texas Journal of Science 7, 405–443; 9, 186–214; 10, 187–230.

Ericksen, M.F., 1991. Histological estimation of age at death using the anterior cortex of the femur. American Journal of Physical Anthropology 84 (2), 171–179.

Ericksen, M.F., Aselrod, D.W., Melsen, F., 1994. Bone Histomorphometry. Raven Press, New York.

Fenton, T., Birkby, W.H., Cornelison, J., 2003. A fast and safe non-bleaching method for forensic skeletal preparation. Journal of Forensic Sciences 48 (2), 274–276.

Frost, H.M., 1958. Preparation of thin undecalcified bone sections by rapid manual method. Stain Technology 33, 271–276.

Frost, H.M., 1963. Bone Remodeling Dynamics. Charles C. Thomas, Springfield, IL.

Frost, H.M., 1964. The Laws of Bone Structure. Thomas, Springfield, IL.

Frost, H.M., 1987. Secondary osteon populations. An algorithm for determining mean bone tissue age. Yearbook of Physical Anthropology 30 (S8), 221–238.

Frost, H.M., 1997. Obesity, and bone strength and "mass": a tutorial based on insights from a new paradigm. Bone 21 (3), 211–214.

Hackett, C.J., 1981. Microscopical focal destruction (tunnels) in exhumed human bones. Medicine, Science, and Law 21, 243−265.

Hall, B.K., 2005. Bones and Cartilage: Developmental and Evolutionary Skeletal Biology. Academic Press, London.

Hammerl, E., 2013. Dental anthropology. In: DiGangi, E.A., Moore, M.K. (Eds.), Research Methods in Human Skeletal Biology. Academic Press, San Diego.

Harsanyi, L., 1990. Differential diagnosis of human and animal bone. In: Grupe, G., Garland, A.N. (Eds.), Histology of Ancient Human Bone: Methods and Diagnosis. Springer, Berlin, pp. 79−94.

Heersche, J.N.M., 1978. Mechanism of osteoclastic bone resorption: A new hypothesis. Calcified Tissue Research 26 (1), 81−84.

Hillson, S., 1996. Dental Anthropology. Cambridge University Press, Cambridge.

Horni, H., 2002. The Forensic Application of Comparative Mammalian Histology. Unpublished Master's Thesis. Texas Tech University, Lubbock, TX.

Hughes-Fulford, M., 2004. Signal transduction and mechanical stress. Science STKE Retrieved from (249), RE12.

Jaffe, H.L., 1929. The structure of bone with particular reference to its fibrillar nature and the relation of function to internal architecture. Archives of Surgery 19 (1), 24−52.

Jans, M.M.E., Nielsen-Marsh, C.M., Smith, C.I., Collins, M.J., Kars, H., 2004. Characterization of microbial attack on archaeological bone. Journal of Archaeological Science 31 (1), 87−95.

Johanson, G., 1971. Age determination from human teeth. Odontologisk Revy 22, 1−126.

Jowsey, J., 1966. Studies of Haversian systems in man and some animals. Journal of Anatomy 100 (4), 857−864.

Jowsey, J., 1977. Metabolic Diseases of Bone. W.B. Saunders, London.

Junqueira, L.C., Carneiro, J., 2003a. Bone. In: Foltin, J., Lebowitz, H., Boyle, P.J. (Eds.), Basic Histology: Text and Atlas, 10th ed. McGraw-Hill Companies, Inc, New York, pp. 141−159.

Junqueira, L., Carneiro, J., 2003b. Basic Histology: Text and Atlas, 11th ed. McGraw-Hill, New York.

Junqueira, L.C., Carneiro, J., Kelley, R.O., 1998. Bone. In: Basic Histology, 9th ed. Appleton & Lange, Stanford, CT, pp. 134−151.

Kerley, E.R., 1965. The microscopic determination of age in human bone. American Journal of Physical Anthropology 23 (2), 149−164.

Kerley, E.R., Ubelaker, D.H., 1978. Revisions in the microscopic method of estimating age at death in human cortical bone. American Journal of Physical Anthropology 49 (4), 545−546.

Kim, Y., Kim, D., Park, D., Lee, J., Chung, N., Lee, W., Han, S., 2007. Assessment of histomorphological features of the sternal end of the fourth rib for age estimation in Koreans. Journal of Forensic Sciences 52 (6), 1237−1241.

Kroman, A.M., Marks, M., 2003. Pink teeth: Postmortem posture and microscopy. Proceedings of the American Academy of Forensic Sciences 9, 180−181.

Kroman, A.M., Symes, S.A., 2013. Investigation of Skeletal trauma. In: DiGangi, E.A., Moore, M.K. (Eds.), Research Methods in Human Skeletal Biology. Academic Press, San Diego.

Lacroix, P., 1971. The internal remodeling of bones. In: Bourne, H.C. (Ed.), The Biochemistry and Physiology of Bone. Academic Press, New York, pp. 119−144.

Leeson, T.S., Leeson, R.C., 1981. Specialized connective tissue: cartilage and bone. In: Histology, 4th ed. W.B. Saunders Company, Philadelphia, Pennsylvania, pp. 137−164.

Lieberman, D., 1993. Life history variables preserved in dental cementum microstructure. Science 261 (5125), 1162−1164.

Lipsinic, F., Paunovitch, E., Hourson, G., Robinson, S., 1986. Correlation of age and incremental lines in the cementum of human teeth. Journal of Forensic Sciences 31 (3), 982−989.

Lucy, D., Pollard, A., 1995. Further comments on the estimation of error associated with the Gustafson dental age estimation method. Journal of Forensic Sciences 40 (2), 222−227.

Maat, G.J., Van Den Bos, R.P., Aarents, M., 2001. Manual preparation of ground sections for the microscopy of natural bone tissue: update and modification of Frost's "rapid manual method". International Journal of Osteoarchaeology 11 (5), 366−374.

Maples, W., 1978. An improved technique using dental histology for the estimation of adult age. Journal of Forensic Sciences 23, 764−770.

Marden, K., Sorg, M., Haglund, W., 2013. Taphonomy. In: DiGangi, E.A., Moore, M.K. (Eds.), Research Methods in Human Skeletal Biology. Academic Press, San Diego.

Martin, D.L., 1991. Bone histology and paleopathology: methodological considerations. In: Ortner, D.J., Aufderheide, A.C. (Eds.), Human Paleopathology. Smithsonian Institution Press, Washington, pp. 55–59.

Martin, R.B., Burr, D.B., 1989. Structure, function, and adaptation of compact bone. Raven Press, New York.

Martin, R.B., Burr, D.B., Sharkey, N.A., 1998. Skeletal Tissue Mechanics. Springer, New York.

Miles, A., Fernhead, R., 1954. Post-mortem color changes in teeth. Journal of Dental Research 33, 735.

Miller, C., Dove, S., Cottone, J., 1988. Failure of use of cemental annulations in teeth to determine the age of humans. Journal of Forensic Sciences 33 (1), 137–143.

Miyabara, Y., Onoe, Y., Harada, A., Kuroda, T., Sasaki, S., Ohta, H., 2007. Effect of physical activity and nutrition on bone mineral density in young Japanese women. Journal of Bone Mineral Metabolism 25 (6), 414–418.

Monro, A., 1776. The anatomy of the human bones, nerves and lacteal sac and duct. Unknown publisher, Dublin.

Moore, M.K., 2008. Body mass estimation from the human skeleton. Unpublished Doctoral Dissertation, The University of Tennessee, Knoxville, TN.

Moore, M.K., 2013. Sex estimation and assessment. In: DiGangi, E.A., Moore, M.K. (Eds.), Research Methods in Human Skeletal Biology. Academic Press, San Diego.

Moore, M.K., 2013. Functional morphology and medical imaging. In: DiGangi, E.A., Moore, M.K. (Eds.), Research Methods in Human Skeletal Biology. Academic Press, San Diego.

Moore, M.K., Ross, A.H., 2013. Stature estimation. In: DiGangi, E.A., Moore, M.K. (Eds.), Research Methods in Human Skeletal Biology. Academic Press, San Diego.

Moore, M.K., Schaefer, E., 2011. A comprehensive regression tree to estimate body weight from the skeleton. Journal of Forensic Sciences 56 (5), 1115–1122.

Morris, P., 1978. The use of teeth for estimating age of wild mammals. In: Butler, P., Joysey, K. (Eds.), Development, Function, and Evolution of Teeth. Academic Press, London, pp. 483–494.

Mulhern, D.M., Ubelaker, D.H., 2001. Differences in osteon banding between human and nonhuman bone. Journal of Forensic Sciences 46 (2), 220–222.

Nawrocki, S., 1997. Cleaning bones. University of Indianapolis Archaeology and Forensics Laboratory. http://archlab.uindy.edu.

Ortner, D.J., 1975. Aging effects on osteon remodeling. Calcified Tissue Research 18, 27–36.

Owsley, D., Miers, A.M., Keith, M.S., 1985. Case involving differentiation of deer and human bone fragments. Journal of Forensic Sciences 30 (2), 572–578.

Paine, R.R., 2007. How to equip a basic histology lab for the anthropological assessment of human bone and teeth. Journal of Anthropological Science 85, 213–219.

Petrtyl, M., Hert, J., Fiala, P., 1996. Spatial organization of the Haversian bone in man. Biomechanics 29 (2), 161–169.

Pfeiffer, S., 1998. Variability in osteon size in recent human populations. American Journal of Physical Anthropology 106 (2), 219–227.

Pfeiffer, S., 2000. Palaeohistology: Health and disease. In: Katzenberg, M.A., Saunders, S.R. (Eds.), Biological Anthropology of the Human Skeleton. Wiley-Liss, New York, pp. 281–296.

Pfeiffer, S., Crowder, C., Harrington, L., Brown, M., 2006. Secondary osteon and Haversian canal diameters as behavioral indicators. American Journal of Physical Anthropology 131, 460–468.

Recker, R.R., 1983. Bone histomorphometry: Techniques and interpretation. CRC Press, Boca Raton.

Ribot, C., Tremollieres, F., Pouilles, J.M., Bonneu, M., Germain, F., Louvet, J.P., 1987. Obesity and postmenopausal bone loss: the influence of obesity on vertebral density and bone turnover in postmenopausal women. Bone 8, 327–331.

Rice, P., Maples, W., 1979. Some difficulties in the Gustafson dental age estimations. Journal of Forensic Sciences 24 (1), 118–172.

Robling, A.G., Stout, S.D., 2008. Histomorphometry of human cortical bone: Applications to age estimation. In: Katzenberg, M.A., Saunders, S.R. (Eds.), Biological Anthropology of the Human Skeleton. Wiley-Liss, New York, pp. 149–183.

Robling, A.G., Castillo, A.B., Turner, C.H., 2006. Biomechanical and molecular regulation of bone remodeling. Annual Review of Biomedical Engineering 8, 455–498.

Sadler, T., 2006. Langman's Medical Embryology, 10th ed. Lippincott Williams and Williams, Philadelphia.

Samson, C., Branigan, K., 1987. A new method of estimating age at death from fragmentary and weathered bone. In: Boodington, A., Garland, A.N., Janaway, R.C. (Eds.), Death, Decay and Reconstruction: Approaches to Archaeology and Forensic Science. Manchester University Press, Manchester, pp. 109–126.

Schenk, R.K., Olah, A.J., Hermann, W., 1984. Preparation of calcified tissues for light microscopy. In: Dickson, G.R. (Ed.), Methods of Calcified Tissue Preparation. Elsevier, New York, pp. 1–56.

Scheuer, L., Black, S., 2000. Developmental Juvenile Osteology. Academic Press, San Diego.

Schultz, M., 2001. Paleohistopathology of bone: A new approach to the study of ancient diseases. Yearbook of Physical Anthropology 44 (S33), 106–147.

Schultz, M., 2003. Light microscopic analysis in skeletal paleopathology. In: Ortner, D.J. (Ed.), Identification of Pathological Conditions in Human Skeletal Remains. Academic Press, San Diego, pp. 73–109.

Schultz, M., 2012. Light microscopic analysis of macerated pathologically changed bones. In: Crowder, C.M., Stout, S.D. (Eds.), Bone Histology, An Anthropological Perspective. CRC Press, Boca Raton.

Scott, G., Turner, C., 1988. Dental anthropology. Annual Review of Anthropology 17, 99–126.

Sharpe, W.D., 1979. Age changes in human bone: an overview. Bulletin of the New York Academy of Medicine 55 (8), 757–773.

Singh, I.J., Gunberg, D.L., 1970. Estimation of age at death in human males from quantitative histology of bone fragments. American Journal of Physical Anthropology 33 (3), 373–382.

Singh, I.J., Tonna, E.A., Gandel, C.P., 1974. A comparative histological study of mammal bones. Journal of Morphology 144 (4), 421–438.

Skinner, M., Anderson, G., 1991. Individualization and enamel histology: a case report in forensic anthropology. Journal of Forensic Sciences 36 (3), 939–948.

Smith, M.O., 2013. Paleopathology. In: DiGangi, E.A., Moore, M.K. (Eds.), Research Methods in Human Skeletal Biology. Academic Press, San Diego.

Stott, G., Sis, R., Levy, B., 1980. Cemental annulation as an age criterion in the common marmoset (*Callithrix jaculus*). Journal of Medical Primatology 9, 274–285.

Stott, G., Sis, R., Levy, B., 1982. Cemental annulation as an age criterion in forensic dentistry. Journal of Dental Research 61 (6), 814–817.

Stout, S.D., 1986. The use of histomorphometry in skeletal identification: the case of Francisco Pizarro. Journal of Forensic Sciences 31 (1), 121–125.

Stout, S.D., 1989. Histomorphometric Analysis of human skeletal remains. In: Kennedy, K.A.R., Iscan, M.Y. (Eds.), Reconstruction of Life from the Skeleton. Alan R. Liss, New York, pp. 41–52.

Stout, S.D., 1992. Methods of determining age at death using bone microstructure. In: Saunders, S.R., Katzenberg, M.A. (Eds.), Skeletal Biology of Past Peoples: Research Methods. Wiley-Liss, New York, pp. 21–25.

Stout, S.D., Paine, R.R., 1992. Brief communication: Histological age estimation using rib and clavicle. American Journal of Physical Anthropology 87, 111–115.

Stout, S.D., Stanley, S.C., 1991. Percent osteonal bone versus osteon counts: the variable of choice for estimating age at death. American Journal of Physical Anthropology 86 (4), 515–519.

Stout, S.D., Porro, M.A., Perotti, B., 1996. Brief communication: a test and correction of the clavicle method of Stout and Paine for histological age estimation of skeletal remains. American Journal of Physical Anthropology 100 (1), 139–142.

Tersigni, M.A., 2005. Serial long bone histology: inter- and intra-bone age estimation. Unpublished Doctoral dissertation. University of Tennessee, Knoxville, TN.

Thompson, D.D., 1979. The core technique in the determination of age at death in skeletons. Journal of Forensic Sciences 24 (4), 902–915.

Thompson, D.D., 1980. Age changes in bone mineralisation, cortical thickness, and Haversian canal area. Calcified Tissue International 31 (1), 5–11.

Thompson, D.D., Gunness-Hey, M., 1981. Bone mineral osteon analysis of Yupikinupiaq skeletons. American Journal of Physical Anthropology 55 (1), 1–7.

Trammell, L.H., 2012. Neurocranial histomorphometrics. Unpublished Doctoral dissertation. University of Tennessee, Knoxville, TN.

Ubelaker, D.H., 1989. Human skeletal remains: excavation, analysis, and interpretation. Taraxacum, Washington DC.

Uhl, N.M., 2013. Age-at-death estimation. In: DiGangi, E.A., , M.K., 2013. Pink teeth of the dead. Journal of Forensic Odontostomatology 5, 41.

Watanabe, Y., Konishi, M., Shimada, M., Ohara, H., Iwamoto, S., 1998. Estimation of age from the femur of Japanese cadavers. Forensic Science International 98 (1-2), 55–65.

Wedl, C., 1864. Uber einen im Zahnbein und Knochen keimenden Pilz. Akademi der Wissenschaften in Vien. Fitzungsberichte Naturwissenschaftliche Klasse A BI. Mineralogi, biologi erdkunde 50, 171–193.

Wheatley, B.P., 2005. An evaluation of sex and body weight determination from the proximal femur using DXA technology and its potential for forensic anthropology. Forensic Sci International 147 (2-3), 141–145.

White, A.A., Panjabi, M.M., Southwick, W.O., 1977. The four biomechanical stages of healing. Journal of Bone and Joint Surgery 59A, 188–192.

Wolff, J., 1892. Das Gesetz der Transformation der Knochen. A. Hirschwald, Berlin.

Yoshino, M., Imaizumi, K., Miyasaka, S., Seta, S., 1994. Histological estimation of age at death using microradiographs of humeral compact bone. Forensic Science International 64 (2-3), 191–198.

Functional Morphology and Medical Imaging

Megan K. Moore

INTRODUCTION

This chapter explores theoretical and methodological considerations of research in functional morphology and bone biomechanics. Washburn (1951) proposed that the "**New Physical Anthropology**"[1] focus more on questions of functional morphology and anatomy as opposed to questions of simple typological classification. The goal of this chapter is to promote that same vision by providing the young researcher with the necessary tool kit for functional morphology research. The chapter begins with a brief overview of the properties of skeletal tissues, bone biomechanics, and the **functional adaptation** of the skeleton. Functional morphology research can be broken down into four general categories: (1) cross-sectional geometry; (2) joint form and pathology; (3) trabecular architecture; and (4) histology (Pearson and Lieberman, 2004). Each category studies different aspects of bone shape, either at the macroscopic or at the microscopic level. This chapter will focus on the first two categories relating to macrostructure. Trammell and Kroman explore bone microstructure in greater detail in the chapter on histology in this volume (Chapter 13).

Many different methods have been used to analyze bone macrostructure. Cross-sectional shape can reveal the bone's ability to resist a variety of forces. A bone's shape is the result of a combination of both **intrinsic** and **extrinsic** variables. Intrinsic or systemic factors act from within the body, such as genetic constraints and hormone levels. Extrinsic factors acting on the skeleton can be due to the environmental influence of nutrition or to the biomechanical influence of different forces acting on the skeleton, such as locomotion and gravity. For example, the neck of the femur is nearly vertical in infancy and only becomes angled as we begin to walk, the result of extrinsic biomechanical variables (Tardieu, 1999).

A variety of different research methods have been developed and implemented to try to understand the functional adaptations of the skeleton. While a two-dimensional radiograph can reveal the internal structure of a bone, it can only provide a rough approximation of the

---

[1]All bolded terms are defined in the glossary at the end of this volume.

functional strength of the bone. Thus, some early research in functional morphology relied on the destructive analyses of cutting transverse sections of the long bone shafts to determine the shape and surface area of the cortical bone cross-section (Burr and Piotrowski, 1982; Harrington et al., 1993). More recent studies take advantage of medical imaging modalities, which are relatively nondestructive for skeletal samples and can provide three-dimensional digital imaging of the internal and external structure, and the material properties of bone density (one measure of bone strength) (Groll et al., 1999; O'Neill and Ruff, 2004; Stojanowski and Buikstra, 2005; Gu et al., 2008; Saeed et al., 2009; Sparacello and Pearson, 2010; Hind et al., 2011; Moore and Schaefer, 2011; Samelson et al., 2012). As medical imaging technologies become less expensive, nondestructive methods are now available to the biological anthropologist to investigate questions of biocultural influences on bone strength and functional adaptation.

The New Physical Anthropology

In 1951, Sherwood Washburn called on physical anthropologists to rethink their research questions (Washburn, 1951). He criticized the discipline for emphasizing data collection of biological traits, only to use them to classify populations, what he called a **typological approach**. Washburn considered this research to have a limited scope with little theoretical development. He proposed that the "New Physical Anthropology" take an interest in understanding human variation and the process of evolution; essentially a "return to Darwinism" (Washburn, 1951). Instead of simply recording a trait, he emphasized the need to understand why the trait is there in the first place, with an emphasis on functional morphology and anatomy. More than 50 years later, Armelagos and Van Gerven (2003) reevaluated the discipline to assess whether we are now successfully addressing Washburn's concerns. They concluded that there is some progress, but it has been slow in terms of the number of studies addressing functional anatomy versus the number that continue to do research using a more typological approach (Armelagos and Van Gerven, 2003). Stojanowski and Buikstra (2004) published a rejoinder to this critique, disagreeing with the conclusion of the former publication about typological studies. Regardless, a functional morphology approach provides a more comprehensive understanding of the human skeletal form. This chapter therefore introduces some of the theory behind functional morphology with advice on how to conduct your own study.

BASIC BONE BIOLOGY

The skeleton appears to be a stable structure, yet the living skeleton is a dynamic system, constantly remodeling in response to both extrinsic mechanical forces and intrinsic metabolic processes. For example, moderate exercise is enough to increase bone mass (Nilsson and Westlin, 1971). Bone acts as a reservoir of calcium to maintain the normal function of the body and muscles. Bone tissue is made up of three different types of cells that maintain bone homeostasis, which are the **osteoclasts**, **osteoblasts**, and **osteocytes**. Osteoclasts are cells that function to resorb existing bone in order to release minerals, remove organic waste, and respond to injury, while osteoblasts synthesize new **bone matrix** or **osteoid** (the unmineralized organic part of bone). Osteoblasts mature into osteocytes, which become intricately woven into the network of calcified bone matrix. Osteocytes maintain the ability to communicate complex information along interconnecting pathways called **canaliculi** (as many as 80 connections per osteocyte), providing information about mechanical forces in order to make necessary modifications to the bone's shape (i.e. macrostructure) (Pearson and Lieberman, 2004). In normal adult aging, the osteoblasts are typically more active at the **periosteum** (external surface of the bone) and osteoclasts more actively resorb bone at the **endosteum** (internal surface of medullary canal). Cell types and function are discussed further in Trammell and Kroman (Chapter 13), this volume.

Bone strength depends on three characteristics: (1) **material properties**, (2) **microstructure**, and (3) **macrostructure** (Ruff, 1981). The material properties include chemical composition and bone density. The chemical composition of bone (percentage of collagen and hydroxyapatite) is the same in both **trabecular** and **cortical** bone in a single individual (Frankel and Nordin, 1980). Bone does, however, change in material properties throughout the life cycle, with a greater percentage of collagen in a juvenile than in an elderly adult (Beck et al., 1993). The **diaphysis** (shaft) of a long bone is predominantly cortical bone and the **epiphyses** (ends of the long bone at the joint) are mostly trabecular bone. The bone macrostructure is a combination of external and internal geometric properties, as well as the trabecular orientation (Ruff, 1981).

Adult bone formation occurs via a process of Haversian remodeling compared to juvenile bone modeling. The long bones of the skeleton in a subadult develop through a process called **endochondral ossification** (i.e., bone formation that starts from a cartilage model). In remodeling, **secondary osteons** (those formed by the replacement of bone) will overlay the **primary lamellar bone** (the original bone layers) (Robling, 1998). Bone remodeling in adults is mostly **subperiosteal expansion** in which the bone shaft grows larger in diameter along with an increase in the medullary canal, which is due to **endosteal resorption** by the osteoclasts. There is some evidence of **endosteal apposition** in individuals, in which the bone grows inward, decreasing the size of the medullary canal, but this is rare (Ruff, et al., 1994; Pearson and Lieberman, 2004; Moore et al., 2007). When the bone is stressed, microfractures can form in the **gap junction** (the space at the surface of each cell) between osteocytes to help dissipate a force. If the stress is beyond a certain threshold, though not enough to cause fracture, **basic multicellular units (BMUs)** will begin to increase bone apposition (i.e., deposition), and decrease resorption to accommodate the increased load. BMUs are made up of a combination of osteoblasts and osteoclasts that coordinate the apposition and resorption. Conversely, when the load threshold has been brought to the lower end of the spectrum for which the bone is well adapted, the remodeling is turned off (Frost, 1997). Microstructure of the bone is characterized by the **modeling** and **remodeling** of **Haversian systems** and trabeculae, and is discussed at length in Trammell and Kroman (Chapter 13), this volume.

BASIC BONE BIOMECHANICS

Bones can sense loads and self-regulate, via the process of **mechanotransduction**, in which cells sense mechanical stimuli. The process is not completely clear, but it appears that the osteocytes act as the **mechanosensory cells** or strain receptors. The process of mechanotransduction is possible because the bone cells have a connected cellular network (CCN) and this network functions like its own nervous system (Aarden et al., 1994; Pearson and Lieberman, 2004). When the bone begins to fail as a result of a minor injury, microfractures form and fluid is forced through the canaliculi and across the gap junctions, which is sensed and interpreted by the cells themselves (Aarden et al., 1994). How the cells interpret this information and respond is unknown (Pearson and Lieberman, 2004). Each skeletal tissue has a microdamage threshold in which normal repair can keep up with the need, but fatigue fracture occurs when the damage overwhelms the repair, which happens when there are repetitive small fractures (Frost, 1993).

During growth and development, bones are extremely plastic to forces of load bearing due to their more elastic material properties (greater percentage of collagen in youth). These forces alter the resultant shape of the bone shaft and its articulations. **Endochondral ossification**[2] occurs primarily through modeling or the depositing of lamellar bone. Because of the higher percentage of collagen present, young bone typically adapts efficiently to normal activities and to the environment (Carter et al., 1991). Mechanical loading early in development may guide endochondral ossification, so that the skeletal form is well designed for its mechanical function (Carter et al., 1991).

As an individual ages, the material properties of bone change from being elastic to more stiff as collagen is gradually lost (Rubin et al., 1990; Frost, 1993). Adult bone therefore responds slightly differently to forces of loading over time. In adult bone, the epiphyses are fused and there is increased mineralization compared to juvenile bone. This gives greater strength and stiffness to adult bone, but it inevitably becomes more brittle. **Young's modulus** (a measure of bone's stiffness) is used to explain material properties of bone (and other materials) in terms of resistance to stress and strain. Bone biomechanics are presented in terms of traumatic bone injury by Kroman and Symes in the chapter on trauma in this volume (Chapter 8).

Long bones can be interpreted as analogous to engineering beams (e.g., in a bridge or a building) when examining the cross-sectional shape properties of the beam (i.e., bone shaft). The cross-sectional cortical area reflects the bone's strength to **axial compression** (for example, the downward force of gravity acting on body mass). The **area moments of inertia** are the cross-sectional property of a beam cross-sectional property (e.g., bone) used to predict its resistance to bending (i.e., **bending strength**). The area moments of inertia are a measure of the distance of the bone surface to the center of the bone (centroid) and are measured in different directions. The direction of greatest bending is represented with the symbol I_{max}, which is perpendicular to the minimum area moment of inertia is signified by I_{min}. The **polar moments of area** are the cross-sectional property of a beam proportional to the torsional rigidity to predict a bone's resistance to twisting or **torsion** (i.e., **torsional strength**, calculated as J is divided by the distance from the subperiosteal surface to the centroid) (Frankel and Nordin, 1980; Ruff, 2000). The symbol "J" is typically used to represent the polar moments of area and equals the sum of any two perpendicular area moments of inertia. Increased surface area provides greater resistance to axial compression, which is

---

[2]Endochondral ossification occurs mostly postcranially in the long bones. In contrast, intramembranous ossification occurs mostly in the skull. See Uhl (Chapter 3) this volume, for more on aging.

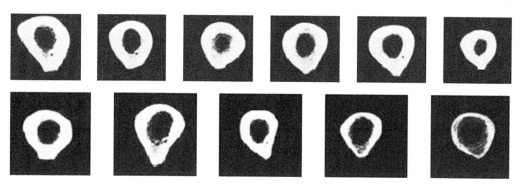

FIGURE 14.1 Image comparing bone cross-sections. The top row depicts male femora and the bottom row depicts female femora from CT scans of individuals from the William M. Bass Donated Skeletal Collection.

the predominant force affecting the epiphyses, but also affects the midshaft cross-sectional area (Frost, 1993; Eckstein et al., 2002). For example, if a bone undergoes extreme axial loading, the bone will accommodate by increasing in cross-sectional area. Lastly, **shear** forces are those that act on the bone in two opposing directions.

Greater bending strength in a certain direction suggests that the bone is loaded more in that direction. Many studies have investigated changing activity patterns reflected in the ratio of maximum (I_{max}) to minimum (I_{min}) bending strength in the femoral midshaft. It has been suggested that a high I_{max}/I_{min} ratio (or **shape index**) correlates strongly with greater levels of activity, especially over rough terrain (Lovejoy et al., 1976; Ruff and Hayes, 1983a, 1984). Dividing the maximum moment of inertia by the minimum (I_{max}/I_{min}) gives a unitless "shape" variable. In the femur, a high shape index reflects more anteroposterior (AP) elongation. If equal to one, the cross-section is more circular; if less than one, the bone cross-section is elongated in the mediolateral (ML) direction (see Figure 14.1). Different types of activities with multiple forces simultaneously (torsion, bending, shear, and compression) can complicate the interpretation of a bone's shape, but it is important to keep in mind that the shape of bone can potentially reflect specific activities. The study of **functional morphology** in skeletal biology explores this relationship between the structure and function of the bones.

FUNCTIONAL MORPHOLOGY

Wolff's Law

The skeleton serves many purposes. It acts as a support system for other organs, it provides levers for action, and it supports the weight of the organism while withstanding forces during locomotion and impact (Schmidt-Nielsen, 1984). Due to the fact that bone is plastic, bone will adapt and model or remodel itself as necessary according to the forces applied. Roux first made the observation in 1881 that bone trabeculae appear to follow engineering principles, a finding later supported by Wolff in 1892. Both researchers recognized a principle of "functional adaptation" in bones, where a bone will reinforce itself along the direction of principal strain (Cowin, 2001). The trabeculae will align themselves along the trajectory of that principal strain, known as the **trajectorial theory of cancellous bone**.

Bone is **anisotropic**, which means that it is resistant to many different types of forces and from many different directions. Bones are extremely complex mechanical systems able to respond simultaneously to multiple forces (compression, bending, shear and torsion, as defined earlier in the biomechanics section). Bones will change in material properties and macrostructure during the stages of growth and development, throughout adulthood and into senescence. The shape of a bone will reflect fluctuating activity and weight bearing throughout life. Intrinsic factors (hormone levels, nutrition, etc.) can also play a role in bone metabolism. Barring any pathology, the skeleton will be strong enough for support and able to withstand impacts from normal activities and locomotion.

The paradox of skeletal function is that it must be simultaneously "strong enough for support, but light enough for locomotion" (Rubin et al., 1990). **Wolff's law** is interpreted as the explanation for this adaptation of bone. Wolff (1892) proposed that a change in a bone's function is followed by a change in the internal structure of the bone according to mathematical laws (Bertram and Swartz, 1991). The ability to maintain the balance between support and locomotion is contained within the bone itself. This balance occurs by a collaborative effort between an extensive network of osteocytes and BMUs. BMUs respond to signals from the osteocytes to initiate bone resorption followed by apposition (Rubin et al., 1990; Frost, 1993; Pearson and Lieberman, 2004). In the BMU, the osteoclasts resorb old bone in a tunnel-like fashion and then the osteoblasts deposit new bone as a secondary osteon (Pearson and Lieberman, 2004).

The three major tenets that have been put forth as Wolff's law are: (1) bone is strong enough for support and light enough for locomotion; (2) the trabeculae align themselves along the direction of principal strain; and (3) the first two tenets above are accomplished through a process of self-regulating mechanisms as the bone responds to mechanical loads (Pearson and Lieberman, 2004). Many skeletal biologists use Wolff's law broadly to explain the bone's ability to adapt to loads, but I personally prefer the term functional adaptation (Bertram and Swartz, 1991; Carter et al., 1991; Cowin, 2001).

Critiques of Wolff's Law

Several researchers have criticized the blanket acceptance of Wolff's law to explain the functional adaptation of bone (Bertram and Swartz, 1991; Cowin, 2001; Pearson and Lieberman, 2004). As Pearson and Lieberman (2004) explain, Wolff's law is neither a "law" nor is it completely true. There are multiple processes occurring simultaneously that are best understood if considered separately (Pearson and Lieberman, 2004). Wolff was also mostly concerned with the trabecular alignment and not the compact bone (Robling, 1998).

Bertram and Schwartz (1991) discuss the four false tenets of Wolff's law. The first tenet is the *trajectorial theory of cancellous bone*, which appears to be true only in growing bone. The second tenet is that of *bone atrophy*, which Bertram and Schwartz (1991) explain has two separate phases of resorption. The sensitivity to resorption is dependent on both age and location within the body. When we are younger, bone resorption can be turned off and reversed. When we are older, bone resorption can exceed apposition and is seemingly irreversible in cases of **osteoporosis**. Furthermore, rates of modeling and remodeling do not appear to be consistent for all locations in the skeleton (Bertram and Swartz, 1991). Third, Wolff's law does not account for *hypertrophy and thresholding*. To explain these terms, bone seems to respond to some aspects of load thresholding, in which a load must reach a certain threshold before the bone responds. Additionally, systemic bone hypertrophy (excessive bone formation throughout the body of some individuals) is not accounted for by Wolff's law (Bertram and Swartz, 1991). Finally, Wolff's law implies that atrophy is equal to the reverse of hypertrophy, which is not true. The localized response of bones in terms of apposition and resorption must reflect the biomechanics of the whole element (Bertram and Swartz, 1991).

Pearson and Lieberman (2004) further caution against assuming a relationship between the direction of loading in long bone **cross-sectional geometry** without experimental testing and validation in terms of cross-sectional geometry, bone density, and musculoskeletal stress markers. Musculoskeletal stress markers are also part of the bones' functional response to varying forces, and are discussed in both Smith (Chapter 7) and Kroman and Symes (Chapter 8), this volume.

Engineering Beam Theory

Living bone is seldom loaded by a single force, which makes bone very complicated to model mathematically. As a result of the nonuniform loading patterns from diverse activities and from body weight, living bone is anisotropic, as mentioned earlier. Bone is ultimately strongest under compression, but is loaded by tension, compression, shear, and bending forces. Muscles create the largest forces on bones (Frost, 1997). Torsional forces are distributed over the entire surface of a bone in a circular fashion (Frankel and Nordin, 1980). The polar moment of inertia is a measure of the torsional strength of a bone, which is directly related to the distance from the surface of the bone to the **neutral axis** (an axis along the shaft in which there are no longitudinal stresses). The neutral axis typically goes through the center of the medullary canal (although this can fluctuate depending on the direction of the force(s) being applied). Increasing surface area or cross-sectional area increases bone's strength to both compression and tension. Area moments of inertia (e.g., I_x, I_y, I_{max}, I_{min}) measure the bending strength of a bone, which is also related to the distance from the **centroid** (the

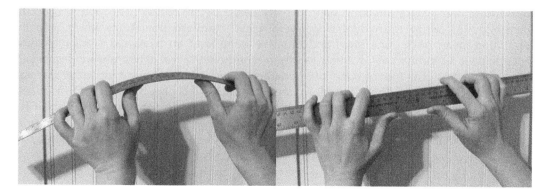

FIGURE 14.2   Ruler analogy for engineering beam theory.

geometric center of a three-dimensional object). If an object is symmetric, the neutral axis and the centroid are one and the same.

A simple demonstration of bending strength can be given with a wooden ruler. Consider the ease of bending a ruler in half along the 2 cm width compared to its 2 mm narrow edge (Larsen, 1997). See Figure 14.2. If you try to bend the ruler along its width, it yields quickly and fails. However, if you try to bend it along the narrow edge of the ruler, it is more difficult to bend and break. The analogy of the ruler is useful when considering the diaphysis of the load-bearing long bones of the lower limb, because bones are typically harder to break in one direction than another, if not circular in cross-section.

Manouvrier first recognized a difference in this cross-sectional ratio in 1888 from nonhuman primates to modern humans, the latter having a more round diaphysis. The purpose of a higher ratio or a more anteroposterior elongated shaft is to resist bending forces in this AP direction. This elongation of the diaphysis has been shown to be the result of greater flexion at the knee, related to crossing over steep or rough terrain (Lovejoy et al., 1976; Larsen, 1997; Ruff, 1987).[3] This ratio is useful because it automatically controls for size differences facilitating comparison between individuals and populations (Ruff and Hayes, 1983a, b).

Bone Density and Osteoporosis

Bone shafts increase in diameter with age, which reduces long bone cortical thickness and gives the appearance of reduced bone density in radiographs. This essentially maintains and increases bending strength into adulthood by increasing the distance from the bone surface to the centroid, while simultaneously decreasing surface area, thus reducing the bone's strength in compression. Women experience an accelerated bone loss following menopause due to a reduction in the hormone estrogen (an intrinsic factor), which has been demonstrated in prehistoric populations as well (Bloom and Laws, 1970; Ericksen, 1976; Ruff and Hayes, 1982, 1984; Nelson et al., 2000).

During growth, osteoblast deposition of osteoid exceeds osteoclast resorption. When the epiphyses fuse, growth ends and consolidation begins. **Consolidation** is the phase in which the bone increases in density until peak bone mass is reached in the early or mid-thirties. **Involution** is then the next stage when bone loss exceeds bone formation. Sex and age are the number one factors affecting bone density cause by involution. Osteoporosis occurs when bone loss in an individual is two and a half **standard deviations** lower than the population mean peak bone mass and thus the bone is at an increased risk of fracture. **Osteopenia** is a condition of low bone density, but without the risk of fracture and less severe than osteoporosis. The rate of bone loss in **osteoporosis** is not the same for trabecular and cortical bone. In general, the rate of loss in bone mineral density (BMD) is approximately 1% per year until the age of 65. The process is accelerated to 2% per year BMD lost for the five years following menopause in women (Zhang-Wong and Seeman, 2002). Trabecular bone can be built up again, but cortical bone loss is relatively irreversible, as mentioned earlier in the discussion on criticisms of Wolff's law. "Overall, women lose 35–50 percent

---

[3]Manouvrier attributed the greater elongation in humans to our being more civilized compared to nonhuman primates (1888).

of trabecular and 25–30 percent of cortical bone mass with advancing age, whilst men lose 15–45 percent of trabecular and 5–15 percent of cortical bone" (Francis, 1998). Cortical bone loss is accelerated following menopause, whereas the trabecular bone loss is relatively constant throughout adult life (Zhang-Wong and Seeman, 2002).

Weight-bearing exercise increases bone density at a slower rate than it increases in muscle mass. Calcium supplementation does not appear to have much of an effect on perimeno-pausal women's bone density and may have other physiologic side effects. The dramatic decrease in estrogen appears to be a more significant factor in maintaining bone metabolism at menopause. Ancestry also plays a significant role in bone density. African American women are less prone to osteoporosis than European American women and tend to have much greater bone density throughout life (Nelson et al., 2000; Saeed et al., 2009). It appears that this distinction is more related to genetics than environment, as another study of individuals from Niger showed increased bone density compared to European and Asian populations despite chronically low intake of calcium in the Niger sample (VanderJagt et al., 2004). Body mass index also plays a role in bone density (Gibson et al., 2004; Looker et al., 2007; Miyabara et al., 2007; Wu et al., 2007; Moore and Schaefer, 2011).

CROSS-SECTIONAL GEOMETRIC SHAPE ANALYSIS

Three decades ago, Ledley et al. (1974) noted that the only noninvasive method for reconstructing cross-sections sufficiently for biomechanical analysis was through **computed tomographic (CT)** scanning. The same is still true today (O'Neill and Ruff, 2004) with even better quality images, faster scanning time, and reduced cost. The resultant 3-D radiographs can be converted into 3-D computer surface models, which facilitate highly sophisticated shape analyses. Three-dimensional computer models enable automation of research, and thus the simultaneous, quantitative interpretation of shape variation in the skeleton. Before medical imaging methods, destructive analysis (or a fortuitous bone fracture in an archaeological specimen) was the only means of directly analyzing the 3-D shape of both the internal and external structures of bone.

Research studies on shape variation in the skeleton that have used cut bone cross-sections have investigated diverse topics ranging from age changes in the skeleton (Burr and Piotrowski, 1982) to the prediction of minimum critical force for fracture risk of the clavicle (Harrington et al., 1993). Bridges (1985) conducted cross-sectional geometric analysis on the humerus and femur of males and females from archaeological samples dating to the Archaic (6000–1000 B.C.) and the Mississipian (1200–1500 A.D.) prehistoric time periods in North America. The results of her research surprisingly revealed that the females actually had larger humeral cross-sections than males during the Mississipian period. This was likely the result of the division of labor in which females manually ground corn—an activity not practiced by the hunters and gatherers of the Archaic period (Bridges, 1985).

Traditional methods for studying the cross-sectional geometry of a bone were to simply cut the bone. An excellent and detailed description of methods for how to determine the location of each slice and to make the cross-sectional cuts for the femur is provided by Ruff (1981). Nagurka and Hayes (1980) developed the computer algorithm SLICE to automatically

TABLE 14.1   Cross-Sectional Measurements

	Measurements
a.	Total cross-sectional area
b.	Cross-sectional area of cortical bone
c.	Cross-sectional area of medullary canal
d.	2nd moments of inertia (area) I_x and I_y perpendicular through centroid—I_x for mediolateral direction, Iy for anteroposterior direction
e.	Product of inertia about x and y axes translated to centroid
f.	Second moments of area about principal axes
g.	Angle between translated x and y axes and principal axes
h.	Maximum distance along major axis from area of centroid to outer perimeter
i.	Maximum distance along minor axis from area of centroid to outer perimeter
j.	Polar moment of area = J or I_p—approximating torsional rigidity
k.	Centroid—center of cortical area

Adapted from SLICE (Nagurka and Hayes, 1980)

analyze the geometric properties of bone cross-sections. All that is needed is an image of the bone cross-section for the analysis. This program is available as a free download from the website of the International Society of Biomechanics (http://isbweb.org/software/imamorph.html). The algorithms used to calculate these properties are available in the publication by Nagurka and Hayes (1980). The geometric shape measurements that are automatically calculated using SLICE are listed in Table 14.1. SLICE can be used to analyze the outline of cut bone or a **DICOM** image (Digital Imaging and Communications in Medicine) from a CT scan.

There is some subjectivity in measurement when deciding whether to include the trabecular bone of the endosteum in the calculation of the cross-sectional properties. Burr and Piotrowski (1982: 341) caution against this: "Including cancellous bone in calculations of structural properties of bone cross-sections may cause the strength and stiffness of the bone to be exaggerated." They have two arguments for why it overestimates strength. First, the trabecular bone is closer to the neutral axis and so has a smaller contribution for overall structural properties in terms of bending and torsion. Second, the trabecular bone has much lower compressive strength than cortical bone, and thus overestimates the overall area (Burr and Piotrowski, 1982).

MEDICAL IMAGING

For research in human skeletal biology, medical imaging provides nondestructive analysis in order to reveal the biomechanical properties of bone, including the internal shape and structure, as well as the material properties of bone density. Medical imaging technologies can be used for additional applications of differential disease diagnosis, for the nondestructive analysis of mummies, or for the imaging of bones from fleshed remains to aid in forensic investigations. There is obviously no radiation risk to individuals who are deceased, thus higher resolution images are possible. Existing medical images of living subjects offer the researcher an opportunity to access data on populations, such as subadults, who are not as well represented in modern skeletal collections. Bones can be imaged easily and these images can be used for nondestructive analysis of functional adaptations, to reveal skeletal pathology and trauma, and provide opportunities to study the skeletons of living subjects. All of these reasons substantiate why you should consider applying medical imaging to research in human skeletal biology.

First discovered in 1895 by the German physicist Rector Wilhelm Conrad Röntgen, X-rays amazed the world with images of the inside of opaque objects, including the body. By presenting an X-ray image of his wife's ringed hand, Röntgen unknowingly founded the practice of medical radiology in January of 1896 (Assmus, 1995). "Men of science in this city [New York] are awaiting with the utmost impatience the arrival of English technical journals which will give them the full particulars of Professor Roentgen's discovery of a method of photographing opaque bodies" (The New York Times, 1896). It took another 30 years for science to even understand the full nature of X-rays (Assmus, 1995). **Traditional X-ray**, computed tomography (CT), and **dual energy X-ray absorptiometry (DEXA)** are all different types of medical imaging that incorporate X-rays, which have the specific wavelength to penetrate the body. **Biplanar radiography** essentially takes a traditional X-ray image of an individual (or bone) from two separate directions (e.g., both AP and ML).

Other types of rays can pass through the body and are used for medical imaging modalities. In **magnetic resonance imaging (MRI)**, radiofrequency waves pass through the body as a large superconducting magnet spins around the subject (Szabo, 2005). Computed tomography and magnetic resonance are two types of cross-sectional tomography. **Tomography** is the process of performing multiple two-dimensional image slices of three-dimensional objects (Szabo, 2005; Brant and Helms, 2007). The idea of tomography was first suggested in 1914, but the principles of axial tomography were developed in the mid 1940s (Seynaeve and Broos, 1995). The clinical use of MRI began in England in 1967. The Englishman Godfrey Hounsfield invented computed tomography in 1972 and his name is still used for the units of measure used to interpret CT images (i.e., Hounsfield units). In 1984, the Food and Drug Administration approved the commercial use of MRI in the United States (Seynaeve and Broos, 1995).

There are additional modalities of computed tomography potentially useful for the skeletal biologist, which include: **peripheral quantitative CT (pQCT)** and **micro-CT**. It is important for our purposes that radiographic technologies (e.g., traditional X-ray, CT, and DEXA) provide a superior image of the internal structures of the more dense skeletal tissues than magnetic resonance imaging (MRI) and **ultrasonography** (Brant and Helms, 2007). Only the various medical imaging methods that are most relevant to the skeletal biologist are described in further detail below. Other medical imaging modalities exist but are outside of the scope of this text.

Traditional X-rays

X-rays, generated by a cathode ray tube, have a specific wavelength that allows them to pass through the body. The X-ray beam is generated when excited by a high-voltage power supply (Bronzino, 2005). All X-ray systems (traditional X-ray, CT, DEXA) have an X-ray source called a *collimator*. The collimator sends the rays that pass through the body. The more dense bone slows down (or attenuates) the beam moreso than the soft tissues. On the other side of the subject is an X-ray detector, which can be X-ray film, an image intensifier, or a set of detectors (Bronzino, 2005). In traditional **radiography**, the X-ray then reacts with a phosphor coating on photographic film (i.e., X-ray film). The difference in the amounts of absorption and attenuation of the X-rays by the different tissues of the body causes the shadowing on the photographic paper (Bronzino, 2005).

Biplanar Radiography

Traditional radiographs (X-rays) provide an image of the cortical thickness of a bone in a single, two-dimensional plane. This can be used to estimate cortical area, but it assumes a circular cross-section of the bone. Combining the breadth measurements of the cortical bone from two separate planes reduces the error and changes the assumption of a circular cross-section to one that is elliptical (Ruff, 1981). Imagine breaking a doughnut in half and seeing the cross-section revealed of the inside of the doughnut. If the doughnut is a perfect sphere, the cross-section you see will well represent the parts that you do not see. Unlike the doughnut, bone is not a perfect sphere nor is it a perfect ellipse. But an ellipse can better approximate the area of a bone's cross-section than if a spherical shape is assumed. By looking at the bone from two separate planes, you are able to view four separate quadrants of the bone area, not just two. In this way, biplanar radiographs are an improvement over traditional X-ray technology and can be used to better approximate the three-dimensional cross-sectional shape of a bone. Biplanar radiographs of a single femur from two different and perpendicular planes can be used to approximate the cortical area at the midshaft and to establish a ratio of I_{max}/I_{min} in order to estimate activity levels.

When using biplanar radiography, the overall shape of the bone must be inferred from two different planes (this is also called ellipse model method (EMM), as explained below). This inevitably introduces a certain amount of error. Validation studies have been undertaken to compare the accuracy of the shape predictions when using biplanar radiography to actual cut cross-sections or CT images. One study found that use of an asymmetrical model from biplanar radiography improves estimates of cross-sectional geometry of the mandible (Biknevicius and Ruff, 1992). Van Gerven (1969), however, found errors of 25% or more when comparing cut cross-sections to estimations of midshaft cortical area from AP radiographs. Another study encountered errors of up to 40% from the cross-sectional areas of the radiographic breadths from several long bones (Ruff, 1981). "Radiographic shadowing" is another problem encountered when using radiographs to infer morphological shape, which results from the overlap of structures (e.g., the tibial crest can obscure the lateral tibial curvature) (Ruff, 1981).

O'Neill and Ruff (2004) compared two different methods for analyzing the biplanar radiographs: the ellipse model method (EMM) and the latex cast method (LCM). EMM, which is simply the standard biplanar method described above, uses the cortical width measured from each of the biplanar radiographs, one radiograph in the AP direction and the other taken perpendicular in the ML direction. LCM also uses biplanar radiographs, but in conjunction with a latex cast taken of the external surface of the bone. With EMM, an assumption is made that the cross-section is elliptical, the general assumption of biplanar radiography. EMM appears to have systematic bias by overestimating the cross-sectional properties when compared to actual cut cross-sections (absolute errors averaging 5–12%) (O'Neill and Ruff, 2004). LCM has a much better correspondence with the actual shape properties from the cut bone section (absolute estimation errors between 3 and 8%) and is thus preferred. The authors applied regression equations to correct for the systematic bias, and were able to improve the accuracy of the EMM on an independent sample (absolute errors reduced to less than 4%) (O'Neill and Ruff, 2004).

Bloom and colleagues conducted radiographic scans using DEXA (which essentially provides a low resolution X-ray) of living individuals and is discussed later in this chapter. They applied a method that combines the cortical thickness measurement from both the medial and lateral thicknesses, which they called "combined cortical thickness" (CCT) (Bloom and Laws, 1970). Ben-Itzhak and colleagues followed the same model to estimate the CCT by using biplanar radiographs to estimate cross-sectional area of the humerus in Neandertals and humans (Ben-Itzhak et al., 1988).

Densitometry

There are four ways to clinically determine bone density: (1) dual energy X-ray absorptiometry (DEXA), (2) quantitative computed tomography (QCT), (3) peripheral quantitative computed tomography (pQCT), and (4) ultrasound. The DEXA scanner is designed to have the patient lie on a table while the arm of the machine with a small pencil beam X-ray passes over the subject, much like the laser image scanner in your home office. The advantages of DEXA are that it looks at integral bone mass and areal density and that it is relatively low radiation, so it is not detrimental to a living patient and it is not limited to the periphery of the bone, as is the case with pQCT, which will be discussed further in this chapter. DEXA exposes the patient to no more radiation than an international flight. DEXA is relatively sensitive to subtle changes in bone density and body composition (the proportion of fat and lean tissue mass).

The disadvantages of DEXA are that it does not determine volumetric density, and can provide only a summary measure of density across a scan path. The DEXA image is a flattened two-dimensional image, like a traditional radiograph, and thus must make assumptions about a three-dimensional object to calculate the bone mineral density (BMD), similar to the analogy of the doughnut from above. Like EMM biplanar radiography, it inaccurately assumes a cylindrical cross-section. It is also unable to distinguish trabeculae from cortex. A volumetric density, as interpreted by the CT scanner, will provide a more accurate density than a two-dimensional interpretation.

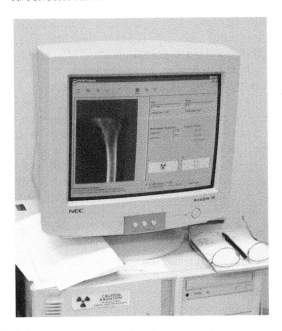

FIGURE 14.3   DEXA console showing a scan of a femur in progress.

Despite some of the problems of DEXA, it is commonly used for bone density calculation and has become the gold standard for living populations. Beck and colleagues used DEXA to determine BMD as well as bone geometry and cortical thickness in a study of living individuals (Beck et al., 2000). They found that areal BMD and bone structural properties were dependent on body size, with body weight as the single best descriptor of skeletal geometry. CT can also provide bone density estimation, but it exposes the patient to much higher levels of radiation than does DEXA. DEXA provides both T- and Z-scores for quickly diagnosing osteoporosis. The **T-score** compares the subject to the optimal bone density of a young healthy individual. The Z-score compares the subject's density to sex, age, height, weight, and ancestry-matched individuals. If the T-score falls below 2.5 standard deviations, the individual is diagnosed with osteoporosis. See Figure 14.3.

Ultrasound

Ultrasonography was developed soon after the sinking of the Titanic in 1912 as a way to use echolocation to find icebergs and other potential underwater hazards; this later became known as SONAR (SOund Navigation And Ranging) (Szabo, 2005). In medical ultrasonography, short pulses of sound waves travel through the body and reflect (i.e., echo) off of the different tissues. When the echo is received, the delay in time for the reflection is mathematically translated into different tissue types interpreted as a grayscale image (Szabo, 2005).

Until the 1960s, pregnant women were radiographed for diagnostic purposes, which was later linked to fetal/infant deaths and cancer (Szabo, 2005). Ultrasounds have replaced this usage and are now standard in living subjects because they carry the lowest risk to a patient (and a fetus *in utero*). Like DEXA, ultrasounds provide both T- and Z-scores for quickly diagnosing osteoporosis.

Ultrasonography has not caught on in skeletal biology, due to the lower quality of images compared to the other imaging methods discussed, but the image quality has now improved. Two disadvantages are that it loses resolution at greater depths within the body and it requires a high level of skill to interpret the images (Szabo, 2005). Existing ultrasounds of living subjects, however, could provide useful information on bone density, comparing the bone density to average young individuals in a population or to sex and age-matched individuals, providing T- and Z-scores, respectively. One study on living subjects used ultrasounds to determine bone density in males and females from Nigeria compared to those of European and Asian ancestry (VanderJagt et al., 2004).

Computed Tomography

Computed tomography is superior to both MRI and ultrasound for imaging the skeleton because it produces superior detail of the dense skeletal tissues. CT performs multiple two-dimensional slices of three-dimensional objects and mathematically reconstructs the cross-sectional image from the X-ray measurement of thin slices (Brant and Helms, 2007). In essence, the CT can create three-dimensional radiographs, but there is an intermediate process called **segmentation** necessary to interpolate the information from one slice to the next to create the 3-D model of a bone.

The advantages of CT are numerous: it (1) allow for rapid data acquisition, (2) is relatively nondestructive (although some DNA degradation is possible as it generates extremely high radiation), (3) provides high-resolution, three-dimensional data of both internal and external bone surfaces, and (4) provides information on bone density. The potential for CT data has been recognized for several decades in anthropology and skeletal biology (Lovejoy et al., 1976; Ruff and Leo, 1986), although its use has mainly been limited to cross-sectional geometry and costs are often prohibitive for large-scale application.

How CT Works

For CT, narrow X-ray beams pass through the subject in a helical fashion as they rotate around the subject. Variation in the tissue densities causes changes in the X-rays' absorption and scatter, which are received by banana-shaped detectors on the opposite side of the subject. The subject is strapped to a table that moves through a doughnut-shaped device in which the X-ray is rotating, enabling the process to be repeated many times automatically. Each time the X-ray makes it 360 degrees around the subject, a new transverse radiograph is created, called a DICOM image. As the image is being interpreted in three dimensions digitally, the data are recorded as **voxels**, which are volumetric (i.e. three dimensional) pixels. The dimensions of a voxel are determined by a chosen algorithm between 1 and 10 mm in resolution. The computer then mathematically reconstructs the cross-sectional DICOM image from the X-ray measurement of the thin slices.

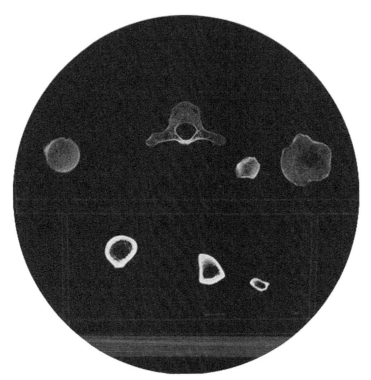

FIGURE 14.4 DICOM slice from the scanning boxes. From the bottom left to right: femur, tibia, and fibula. From the top left to right: left humerus, thoracic vertebra, right ulna, and right humerus.

Image Segmentation

Segmentation is the process of selecting regions or surfaces from three-dimensional images and then separating the objects into three-dimensional surface models based on specific grayscale threshold values. DICOM images are the individual transverse 2-D images created during a CT scan. DICOMs require specialized imaging software to be opened, and there are shareware computer programs available free on the Internet to simply open and read the DICOMs.[4] There are other programs designed to create three-dimensional models from the DICOM. One such computer program is the commercially available program Amira®, which can segment the high-resolution DICOM images to create 3-D models. See Figure 14.4.

There are two types of image segmentation: manual and automatic. For manual segmentation, the researcher opens a series of DICOM images in a 3-D imaging program like Amira. Starting at one end of the bone, the researcher opens a single DICOM slice. Cortical bone is dense and appears as voxel values that are very light gray to white, trabecular bone appears as a range of darker gray, and the background appears black. The grayscale value of the region of interest (i.e., the cortical bone) is selected, using maximum and minimum threshold

---

[4]Free DICOM readers are available from many Internet sites. Two such sites are OsiriX at http://www.osirix-viewer.com/, and Cad/Cam Services, Inc. at http://xrayscan.com/software/free-dicom-viewers.php.

FIGURE 14.5 Segmentation of a femur in Amira® with a segmented femur model.

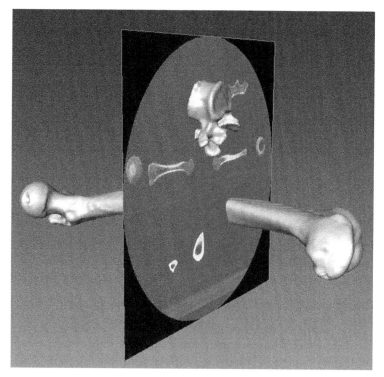

FIGURE 14.5 Segmentation of a femur in Amira® with a segmented femur model.

values of gray (which are measured in Hounsfield units after the inventor, as mentioned previously) as a criterion. This shades in the selected area of interest, similar to the "fill" command in most photo editing programs. The voxel grayscale values therefore correspond to the different densities of the object scanned. See Figure 14.5.

In Amira®, the entire shaded area can then be selected and enclosed in a colored outline. This area of interest is termed a "label." Because bone densities between the diaphysis and the epiphyses are very different in densities and thus have different gray values, it may leave open holes in the surface of the model if the threshold is set too narrowly. If the threshold is set too broadly, it may interpret any adhering soft tissues as part of the bone, for example. The researcher can therefore manually segment each epiphysis. Once both proximal and distal slices are given the same label, a simple click on the same gray value anywhere in between will automatically detect the rest of the cortical bone. It is necessary to check through each DICOM slice of your new model to verify that the entire bone was accurately selected. Automatic segmentation follows a similar format. The main distinction is that the maximum and minimum thresholds for every slice are set simultaneously. This saves a great deal of time, but renders poorer models, due to the vastly different densities in compact and trabecular bone. This process of segmentation will likely become more sophisticated and completely automatic in CT scans in the near future. For now, it is a crucial step in the process of creating computer bone models.

CT and Geometric Morphometrics

Geometric morphometric techniques based on bony landmarks are replacing traditional linear measurement as the preferred method of capturing cranial shape and size. This can be accomplished by using a 3-D digitizer to capture the landmarks in a Cartesian coordinate system (i.e., x, y, z) or by using laser surface scans. The advantages to a landmark approach are that it can be much less expensive than using medical imaging and the methods therein are more readily available to most skeletal biologists. Studies have used a geometric morphometric approach to analyze the three-dimensional form of the vertebrae, os coxa, and femur, to mention just a few (Manfreda et al., 2006; Gu et al., 2008; De Groote et al., 2010). The requirement of corresponding landmarks, however, has made the application of these techniques to the post-crania difficult since most long bones lack sufficient, well-defined landmarks. See McKeown and Schmidt (Chapter 12), this volume, for more information on geometric morphometrics. Computed tomography scanning provides data potentially suitable for the application of geometric morphometric techniques to post-cranial elements, but has the added benefit of visualizing the internal structure, which is not possible from most geometric morphometric methods.

Peripheral Quantitative Computed Tomography (pQCT) and Micro-CT

Two different variations of CT that may be of interest to the skeletal biologist are micro-CT and pQCT. Micro-CT provides extremely high resolution, as small as 1 μm, but the level of radiation at this resolution is lethal to living subjects. This method could be extremely valuable for nondestructive histological analysis of skeletal samples. One study compared micro-CT to histological analysis of osteochondritis dissecans (a disease in a joint caused by avascular necrosis or loss of blood supply) in three subjects and found it of great speed and utility, though they were not able to image cells or different tissue types (Mohr et al., 2003).

Compared to DEXA, peripheral quantitative computed tomography (pQCT) allows for the assessment of trabecular and cortical bone separately, and the ability to measure the volumetric density. The pQCT is often used to take bone mineral density readings of the smaller peripheral parts of the body (e.g., arms, hands, and feet). The pQCT has lower radiation than CT, but with higher precision and higher predictive capabilities for peripheral fractures (Groll et al., 1999). The pQCT is only able to measure the smaller peripheral appendages of a living individual or just a portion of a dry long bone. This method works well for comparing shape variation of the hands and feet in living subjects. Briggs and colleagues (2010) compare the quality and the advantages and disadvantages of bone mineral density calculations of the vertebrae from DEXA, pQCT, and micro-CT.

CASE STUDY: FUNCTIONAL MORPHOLOGY, CT, AND BONE DENSITY IN ACTION

Research questions from a perspective of functional morphology tend to be considerable undertakings. The researcher should have an understanding of biomechanics, bone biology, and the different medical imaging methods available to best suit the study. A study that intends to investigate the mechanical properties of bone from multiple perspectives (e.g., both macrostructure and the material property of bone density) is able to offer a more holistic perspective of the functional adaptation of the human skeleton. For my dissertation, I was interested in the functional morphology of body mass, especially the effects of obesity. My first step in this process was to take courses in biomechanics to gain a better understanding of human movement and the different forces that can affect bones. If you are also interested in functional morphology, this is an essential first step in graduate school. My goal was to analyze the shape changes of the weight-bearing bones of the lower limb, so I investigated the differences in the biomechanics of movement in normal weight and obese subjects. There are significant variations in gait patterns between the two groups as a result of weight, so my predictions about how the bone would alter as a result of this difference in gait developed out of the knowledge gained during my graduate level biomechanics coursework.

At the University of Tennessee, I had access to the William M. Bass Donated Human Skeletal Collection, which is a very large and documented collection of skeletons of modern individuals with known age, sex, height, weight, and other **antemortem** data. This collection represents a broad spectrum of body size from a body mass index (BMI=kg/m^2) of only 16 (severely underweight) to a BMI of 87 (an individual who weighed over 600 pounds).

The next step in my research logistics was to decide on a methodology. I wanted to develop a holistic perspective of the functional effects of body mass on the skeleton, looking at both the material properties of bone density and the macrostructural properties of bone, so I chose to pursue both DEXA and CT. I then developed partnerships with the Radiology Department at the University of Tennessee Medical Center, the Department of Exercise Science, and the Department of Biomedical Engineering, in addition to my existing affiliation with the Department of Anthropology, which houses the skeletal collection. The Department of Exercise Science houses a DEXA scanner and the Radiology Department has several CT machines. The Biomedical Engineering Department provided research funding and expertise in the three-dimensional analysis of the DICOM images. In addition to the actual data collection and analysis, my role was to act as a liaison between these departments, to be responsible for the care and analysis of the skeletal remains during the scanning procedure, to negotiate the necessary costs, and to coordinate the scanning logistics.

Bone Density Scanning

To conduct the bone density scans, I focused on just the femur. I chose the femur specifically because it is a weight-bearing bone of the lower leg, which would presumably exhibit the greatest changes in bone density in response to body mass. Each dry femur was placed in a plastic container 65 cm long, 14 cm tall, and 11 cm wide. A 2 cm thick cube of low-density foam was placed under the lesser trochanter to make the shaft approximately parallel to the table surface (as recommended by Ruff, 1981). Both distal condyles were set directly on the bottom of the box. Leveling the femur in this way better approximates anatomical position. There is a slight natural rotation of the proximal femur in the living body that this method does not account for. As a result, the lesser trochanter is visible in the density scans, which would not be the case in living individuals.

The DEXA machine is designed to recognize living individuals, so an individual's age is calculated by entering their birth date in the user interface. To compensate for this, we

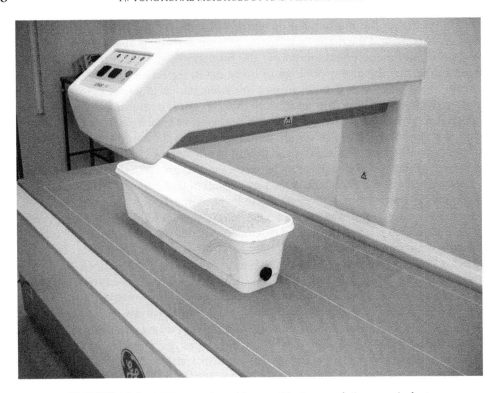

FIGURE 14.6   DEXA scanning of femur with rice as soft-tissue equivalent.

subtracted the age of the decedent from the scanning date to arrive at a birth date that was entered into the computer. To standardize the amount of radiation in each scan, the weight of the individual was set to 90 pounds, thus using the "thin mode" setting of the machine. This is consistent with a soft-tissue thickness of 12 cm, as suggested by the manufacturer. See Figure 14.6. If we reported a higher body weight, the machine would expect more soft-tissue equivalent material over the bone and would abort the scan. This had no bearing on the results except for Z-scores because the Z-scores are calculated in comparison to individuals of the same age, sex, height, and weight. This method, however, maintained a constant level of radiation to ensure an accurate reading through each scan. This aspect of the research differs from previous research with living subjects because the DEXA scanner must accommodate different tissue thicknesses for obese and emaciated individuals, which may reduce the accuracy of comparisons in living individuals between these two body mass extremes.

Dual energy X-ray absorptiometry machines are designed to scan living individuals with both soft and hard tissues. If only bone is present, the machine would abort a scan. To avoid this, the bone was placed at the bottom of a plastic container that was filled with dry white rice to a depth of approximately 12 cm over the proximal end of the bone only. The rice serves as a human soft-tissue density equivalent for the DEXA scans, as per GE, the manufacturer of the DEXA Lunar scanner®. The average density of human soft tissues, both lean and fat combined, is approximately equivalent to dry rice. A precedent for this method was created in an earlier study that compared a commercial density phantom to rice as a soft-tissue equivalent (Cohen and Rushton, 1995).

The box was positioned on the table so that the femur (right or left) was also in the approximate anatomical position (about two-thirds down the table, mimicking a patient lying on the table). In this way, the machine interprets a complete individual. Consequently, we could use the standard DEXA software. The arm of the machine was brought to a level just superior to midshaft. The areas of interest were manually selected on the computer by moving the rectangular field of view over the femoral neck. Two triangular fields of view were placed over the greater and lesser trochanters. The standard DEXA measurements of bone mineral density (BMD) (g/cm^2) were calculated automatically for four anatomical areas: (1) the femoral neck, (2) Ward's triangle, (3) the greater trochanter, and (4) the proximal shaft, in addition to the calculation of total BMD.

CT Scanning

To facilitate CT data acquisition I worked with another anthropologist and biomedical engineer to develop a system that permitted rapid data collection. Six identical sets of two boxes (one 125 cm × 32 cm × 3 cm and the other 150 cm × 22 cm × 5 cm) were built from foam core board. Each set of two boxes was large enough to hold all the skeletal elements

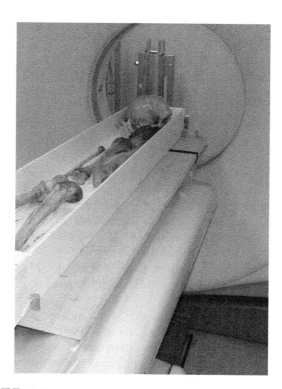

FIGURE 14.7   CT scanning boxes to standardize scanning positions.

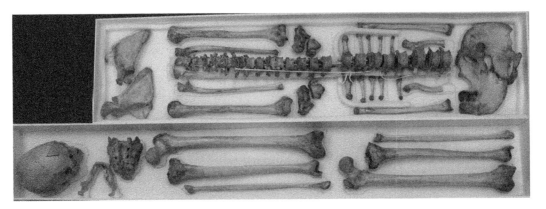

FIGURE 14.8   CT scanning with board and dowels to standardize scans.

TABLE 14.2   CT Specifications for Scanning Bones for GE Light-
speed® 16 Slice CT Scanner

Parameters	Specs
Table size	1.5 m length
Mass	150 at 0.8 seconds
Field of view (FOV)	32 cm
Resolution	0.625 mm slices
Peak kilovoltage (kVp)	100 KV
Bone algorithm	512/512 mm

of one large individual except for ribs, metacarpals, and phalanges. Each box was lined with low-density polyurethane foam with an outline drawn for each bone to standardize positioning. I made a slice down the center of a strip of foam in which to place the vertebral spinous processes in sequence. All foam elements were glued into position in the boxes. All bones were positioned so that they touched neither another bone nor the foam core board, only the foam liner. We then standardized the positioning of the boxes in the CT scanner by strapping a piece of plywood to the scanner table. The plywood had eight dowels that were used as reference markers to maintain the same position of the boxes in each scan. See Figures 14.7 and 14.8.

All individuals were scanned at the University of Tennessee Medical Center Outpatient Diagnostic Center. Scanning was conducted using a GE Lightspeed® 16 slice computed tomography scanner. The CT specifications used are shown in Table 14.2. The voxel dimensions were chosen as 512 × 512 mm on the advice of the radiologist to ensure the accuracy of the measurements in the reconstructed DICOM image, with slices being 0.625 mm apart.

Analyzing the Data

In statistical regression, it is suggested to not have as many variables in the calculations as there are individuals in the study. To reduce the number of variables, a statistical variable selection method called McHenry's algorithm (1978) was used independently for the cross-sectional CT variables and DEXA density variables in order to choose the best variables to develop the multiple regression equations. The best variables for each sex were then subjected to a second variable selection. The best two or three variables were used to create robust multiple regression equations in NCSS (Number Crunching Statistical Software, 1997). To avoid problems with multicollinearity, only the strongest density variable was included to develop each multiple regression equation. Multicollinearity is the statistical problem of two variables reflecting the exact same effect, thus overemphasizing its influence on the end result.

The results of this study demonstrate that bone mineral density has a strong correlation with body mass in the proximal human femur for both European American males and females. Furthermore, there are significant differences in bone mineral density between different weight classifications in both males and females. This correlation is not as strong in males as it is for females between the average weight and obese individuals. From the CT scans, the shape variables that were important for body mass in both males and females were the cross-sectional area at most proximal cross-section, polar moments of area (i.e., torsional strength) at several locations, and the area moments of inertia in various directions. The shape indices (I_{max}/I_{min} and I_y/I_x) surprisingly do not show any clear relationship with body mass, but may still in fact reflect activity. Further, there does not appear to be a clear correlation between the canal area and body mass, as was predicted by the fact that endosteal apposition occurred at a higher rate in obese individuals in other studies (Ruff, et al., 1994; Pearson and Lieberman, 2004; Moore et al., 2007).

One advantage of this study over previous studies was that by using skeletal femora with a uniform depth of soft-tissue equivalent material, any inconsistencies that arose from different thicknesses of living tissue were removed. Another advantage was the ability to directly compare the results from DEXA with the cross-sectional geometry of the same bones gathered from CT scanned data.[5] In a living population, this would have required exposing patients to excessive amounts of radiation. By using a skeletal sample, the resolution of the images could be increased to provide more accurate models. This allowed the addition of a cross-sectional analysis to better predict body mass, which improved upon previous research and increased the power of the model. Both CT and DEXA use X-rays to develop an image of the internal and external structure of bone for better interpretation of the material properties (bone density) and macrostructure to provide a more holistic view of the functional adaptation that results from variations in body mass.

There were many logistical obstacles to overcome during this multidisciplinary dissertation project. Through collaboration with multiple departments, valuable resources were shared to that mutual benefit of all parties concerned. The CT scans that I helped produce

---

[5]The CT scans are now part of the UT collection, and can be made available for many potential research projects. Contact the Forensic Anthropology Center at UT for information: www.utk.edu.

now provide a digital archive of the William M. Bass Donated Skeletal Collection, preserved for many researchers in the future.

For access to any skeletal collection, make sure you go through the standard process of requesting permission. E-mail the curator of the collection of interest to determine the necessary protocol. There is no need to reinvent the wheel, nor should you rescan the whole collection, if the data already exist. My research had applications for forensic anthropology and I was able to secure funding from the National Institute of Justice. Biomedical applications abound for studies involving human skeletal collections, with the potential for collaborations and funding from many different sources.

Academic insecurity is normal in the young researcher, so never fear. You may feel that your lack of expertise in one area will prevent you from conducting a certain project. Anthropologists notoriously work independently on projects and, as a result, have a much lower output than researchers in the natural or other social sciences. Remember that you will never be an expert in every subject, but you can be productive by working with peers in anthropology and in other disciplines. Consider how your research question overlaps with other disciplines and attempt to develop collaborations. Working with scientists in other fields can make for an ideal collaboration, as everyone benefits from greater output and from diversifying their skillsets.

CONCLUSION

Biological anthropologists ask questions differently than do clinicians. We place a strong emphasis on population variation when studying the human skeleton. Our access to and involvement with skeletal collections can be one of our great assets when collaborating with researchers from other disciplines. Pietrusewsky (2000) claimed that for anthropology, "the discipline's most notable contributions to science" are anthropometry (measurement of the living) and osteometry (measurement of the skeleton). I would like to add one more contribution, the legacy of existing skeletal collections that preserve past and contemporary human biological and cultural variation. If we have learned anything from Sherwood Washburn (1951), we understand the importance of looking at the bigger questions related to the continuous human variation that results from both biological and cultural factors.

Medical imaging technology offers a variety of methods to study questions of functional morphology. Computed tomography and biplanar radiography are two modalities for studying the macrostructural properties of bone. The investigation of the internal structural changes from three-dimensional CT models can test hypotheses developed from traditional osteological analysis. The material properties of bone density can be analyzed using CT, DEXA, or pQCT. By investigating the functional adaptation of bone using multiple approaches, we are able to gain a more holistic perspective of the intrinsic and extrinsic properties that affect bone. Quantifying bone size and shape to study the functional adaptation of the human skeleton remains a fundamental task for many anthropological research questions pertaining to human variation and the reconstruction of contemporary and past activity patterns as well as numerous other bioarchaeological and forensic questions.

ACKNOWLEDGMENTS

I would like to acknowledge the amazing editorial skills of Elizabeth DiGangi and thank her for all of her hard work on this textbook. I would also like to thank those individuals who contributed to my dissertation research: My advisor Lyle Konigsberg, Mohamamed Mahfouz and Emam Fattah from Biomedical Engineering, Kent Hutson from the Department of Radiology, Dixie Thompson from Exercise Sciences, and all of the graduate students from Biomedical Engineering and Anthropology who contributed many hours of work to gather the CT data at the UT Medical Center.

REFERENCES

Aarden, E.M., Burger, E.H., Nijweide, P.J., 1994. Function of osteocytes in bone. Journal of Cellular Biochemistry 55 (3), 287–299.

Armelagos, G.J., Van Gerven, D.P., 2003. A century of skeletal biology and paleopathology: contrasts, contradictions, and conflicts. American Anthropologist (1), 53–64.

Assmus, A., 1995. Early history of X rays. Beam Line Summer 1995, 25 (2), 10–24.

Beck, T.J., Ruff, C.B., Bissessur, K., 1993. Age-related changes in female femoral neck geometry: implications for bone strength. Calcified Tissue International 53 (Suppl. 1), S41–46.

Beck, T.J., Ruff, C.B., Shaffer, R.A., Betsinger, K., Trone, D.W., Brodine, S.K., 2000. Stress fracture in military recruits: gender differences in muscle and bone susceptibility factors. Bone 27 (3), 437–444.

Ben-Itzhak, S., Smith, P., Bloom, R.A., 1988. Radiographic study of the humerus in Neandertals and *Homo sapiens*. American Journal of Physical Anthropology 77 (2), 231–242.

Bertram, J.E., Swartz, S.M., 1991. The "law of bone transformation": a case of crying Wolff? Biological Reviews of the Cambridge Philosphical Society 66 (3), 245–273.

Biknevicius, A.R., Ruff, C.B., 1992. Use of biplanar radiographs for estimating cross-sectional geometric properties of mandibles. Anatomical Record 232 (1), 157–163.

Bloom, R.A., Laws, J.W., 1970. Humeral cortical thickness as an index of osteoporosis in women. British Journal of Radiology 43 (512), 522–527.

Brant, W.E., Helms, C.A., 2007. Fundamentals of Diagnostic Radiology. Lippincott, Williams & Wilkins, Philadelphia.

Bridges, P.S., 1985. Changes in Long Bone Structure with the Transition to Agriculture: Implications for Prehistoric Activities. PhD thesis. University of Michigan Dissertation, Ann Arbor.

Briggs, A.M., Perilli, E., Parkinson, I.H., Wrigley, T.V., Fazzalari, N.L., Kantor, S., et al., 2010. Novel assessment of subregional bone mineral density using DXA and pQCT and subregional microarchitecture using micro-CT in whole human vertebrae: applications, methods, and correspondence between technologies. Journal of Clinical Densitometry 13 (2), 161–174.

Bronzino, J.D., 2005. Radiation imaging. In: Enderle, J.D., Bronzino, J.D., Blanchard, S.M. (Eds.), Introduction to Biomedical Engineering. Elsevier Academic Press, Amsterdam, pp. 882–899.

Burr, D.B., Piotrowski, G., 1982. How do trabeculae affect the calculation of structural properties of bone? American Journal of Physical Anthropology 57 (3), 341–352.

Carter, D.R., Wong, M., Orr, T.E., 1991. Musculoskeletal ontogeny, phylogeny, and functional adaptation. Journal of Biomechanics 24 (Suppl. 1), 3–16.

Cohen, B., Rushton, N., 1995. Accuracy of DEXA measurement of bone mineral density after total hip arthroplasty. Journal of Bone and Joint Surgery. British Volume 77 (3), 479–483.

Cowin, S.C., 2001. Bone Mechanics Handbook. CRC Press, Boca Raton, FL.

De Groote, I., Lockwood, C.A., Aiello, L.C., 2010. Technical note: A new method for measuring long bone curvature using 3D landmarks and semi-landmarks. American Journal of Physical Anthropology 141 (4), 658–664.

Eckstein, F., Faber, S., Muhlbauer, R., Hohe, J., Englmeier, K.H., Reiser, M., et al., 2002. Functional adaptation of human joints to mechanical stimuli. Osteoarthritis and Cartilage 10 (1), 44–50.

Ericksen, M.F., 1976. Cortical bone loss with age in three native American populations. American Journal of Physical Anthropology 45 (3 pt. 1), 443−452.

Francis, R.M., Sutcliffe, A.M., Scane, A.C., 1998. Pathogenesis of osteoporosis. In: Stevenson, J.C., Lindsay, R. (Eds.), Osteoporosis. Chapman & Hall, London, pp. 29−52.

Frankel, V.H., Nordin, M., 1980. Basic Biomechanics of the Skeletal System. Lea & Febiger, Philadelphia.

Frost, H.M., 1993. Suggested fundamental concepts in skeletal physiology. Calcified Tissue International 52 (1), 1−4.

Frost, H.M., 1997. Obesity, and bone strength and "mass": a tutorial based on insights from a new paradigm. Bone 21 (3), 211−214.

Gibson, J.H., Mitchell, A., Harries, M.G., Reeve, J., 2004. Nutritional and exercise-related determinants of bone density in elite female runners. Osteoporos is International 15 (8), 611−618.

Groll, O., Lochmuller, E.M., Bachmeier, M., Willnecker, J., Eckstein, F., 1999. Precision and intersite correlation of bone densitometry at the radius, tibia and femur with peripheral quantitative CT. Skeletal Radiology 28 (12), 696−702.

Gu, D., Chen, Y., Dai, K., Zhang, S., Yuan, J., 2008. The shape of the acetabular cartilage surface: A geometric morphometric study using three-dimensional scanning. Medical Engineering and Physics 30 (8), 1024−1031.

Harrington Jr., M.A., Keller, T.S., Seiler 3rd, J.G., Weikert, D.R., Moeljanto, E., Schwartz, H.S., 1993. Geometric properties and the predicted mechanical behavior of adult human clavicles. Journal of Biomechanics 26 (4−5), 417−426.

Hind, K., Gannon, L., Whatley, E., Cooke, C., 2011. Sexual dimorphism of femoral neck cross-sectional bone geometry in athletes and non-athletes: a hip structural analysis study. Journal of Bone and Mineral Metabolism, published online 13 December 2011.

Kroman, A.M., Symes, S., 2013. Investigation of Skeletal trauma. In: DiGangi, E.A., Moore, M.K. (Eds.), Research Methods in Human Skeletal Biology. Academic Press, San Diego.

Larsen, C.S., 1997. Bioarchaeology: Interpreting Behavior from the Human Skeleton. Cambridge University Press, New York.

Ledley, R.S., 1974. Innovation and creativeness in scientific research: my experiences in developing computerized axial tomography. Computers in Biology and Medicine 4 (2), 133−136.

Looker, A.C., Flegal, K.M., Melton 3rd, L.J., 2007. Impact of increased overweight on the projected prevalence of osteoporosis in older women. Osteoporos is International 18 (3), 307−313.

Lovejoy, C.O., Burstein, A.H., Heiple, K.G., 1976. The biomechanical analysis of bone strength: a method and its application to platycnemia. American Journal of Physical Anthropology 44 (3), 489−505.

Manfreda, E., Mitteroecker, P., Bookstein, F.L., Schaefer, K., 2006. Functional morphology of the first cervical vertebra in humans and nonhuman primates. Anatomical Record. Part B, New Anatomist 289 (5), 184−194.

McHenry, C., 1978. Multivariate subset selection. Journal of the Royal Statistical Society Series C 27, 291−296.

McKeown, A.H., Schmidt, R.W., 2013. Geometric morphometrics. In: DiGangi, E.A., Moore, M.K. (Eds.), Research Methods in Human Skeletal Biology. Academic Press, San Diego.

Miyabara, Y., Onoe, Y., Harada, A., Kuroda, T., Sasaki, S., Ohta, H., 2007. Effect of physical activity and nutrition on bone mineral density in young Japanese women. Journal of Bone and Mineral Metabolism 25 (6), 414−418.

Mohr, A., Heiss, C., Bergmann, I., Schrader, C., Roemer, F.W., Lynch, J.A., et al., 2003. Value of micro-CT as an investigative tool for osteochondritis dissecans. Acta Radiologica 44 (5), 532−537.

Moore, M.K., Schaefer, E., 2011. A comprehensive regression tree to estimate body weight from the skeleton. Journal of Forensic Sciences 56 (5), 1115−1122.

Moore, M.K., Fatah, E.A., Mahfouz, M.R., 2007. Body mass estimation from human femoral midshaft cross-sectional area. Am J. Phys. Anthropol. 132 (S44) 173.

Nagurka, M.L., Hayes, W.C., 1980. An interactive graphics package for calculating cross-sectional properties of complex shapes. Journal of Biomechanics 13, 59−64.

Nelson, D.A., Barondess, D.A., Hendrix, S.L., Beck, T.J., 2000. Cross-sectional geometry, bone strength, and bone mass in the proximal femur in black and white postmenopausal women. Journal of Bone and Mineral Research 15 (10), 1992−1997.

Nilsson, B.E., Westlin, N.E., 1971. Bone density in athletes. Clinical Orthopaedics and Related Research 77, 179−182.

O'Neill, M.C., Ruff, C.B., 2004. Estimating human long bone cross-sectional geometric properties: a comparison of noninvasive methods. Journal of Human Evolution 47 (4), 221−235.

Pearson, O.M., Lieberman, D.E., 2004. The aging of Wolff's "law": Ontogeny and responses to mechanical loading in cortical bone. American Journal of Physical Anthropology (Suppl. 39), 63–99.

Pietrusewsky, M., 2000. Metric analysis of skeletal remains: methods and applications. In: Katzenberg, M.A., Saunders, S.R. (Eds.), Biological Anthropology of the Human Skeleton. Wiley, New York, pp. 487–532.

Robling, A.G., 1998. Histomorphometric Assessment of Mechanical Loading History from Human Skeletal Remains: The Relation Between Micromorphology and Macromorphology at the Femoral Midshaft. PhD thesis. University of Missouri, Dissertation, Columbia, pp. 174.

Rubin, C.T., McLeod, K.J., Bain, S.D., 1990. Functional strains and cortical bone adaptation: epigenetic assurance of skeletal integrity. Journal of Biomechanics 23 (Suppl. 1), 43–54.

Ruff, C.B., 1981. Structural Changes in the Lower Limb Bones with Aging at Pecos Pueblo. PhD thesis. Dissertation. University of Pennsylvania.

Ruff, C.B., Hayes, W.C., 1982. Subperiosteal expansion and cortical remodeling of the human femur and tibia with aging. Science 217 (4563), 945–948.

Ruff, C.B., Hayes, W.C., 1983a. Cross-sectional geometry of Pecos Pueblo femora and tibiae—a biomechanical investigation: I. Method and general patterns of variation. American Journal of Physical Anthropology 60 (3), 359–381.

Ruff, C.B., Hayes, W.C., 1983b. Cross-sectional geometry of Pecos Pueblo femora and tibiae—a biomechanical investigation: II. Sex, age, side differences. American Journal of Physical Anthropology 60 (3), 383–400.

Ruff, C.B., Hayes, W.C., 1984. Bone-mineral content in the lower limb. Relationship to cross-sectional geometry. Journal of Bone and Joint Surgery. American Volume 66 (7), 1024–1031.

Ruff, C.B., Leo, F.P., 1986. Use of computed tomography in skeletal structure research. Yearbook of Physical Anthropology 29 (S1), 181–195.

Ruff, C.B., Walker, A., Trinkaus, E., 1994. Postcranial robusticity in Homo. III: Ontogeny. American Journal of Physical Anthropology 93 (1), 35–54.

Saeed, I., Carpenter, R.D., Leblanc, A.D., Li, J., Keyak, J.H., Sibonga, J.D., et al., 2009. Quantitative computed tomography reveals the effects of race and sex on bone size and trabecular and cortical bone density. Journal of Clinical Densitometry 12 (3), 330–336.

Samelson, E.J., Christiansen, B.A., Demissie, S., Broe, K.E., Louie-Gao, Q., Cupples, L.A., et al., 2012. QCT measures of bone strength at the thoracic and lumbar spine: the Framingham Study. Journal of Bone and Mineral Research 27, 654–663.

Schmidt-Nielsen, K., 1984. Scaling, Why is Animal Size so Important? Cambridge University Press, Cambridge; New York.

Seynaeve, P.C., Broos, J.I., 1995. [The history of tomography]. Journal Belge de Radiologie 78 (5), 284–288.

Smith, M.O., 2013. Paleopathology. In: DiGangi, E.A., Moore, M.K. (Eds.), Research Methods in Human Skeletal Biology. Academic Press, San Diego.

Sparacello, V.S., Pearson, O.M., 2010. The importance of accounting for the area of the medullary cavity in cross-sectional geometry: A test based on the femoral midshaft. American Journal of Physical Anthropology 143 (4), 612–624.

Stojanowski, C.M., Buikstra, J.E., 2005. Research trends in human osteology: a content analysis of papers published in the American Journal of Physical Anthropology. American Journal of Physical Anthropology 128 (1), 98–109.

Szabo, T., 2005. Medical Imaging. In: Enderle, J.D., Bronzino, J.D., Blanchard, S.M. (Eds.), Introduction to Biomedical Engineering. Elsevier Academic Press, Amsterdam; Boston, pp. 908–972.

Tardieu, C., 1999. Ontogeny and phylogeny of femoro-tibial characters in humans and hominid fossils: functional influence and genetic determinism. American Journal of Physical Anthropology 110 (3), 365–377.

The New York Times Jan. 16, 1896, p. 9.

Trammell, L., Kroman, A.M., 2013. Bone and Dental Histology. In: DiGangi, E.A., Moore, M.K. (Eds.), Research Methods in Human Skeletal Biology. Academic Press, San Diego.

VanderJagt, D.J., Damiani, L.A., Goodman, T.M., Ujah, I.O., Obadofin, M.O., Imade, G.E., et al., 2004. Assessment of the skeletal health of healthy Nigerian men and women using quantitative ultrasound. Bone 35 (2), 387–394.

Van Gerven, D.P., Armelagos, G.J., 1969. Roentgenographic and direct measurement of femoral cortical involution in a prehistoric Mississippian population. American Journal of Physical Anthropology 31 (1), 23–38.

Washburn, S.L., 1951. The new physical anthropology. Transactions of the New York Academy of Sciences 13, 298–304.

Wolffe, J., 1892. [The law of bone remodeling]. A. Hirschwald, Berlin.

Wu, W., Zhi, X.M., Li, D.F., Lin, K., Xu, L., Yang, Y.H., 2007. [Vitamin D receptor gene polymorphism is not associated with bone mineral density of pre-menopausal women in Guangzhou]. Nan Fang Yi Ke Da Xue Xue Bao 27 (3), 364–366.

Zhang-Wong, J.H., Seeman, M.V., 2002. Antipsychotic drugs, menstrual regularity and osteoporosis risk. Archives of Women's Mental Health 5 (3), 93–98.

Isotopes

Jonathan D. Bethard

INTRODUCTION

In scholarship concerning modern human skeletal biology, novel methodological milestones have occasionally been introduced to the field with unmatched potential for tackling the previously unanswerable. Such was the case when Vogel and van der Merwe (1977) published the first paper linking evidence for maize agriculture with the isotopic composition of human bone. In her recent review, Katzenberg (2008) described the initial application of isotopic chemistry to anthropological questions as a kind of real-life science fiction. In this description, Katzenberg aptly described the anthropological "buzz" surrounding stable isotope analysis when it was first introduced to the field in the late 1970s, as scholars realized that a powerful new tool for unlocking information about the past had been introduced. The application of isotope analysis to research questions in skeletal biology underscores the importance of creative, interdisciplinary scholarship.

After the discovery of stable isotopes in 1913 by the Nobel Laureate Joseph John Thomson, decades of research in the natural sciences followed (Craig, 1954; Gavelin, 1957; Compston, 1960). Archaeological uses of the radiocarbon isotope (^{14}C) followed suit after its application to radiometric dating was discovered in 1949 and questions turned to calculating chronology and temporal context (Hall, 1967; Bender, 1968). Since these initial breakthroughs, stable isotope analysis has become a mainstay in the skeletal biologist's methodological toolkit, primarily due to widespread adoption of automated mass spectrometers (the instrumentation that analyzes isotopes) in the biological, ecological, and geological sciences. In the twenty-first century, scholars who wish to answer anthropological questions with stable isotope data have numerous well-qualified laboratories to choose from, even if their own institutions do not house dedicated stable isotope core facilities. In this chapter, I will outline the kinds of research questions to which stable isotope analyses can be applied, introduce the technical aspects of stable isotope analyses, discuss methodological issues related to the preparation of bones and teeth for isotope analysis, and conclude with a case study illustrating the application of stable isotope analysis to a bioarchaeological context from pre-Columbian Peru. Like Cabana and colleagues (Chapter 16, this volume), this chapter is intended to equip the interested skeletal biologist with an overview of stable isotope analysis while simultaneously emphasizing the importance of <u>hands-on</u> instruction with experienced scholars familiar with the intricacies of this research.

WHAT QUESTIONS CAN BE ANSWERED WITH STABLE ISOTOPE ANALYSIS?

As has been described in this volume (see DiGangi and Moore [Chapter 2]), it is imperative that researchers understand the link between their research questions and the types of methodological approaches that might assist them. For example, skeletal biologists interested in subsistence might consider analyzing the frequency of dental caries, or the composition of dental calculus (see Hammerl [Chapter 10], this volume); or they might decide to analyze the isotopic composition of various human tissues. Ultimately, it is incumbent upon the researcher to make clear connections between their research questions, theoretical framework, and methodological approach. Given that the focus of this chapter is on stable isotope analysis, skeletal biologists should seek to understand the connection between human behavior and bone chemistry.

While most university composition instructors, and indeed numerous anthropology faculty, might deduct points from their students' essays for the overuse of trite clichés in formal writing, I am going to break that rule-of-thumb here by emphasizing one adage that highlights the primary reason that skeletal biologists are interested in stable isotope analysis in the first place: you are what you eat! In essence, it is well known that through numerous physiological processes the chemical elements consumed and imbibed by *Homo sapiens* sometimes become directly incorporated into skeletal and dental tissues through complex processes such as bone remodeling (Agarwal, 2008; Trammell and Kroman [Chapter 13], this volume) or ion substitution (see Burton (2008)). As will be described in this chapter, the isotopic signature of various foodstuffs also provides clear insight into the types of subsistence strategies that humans have utilized (as well as when major shifts in plant exploitation occurred), clues regarding an individual's geological origin, and nuanced insight into status and estimates of social hierarchy. These areas are of major interest to skeletal biologists and other scholars with research interests in biological anthropology and archaeology.

Perhaps no topic utilizing stable isotopes has been of greater interest than that of subsistence, on both individual and population levels. In particular, researchers have correlated the development of large-scale social transformations with marked shifts in subsistence strategies. Taking the Southeastern United States as an example, scholars have long recognized that adoption of maize agriculture was one component of Mississippian cultural developments that set this period of time apart from earlier epochs (Griffin, 1967; Doolittle, 2004; Blitz, 2010). In an early study, Lynott and colleagues (1986) were able to apply stable isotope analyses and radiocarbon dating to a sample of 20 individuals from 14 archaeological sites throughout the Ozark region of Missouri and Arkansas that spanned a timeframe from 3200 B.C. to approximately 1880 A.D. Ultimately, the analysis of carbon isotopes in this study demonstrated a marked shift to maize-based agriculture after 1000 A.D., which was correlated with the emergence of politically centralized ceremonial centers.

While archaeological data are important tools for the reconstruction of prehistoric social hierarchies, stable isotope analyses also represent a unique lens in which to view social relationships. In an elegant example, Ambrose and colleagues (2003) utilized stable isotope data of both carbon and nitrogen isotopes to investigate status differences between a subsample of 272 individuals interred in Mound 72 at Cahokia (just outside present-day St. Louis, Missouri). Of these individuals, archaeological evidence suggested at least two distinct social groups were interred at the site. These distinctions were based upon the presence of extra-local artifacts that had been buried with some individuals and not others. Moreover, bioarchaeological analyses of the two groups indicated differences in the frequency of paleopathological lesions, with lower status individuals described as having higher frequencies of **nonspecific indicators of stress**[1] (see Smith [Chapter 7], this volume, for a review of stress indicators).

Isotopic data revealed several interesting characteristics about the mortuary sample from Mound 72. Data from bone collagen (the organic component of bone) yielded nitrogen signatures that suggested the diet of high-status individuals was more enriched from animal protein sources. Further, analysis of carbon from biological apatite (the mineral part of bone) indicated an even more marked disparity between the high-status and low-status groups. Given that carbon isotopes derived from biological apatite provide an indicator of whole or bulk diet, differences in maize consumption between groups were even more apparent. Overall, these isotopic data suggest that the high-status individuals had access to additional food sources while the lower status individuals did not (Ambrose et al., 2003).

WHAT ARE ISOTOPES?

As many skeletal biologists may have limited experience in chemistry, a rudimentary understanding of the concepts involved is necessary before proceeding further. **Isotopes** are variations of chemical elements that differ in the number of neutrons but have the same number of protons. As a result, isotopes of the same element will differ in their **atomic mass,** or the sum of the number of protons and neutrons. For example, strontium-86 (written ^{86}Sr) is one isotope of the element strontium with a mass number of 86. The **atomic number** of strontium is 38, indicating that every strontium atom has 38 protons, so that the **neutron number** of this isotope is 48 (38 protons + 48 neutrons = 86 mass number). A list of isotopes and their masses is presented in Table 15.1. The isotopes presented in this table are all defined as *stable isotopes*, (as opposed to unstable or *radioactive isotopes*, i.e., those that decay over time), and are commonly analyzed by skeletal biologists.

While each of the isotopes of an element have had the same atomic number, their different atomic masses influence the ways in which they behave during physical and chemical processes (Brown and Brown, 2011). For example, ^{13}C is 8.3% heavier than ^{12}C, which means that it reacts more slowly in biochemical reactions such as photosynthesis (the process plants use to convert atmospheric carbon dioxide to glucose for energy). During photosynthesis, the lighter isotope becomes enriched more rapidly than the heavier isotope, resulting in **isotope fractionation,** or a change in isotope ratios due to chemical processes (i.e., the ratio of ^{13}C compared to ^{12}C). The degree of isotope fractionation is plant-specific and ultimately

---

[1]All bolded terms are defined in the glossary at the end of this volume.

TABLE 15.1   Stable Isotopes of Interest to Skeletal Biologists and Their Abundances in Nature. Extracted from Katzenberg (2008) and Brown and Brown (2011).

Element	Isotope	Abundance in Nature
Carbon	^{12}C	98.93%
	^{13}C	1.07%
Hydrogen	^{1}H	99.985%
	^{2}H	0.015%
Nitrogen	^{14}N	99.64%
	^{15}N	0.36%
Oxygen	^{16}O	99.76%
	^{17}O	0.04%
	^{18}O	0.20%
Sulfur	^{32}S	95.0%
	^{33}S	0.76%
	^{34}S	4.22%
	^{36}S	0.014%
Strontium	^{84}Sr	0.56%
	^{86}Sr	9.86%
	^{87}Sr	7.02%
	^{88}Sr	82.56%

separates plant species into three distinct groups with varying carbon isotope ratios. Specific isotopes used in skeletal biology projects will be discussed after the following section.

RESEARCH DESIGN OF STABLE ISOTOPE PROJECTS

When initiating a stable isotope analysis project, I suggest breaking down the methodological component of a research design into three distinct parts: (1) obtaining samples; (2) extracting tissues from those samples; and (3) analyzing the extracted tissues on a mass spectrometer.

Sample Procurement

Let's first discuss the issue of sample procurement. Given the focus of many skeletal biologists on research in the United States, the Native American Graves Protection and Repatriation Act (NAGPRA) legislation might very well provide the first stumbling block to a project dedicated to stable isotope analysis of human bones and teeth (see discussion in DiGangi and Moore [Chapter 1], this volume). In other words, interested researchers should determine if stable isotope analyses are permissible on human samples derived from archaeological contexts in the United States. Ultimately, numerous skeletal collections in the United States will be unavailable for stable isotope projects; therefore, researchers should take care to ascertain this from the outset.

For those researchers who are engaged in research outside of the United States, analysis of stable isotopes from mineralized tissues may pose equally challenging obstacles, as sampling and exporting permission processes are diverse and variable. For thorough treatment of issues related to international research programs in skeletal biology, interested readers should consult Turner and Andruskho (2011) for practical guidelines related to international collaboration. In my own experience, a minimum of six months was required to obtain permits to sample an archaeological collection for a stable isotope project. This adds an important logistical concern for projects.

Regardless of where samples come from, it should be mentioned that current methodological protocols only require minimum amounts of samples. For example, extraction of collagen only requires ~10 g of bone and extraction of apatite from tooth enamel only requires ~15 mg of enamel. Moreover, cutting-edge methods involving *laser ablation* have been utilized by some researchers interested in strontium isotope analysis. Laser ablation has been applied to Neandertal samples and was described as a relatively nondestructive method by the authors and ultimately required much less sample than traditional methodologies (Richards et al., 2008). Regardless, researchers should confirm minimum sample standards with their collaborating laboratories.

Tissue Extraction: Collagen

The issue of sample preparation requires some discussion of the types of tissues that can be analyzed by stable isotope analysis. The first tissue to be studied was bone collagen, as researchers had been using this tissue for radiocarbon dating prior to the late 1970s. As other authors in this volume have highlighted (see Trammell and Kroman [Chapter 13]), bone is comprised of both organic and inorganic compounds. The organic component, called Type-1 collagen, comprises approximately 30% of dry bone. In its pure form, Type-1 collagen is approximately 35% carbon and 11–16% nitrogen by weight (van Klinken, 1999), making it the ideal tissue for stable isotope analysis of these two elements.

Researchers interested in collagen isolation should review the various approaches that are available (Longin, 1971; Schoeninger and DeNiro, 1984; Brown et al., 1988; Tuross et al., 1988; Ambrose, 1990). Each of these procedures has been used with success and involves wet chemistry protocols that demineralize the bone and separate out the collagen component. Researchers should keep in mind that taphonomic processes (see Marden et al. [Chapter 9], this volume) might result in poorly preserved bone, and therefore poorly preserved bone collagen. Consequently, one should choose an appropriate extraction protocol tailored to these circumstances (Brown et al., 1988).

As Katzenberg (2008) aptly points out, it is of utmost importance for a skeletal biologist interested in analyzing bone collagen to demonstrate that the final product under analysis is actually bone collagen and not some other chemically altered, taphonomic byproduct. DeNiro (1985) was the first to suggest that researchers should evaluate the ratio of carbon-to-nitrogen (C/N) in their collagen samples. In "good" samples of collagen, the C/N ratio will fall somewhere between the values of 2.9 and 3.6, which reflects the C/N ratio of 3.2 typically found in modern, taphonomically unaffected bone samples. In performing literature searches on stable isotope analyses of bone collagen, researchers should certainly take note of those studies that report C/N ratios and those that do not, as a failure to report this ratio does not allow for authentication of the results.

Tissue Extraction: Biological Apatite

Besides bone collagen, researchers have recognized that the mineral portion of bone, as well as tooth enamel, also contains useful isotopic information, particularly for the analysis of carbon, strontium, and oxygen isotopes. This inorganic component of bone, comprising approximately 70% of dry bone weight, is dominated by a mineral called *hydroxyapatite* (see Trammell and Kroman [Chapter 13], this volume). The mineral component of tooth enamel is even higher, as nearly 96% is hydroxyapatite. Often termed bioapatite, apatite carbonate, or bone carbonate, scholars agree that biological apatite has a propensity to survive various depositional contexts, even when bone collagen is too far degraded to be of much use for isotopic analysis. For example, Sponheimer and colleagues (2006) reported isotopic results derived from biological apatite in 1.8-million-year-old *Paranthropus robustus* teeth. Such findings reiterate the importance of the mineral component of bones and teeth in isotopic analysis. Techniques for isolating biological apatite are widely known and have been reported by numerous authors (e.g., Lee-Thorp et al., 1989; Lee-Thorp and van der Merwe, 1991; Balasse et al., 2002; Garvie-Lok et al., 2004). In these methods, samples are soaked in sodium hypochlorite (household bleach) and then treated with an acetic acid solution to remove external carbonate. Moreover, skeletal biologists have recognized that biological apatite derived from tooth enamel provides a unique snapshot of enamel formation during childhood while biological apatite extracted from bone is indicative of an individual's last few years of life (Knudson et al., 2009).

If researchers' questions involve carbon, nitrogen, or oxygen isotopes, then no further processing is necessary once biological apatite has been extracted. Workers interested in strontium isotopes, on the other hand, are required to complete an additional step before those isotopes can be analyzed. This step requires the separation of strontium under clean-lab circumstances. In my experience, few skeletal biologists maintain such laboratories (with the exception of ancient **DNA** labs) and often are required to collaborate with experts from the geological sciences. While many skeletal biologists often ship samples of extracted biological apatite to these experts for strontium isotope analysis, it should be noted that many colleagues in geology are eager to work with skeletal biologists and will gladly provide training on strontium extraction procedures. Regardless, skeletal biologists must keep these special considerations in mind when planning any project on strontium isotope analysis.

Laboratory Considerations

In ideal circumstances, skeletal biologists would be equipped with the laboratory capabilities to extract both collagen and biological apatite. Both extraction methodologies can be applied in standard laboratories equipped with one or more fume hoods, chemical storage capabilities, and a source of distilled water. Collagen extraction typically requires glassware, so interested skeletal biologists should consider the number of samples they hope to analyze when preparing equipment orders or budgeting for grant proposals. An important consideration for collagen preparation involves residual carbon that may adhere to glassware between samples. Because it is important to ensure that all collagen-preparation glassware is free of carbon from one sample to the next, it is important to thoroughly clean each piece after each use. While multiple approaches for mitigating reuse exist, an effective method involves rinsing each piece of glassware in a sulfuric acid bath and then heating each piece in a commercial kiln used for firing ceramics (S. Ambrose, personal communication, 2007).

An ideal laboratory setup might involve dedicating two distinct spaces for staging collagen and biological apatite extractions. In this setting, a "dry lab" would be dedicated for preliminary processing of samples. For example, if archaeological matrix is present, it is removed in the dry lab under a dedicated fume hood. Samples might be ground or drilled to a powder in this space and then removed to the "wet lab" for chemical treatment.

Once all wet chemistry is complete, all samples must be analyzed on a mass spectrometer, typically in dedicated core facilities having specialists with expertise in **mass spectrometry.**

Stable Isotopes and Mass Spectrometry

In typical projects that involve analysis of stable isotopes, the step following collagen and biological apatite extraction utilizes instrumentation called **isotope ratio mass spectrometers (IRMS).** The IRMS typically have four components: a combustion chamber, an ion source, a mass analyzer, and series of ion detectors. These components act to detect subtle differences in various isotopes, for example ^{13}C and ^{12}C, by initially combusting the sample and then automatically transferring the converted gas into the mass spectrometer for analysis. Upon entering the mass spectrometer, the gas is ionized so that it can be directed into the mass analyzer where it is measured against known standards in the ion detectors (sometimes called Faraday collectors). Interested skeletal biologists are encouraged to consult other sources for more detailed descriptions of the process of analyzing samples via IRMS (i.e., Barrie and Prosser, 1996; Katzenberg, 2008; Brown and Brown, 2011). Moreover, to fully understand the complexities of the instrumentation, and to perhaps gain experience operating this type of laboratory equipment, individuals are encouraged to seek out specialists to gain practical skills in this area, even if this means temporarily relocating, taking an additional course outside of the traditional skeletal biology curriculum, or volunteering as a laboratory assistant at any IRMS core facility.

In addition to understanding the basic principles of the IRMS, skeletal biologists should have some awareness about how stable isotope ratios are calculated on the mass spectrometer. As mentioned above, the mass spectrometer analyzes both the sample and a known standard. The standards are regulated on an international level by such agencies as the United States National Institute of Standards and Technology (NIST), sometimes referred to as the National Bureau of Standards (NBS), and by the International Atomic Energy Agency (IAEA). A list of common standards can be found by accessing the following website: http://nucleus.iaea.org/rpst/ReferenceProducts/ReferenceMaterials/index.htm. Ultimately, any IRMS core facility will be well versed in NIST/IAEA standards and interested researchers should familiarize themselves with the protocols of their particular laboratory. As research projects progress beyond the analytical stage to scientific presentations and publications, explicitly discussing which standards were used in any stable isotope project is compulsory.

Understanding that stable isotope analyses require comparison of isotopic values in unknown samples to reference standards clarifies how results from the mass spectrometer are calculated and reported. Taking carbon as an example, the following notation is used:

$$\delta^{13}C = (R_{sample}/R_{standard} - 1) \times 1000\%$$

where R is the ratio of the heavier to the lighter isotope (e.g., $^{13}C/^{12}C$) and the δ (delta) notation expresses this ratio as parts per thousand (‰, per mil). For all stable carbon isotopes, the original standard material was a sample of marine limestone called the *Peedee belemnite* (PDB). Though PDB has been exhausted in its original form, other standards whose $\delta^{13}C$ values have been calibrated against it are readily available (Hoefs, 2009). A positive $\delta^{13}C$ value indicates that ^{13}C is enriched compared to the standard and depleted for ^{12}C, or as is the case with human tissues, negative $\delta^{13}C$ values are depleted for ^{13}C and enriched in ^{12}C (Brown and Brown, 2011).

Stable Isotopes and Diet: Carbon and Nitrogen

In particular, skeletal biologists have concentrated a tremendous amount of effort on studying carbon and nitrogen isotopes to answer questions regarding subsistence and paleodiet, and typically analyze these isotopes in tandem. Fortunately for the researcher, both carbon and nitrogen can be analyzed simultaneously from a single sample of prepared collagen. Today's mass spectrometers are capable of analyzing both isotopes concurrently; therefore, two distinct datasets can be generated at once.

Carbon

The first stable isotope to receive attention in anthropological literature was carbon. Initially, pioneering researchers realized that maize was often more difficult to date with radiocarbon than other types of organic material like charcoal (Katzenberg, 2008). Second, during this initial time researchers were continuing to differentiate the three photosynthetic pathways that now form the basis of $\delta^{13}C$ interpretations.

To sum, each of these photosynthetic pathways is represented by a distinct group of plants that are differentiated by the way in which they convert atmospheric carbon dioxide (CO_2) into glucose. Ultimately, it is this process of CO_2 conversion to sugar (referred to as carbon fixation) that results in distinct $\delta^{13}C$ signatures, as the type of plant dictates the degree of carbon fixation that occurs (O'Leary, 1988; Brown and Brown, 2011). The C_3, or *Calvin photosynthetic pathway*, is found in plants common to temperate climatic regions and their $\delta^{13}C$ values average -26.5% (Tykot, 2006). Cultigens such as wheat, barley, and quinoa are examples of C_3 cultigens. The *Hatch-Slack photosynthetic pathway*, represented by C_4 plants, fixes carbon in an entirely different way. Maize, sorghum, millet, and sugarcane are examples of C_4 plants and these plants are known to come from more tropical climates—their $\delta^{13}C$ values average -12.5% (Tykot, 2006). Succulent species (e.g., cacti), plants that follow the **CAM** (*crassulacean acid metabolism*) pathway, yield $\delta^{13}C$ values that fall between C_3 and C_4 plants.

Skeletal biologists interested in analyses of carbon isotopes should recognize that the tissue type (e.g., biological apatite or collagen) under analysis plays an important part in dietary reconstruction. This phenomenon was first realized after various controlled feeding experiments with laboratory animals (Ambrose and Norr, 1993; Tieszen and Fagre, 1993; Howland et al., 2003). As a result, it is well known that $\delta^{13}C$ data derived from biological apatite are more reflective of an individual's whole diet (or dietary energy) while $\delta^{13}C$ data gleaned from bone collagen are more reflective of protein sources (Harrison and Katzenberg, 2003; Tykot, 2006). Moreover, Ambrose and Norr (1993) demonstrated that $\delta^{13}C$ values differed by 9.4‰ between collagen ($\delta^{13}C_{CO}$) and biological apatite ($\delta^{13}C_{AP}$), primarily due to the complex physiological differences by which these tissues take up carbon. Such dissimilarities had been suggested by earlier scholars (Krueger and Sullivan, 1984; Lee-Thorp et al., 1989) and have ultimately demonstrated that skeletal biologists can reconstruct a more nuanced dietary interpretation by analyzing differences between $\delta^{13}C_{CO}$ and $\delta^{13}C_{AP}$, otherwise known as *dietary spacing* (Ambrose et al., 1997).[2] Recent work by Kellner and Schoeninger (2007) and Froehle et al. (2012) produced several dietary models that further indicate analyzing $\delta^{13}C_{CO}$ and $\delta^{13}C_{AP}$ together allow for further elucidation of C_3 and C_4 dietary strategies.

Nitrogen

Shortly after the first studies on carbon isotopes were published, other researchers began publishing work on nitrogen isotopes ($\delta^{15}N$) (DeNiro and Epstein, 1981). Initially, these studies were initiated to investigate *trophic level* distinctions within the food chain, with particular emphasis on marine systems (DeNiro and Schoeninger, 1983; Schoeninger and DeNiro, 1983, 1984). Generally, nitrogen isotope values are correlated with an organism's position in the food chain and typically increase by 2–3‰ per trophic level (Tykot, 2006). For example, in a study sampling species from numerous trophic positions, Katzenberg and Kelly (1991) demonstrated distinct differences in ^{15}N levels between humans and lower-position animals from the Sierra Blanca region of New Mexico. Trophic level distinctions were also apparent in a similar study from Lake Baikal, Siberia (Katzenberg and Weber, 1999), as freshwater seals (animals close to the top position of the food web) had the highest $\delta^{15}N$ values of all species sampled at approximately 14‰.

In addition to questions surrounding trophic levels, researchers utilize nitrogen isotopes to differentiate between plant and animal protein sources, as well as to separate terrestrial from marine protein. In the case of differentiating between terrestrial and marine protein sources (and human consumers), it is well known that marine plants are more enriched for $\delta^{15}N$ than their terrestrial counterparts. As a result, $\delta^{15}N$ values increase with each subsequent trophic level; therefore, human consumers of marine protein sources present significantly enriched $\delta^{15}N$ values when compared to their terrestrial resource consuming counterparts.

Finally, several researchers have indicated that $\delta^{15}N$ is variable in hot, dry climates (Heaton et al., 1986; Ambrose, 1991). This phenomenon is in part due to the way in which nitrogen is excreted by mammals through urination. In essence, in parts of the world where water is (or at times becomes) scarce, mammals excrete nitrogen in their urine at higher levels. At the same time, however, this higher level of excretion must be balanced by the retention of $\delta^{15}N$ in the organism's tissues. As a result, Ambrose (1991) demonstrated that water-stressed

---

[2]Dietary spacing is represented by the notation $\Delta^{13}C_{CO-AP}$. The Δ symbol indicates a change (i.e., difference) between $\delta^{13}C_{CO}$ and $\delta^{13}C_{AP}$ (see Hedges, 2003 for a review).

individuals have elevated $\delta^{15}N$ levels compared to nonstressed individuals. These data caution researchers against making interpretations related to diet in populations from arid regions. In these instances, $\delta^{15}N$ levels may be enriched for reasons other than dietary choice.

Strontium

In 1985, Ericson published the first example of the anthropological use of strontium isotopes ($^{87}Sr/^{86}Sr$). The application of strontium isotope analysis to problems in skeletal biology is straightforward. In essence, strontium is a trace element that exists in geological bedrock. The concentration or abundance of strontium in geological substrate is variable and depends on the type of bedrock present. Numerous authors (see Bentley (2006) for a review) have discussed the way in which strontium is transferred throughout an ecosystem. Essentially, the geological composition of bedrock subsequently influences the concentrations of strontium in groundwater and soil, which are taken up or absorbed by local flora and fauna. In other words, the concentration in local flora and fauna mimics the underlying strontium concentration contained in local bedrock.

Strontium becomes incorporated into the body's skeletal and dental tissues through the ingestion of water, plants, and animals. It then replaces some calcium in the hydroxyapatite in bones and teeth. Unlike other isotopes, such as $\delta^{15}N$, no change or fractionation occurs as the isotopes move from water, plants, and animals to humans. As a result, an individual's skeletal and dental tissues mirror the strontium concentration in soil and groundwater of their local area. It is important to note here, however, that numerous scholars (Knudson et al. (2005) for example) emphasize that strontium isotopes in tooth enamel reflect the geological bedrock of the local area that the individual lived in while their teeth were developing (because unlike bone, once the teeth are formed, they do not remodel), predominantly during the first 12 years of life. As a result, $^{87}Sr/^{86}Sr$ is often construed to indicate an individual's place of origin. See Hammerl (Chapter 10), this volume, for an example of how strontium analysis has been used with teeth.

Strontium isotope analysis is therefore used to detect residential mobility or migration in the archaeological record, as those individuals who are migrants oftentimes present $^{87}Sr/^{86}Sr$ ratios that are outside of the expected local level where their remains were recovered. Local "baseline" levels have traditionally been calculated by first surveying geological literature for previously reported $^{87}Sr/^{86}Sr$ ratios. Those levels are then compared to "baseline" data that are created by analyzing archaeological local fauna, or by taking modern examples from wherever the local area might be. Regarding calculation of the local $^{87}Sr/^{86}Sr$ level, it is important to note that researchers are encouraged to choose locally raised fauna. In the corpus of work from the Andean region of South America, scholars have utilized guinea pigs or *cuy* (in Spanish) to serve as baseline data for their respective areas of study. *Cuy* are ubiquitous throughout the Andes and are an excellent example of a locally raised species, both from prehistory and the present day. As a result, samples from *cuy* are preferential to highly migratory camelids (i.e., llamas, alpacas, vicuña). Once local samples are obtained, calculating a local signature requires the researcher to calculate the mean ± two standard deviations of the entire local faunal sample. Any human that falls outside of this local range is considered a migrant or nonlocal individual.

One example that illustrates the role of strontium isotopes in identifying nonlocal individuals comes from the work of Knudson and colleagues (2005). In this paper, Knudson et al.

describe an assemblage of naturally mummified human remains recovered from a cave in southern Bolivia. These individuals were recovered with artifacts in the Tiwanaku style, which is centered some 600 km away from the cave site in northern Bolivia. The presence of extra-local artifacts suggested nonlocal individuals; however, $^{87}Sr/^{86}Sr$ analyses demonstrated that these individuals were in fact from the local area in southern Bolivia. Such findings led the workers in this study to question the sphere of influence of Tiwanaku in southern Bolivia.

Oxygen

Like strontium, oxygen isotopes have been used by skeletal biologists to reconstruct mobility in prehistoric populations (Sponheimer and Lee-Thorp, 1999; Knudson, 2009; Knudson et al., 2012). Stable oxygen isotopes ($\delta^{18}O$) in biological apatite echo the isotopic composition of water in the body, $\delta^{18}O$ at 37°C. In turn, body water $\delta^{18}O$ itself is influenced by the isotopic composition of imbibed water, as well as the oxygen in the air and food sources (Sponheimer and Lee-Thorp, 1999; Turner et al., 2009). The isotopic composition of imbibed water is influenced by a host of ecological variables including latitude, altitude, aridity, seasonal temperature fluctuations, and rainfall (Gil et al., 2011). Under this assumption, skeletal biologists have used $\delta^{18}O$ values from biological apatite to infer an individual's geographic location at the time that the apatite was laid down (White et al., 1998; Prowse et al., 2007). Similar to strontium isotope analysis, skeletal biologists must also understand the $\delta^{18}O$ variation of potential water sources before making inferences about an individual's migratory status. Utilizing examples from the Andes, Knudson (2009) cautions that the complex movement of water through diverse ecological zones might complicate or even prevent interpretations derived from $\delta^{18}O$ data.

CASE STUDY: ARCHAEOLOGICAL RESEARCH QUESTIONS WITH STABLE ISOTOPE DATA

Echoing my earlier comments, as well as those of Cabana and co-workers (Chapter 16), this volume, the intention of this case study is to provide a general overview of how an interested skeletal biologist might actually perform stable isotope analyses on bones and teeth. As has been mentioned, numerous steps are involved with both sample procurement and analysis. Once samples are physically located in the laboratory, researchers must first extract collagen and/or biological apatite from them. After this has been accomplished, those samples are analyzed on the mass spectrometers. It should be emphasized here that both wet chemistry extractions and mass spectrometer work should only be initiated under the supervision of highly experienced personnel. In my experience, it was necessary to travel to another institution and learn from a mentor who was exceptionally generous with his time. Extensive treatment of methodological techniques can be found by reviewing articles in the *Journal of Archaeological Sciences, Archaeometry,* and *Archaeological and Anthropological Sciences.* The Society for Archaeological Sciences' (http://www.socarchsci.org/) triannual publication might prove useful, as would resources gathered from attending the yearly International Symposium on Archaeometry. In the remaining portions of this section, I will highlight how stable isotope analysis of carbon, nitrogen, and strontium was utilized to investigate archaeological questions regarding diet and residential mobility at the site of Santa Rita B on the north coast of Peru.

Archaeological Context—Santa Rita B

As has been discussed throughout this chapter, analyses of stable isotopes of the organic and inorganic components of human skeletal and dental tissues have been reported from numerous archaeological regions throughout the world, including the Andes (Burger and van der Merwe, 1990; Tomczak, 2003; Knudson et al., 2007). While numerous researchers have reported stable isotopic data from archaeological contexts throughout the Andean Cordillera, few have presented data from the north coast of Peru. This is surprising, given the amount of scholarly attention paid to archaeological cultures such as Moche and Chimu and monumental archaeological sites like Huacas de Moche and Chan Chan (Pillsbury, 2001). The work presented in this case study adds to the few studies published from the north coast by presenting stable isotopic results from the Santa Rita B archaeological project.

The Santa Rita B archaeological site is located on the western slopes of the Andes in northern Peru. It can be found in the lower portion of the middle Chao Valley at an average elevation of 484 m above mean sea level, approximately 25 km from the Pacific Ocean (Figure 15.1). For over ten years, the Santa Rita B Archaeological Project was involved with defining the nature of the human occupation of the site and investigating selected aspects of its economic, social, political, and ideological history. Most recently, excavations were targeted in areas of apparent domestic architecture, representing complexes or rooms. One of these, known as "Archaeological Complex No. 3" (or CA3), is a rock-walled compound measuring about 29 m × 25 m, and is subdivided into numerous rooms. Rich archaeological deposits were recovered from CA3 and include numerous classes of artifacts such as ceramics and lithics, as well as zooarchaeological and botanical remains. Moreover, several *Spondylus* shell caches (including complete bivalves and worked shell) have been recovered, along with numerous articulated camelid (llama or alpaca) skeletons (Gaither et al., 2008, 2009).

Beginning in 2002, excavators at Santa Rita B began recovering human skeletal remains from CA3 (Figure 15.2). All individuals were buried 30–40 cm below the ground surface in alluvial strata superimposed on top of other culturally derived deposits. Though some looting has occurred at CA3, the majority of individuals have been excavated from sealed contexts and little **postmortem** commingling has occurred. The upper strata containing human skeletal remains were deposited sometime between 1050 and 1280 A.D., based on calibrated radiocarbon dates derived from bone collagen.

Interestingly, several individuals from Santa Rita B present **perimortem trauma** (i.e., cutmarks and blunt force injuries) and burial positions indicative of the pan-Andean practice of human sacrifice (Gaither et al., 2009). Figure 15.3 illustrates atypical body positioning of one individual who presented with perimortem trauma (for a detailed discussion of trauma see Kroman and Symes [Chapter 8], this volume). In addition, two individuals recovered from CA3 represent what might be classified as principal burials. Entierro (Burial) 4, a child aged 5–9, was buried with a young camelid and presented no perimortem trauma and Entierro 8, an adult male, was buried in an extended, supine position. Though this burial

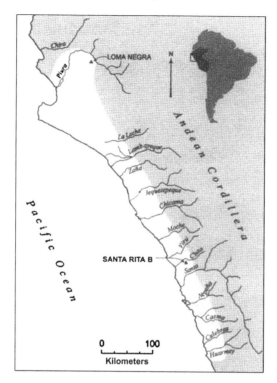

FIGURE 15.1   Location of the archaeological site Santa Rita B described in the case study example. Adapted from Gaither et al. (2008).

had been looted prior to excavation, Gaither and colleagues (2009) suggest differential mortuary treatment when compared to those individuals with clear perimortem trauma.

Such bioarchaeological evidence, coupled with the high number of *Spondylus* shells and articulated camelid remains, suggests that CA3 was utilized for highly specialized activities. When taken in context, three primary questions surrounding the **life histories** of the individuals recovered from CA3 emerged:

1. Given the differential mortuary treatment between individuals, would isotopic analysis of carbon and nitrogen isotopes indicate discrepancies in access to dietary resources?
2. Might some individuals present signatures of a more terrestrially sourced diet while others exploited marine resources?
3. Given the differential mortuary treatment between individuals, would analysis of strontium isotopes indicate that the individuals interred at CA3 were local to the Chao valley? If not, where might these individuals have come from?

Archaeological Materials and Sampling

As is the case with many archaeological projects, permits were an absolute requirement so that our team could legally remove bone and tooth samples from each skeleton and export

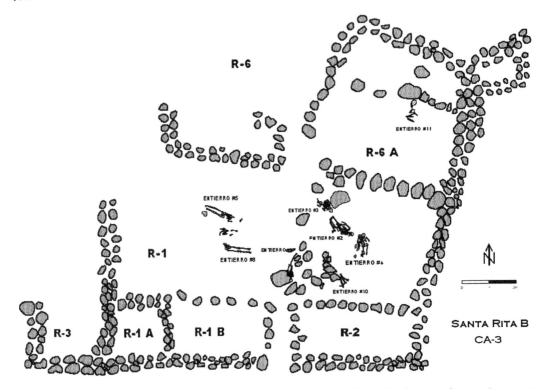

FIGURE 15.2 Detailed plan view of CA3 depicting the spatial relationship between human interments. Adapted from Gaither et al. (2009).

them for analysis. This process was initiated well in advance of my arrival in Peru for the 2006 field season with the help of colleagues from the Peruvian National Institute of Culture-La Libertad.[3] Once permits were granted, samples of skeletal and dental tissues were obtained from each individual recovered from CA3 and transported to the United States for analysis. In this instance, approximately 15 mg of bone was sampled from long bones and permanent first molars were retained. In addition, six modern *cuy* were obtained for the purpose of establishing a "local" strontium baseline. Four of these animals were raised in the Chao Valley approximately 3.5 km from the site, while two were purchased from a local market in the upper Chao Valley where commodities are exchanged between valley and highland inhabitants.

Wet Chemistry and Use of the Mass Spectrometer

All samples were prepared and analyzed in the Environmental Isotope Paleobiogeochemistry Laboratory at the University of Illinois at Urbana-Champaign. Bone collagen was prepared following Ambrose (1990) while bone and tooth carbonate was purified

[3]Archaeological permits in Peru are now administered by the Ministry of Culture.

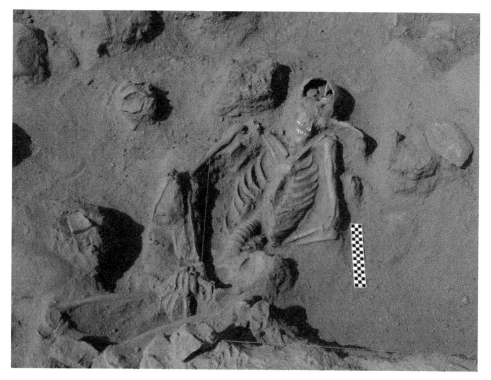

FIGURE 15.3   *In situ* photograph of Entierro 2. Note the semiflexed burial position, as well as the position of the individual's left arm. Perimortem trauma of numerous skeletal elements was observed.

following Balasse et al. (2002). A Finnegan MAT 252 isotope mass spectrometer coupled with an elemental analyzer and cryogenic distillation system (Kiel III device) was utilized to analyze bone collagen and bioapatite, respectively. Bone collagen samples were evaluated for diagenesis (i.e., degradation) using percent nitrogen, carbon, and atomic C:N ratios (DeNiro, 1985).

Strontium was separated from purified human and *cuy* biological apatite utilizing EiChrom SrSpec resin and analyzed on a Nu Plasma HR multicollector inductively coupled plasma mass spectrometer (MC-ICPMS) in the Department of Geology at the University of Illinois at Urbana-Champaign.

Nitrogen and Carbon Isotope Results

Values of $\delta^{15}N$ and $\delta^{13}C$ are presented in Table 15.2. Four individuals' atomic C:N ratio fell outside the acceptable range of 2.9–3.6; therefore, those data were excluded from subsequent anthropological analyses. It should be reiterated here that researchers must be exceptionally cautious in interpreting raw isotopic data. If, for example, the atomic C:N ratio was not taken into account in this case study, I may have interpreted the diet of Entierro 1 as an anomalous **outlier** from the clustered dietary signature of the other individuals (Figure 15.4).

TABLE 15.2   Demographic and Isotopic Data from Archaeological Human Samples from Santa Rita B

Entierro	Sex	Age	C:N	δ^{15}N	δ^{13}C	$\Delta^{13}C_{CO\text{-}AP}$
1	F	13–15	3.84	5.44	−15.66	7.37
2	M	25–30	5.00	0.36	−21.509	15.21
3	?	10–12	3.47	7.369	−13.063	6.69
4	?	5–9	3.24	8.988	−11.772	5.05
5	?	10–12	3.27	8.02	−14.266	5.00
8	M	35–40	3.34	7.237	−11.092	4.87
9	M?	12–16	6.30	6.479	−19.881	13.47
10	?	8–10	3.35	7.235	−10.994	5.72
11	?	9–11	4.17	2.055	−20.285	13.95

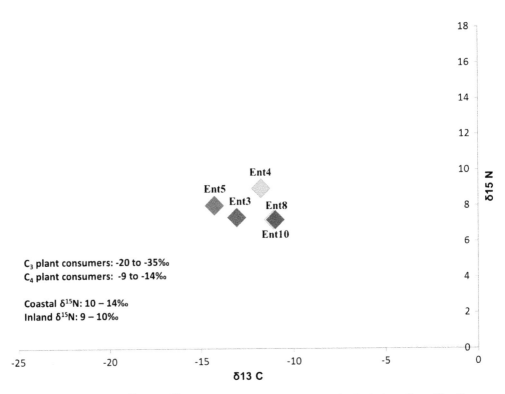

FIGURE 15.4 δ^{13}C and δ^{15}N values for bone collagen for individuals from Santa Rita B.

After excluding problematic data, a clear dietary pattern of the individuals interred at CA3 emerged. First, $\delta^{13}C$ results suggest that individuals were C_4 maize consumers. Given that maize had been utilized as an agricultural staple on the north coast of Peru for several centuries prior to the temporal context under investigation, this conclusion is not entirely surprising. However, $\delta^{15}N$ results indicate moderately low marine protein consumption even though Santa Rita B is located just 25 km from the Pacific Ocean.

Though few researchers have applied stable isotope analyses to archaeological contexts from the north coast of Peru, Ericson and colleagues' (1989) analysis of samples from the Viru Valley (the valley directly north of the Chao Valley) serves as an excellent body of work for which to compare results from Santa Rita B. In their study, Ericson et al. (1989) investigated the development of maize agriculture in the Viru Valley over a 1500 year period (400 B.C.–1000 A.D.). These researchers found that maize exploitation was widespread for centuries prior to the time period under investigation at CA3 and comprised at least 40–50% of the diet (Ericson et al., 1989). Furthermore, $\delta^{15}N$ isotopes indicate that marine resource utilization dropped off as individuals moved from the coast and into the Viru Valley, as coastal nitrogen values ranged from 10 to 14‰ while inland values ranged from 9 to 10‰ (Schoeninger and Moore, 1992).

Such interpretations are corroborated by evaluating the difference in isotope values of bone apatite and collagen ($\Delta^{13}C_{CO-AP}$) or apatite–collagen spacing. Numerous researchers have found that apatite–collagen spacing values >4.4‰ indicate populations that extensively consumed maize and received their protein from terrestrial sources (Ambrose and Norr, 1993; Ambrose et al., 1997; Finucane et al., 2006). Data from individuals recovered from CA3 present mean apatite–collagen spacing of 5.466, clearly indicating that these individuals were maize and terrestrial protein consumers.

Strontium Isotope Results

As discussed previously, numerous individuals excavated from CA3 presented perimortem trauma and body positions consistent with human sacrifice. Hypotheses regarding the geographic origin of these individuals are numerous, as differentiating locals from nonlocals in bioarchaeological contexts of sacrifice have recently been suggested in the literature (Sutter and Cortez, 2005). In order to gain insight into these questions, as well as to contribute to a growing body of literature regarding strontium isotope analysis in the Andes, the teeth of six individuals from CA3 were analyzed.

In order to utilize strontium isotope analysis for the purposes of documenting residential mobility, "local" signatures must be generated first. As a result, interested scholars need to characterize the geology for the region under study and supplement those data with local fauna in order to get the most comprehensive "local" signature (Knudson et al., 2005; Bentley, 2006; Knudson and Tung, 2007). To date, few studies have characterized strontium isotopes of the north coast of Peru; however, Petford and colleagues (1996) define an area of Cordillera Blanca batholith (from 9 to 11˚S) with a strontium isotope range of 0.70410–0.70571. While the samples from this study are derived from an area south of the Chao Valley, they are the geographically closest data currently available.

The geology of the middle Chao Valley is dominated by an alluvial outwash fan (i.e., a geological area that has been extensively mixed by water), along with outcrops of

Cretaceous period sedimentary and intrusive deposits. Santa Rita B is located on the alluvial deposit, a reality that makes characterizing a local strontium signature from geological formations more difficult and underscores the importance of utilizing local fauna to obtain a signature. In this instance, the "local" signature for the middle Chao Valley was calculated as the mean of *cuy* strontium isotope results, plus or minus two standard deviations. Using this methodology, the local range for Santa Rita B is 0.70502–0.70557—a range that loosely matches results published by Petford and colleagues (Figure 15.5).

Upon examining strontium isotope data from six individuals with viable strontium isotope ratios, several conclusions can be drawn. First, it is apparent that the local signature for Santa Rita B can be revealed by evaluating geological data and locally raised faunal sources. In addition, it appears as if two of the individuals included in this case study were not born in the middle Chao Valley (Figure 15.5). These results indicate that individuals interred at CA3 were from multiple locations and that several of the individuals presenting perimortem trauma were most likely interred a short distance from their place of birth. The geographic origin of Entierros 4 and 11 is still poorly understood, as data from other north coast localities are currently unavailable. While strontium isotope analysis presents

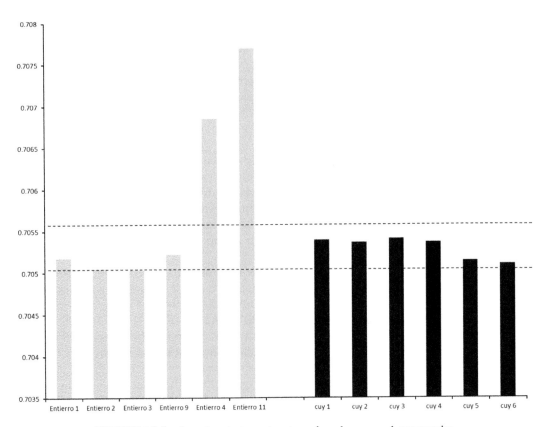

FIGURE 15.5 Strontium isotope signatures from human and *cuy* samples.

a powerful tool for investigating residential mobility, it is clear that more work needs to be done to characterize local signatures on the north coast and throughout the Andes in general. In essence, the geological birthplace of these two individuals remains unknown, and more importantly, we continue to investigate why they were interred at CA3 in the first place.

This case study demonstrates that stable isotope analysis is a powerful addition to the toolkit of Andean bioarchaeologists. It is evident that maize consumption was widespread throughout the north coast, and the pattern observed at Santa Rita B corroborates previous evidence and shows the inhabitants were maize consumers who relied on terrestrial protein sources. Moreover, we have learned that several individuals interred at CA3 were most likely not born in the middle Chao Valley. We are hopeful that our results will add to a growing dataset regarding the subsistence and residential mobility of people who inhabited the north coast of Peru. As with all research, new results often lead to new questions, and my colleagues and I look forward to tackling those in the near future.

CONCLUSION

In the nearly four decades since the first pioneering work on stable isotope analysis emerged, skeletal biologists have seen a tremendous increase in the application of the technique across the various constituencies of the discipline. Contemporary bioarchaeologists have generated remarkably nuanced biocultural interpretations by carefully coupling isotopic data with archaeological and ethnographic information. Of course, these developments could not have occurred without those dedicated researchers who toiled in their laboratories for countless hours perfecting extraction procedures, troubleshooting mass spectrometer problems, and critically considering the role of analytical (and sometimes destructive) techniques in human skeletal biology (see DiGangi and Moore [Chapter 2], this volume for a discussion of ethical issues). It cannot be understated that researchers in the twenty-first century must not take for granted the contributions of earlier scholars who originally perfected the ideas and procedures that now seem commonplace. Moreover, researchers must take exceptional care to thoroughly understand each step of a stable isotope project rather than proceeding with a rushed research design that does not take into account each step in the process. As other authors in this volume have stressed, perhaps the most important next step in planning a potential project is reading as much literature as one can so that each complex part of a stable isotopic project is well thought out from the beginning. Throughout the entire process, experienced mentors are invaluable; therefore, all interested skeletal biologists are urged to ally themselves with an experienced practitioner early on in the process.

In closing, stimulating new developments in stable isotope analysis have expanded to the forensic realm of skeletal biology, as investigators have employed these data to aid in the identification of unidentified individuals (Meier-Augenstein and Liu, 2004; Juarez, 2008; Meier-Augenstein and Fraser, 2008; Ehleringer et al., 2010). Certainly, as forensic applications of skeletal biology continue to mature around the globe, I suspect that uses of stable isotope analysis will continue to be tested so that benefits and limitations in forensic contexts are fully understood. Given the handful of skeletal biologists actively researching this topic in the United States, it stands to reason that much more work remains to be done. Regardless of one's specific interest in stable isotope analysis, it appears to me an ideal moment in our discipline's history to be getting started!

ACKNOWLEDGMENTS

I would like to thank the editors of this volume, Elizabeth A. DiGangi and Megan K. Moore, for the invitation to contribute this chapter. I would also like to thank Teresa Rosales, Victor Vasquez, Jonathan Kent, and Cathy Gaither for their collaboration on the Santa Rita B project. Stanley Ambrose's mentorship was invaluable while I was first learning about stable isotopes and Justin Glessner's cheerful explanations about the ICPMS were invaluable as well. The William M. Bass Endowment funded the analytical costs related to the case study presented here.

REFERENCES

Agarwal, S.C., 2008. Light and broken bones: examining and interpreting bone loss and osteoporosis in past populations. In: Katzenberg, M.A., Saunders, S.R. (Eds.), Biological Anthropology of the Human Skeleton, 2nd ed. Wiley-Liss, New York, pp. 387–410.

Ambrose, S.H., 1990. Preparation and characterization of bone and tooth collagen for isotopic analysis. Journal of Archaeological Science 17 (4), 431–451.

Ambrose, S.H., 1991. Effects of diet, climate, and physiology on nitrogen isotope abundances in terrestrial food-webs. Journal of Archaeological Science 18 (3), 293–317.

Ambrose, S.H., Norr, L., 1993. Experimental evidence for the relationship of the carbon isotope ratios of whole diet and dietary protein to those of bone collagen and carbonate. In: Lambert, J.B., Grupe, G. (Eds.), Prehistoric Human Bone: Archaeology at the Molecular Level. Springer-Verlag, Berlin, pp. 1–37.

Ambrose, S.H., Butler, B.M., Hanson, D.B., Hunter-Anderson, R.L., Krueger, H.W., 1997. Stable isotopic analysis of human diet in the Marianas archipelago, Western Pacific. American Journal of Physical Anthropology 104 (3), 343–361.

Ambrose, S.H., Buikstra, J.E., Krueger, H.W., 2003. Status and gender differences in diet at Mound 72, Cahokia, revealed by isotopic analysis of bone. Journal of Anthropological Archaeology 22 (3), 217–226.

Balasse, M., Ambrose, S.H., Smith, A.B., Price, T.D., 2002. The seasonal mobility model for prehistoric herders in the South-western Cape of South Africa assessed by isotopic analysis of sheep tooth enamel. Journal of Archaeological Science 29 (9), 917–932.

Barrie, A., Prosser, S.J., 1996. Automated analysis of light-element stable isotopes by isotope ratio mass spectrometry. In: Boutton, T.W., Yamasaki, S. (Eds.), Mass Spectrometry of Soils. Marcel Dekker, New York, pp. 1–46.

Bender, M.M., 1968. Mass spectrometric studies of carbon 13 variation in corn and other grasses. Radiocarbon 10 (2), 468–472.

Bentley, R.A., 2006. Strontium isotopes from the Earth to the archaeological skeleton: A review. Journal of Archaeological Method and Theory 35 (3), 82–91.

Blitz, J.H., 2010. New perspectives in Mississippian archaeology. Journal of Archaeological Research 18 (1), 1–39.

Brown, T., Brown, K., 2011. Stable Isotopes. Biomolecular Archaeology: An Introduction. Wiley-Blackwell, Malden, pp. 79–88.

Brown, T.A., Nelson, D.E., Vogel, J.S., Southon, J.R., 1988. Improved collagen extraction by modified Longin method. Radiocarbon 30 (2), 171–177.

Burger, R.L., Lee-Thorp, J.A., van der Merwe, N.J., 1990. Maize and the origin of highland Chavín civilization: an isotopic perspective. American Anthropologist 92 (1), 85–95.

Burton, J., 2008. Bone chemistry and trace element analysis. In: Katzenberg, M.A., Saunders, S.R. (Eds.), Biological Anthropology of the Human Skeleton, 2nd ed. Wiley-Liss, New York, pp. 443–460.

Cabana, G.S., Hulsey, B.I., Pack, F.L., 2013. Molecular methods. In: DiGangi, E.A., Moore, M.K. (Eds.), Research Methods in Human Skeletal Biology. Academic Press, San Diego.

Compston, W., 1960. The carbon isotopic composition of certain marine invertebrates and corals from the Australian Permian. Geochimica et Cosmochimica Acta 18 (1-2), 1–22.

Craig, H., 1954. Carbon 13 in plants and the relationships between carbon 13 and carbon 14 variations in nature. Journal of Geology 62 (2), 115–1149.

Deines, P., 1980. The isotopic composition of reduced organic carbon. In: Fritz, P., Fontes, J.C. (Eds.), Handbook of Environmental Isotope Geochemistry (The Terrestrial Environment). Elsevier, Amsterdam, pp. 329–406.

DeNiro, M.J., 1985. Postmortem preservation and alteration of *in vivo* bone collagen isotope ratios in relation to palaeodietary reconstruction. Nature 317 (6040), 806–809.

DeNiro, M.J., Epstein, S., 1981. Influence of diet on the distribution of nitrogen isotopes in animals. Geochimica et Cosmochimica Acta 45 (3), 341–351.

DeNiro, M.J., Schoeninger, M.J., 1983. Stable carbon and nitrogen isotope ratios of bone collagen: Variations within individuals, between sexes, and within populations raised on monotonous diets. Journal of Archaeological Science 10 (3), 199–203.

DiGangi, E.A., Moore, M.K., 2013. Introduction to skeletal biology. In: DiGangi, E.A., Moore, M.K. (Eds.), Research Methods in Human Skeletal Biology. Academic Press, San Diego.

DiGangi, E.A., Moore, M.K., 2013. Application of the scientific method to skeletal biology. In: DiGangi, E.A., Moore, M.K. (Eds.), Research Methods in Human Skeletal Biology. Academic Press, San Diego.

Doolittle, W.E., 2004. Permanent vs. shifting cultivation in the Eastern Woodlands of North America prior to European contact. Agriculture and Human Values 21 (2-3), 181–189.

Ehleringer, J.R., Thompson, A.H., Podlesak, D.W., Bowen, G.J., Chesson, L.A., Cerling, T.E., Park, T., Dostie, P., Schwarcz, H., 2010. A framework for the incorporation of isotopes and isoscapes in geospatial forensic investigations. In: West, J.B., Brown, G.J., Dawson, T.E., Tu, K.P. (Eds.), Isocapes: Understanding Movement, Pattern, and Process on Earth Through Isotope Mapping. Springer, Dordrecht, pp. 357–387.

Ericson, J.E., 1985. Strontium isotope characterization in the study of prehistoric human ecology. Journal of Human Evolution 14 (5), 503–514.

Ericson, J.E., West, M., Sullivan, C.H., Krueger, H.W., 1989. The development of maize agriculture in the Viru Valley of Peru. In: Price, T.D. (Ed.), The Chemistry of Prehistoric Human Bone. Cambridge University Press, Cambridge, pp. 68–104.

Finucane, B., Agurto, P.M., Isbell, W.H., 2006. Human and animal diet at Conchopata, Peru: stable isotope evidence for maize agriculture and animal management practices during the Middle Horizon. Journal of Archaeological Science 33 (12), 1766–1776.

Froehle, A.W., Kellner, C.M., Schoeninger, M.J., 2012. Multivariate carbon and nitrogen stable isotope model for the reconstruction of prehistoric human diet. American Journal of Physical Anthropology 147 (3), 352–369.

Gaither, C.M., Kent, J., Vásquez Sánchez, V., Rosales Tham, T., 2008. Mortuary practices in human sacrifice in the middle Chao valley of Peru: their interpretation in the context of Andean mortuary patterning. Latin American Antiquity 19 (2), 107–121.

Gaither, C.M., Bethard, J.D., Kent, J., Vásquez Sánchez, V., Rosales Tham, T., Busch, R., 2009. Strange harvest: a discussion of sacrifice and missing body parts on the north coast of Peru. Andean Past 9, 177–194.

Garvie-Lok, S.J., Varney, T.L., Katzenberg, M.A., 2004. Preparation of bone carbonate for stable isotope analysis: the effects of treatment time and acid concentration. Journal of Archaeological Science 31 (6), 763–776.

Gavelin, S., 1957. Variations in isotopic composition of carbon from metamorphic rocks in Northern Sweden and their geological significance. Geochimica et Cosmochimica Acta 12 (4), 297–314.

Gil, A.F., Neme, G.A., Ugan, A., Tykot, R.H., 2011. Oxygen isotopes and human residential mobility in central western Argentina. Journal of Archaeological Science. http://dx.doi.org/10.1002/oa.1304.

Griffin, J.B., 1967. Eastern North American archaeology: a summary. Science 156 (3772), 175–191.

Hall, R.L., 1967. Those late corn dates: isotopic fractionation as a source of error in carbon-14 dates. Michigan Archaeologist 13 (4), 171–180.

Hammerl, E., 2013. Dental anthropology. In: DiGangi, E.A., Moore, M.K. (Eds.), Research Methods in Human Skeletal Biology. Academic Press, San Diego.

Harrison, R.G., Katzenberg, M.A., 2003. Paleodiet studies using stable carbon isotopes from bone apatite and collagen: examples from Southern Ontario and San Nicolas Island, California. Journal of Anthropological Archaeology 22 (3), 227–244.

Heaton, T.H.E., Vogel, J.C., von la Chevallerie, Collet, G., 1986. Climatic influence on the isotopic composition of bone nitrogen. Nature 322 (6082), 822–823.

Hedges, R.E.M., 2003. On bone collagen—apatite—carbonate isotopic relationships. International Journal of Osteoarchaeology 13 (1-2), 66–79.

Hoefs, J., 2009. Stable Isotope Geochemistry, 6th ed. Springer-Verlag, Berlin.

Howland, M.R., Corr, L.T., Young, S.M.M., Jones, V., Jim, S., van der Merwe, N.J., Mitchell, A.D., Evershed, R.P., 2003. Expression of the dietary isotope signal in the compound-specific $\delta^{13}C$ value of pig bone lipids and amino acids. International Journal of Osteoarchaeology 13 (1-2), 54–65.

Juarez, C.A., 2008. Strontium and geolocation, the pathway to identification for deceased undocumented Mexican border-crossers: a preliminary report. Journal of Forensic Sciences 53 (1), 46–49.

Katzenberg, M.A., 2008. Stable isotope analysis: A tool for studying past diet, demography, and life history. In: Katzenberg, M.A., Saunders, S.R. (Eds.), Biological Anthropology of the Human Skeleton, 2nd ed. Wiley-Liss, New York, pp. 413–442.

Katzenberg, M.A., Kelly, J.H., 1991. Stable isotope analysis of prehistoric bone from the Sierra Blanca region of New Mexico. In: Beckett, P.H. (Ed.), Mogollon V: Proceedings of the 1988 Mogollon Conference. COAS Publishing and Research, Las Cruces, NM, pp. 207–209.

Katzenberg, M.A., Weber, A., 1999. Stable isotope ecology and paleodiet in the Lake Baikal Region of Siberia. Journal of Archaeological Science 26 (6), 651–659.

Kellner, C.M., Schoeninger, M.J., 2007. A simple carbon isotope model for reconstructing prehistoric human diet. American Journal of Physical Anthropology 133 (4), 1112–1127.

Knudson, K.J., Tung, T.A., 2007. Using archaeological chemistry to investigate the geographic origin of trophy heads in the Central Andes. In: Glascock, M.D., Speakman, R.J., Popelka-Filcoff, R. (Eds.), Archaeological Chemistry: Analytical Techniques and Archaeological Interpretation. American Chemical Society, Washington, D.C., pp. 99–113.

Knudson, K.J., 2009. Oxygen isotope analysis in a land of environmental extremes: the complexities of isotopic work in the Andes. International Journal of Osteoarchaeology 19, 171–191.

Knudson, K.J., Tung, T.A., Nystrom, K.C., Price, T.D., Fullagar, P.D., 2005. The origin of the Juch'uypampa Cave mummies: strontium isotope analysis of archaeological human remains from Bolivia. Journal of Archaeological Science 32 (6), 903–913.

Knudson, K.J., Aufderheide, A.C., Buikstra, J.E., 2007. Seasonality and paleodiet in the Chiribaya polity of southern Peru. Journal of Archaeological Science 34 (3), 1–12.

Knudson, K.J., Williams, S.R., Osborn, R., Forgey, K., Williams, P.R., 2009. The geographic origins of Nasca trophy heads using strontium, oxygen, and carbon isotope data. Journal of Archaeological Science 28 (2), 244–257.

Knudson, K.J., O'Donnabhain, B., Carver, C., Cleland, R., Price, T.D., 2012. Migration and Viking Dublin: paleo-mobility and paleodiet through isotopic analyses. Journal of Archaeological Science 39 (2), 308–320.

Kroman, A.M., Symes, S.A., 2013. Investigation of Skeletal trauma. In: DiGangi, E.A., Moore, M.K. (Eds.), Research Methods in Human Skeletal Biology. Academic Press, San Diego.

Krueger, H.W., Sullivan, C.H., 1984. Models for carbon isotope fractionation between diet and bone. In: Turnlund, J.E., Johnson, P.E. (Eds.), Stable Isotopes and Nutrition. American Chemical Society, Washington, D.C.

Lee-Thorp, J.A., van der Merwe, N.J., 1991. Aspects of the chemistry of modern and fossil biological apatites. Journal of Archaeological Science 18 (3), 343–354.

Lee-Thorp, J.A., Sealy, J.C., 1989. van der Merwe, N.J., 1989. Stable carbon isotope ratio differences between bone collagen and bone apatite, and their relationship to diet. Journal of Archaeological Science 16 (6), 585–599.

Longin, R., 1971. New method of collagen extraction for radiocarbon dating. Nature 230 (5291), 241–242.

Lynott, M.J., Boutton, T.W., Price, J.E., Nelson, D.W., 1986. Stable carbon isotopic evidence for maize agriculture in southeast Missouri and northeast Arkansas. American Antiquity 51 (1), 51–65.

Marden, K., Sorg, M.H., Haglund, W.D., 2013. Taphonomy. In: DiGangi, E.A., Moore, M.K. (Eds.), Research Methods in Human Skeletal Biology. Academic Press, San Diego.

Meier-Augenstein, W., Fraser, I., 2008. Forensic isotope analysis leads to identification of a mutilated murder victim. Science & Justice 48 (3), 153–159.

Meier-Augenstein, W., Liu, R.H., 2004. Forensic applications of isotope ratio mass spectrometry. In: Yinon, J. (Ed.), Advances in Forensic Applications of Mass Spectrometry. CRC Press, Boca Raton, pp. 149–180.

Moseley, M.E., Cordy-Collins, A., 1991. The Northern Dynasties: Kingship and Statecraft in Chimor. Dumbarton Oaks, Washington, D.C.

O'Leary, M.H., 1988. Carbon isotopes in photosynthesis. Bioscience 38 (5), 328–336.

Petford, N., Atherton, M.P., Halliday, A.N., 1996. Rapid magma production rates, underplating and remelting in the Andes: isotopic evidence from northern-central Peru (9—11°S). Journal of South American Earth Sciences 9 (1/2), 69—78.

Pillsbury, J., 2001. Moche Art and Archaeology in Ancient PeruNational Gallery of Art, Washington, D.C.

Prowse, T.L., Schwarcz, H.P., Garnsey, P., Knyr, M., Macchiarelli, R., Bondioli, L., 2007. Isotopic evidence for age-related immigration to imperial Rome. American Journal of Physical Anthropology 132 (4), 510—519.

Richards, M., Harvati, K., Grimes, V., Smith, C., Smith, T., Hublin, J., Karkanas, P., Panagopoulou, E., 2008. Strontium isotope evidence of Neanderthal mobility at the site Lakonis, Greece using laser-ablation PIMMS. Journal of Archaeological Science 35 (5), 1251—1256.

Schoeninger, M.J., DeNiro, M.J., 1983. Stable nitrogen isotope ratios of bone collagen reflect marine and terrestrial components of prehistoric human diet. Science 220 (4604), 1381—1383.

Schoeninger, M.J., DeNiro, M.J., 1984. Nitrogen and carbon isotopic composition of bone collagen from marine and terrestrial animals. Geochimica et Cosmochimica Acta 48 (4), 625—639.

Schoeninger, M.J., Moore, K.M., 1992. Bone stable isotope studies in archaeology. Journal of World Prehistory 6 (2), 247—296.

Sealy, J.C., 1986. Stable carbon isotopes and prehistoric diets in the southwestern Cape Province. South Africa. British Archaeological Reports International Series 293, Oxford.

Smith, M.O., 2013. Paleopathology. In: DiGangi, E.A., Moore, M.K. (Eds.), Research Methods in Human Skeletal Biology. Academic Press, San Diego.

Sponheimer, M., Lee-Thorp, J.A., 1999. Isotopic evidence for the diet of an early hominid, *Australopithecus africanus*. Science 283 (5400), 368—370.

Sponheimer, M., Passey, B., de Ruiter, D., Guatelli-Sternberg, D., Cerling, T., Lee-Thorp, J., 2006. Isotopic evidence for dietary flexibility in the early hominin. *Paranthropus robustus*. Science 314 (5801), 980—982.

Sutter, R.C., Cortez, R.J., 2005. The nature of Moche human sacrifice: a bio-archaeological perspective. Current Anthropology 46 (4), 521—549.

Sutter, R.C., Verano, J.W., 2007. Biodistance analysis of the Moche scarification victims from Huaca de la Luna plaza 3C: matrix method test of their origins. American Journal of Physical Anthropology 132 (2), 193—206.

Tieszen, L.L., Fagre, T., 1993. Effect of diet quality and composition on the isotopic composition of respiratory CO_2, bone collagen, bioapatite and soft tissues. In: Lambert, J.B., Grupe, G. (Eds.), Prehistoric Human Bone: Archaeology at the Molecular Level. Springer-Verlag, Berlin, pp. 121—155.

Tomczak, P.D., 2003. Prehistoric diet and socioeconomic relationships within the Osmore Valley of southern Peru. Journal of Anthropological Archaeology 22 (3), 262—278.

Trammell, L.H., Kroman, A.M., 2013. Bone and dental histology. In: DiGangi, E.A., Moore, M.K. (Eds.), Research Methods in Human Skeletal Biology. Academic Press, San Diego.

Turner, B.L., Andrushko, V.A., 2011. Partnerships, pitfalls, and ethical concerns in international bioarchaeology. In: Agarwal, S.C., Glencross, B.A. (Eds.), Social Bioarchaeology. John Wiley & Sons, Malden, pp. 44—67.

Turner, B.L., Kamenov, G.D., Kingston, J.D., Armelagos, G.J., 2009. Insights into immigration and social class at Machu Picchu, Perú based on oxygen, strontium, and lead analysis. Journal of Archaeological Science 36 (2), 317—332.

Tuross, N., Fogel, M.L., Hare, P.E., 1988. Variability in the preservation of the isotopic composition of collagen from fossil bone. Geochimica et Cosmochimica Acta 52 (4), 929—935.

Tykot, R.H., 2006. Isotope analyses and the histories of maize. In: Staller, J., Tykot, R., Benz, B. (Eds.), Histories of Maize: Multidisciplinary Approaches to the Prehistory, Linguistics, Biogeography, Domestication, and Evolution of Maize. Academic Press, San Diego, pp. 130—141.

van Klinken, G.J., 1999. Bone collagen quality indicators for palaeodietary and radiocarbon measurements. Journal of Archaeological Science 26 (6), 687—695.

Vogel, J.C., van der Merwe, N.J., 1977. Isotopic evidence for early maize cultivation in New York State. American Antiquity 42 (2), 238—242.

White, C.D., Spence, M.W., Stuart-Williams, H.L.Q., Schwarcz, H.P., 1998. Oxygen isotopes and the identification of geographical origins: the Valley of Oaxaca versus the Valley of Mexico. Journal of Archaeological Sciences 25 (7), 643—655.

Molecular Methods

Graciela S. Cabana, Brannon I. Hulsey, Frankie L. Pack

INTRODUCTION

Anthropological use of molecular data has grown tremendously in the last decade. This phenomenon has contributed to an increased enthusiasm towards long-standing anthropological debates, such as human origins, our relationship to extant and extinct human and nonhuman primates, and the pattern and meaning behind global and local human variation.

More than simply adding another corroborating line of evidence (à la Chamberlin, 1965), recent molecular methods have added to, and even upturned, previous knowledge. Perhaps the most prominent example is in the Neandertal—modern human debate. From the 1990s onward, the consensus among scientists was that Neandertals effectively contributed nothing, genetically speaking, to modern human variation. However, because of technological breakthroughs of the last decade, we now have genetic evidence not only for the interbreeding of Neandertals and modern humans (Green et al., 2010), but also for interbreeding among other archaic humans, Neandertals, and modern humans in differing proportions in different parts of the Old World (Reich et al., 2010).

As this chapter will show, the use of molecular methods in anthropology has been around since at least the early twentieth century. In the last decade, we have been witnessing an unprecedented shift in our ability to access much more of the genome due to rapid technological advances, large-scale initiatives for data collection, and a parallel development of population databases, many of which are freely accessible and ever-growing. Accessing more of the genome combined with the mathematical and computational power to draw significant associations means that those questions that have been plaguing us for the better part of a century can now be feasibly addressed.

This chapter is intended to function as a practical guide to incorporating molecular methods into the skeletal biologist's research program. How are molecular methods relevant, and how does the aspiring skeletal biologist/geneticist use them? The chapter begins with a brief history of the use and role of genetics in anthropology from the 1900s to the present. The chapter moves on to provide some of the key theoretical, methodological, and interpretive understandings needed to develop a molecular complement to skeletal biological research. At that point the chapter turns to the practicalities of initiating a molecular study

E.A. DiGangi and M.K. Moore: Research Methods in Human Skeletal Biology

based on bones and teeth as data sources. The chapter wraps up with a vision for future research directions in the combined field of genetics and skeletal biology.

GENETICS AND GENOMICS

The word **genetics**[1] was first coined in 1906 by William Batson, a British biologist, to refer to the study of heredity and the science of variation; the word comes from a set of related Greek words referring to "birth" or "origin." Following this original sense, "genetics" is currently used, first and foremost, as an overarching term for the study of biological inheritance, which can cover the pattern, structure, function, and behavior of genes within an organism's **genome** (the entirety of an organism's hereditary information) and their transfer to new generations of organisms. Numerous definitions of "gene" exist, but George C. Williams' (1996) general definition best meets the purposes of this chapter: a **gene** is "any portion of chromosomal material that potentially lasts for enough generations to serve as a unit of natural selection."

Today, scientists are using powerful new tools for sequencing the genomes of entire organisms, including humans. These advances are expected to improve our understanding of how multiple genes and gene products interact with other genes and environmental factors. The term **genomics** is often used to denote both these advanced sequencing capabilities and a more complex model interaction. Many times researchers will use the term "genomics" instead of "genetics," yet "genomics" should be formally subsumed under "genetics." What is meant by this separation of terms? Many people associate the term "genetics" with a singular focus on single genes along with the application of classic Mendelian principles of inheritance in which one gene represents one trait. From this perspective, genetics is the study of single genes and their effects, and genomics is the study of the functions and interactions of all the genetic material in the genome, including interactions with environmental factors.

Anthropologists in general have not been concerned with the study of genes *per se*, but rather with single or a few markers to reconstruct those biological and social processes that have contributed to the history of human groups. Today, we find ourselves in the so-called "genomic era," which has brought to anthropological inquiry a tremendous explosion in the number of available markers (hundreds of thousands), with the potential to look at the entire genome (all 3 billion base pairs) at little cost[2] in the next few years.

GENETICS IN ANTHROPOLOGY

The use of genetics in anthropology gained traction with the early discovery of **monogenic traits** in blood, so called because their inheritance was presumed to be due to the action of single or very few genes. The early twentieth century saw the discovery of blood types

---

[1] All bolded terms are defined in the glossary at the end of this volume.

[2] As of this writing, it is possible to sequence a genome for as little as $1000. It is probable that in the next five to ten years that cost will go down even further. This is astounding considering that the first low-resolution draft of the human genome came in at a final cost of $3 billion!

(also known as blood groups). A blood type is a classification of blood based on the presence or absence of inherited molecular substances (called **antigens**) on the surface of red blood cells. By the mid-1900s, multiple blood group types had been discovered, as had similar protein systems. Anthropologists quickly recognized the potential of blood and protein groups for the study of variation within and among human groups. Because monogenic blood groups and proteins were considered to be more fundamental substances than gross anatomical polygenic features (such as any found on the skeleton), they were also considered to be more useful for the overt classification of human variation; they subsequently formed the basis of the "genetical method" of early to mid-twentieth century physical anthropology (Boyd, 1939, 1963).

The field of "anthropological genetics" had its effective beginnings in the 1950s, though it truly began to assert itself in the 1970s (see Crawford and Workman, 1973). While some physical anthropologists continued to focus their research on the classificatory potential of blood groups and proteins (now known as **classical markers**), others kept their eye on theoretical developments in mathematical theory as applied to evolution (also known as **population genetics**), as well as in genetics, biology, and computer science. These fields, combined with the classical anthropological concern of local and regional biological variation and adaptation led to the new research program of **anthropological genetics**, aptly defined in 1980 by Derek F. Roberts as "the study of the genetic variation that occurs within and between human populations, its origin, and the factors and processes that maintain it" (1980:419). Indeed, the anthropological genetics research agenda from the 1950s through the 1990s was to document evolutionary process in small, highly isolated, non-Western human groups. In addition, anthropological geneticists began to engage in the mathematical modeling of **polygenic traits**, or traits presumed to be controlled by multiple genes (also, "complex" traits). These include disease traits as well as skeletal and other anatomical features.

Advances in genetic technology first spurred the onset of a "molecular revolution" in the 1990s, and later, the "genomic revolution" of the 2000s. In response, the field of anthropological genetics has been shifting in emphasis from the characterization of **population structure** (how populations are subdivided, if at all, into local or subpopulations) to the study of human origins and diaspora. In addition, the trend now is movement from indirect inference to direct analysis of the genetic component of traits by actual mapping of genes and associated genomic regions. This most recent trend is reflected in the most current definition of anthropological genetics as "a synthetic discipline that applies the methods and theories of genetics to evolutionary questions posed by anthropologists" (Crawford, 2007:1). See Table 16.1.

For More Information …

The history of the field of anthropological genetics from the 1950s/70s onwards can be easily tracked by reading through the successive series of edited volumes by Michael Crawford (University of Kansas) and colleagues. These are, in chronological order: *Methods and Theories of Anthropological Genetics* (Crawford and Workman, 1973), *Current Developments in Anthropological Genetics, Volume I, Theory and Methods* (Mielke and Crawford, 1980), *Current Developments in Anthropological Genetics, Volume II, Ecology and Population Structure* (Crawford

TABLE 16.1   Genetics in Anthropology: Historical Time Table

Time Period	Development
1900s–1950s	Development of blood and protein groups for the purposes of typological classification
1950s–1980s	The field of "anthropological genetics" takes off, with emphasis on evolutionary principles. Researchers begin to document evolutionary processes in small, highly isolated, non-Western human groups. They also become interested in complex traits
1980s–1990s	Development of PCR (polymerase chain reaction) launches "molecular revolution." Interest shifts to question of human origins and migrations, as well as gene mapping
2000s–present	Development of high-throughput sequencing launches "genomic era"

and Mielke, 1980), and *Anthropological Genetics: Theory, Methods and Applications* (Crawford, 2007).

INCORPORATING GENETICS INTO ANTHROPOLOGICAL RESEARCH: WHAT DO I NEED TO KNOW?

As an aspiring user of genetic tools to address anthropological questions, you will need an understanding of the theoretical, methodological, and interpretive aspects of anthropological genetics. Essentially, what you will be looking to do is use genetic data to evaluate similarities and differences, through time and space, between two or more samples. This section will review theory, method, and interpretation of genetic data.

1. Theory

First, you will need a basis for "similarity" and "difference" as it relates to genetic data. This basis relies on the concept of **population**. Regardless how much genetic information you have about any particular individual(s), all that information is meaningless without context. For example, if an individual demonstrates a particular genetic variant,[3] should we consider that variant to be rare or frequent? Does its presence help differentiate that individual from any other? Is that variant clearly associated with a particular trait of interest, such as a disease state? Is it functional? Alternatively, does it mean nothing? To address these questions, we use the concept of "population"—the one from which the individual (and her genome) was drawn, and/or other populations. The answer to the question "What defines a population?" depends on the research question, and for this reason, it is easier to think

---

[3]For example, that person may have the DNA base "A" in a certain location (or **locus**) on the genome, while others may have a "T." Here, the relatively generic term "genetic variant" is taking the place of the more specialized term "allele" that is defined in the glossary and also defined later in the chapter.

of the concept of "population" as simply the "sample" being used (see also DiGangi and Moore [Chapter 1], this volume).

Evolutionary theory comes into play for understanding the context of genetic data through time. **Evolution** simply refers to change over time in one or more inherited traits found in populations of organisms, and evolutionary theory attempts to provide explanatory mechanisms for that change. Four classic explanatory mechanisms—(1) mutation, (2) genetic drift, (3) gene flow, and (4) natural selection—are often referred to as the "forces of evolution."

The Four Forces of Evolution

Although any of the four forces alone, or in combination, can act to change frequencies of genetic variants in populations from one generation to the next, **mutation** is the ultimate source of new genetic variation. A mutation is a change in the DNA sequence of an organism, and is only of potential evolutionary importance if it is inherited by one or more offspring. This means that even though an individual may develop a mutation, and is somehow affected by it (for better or for worse), if it is not passed on to future generations, it will not have an impact on the population.

Genetic drift refers to changes in the frequency of gene variants, or **alleles**, in a population due to random sampling. Random sampling of alleles in a population context can occur in multiple ways. For example, alleles present in offspring are a random sample of those in the parents. Whether a given individual survives long enough to reproduce could be determined by chance events, such as a fatal car crash or a natural disaster. From one generation to the next, the combined and accumulated effect of these random processes may be to drive one or more alleles to the point of disappearing entirely from a population, thereby reducing overall population genetic variation.

Mutational changes can counteract the variation-reducing effect of genetic drift in a population by introducing new variation, as can **gene flow**. Gene flow is simply the movement of alleles from one population to another via people mating with individuals outside of their own group. Even though genetic drift may be culling variants from a population over time, gene flow provides a constant replenishment of alleles, depending on its rate (i.e. how many individuals, along with their gene variants, mate between populations every generation). On the whole, gene flow introduces new genetic variation into a population at a much faster rate than does mutation.

The last evolutionary force is **natural selection**. Natural selection is the process by which alleles become more or less common in a population because of factors impinging on the survival and reproduction of their bearers. Natural selection acts on the expressed characteristics (i.e., the **phenotype**) of an organism, such as all the factors that help a hare outrun a hungry cheetah, including long legs, fast twitch muscle fibers in the right places, and small size for hiding in hard-to-reach places. Only those heritable aspects of any phenotype (i.e., the **genotype**) that confer advantages in survival and reproduction will ultimately become more common in a population. Over time, this process can result in adaptations that specialize populations for particular environments (be they ecological or social) and may eventually result in the development of a new species.

Box 16.1 gives some examples of how each of these four forces has impacted human evolution and variation.

BOX 16.1
_____

EVOLUTIONARY FORCES IN HUMAN HISTORY

As explained in the main text, the four classic evolutionary forces—mutation, gene flow, genetic drift, and natural selection work in concert with each other, though the evolutionary history of a trait or traits can be shaped primarily by one or two of these "forces" relative to the rest. Here are some examples of how this can happen.

Mutation and Natural Selection: The Case of Lactase Persistence

Lactase is the enzyme responsible for the digestion of the milk sugar called lactose. Lactase production decreases after the weaning phase in most humans, at which point the typical individual becomes lactose intolerant and experiences digestive upset (gas, bloating, and/or diarrhea) upon the consumption of fresh milk. Some people, however, continue to produce lactase into adulthood, a trait known as lactase persistence, or LP. LP is a genetically controlled trait that is found at moderate to high frequencies in European (particularly northern), some African, Middle Eastern, and Southern Asian populations.[4]

It turns out that the condition has evolved independently in at least four places around the globe and a number of different mutations have been found in association with the LP trait. What explains the high frequency of LP alleles in only certain populations? Genetic drift and gene flow have probably played a role, but here is a case in which natural selection is a more compelling candidate. Age estimates in terms of the antiquity of lactase persistence-associated alleles coincide with those for the origins of animal domestication and the cultural practice of dairying.[5] Though humans were likely consuming milk products

before these LP gene variants arose, they had to remove the milk's lactose through fermentation and at the same time lose 20–50% of its calories. In situations of sporadic famines, those additional calories obtained through LP could aid tremendously in survival and reproduction. This appears to not be coincidental, as lactase persistence can be evolutionarily advantageous.[6]

Genetic Drift: The Case of the Initial Peopling of the Americas

The topic of the peopling of the Americas has captivated anthropological audiences for decades now, and not without numerous points of contention. Anthropologists do tend to agree on one thing, however: that the primary original entry point of humans onto the American continents was likely through the Bering Strait in northern Alaska. This suggests that humans experienced a **founder effect**, or a loss of genetic variation that occurs when a very small number of individuals from a larger population establish a new population, in this case, in a new continent. This could have profound implications on the pattern of morphological and genetic variation in the Americas.

In the past decade and a half, genetic studies have provided some evidence for a strong founder effect. Broad, worldwide surveys of genetic variation have demonstrated that both ancient and modern Native Americans harbor a subset of the variation found in Asia. MtDNA provides the clearest example: currently, populations in Asia demonstrate ca. eight to ten broad mtDNA lineages, whereas Native Americans show five of those. For a recent review, see Kemp and Schurr (2010).[7]

(Continued)

BOX 16.1   *(cont'd)*

Gene Flow: A Hypothetical-but-Easy-to-Imagine-in-Real-Life Case Study

Imagine that a group of blue-eyed Danes moves to a small village in Zaire, in which all Zairians without exception have brown eyes. This sudden influx of gene variants that lead to blue eyes being present in the Zairian village is gene flow. The blue eye version (or allele) of an eye color gene has flowed into the population. Before the movement of blue-eyed people into the village, the Zairian village population had 100% brown alleles, whereas afterwards, it becomes more like 30% blue to 70% brown alleles. The gene frequency of the blue allele

has increased in this village population due to gene flow.

[4]Itan, Y., Jones, B.L., Ingram, C.J., Swallow, D.M., Thomas, M.G., 2010. A worldwide correlation of lactase persistence phenotype and genotypes. BMC Evolutionary Biology 10, 36, online publication.
[5]Gerbault, P., Liebert, A., Itan, Y., Powell, A., Burger, J., Swallow, D.M., Thomas, M.G., 2011. Evolution of lactase persistence: an example of human niche construction. Philosophical Transactions of the Royal Society London, B, Biological Sciences 366, 863-877.
[6]Cochran, G., Harpending, H., 2009. The 10,000 Year Explosion: How Civilization Accelerated Human Evolution. Basic Books, New York.
[7]Kemp, B.K., Schurr, T.G., 2010. Ancient and modern genetic variation in the Americas. In Auerbach, B.M. (Ed.), Human Variation in the Americas: The Integration of Archaeology and Biological Anthropology. Center for Archaeological Investigations, Carbondale, IL, pp. 12–50.

Population Genetics

The field of population genetics concerns itself with understanding how these evolutionary forces combine with population demography to ultimately produce evolutionary change short and long term. Since about the 1920s, population geneticists have been developing analytical (mathematical) and simulation models that are used to evaluate actual, observed genetic data vis-à-vis hypothetical evolutionary scenarios. Many of the interpretive tools presented below are based on innovations in population genetic theory.

Population genetic theory is important to understanding **population structure** and its history. Population structure is the study of the relationship between group composition (including size), mating practices, and genetic drift. Studies of population structure ask what mechanisms impact the observed pattern in the genetic variation of populations. Studies of **population history** ask whether any similarities or differences in population structure between two or more populations are due to a shared ancestry or mate exchange (Harpending and Jenkins, 1973).

This concept of "**population history**" is often contrasted with that of "**adaptive history**." When embarking on an investigation of population history, you are essentially attempting to understand what factors have shaped genetic variation in your sample, except for natural selection. In contrast, an investigation of adaptive history is a study of the history of natural selection on one or more traits exhibited by the population sample in question.

To conduct a population history study, the most straightforward way is to deliberately search out genomic regions that have not been affected by natural selection, that is, regions that are "selectively neutral." A classic study by Cann and colleagues (1987) provides a good example: These authors were the first to use mitochondrial DNA (See What Constitutes Genetic Data?, below) to argue that modern humans must have arisen in Africa about 200,000 years ago. They did this by looking at variation within the mitochondrial genomes of 147 people distributed worldwide, and found that individuals from the sub-Saharan part of Africa exhibited the most amount of genetic variation. More variation requires more time to accumulate. From an estimate of the average mitochondrial DNA mutation rate, the authors were able to say something about how long that variation must have taken to accumulate—about 200,000 years.

In contrast, for a study of adaptive history, researchers target genomic regions thought to be in some way largely genetically responsible for specific trait(s). A recent example is the study by Perry and colleagues (2007), which tapped into the idea that individuals can (and do) have multiple copies of a gene, and that population differences can exist in the average number of copies that individuals will have. In their study, the researchers looked at the number of copies of the particular gene responsible for the production of salivary amylase proteins among individuals in different populations. It turns out that higher numbers of copies of the salivary amylase gene tend to be found in populations that have historically relied on high starch diets, and lower numbers of copies in those that have not. The inference here is that natural selection has favored higher numbers of copies in those groups relying on starchy foods.

Genotype and Phenotype

Genotype refers to the heritable information carried by all living organisms. Phenotype is the product of the interaction between genotype and "environmental" factors. Some phenotypes are almost completely determined by heredity, such as blood groups (discussed earlier), but most, such as human height, are also greatly impacted by nonhereditary factors, such as nutrition.

At a fundamental level we are concerned with changes in the genotypes that make up a population from generation to generation when talking about evolution. Additionally, since an organism's genotype generally affects its phenotype, the phenotypes that make up the population are also likely to change.

To Learn More …

There is much, much more to learn about the topics of evolution and evolutionary theory, including population genetics. Unfortunately this cannot all be covered within a subsection of a single book chapter. Please consult the myriad of existing textbooks on evolution (such as Futuyma, 2009 or Ridley, 2004) and population genetics (for example, Hartl and Clark, 2006).

2. Method

What Constitutes Genetic Data?

What follows is a detailed explanation of those aspects of the human genome on which researchers are currently focused. This explanation applies to researchers who deal with DNA from living, recently deceased, and ancient organisms.

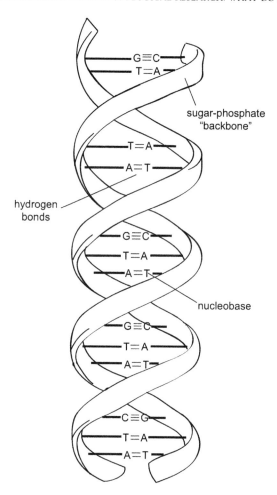

FIGURE 16.1 Stylized DNA double helix.

At the most basic level, genetic data consist of one or more DNA **bases**. **DNA**,[8] or DeoxyriboNucleic Acid, is structured like a twisted ladder, with paired bases comprising the rungs, and a repetitive chain of a sugar (deoxyribose) and a phosphate forming the ladder's sides (Figure 16.1). The bases are **nucleobases** known as Adenine (A), Guanine (G), Cytosine (C), and Thymine (T). In a DNA molecule, these will bond in complementary pairs, with A always pairing with T via two hydrogen bonds, and C always pairing with G via three hydrogen bonds. The combination of a sugar, phosphate, and a single base is known as a **nucleotide**.

In all eukaryotic cells, such as those of humans, DNA can be found in two locations—in the nucleus and in the mitochondria of the cell (Figure 16.2). The nucleus is defined as simply

---

[8]Table 16.2 provides a listing of all the acronyms used in this chapter.

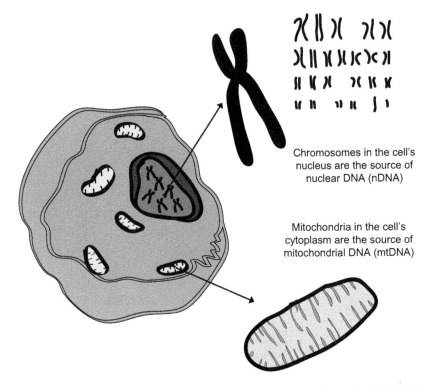

Chromosomes in the cell's
nucleus are the source of
nuclear DNA (nDNA)

Mitochondria in the cell's
cytoplasm are the source of
mitochondrial DNA (mtDNA)

FIGURE 16.2   Eukaryotic cell showing locations of nuclear and mitochondrial DNA.

that structure within the cell that houses the bulk of an organism's hereditary information, or DNA. Mitochondria (singular, mitochondrion), as the "powerhouses" of the cell, are located within the bounds of the cell membrane in the thick liquid called cytoplasm, but outside of the nucleus. DNA housed in the nucleus is called nuclear DNA, or **nDNA**, while DNA housed in mitochondria is called mitochondrial DNA, or **mtDNA**.

In humans, nuclear DNA is packaged into 23 pairs of **chromosomes**, including a pair of sex chromosomes. Nuclear DNA is, for the most part, biparentally inherited: each of your biological parents contributed approximately half of your DNA. The only exception to this is a significant portion of the male sex chromosome, the Y chromosome. Over 95% of the Y chromosome is inherited relatively intact from the biological father and is referred to as the **NRY**, or NonRecombining Y (also **MSY**, or Male-Specific Y) (Figure 16.3).

Mitochondrial DNA is inherited exclusively from the mother; males do not contribute mitochondria to offspring. A female's reproductive cell, the ovum (egg), contains within it a set of 23 chromosomes in a nucleus, plus copies of maternal mitochondria. Though the male reproductive cell, or sperm, does have mitochondria (mostly wrapped around the tail to power its movement), its mitochondria fail to enter and are quickly degraded upon contact with the egg.

In sum, while most nuclear DNA is biparentally inherited, the NRY and mtDNA are uniparentally inherited. Only sons inherit the NRY from their fathers, but both sons and

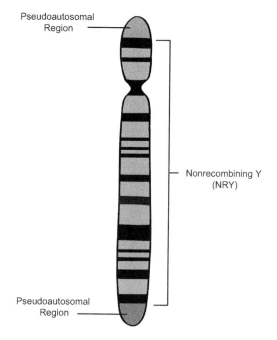

FIGURE 16.3   Basic structure of the human Y chromosome.

TABLE 16.2   Molecular Acronyms

Acronym	Full Name
DNA	Deoxyribonucleic Acid
mtDNA	Mitochondrial DNA
MSY	Male-Specific Y (chromosome)
nDNA	Nuclear DNA
NRY	Nonrecombining Y (chromosome)
PCR	Polymerase Chain Reaction
RNA	Ribonucleic Acid
SNP	Single Nucleotide Polymorphism
STR	Short Tandem Repeat

daughters inherit their mitochondrial DNA from their mothers (but only daughters can pass on their mtDNA to offspring).

These different modes of inheritance have important implications for genetic analysis. Nuclear DNA contains within it the genomic information of all your ancestors, but it is not possible to track which exact bits of DNA came from which specific ancestors because it has gone through so much reshuffling. Because the NRY and mtDNA genome are inherited virtually intact from each parent, genetic information can be clearly assigned to either the paternal or maternal lineage, respectively.

Molecular Markers

DNA consists of two strands connected by "rungs" of complementary bases (i.e., it is double stranded). Each strand contains approximately 3 billion bases. If we consider the total number of bases contained in both strands, the count doubles to 6 billion.

Probably within the next five to ten years, it will be possible to analyze all 6 billion bases contained within a single human individual's genome at once. However, at present, both cost and technology are limiting factors, so we take shortcuts to obtaining genetic information by targeting molecular **markers** instead. A "marker" is any informative region of the genome that is either nonprotein coding and therefore selectively neutral, or is protein coding and therefore potentially subject to selection. The particular research interests dictate whether or not any particular region of the genome is informative, and therefore if it may qualify as a "marker."

Currently, researchers regularly utilize three types of markers—**SNPs**, **STRs**, and more rarely, *Alu* elements—each of which will be explained further in this section. Though the human genome literally consists of linear arrays of bases arranged into chromosomes, this doesn't mean that all genomic regions behave in the same way, or that they impart the same kind of information. Some genomic sites develop mutational changes frequently (i.e., from one generation to the next) and others do not; the difference has to do with the biochemistry of the genomic regions themselves. Some genomic regions even contain molecular tools to virtually "cut and paste" themselves from one part of the genome to another!

SINGLE NUCLEOTIDE POLYMORPHISM (SNP)

The simplest form of genetic variant is a Single Nucleotide Polymorphism, or SNP (pronounced "snip"). An SNP is a difference in a single base in a particular location on the genome (i.e., at a particular nucleotide position). At the moment, researchers are not interested in *unique* SNPs (those present only in a single or in a very few individuals) precisely because they cannot be used to provide information about any random individual drawn from a population sample. This may change as the cost of obtaining and storing information on whole genomes decreases.

SNPs can take one of three forms: a single base change (for example, some individuals have an A at a genomic site while others may have a C, G, or T), an insertion of base, or a deletion of a base in a DNA sequence. SNPs are common throughout both nuclear and mitochondrial genomes.

Though they are common, the chances of a SNP developing as the result of a mutation is low; it is estimated that an SNP will occur once in every 10^8 bases per generation (Kruglyak, 1999). Because it is relatively unusual for a new mutational change to occur in any particular genomic location in an individual, and for it to become prevalent in a population over time, SNPs tend to be most useful in addressing questions of long-term evolutionary significance. For example, if researchers were to find two individuals in a population sharing an A at a particular genomic site, we would assume that they likely share that A because at some point back in time they shared an ancestor who had developed the "A" mutation, and not because they both happened to develop the mutation independently.

Also, because SNP differences are so rare relative to other DNA markers, and because any single individual will only present at most one of four possibilities at that SNP site (an A, G,

C, or T), it is not feasible to use one or a handful of known SNPs to discriminate among individuals in any given population. However, technological advances have progressed to the point that it is now possible to type several hundreds of thousands of SNPs in any one individual so that we can use this technology to distinguish one individual from any other (because the probability that any other individual will have exactly the same combination of SNP variants is at or close to zero).

As of this writing, anthropological researchers interested in questions of evolutionary significance tend to use SNPs regularly, while at present, forensic geneticists do not (though this might change in the next five years or so, due to the possibility of using large numbers of SNPs for individuating purposes).

SHORT TANDEM REPEAT (STR)

A $\underline{S}$hort $\underline{T}$andem $\underline{R}$epeat, or STR (pronounced s-t-r), is a genetic variant consisting of a linear repetition of a characteristic sequence motif. For example, at the same genomic region, one individual's genome may read AGTCAGTCAGTCAGTC, while another's genome may read AGTCAGTCAGTCAGTCAGTC. Here the repeat motif is "AGTC," with the former individual exhibiting four repeats of the motif—denoted as $(AGTC)_4$—and the latter, five $[(AGTC)_5]$. An STR typically contains a repeated unit of between two and six bases, and can form series of up to 100 bases in length.

A difference in the number of repeats between parents and offspring is fairly common—much more common than for SNPs (as above) or transposable elements (as below). It is not really known why this is the case, but it probably has something to do with a "slippage" of strands occurring during the replication of DNA prior to cell division.

Unlike the estimated low mutation rate for SNPs, STRs have relatively high estimated mutation rates, ranging from 10^{-6} to 10^{-2} bases per generation (Fan and Chu, 2007).

STRs are only found in the nuclear genome; the mitochondrial genome is devoid of them.

ALU ELEMENTS

An *Alu* element (or simply, "*Alu*") is a transposable element, also known as a "jumping gene." Transposable elements are rare sequences of DNA that can move (or transpose) themselves to new positions within the genome of a single cell. *Alu* elements are about 300 bases long and are found throughout the human genome. Their sheer size combined with their unusual "copy and paste" mechanism means that an *Alu* element insertion in any particular genomic region is unusual and therefore very unlikely to happen more than once. Therefore, we can assume when any two individuals share a specific *Alu* element insertion, it is likely due to common ancestry.

As with STRs, *Alu* elements are only found in the nuclear genome.

Obtaining DNA Data

A relatively straightforward way to obtain DNA data is to use data already generated by other researchers. Sometimes researchers publish journal articles or book chapters with summary results and interpretations based on DNA data that they generated themselves, but the data themselves are not immediately accessible. In that case, writing to the corresponding author of the publication with a request for the data is in order. However, it is becoming more common for researchers to make data available as downloadable digital files, either on research websites or on public database websites. See Box 16.2 for a list of some of the more popularly used database sites.

Generating DNA data can also be straightforward, particularly if you are dealing with DNA that has not yet decayed substantially. Regardless of DNA quality, basic and standardized methods exist for retrieving it. These are summarized below in four steps and in Figure 16.4.

STEP 1: SAMPLE PREPARATION

If your DNA source is bone or teeth, your sample will need to be prepared for DNA extraction by first decontaminating the sample of exogenous DNA (i.e. that not from the individual). This involves removing exposed surfaces followed by successive washes in

---

BOX 16.2

COMMONLY USED PUBLIC DNA DATABASES

National Center for Biotechnology Information (NCBI) Databases: Provides a more-or-less comprehensive listing of major databases, including references, nucleotide and protein sequences, protein structures, complete genomes, etc. **Access**: http://www.ncbi.nlm.nih.gov/Database/index.html

dbGaP: The database of Genotypes and Phenotypes (dbGaP) was developed to archive and distribute the results of studies that have investigated the interaction of genotype and phenotype.
Access: http://www.ncbi.nlm.nih.gov/gap

GenBank: National Institutes of Health (NIH) genetic sequence database, an annotated collection of all publicly available DNA sequences. **Access**: http://www.ncbi.nlm.nih.gov/genbank

SPSmart: This is a reprocessing engine for any given population-based genotype database that is able to deal even with billions of genotypes, and that is also capable of summarizing all that information into the most common population genetics indices. **Access**: http://spsmart.cesga.es

The Genographic Project Public Participation Mitochondrial DNA Database: The Genographic Project is studying the genetic signatures of ancient human migrations and creating an open-source research database. It allows members of the public to participate in a real-time anthropological genetics study by submitting personal samples for analysis and donating the genetic results to the database. The first 18 months of public participation in the Genographic Project can be currently accessed as the largest standardized human mitochondrial DNA (mtDNA) database ever collected, comprising 78,590 genotypes.[9] **Access**: http://www.plosgenetics.org/article/info:doi/10.1371/journal.pgen.0030104

Y Chromosome Haplotype Reference Database (YHRD): A free searchable Y-STR database. **Access**: http://www.yhrd.org

[9]Behar, D.M., Rosset, S., Blue-Smith, J., Balanovsky, O., Tzur, S., Comas, D., Mitchell, R.J., Quintana-Murci, L., Tyler-Smith, C., Wells, R.S., Genographic Consortium. The Genographic Project public participation mitochondrial DNA database. PLoS Genetics 2007, 3(6), e104.

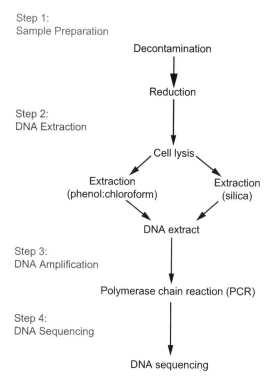

FIGURE 16.4   Simplified steps for DNA extraction and sequence analysis from hard tissue.

a DNA "eliminating" product, such as household bleach. Second, the sample is reduced to the smallest bits possible with the purpose of exposing as much surface area as possible. This can be done by dipping the sample in liquid nitrogen to flash freeze it and then shattering the sample, particularly if the sample is soft tissue. Another option is to mechanically reduce the sample using sandpaper, a rotary grinding tool, a hammer, or even a coffee grinder (depending on the tissue source). A final option is to chemically reduce the sample using a demineralization protocol.

STEP 2: DNA EXTRACTION

With the DNA sample now reduced to small particle sizes, it is ready to undergo a series of chemical reactions designed to break open cell membranes and isolate DNA from all other cellular components. The two most common DNA extraction methods are based on the use of phenol and chloroform, or silica (or both). Standardized protocols for DNA extraction exist and are widely published; an authoritative source is Ausbel et al. (2002).

The process of DNA extraction produces a good amount of DNA, but that quantity is not really sufficient for many subsequent procedures. This is the case particularly if only a trace amount of DNA was present in the sample in the first place, such as with ancient or forensic DNA. Therefore it has become almost routine procedure to augment the sample through an "amplification" process.

STEP 3: DNA AMPLIFICATION

"Amplification" refers to the process of making many, many copies of a sequence of DNA. Currently multiple amplification methods exist, including **cell cloning** where host cells are manipulated to carry and replicate a foreign DNA sequence.

One particular method of DNA amplification has proved very important: polymerase chain reaction, or **PCR** (Figure 16.5). This method is used to target limited sections of DNA. The method relies on temperature cycling, consisting of cycles of repeated heating and cooling of the reaction in order to "melt" the DNA (releasing of hydrogen bonds), and replication of the DNA through the help of special biomolecules. Primers (short DNA fragments) containing sequences complementary to the target region along with a DNA *polymerase* are key components to enable selective and repeated amplification. A DNA polymerase is a special kind of protein molecule, called an enzyme, which works to add complementary bases to a single-stranded DNA chain. As PCR progresses, the DNA generated is itself used as a template for replication, setting in motion a chain reaction in which the DNA is exponentially amplified. So, in the first PCR cycle, a single target double-stranded DNA molecule will be copied into two such molecules. In the second PCR cycle, those two molecules will both be copied, making four copies, and the next cycle will produce eight, then 16, then 32, and so on. The more cycles, the more copies. The reaction ultimately stops when the chemicals in the reaction are used up.

PCR was developed in the early 1980s and was the first accessible form of DNA amplification. Its development was responsible for the launching of the "molecular revolution" of the late 1980s—1990s mentioned earlier. The method was liberating in that it allowed researchers to easily target and analyze DNA from both living and long-dead organisms. It does have some drawbacks, however. For example, the method potentially amplifies any and all DNA in the extract. The method also requires you to target one or a few genomic regions through the use of specific primers. Lastly, PCR tends to favor undamaged DNA, which can be a problem if the DNA that you are hoping to target is damaged, as would be the case with DNA from ancient or forensic contexts.

To give you an idea of what PCR can do, imagine that that you are interested in amplifying DNA from a Neandertal specimen. At the end of any of your PCR runs, you will likely end up with a mix of DNA from the Neandertal specimen (the endogenous DNA), plus that of any excavators and museum curators (exogenous, or "contaminating" DNA) who may have touched the samples or even shared the same space as the samples. Additionally, though you will have thousands of copies of that DNA mixture, it will consist of short representative sequences of the Neandertal—modern human mixture, and not the entirety of DNA that is available, because classical PCR forces you to target select regions of the genome.

DNA amplification is a necessary step for providing enough DNA for further downstream applications. After amplification, researchers can choose among various data-generating options; a common next step is to sequence the amplification products.

STEP 4: DNA SEQUENCING

DNA sequencing involves several technologies used to determine the order of the nucleotide bases in a molecule of DNA. Often we view sequencing results in the form of a sequence file (Figure 16.6). DNA sequencers tend to be located in core laboratories with dedicated staff.

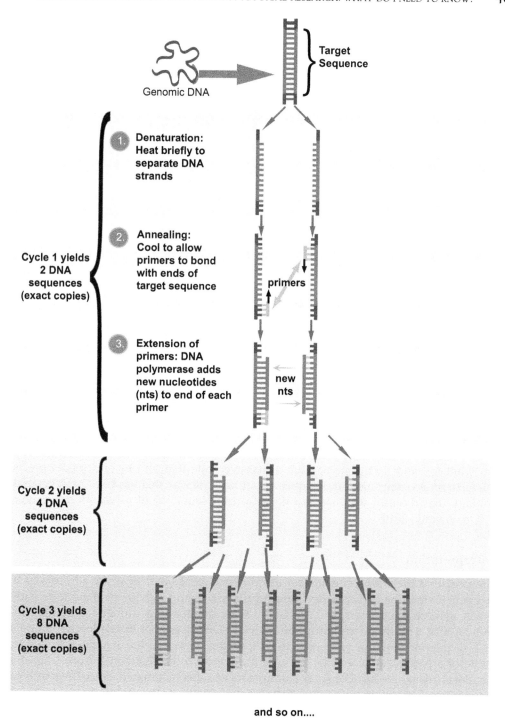

FIGURE 16.5 Polymerase chain reaction (PCR) steps.

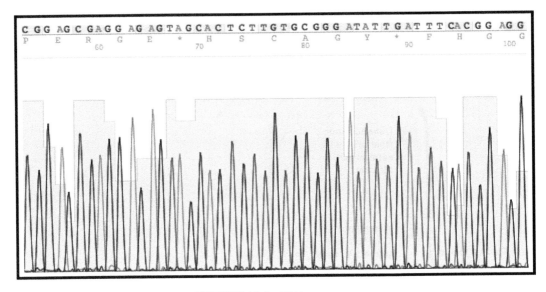

FIGURE 16.6   DNA sequence.

New Developments

In the past five to ten years, new developments in genetic technologies have allowed the steps of amplification and sequencing to be combined into so-called "high-throughput" methodologies. These methods use technologies that "parallelize" the amplification/sequencing process, meaning that thousands or millions of sequences are produced at once. The advantages are multiple: the amplification/sequencing protocol does not require you to target select bits and pieces of the genome as classical PCR does—though you can if you want to—and it is done at such a massive scale that all bits and pieces present in a DNA extract are amplified and sequenced at once. It was this kind of "next generation" technology that recently was used to finish a draft sequence of a Neandertal genome in 2010 (Green et al., 2010).

3. Interpretation

Interpretative tools for genetic data are mathematical (statistical) in nature and allow researchers to describe and compare their results to real and hypothetical models. Statistical methods involve parameters and statistics. A **parameter** is a numeric quantity, usually unknown, that describes a certain population characteristic. For example, the "population mean" is a parameter that is often used to indicate the average value of a quantity. A concrete example of a parameter would be the true number of individuals in Europe who died of tuberculosis during the Middle Ages. Parameters are often estimated, since their true values are generally unknown, in particular when the population is large enough for it to be impossible to obtain data from all population members (e.g., all Europeans). A **statistic** is a quantity that is calculated from a sample that is used to estimate a parameter.

Descriptive statistics are used to summarize a set of observations, with the purpose of communicating as much as possible and as simply as possible about a sample. No models or hypotheses are necessarily being tested. For example, take the hypothetical statement, "95% of survey takers in California claim to like chocolate." The use of a percentage immediately leads one to understand that an overwhelming proportion of individuals in the hypothetical sample are chocolate fans.

Let's say that we want to know whether or not such a response is unusual. To begin with, we want to know what the likelihood is that that response result could have been observed from any random set of observations. We might also want to know if that response result is unusual with respect to worldwide data on chocolate preferences, for example. Addressing both these and similar questions requires the construction of models—including models of randomness—against which to compare the data. Many of the statistical methods currently in use have already developed robust comparative models, and can be used to generate indices of statistical **significance**—that is, a value (known as a **probability** or **p-value**) that expresses how unusual or unexpected the research result is, given the statistical model.

Researchers often incorporate statistics into simulation-based methodologies. Simulation modeling is an approach that predicts probability distributions based on given hypotheses. This approach allows researchers to take into account the complexity of multiple interacting variables. In general, modeling methods force researchers to formalize their assumptions, allow researchers to explore the interactions of the parameters structuring their models, and help convert models of process into patterns that can be compared with real world, observed data.

To help researchers in the task of developing interpretive statements of genetics-based data, software packages are now available, many of which are freely downloadable. Depending on the software, you will be able to generate descriptive statistics for your data, and evaluate your data against various models, including population genetic models. For example, a popular and widely used software package for use with genetic data is *Arlequin*, developed by Laurent Excoffier and colleagues (the latest version, *Arlequin* v. 3.5.1.2, is described in Excoffier and Lischer, 2010). *Arlequin* is designed to provide the average user with a large set of basic methods and statistical tests to derive population genetic information on a collection of population samples. For a listing of more of the widely utilized software packages, see the review article by Excoffier and Heckel (2006).

DEGRADED DNA

How does DNA Decay?

All organisms, whether living or dead, sustain damage to their DNA. In life, an organism has active biomolecules that repair DNA as needed. That repair necessarily involves biomolecules that both excise and stitch together nucleotides, as damaged nucleotides need to be removed and then replaced. In death, these repair molecules stop working but the excising molecules continue to function, chopping up DNA into fragments. This process is called **autolysis**, and is capable of completely degrading an organism's DNA unless hindered by extreme desiccation or freezing.

Biomolecules can undergo further degradative activity through environmental elements and microbial activity. Water and oxygen are highly reactive compounds, meaning they will readily interact with other molecules. In the case of DNA, these compounds will break bonds apart through hydrolysis and oxidation, respectively. Several sources of radiation (cosmic, ultraviolet (from the sun), and geological) affect DNA integrity. Finally, microorganisms feed on the decaying organic material of organisms and utilize their own biomolecules to break it down for consumption (your own saliva performs the same function).

The ultimate effect of all the above factors on DNA preservation depends heavily on the environmental conditions in which the deceased organism ultimately winds up. Warm and humid conditions favor autolytic, hydrolytic, oxidative, and microbial activity. Whether the organism is exposed on the surface or buried also impacts biomolecular degradation, though even a buried organism can suffer DNA damage, depending on how deeply buried it is, or whether ground water is running through the soil, for example. Generally speaking, the longer an organism has been dead, the more DNA damage and decay is expected. However, environmental conditions play a very large role in whether DNA ultimately preserves or not.

Research Involving Degraded DNA

Two categories of research exist to deal with degraded biomolecules: **ancient DNA**, or the DNA analysis of long-deceased organisms (generally 100 or more years), and **forensic DNA**, or the DNA analysis of recently deceased organisms for medicolegal purposes. The only important difference between them is the expectation for the degree of DNA decay.

Generally, the relative decay rate of DNA from the nucleus (nDNA) is faster than of the mitochondrion. This is true for two reasons. The first is because nDNA, relative to mtDNA, is more vulnerable to autolysis, given that only a single membrane bounds the cell nucleus while a double membrane bounds the entire mitochondrion and its genomic material. The second reason is because mtDNA exists in a higher copy number per cell relative to nDNA. Every mitochondrion has on average two and half copies of its genome, and cells can contain up to 1000 to 2000 mitochondria! It is because of this overall difference in decay rates that most ancient DNA research rests on mtDNA data, which, though more abundant, contains less potential information due to the fact that it has only ca. 16,000 bases relative to the 3 billion bases found in the nuclear genome. In contrast, forensic DNA research focuses almost exclusively on data derived from nDNA for the purposes of individual identification. Because the degree of expected decay should be less than that of ancient DNA, the successful extraction of nDNA in forensic contexts is more of a possibility.

Controlling for Contamination

Because degraded DNA is by definition DNA that is subpar in quality, contamination from sources containing higher quality DNA is a persistent problem. All the existing chemical reactions designed to isolate DNA from other cell components (DNA extraction) and to make copies of targeted sections of DNA (DNA amplification) will work better when the DNA is of high quality (i.e., not decayed or damaged) because it is abundant and intact, so chemicals can easily bind where they need to.

The first way to control for contamination is to minimize a sample's exposure to the DNA of any organisms, but especially the DNA of organisms in the species that is closely related to the sample. Why is this? Recall that PCR works by targeting genomic regions of interest using short sequences of about 20 bases called **primers** (so called because these short sequences *prime* the reaction, or set it up). Most individuals within a species are probably going to have the exact same sequence within these 20 bases, or at most, a single base difference only. This is especially true for *Homo sapiens*, members of which show 99.8% sequence similarity. This means that a PCR will pick up all sequences of individuals within that species.[10] In the case of a human sample, the number of archaeological excavators, curators, and any others should be minimized. Samples expected to undergo DNA analysis should be carefully retrieved. In archaeological contexts, this means wearing a protective suit, a hair cover, a facemask, and gloves. Samples should be transferred to a specialized laboratory in DNA-free containers.

A specialized laboratory for the analysis of degraded DNA is a clean room laboratory (Figure 16.7). Clean rooms have controlled airflow: the intake of air is controlled so that it is filtered of particles that might bear bits of DNA copies. The room itself has positive pressure, so that once air comes in, it can only move out through a single exit. Rooms are regularly cleaned with chemicals that will immediately break up contaminating DNA. Everyone who works in the clean room has a copy of their DNA markers and/or sequences on file to be compared to the degraded DNA results, just in case. Finally, any researchers going into the room wear protective suits, shoe covers, facemasks, and hair covers.

CASE STUDY: SETTING UP A DEGRADED DNA ANALYSIS

This case study will take you through the trials and tribulations of setting up a DNA-based analysis of skeletonized remains, which can include either bones or teeth. By definition, you will be embarking on an analysis of degraded DNA.

What is Your Question?

Before embarking on your project, you will need to know what question you are addressing. To frame the question, you will need to decide what your theoretical approach is. For example, are you addressing a long-debated issue within evolutionary studies, or one within the medicolegal community? You will need to develop a hypothesis (or hypotheses), and predictions for those hypotheses, that are based on whatever theoretical approach you will use (see DiGangi and Moore [Chapter 2], this volume). Then, your theory, hypotheses, and

---

[10]To explain this in more detail, consider the following situation: Let's say that your dog chews a human bone from which you want to extract DNA. Would PCR pick up the dog DNA and the human DNA, or only the dog or only the human DNA? The long answer to that is that it depends on the genomic region you target using PCR. It is possible to target a region that is evolutionarily conserved (meaning it is the same) between dogs and humans, such that PCR cannot discriminate between the human and dog DNA. Conversely, it is possible to target regions that we know to be different between dogs and humans, in which case we can use PCR to amplify only dog or only human DNA.

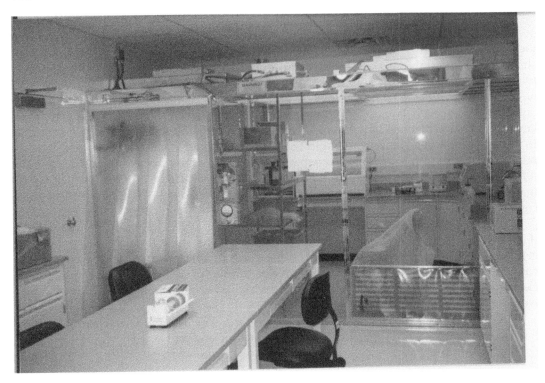

FIGURE 16.7 Example of a modular clean room laboratory. Note that the laboratory has its own air filtration system at the top of the unit; the inside of the room is positive pressured. All air, therefore, only comes in through the ceiling filtration units and only goes out one door (seen to the very left). The room's inside is equipped with UV lights that are turned on to "decontaminate" the room when not in use. Photo courtesy of Dr. Anne C. Stone, Arizona State University.

predictions will help guide you towards the appropriate data source: Do you need biparentally inherited nuclear DNA, or uniparentally inherited mtDNA and/or NRY? What level of resolution do you need? That is, do you need broad evolutionary lineages, or do you want to be able to be as individually identifying as possible? The answers to these questions will help you decide what regions of the genome and kind of **genetic marker(s)** you should study and how many markers you will need to best address your hypotheses.

Before Considering a Project Using Degraded DNA …

… make sure you have access to two very important things: (1) someone with extensive experience working with degraded DNA and (2) a clean room laboratory. These two factors are very important because while "modern DNA" techniques (i.e., DNA techniques oriented towards high-quality DNA) appear the same as those applied to degraded DNA, they differ extensively in the details. The following are just a very few examples of the differences between working with modern versus degraded DNA: instead of standard chemical reagents (that are sold with a certain degree of purity and sterility), you must order DNA-free

TABLE 16.3   Differences between "Modern" and "Degraded" DNA Analysis

"Modern"	"Degraded" (ancient or forensic)
Standard DNA laboratory; can contain PCR machines	Clean room laboratory with filtered air, positive pressure, and UV lights; no PCR machines
Purified and sterile chemical reagents; DNA-free	Molecular grade, certified DNA-free chemical reagents
Sterilized equipment	Equipment treated with DNA-eliminating chemicals and/or UV light
Purified and sterile disposables	Certified DNA-free disposables
Personnel wear reusable cloth lab coat and disposable gloves	Personnel wear disposable jumpsuits, headgear, facemasks, and gloves

molecular grade reagents and disposables; instead of reusing the same lab coat over street clothes, you wear a disposable "bunny suit"; instead of freely touching and moving any object as you would in a modern DNA lab, in a clean room lab, you would minimize every movement to avoid drafting DNA-containing cells over samples (see Table 16.3). Only a person with experience in this area can help you navigate through the myriad of specific requirements successfully.

I Have Access to Adequate Training and a Clean Room Lab. Now What?

A study that relies on degraded DNA is a high-risk project. For any sample, you will not know if it is possible to obtain any DNA at all. Therefore, the first thing to do is a trial run on your chosen sample to ascertain (1) whether you obtain any DNA, (2) what kind of DNA, (3) in what quantities, and (4) at what quality.

Take a small set of samples (about ten) from the population or set of remains of interest. Go through all the appropriate decontamination and DNA extraction steps. Then, attempt to amplify mtDNA first. If you cannot, then you know that attempting to amplify nDNA is almost pointless, because it is present in far less copy number per cell than mtDNA. If you are successful in amplifying mtDNA, take the analysis a step further, such as sequencing. The clarity of the sequence(s) will indicate the degree of DNA damage, if any. If all these steps work out, you can move on to amplify nDNA and sequence it, again, to assess DNA quality. If it all checks out, you are ready to obtain more samples for analysis. If not, move on to a different sample.

How and What do I Sample?

The best sources from which to obtain DNA are thick cortical bone and whole teeth. You will need to collect samples in as sterile conditions as possible. First, take a sample large enough so that you have enough left over after you go through the decontamination procedures (see below). If you can, sample an entire bone (for example, an entire metatarsal) or a whole tooth, preferably a molar.

If your sample will be coming directly from an excavation, the ideal situation is for only one person to excavate the sample in protective gear to minimize any skin or hair exposure. The gear is to protect the sample from you (and your DNA), not the reverse. If you are sampling already excavated and curated remains, you should at least wear a facemask, hair cover, and gloves. Make sure to also take DNA samples (cheek swab samples are fine) from anybody who has been in contact with the remains to control for the presence of their DNA on the sample as possible contaminants.

The primary sample should be stored in a DNA-free bag or container (use full-strength household bleach to clean the inside of a plastic bag, rinse with DNA-free sterile water, and dry; or use DNA-free tubes). Transfer the sample to the clean room lab.

Just inside the clean room lab, the external part of the storage receptacle will need to be decontaminated (use a solution of 10–30% household bleach). By this point you will be encased in protective gear and will remove the sample from the receptacle and prepare to take your secondary sample. If you have sampled a bone, the first step is to decontaminate the external surface. As per above, this can be done mechanically by physically removing the outer layer as well as any trabeculae (trabecular bone is notoriously hard to clean and decontaminate), followed by a rinse in 10–30% household bleach, followed by sterile, DNA-free water. If you are dealing with a tooth, the tooth can be submerged in household bleach for about ten minutes, then rinsed with sterile DNA-free water. You may decide to use the entire tooth, or just a section of it.

Most ancient DNA protocols ask for between a quarter and one gram of sample in a typical extraction (see for example Rohland and Hofreiter, 2007).

Please keep in mind that the intention here is to give very general indications for how to conduct an analysis of degraded DNA. In practice, these steps are much more specific and detailed. They also tend to be sample specific. You should consult optimized protocols for extraction of degraded DNA, which can be found in the methods section of any published paper on ancient or forensic DNA. The scientific journals *Forensic Science International*, *Genetics*, *BioTechniques*, and *Electrophoresis*, to list some examples, tend to publish useful methods articles on a regular basis. All protocols will tend to use some variation of the standard protocols that are either silica- or phenol-chloroform-based (or both), as mentioned earlier in the chapter.

At this point you are ready to reduce your sample in preparation for DNA extraction (as per earlier discussion).

What Kind of Questions can I Feasibly Address Using Degraded DNA?

In most analyses relying on degraded DNA, you will be dealing with small sample sizes, meaning few individual specimens will yield any DNA at all, and for those that do, fragment sizes will be very small. This means that sequence lengths will be short, and you may need to further limit your analysis to very informative SNPs.

Despite its limitations, working with degraded DNA has a huge advantage: it enables the access of *direct* information about individual and populational genetic variation, past or present. Below we discuss some typical kinds of studies, all of which represent successful examples of the utility of degraded DNA analysis for anthropology.

Population Relationships, Past and Present

How are individuals buried at a single site related to each other? How are individuals buried at one site related to those at another site? What if those burial sites date to very different time periods? Biologically speaking, could we argue that they are from the same or a similar population? An early and iconic set of papers addressing these questions come from Anne C. Stone's 1996 dissertation work on the Norris Farms #36 site located in the U.S. state of Illinois (Stone, 1996; Stone and Stoneking, 1993, 1998), though many others have since followed suit (e.g., Ottoni et al., 2011, among others).

Ultimate Origins

Questions about ultimate origins concern the initial appearance of new species: for example, studies on the origins of Neandertals and their relationship to modern humans (are they a different species from *Homo sapiens*?) abound. The direct analysis of Neandertal DNA has brought tremendous insight into this question, as mentioned in the introduction to this chapter (Green et al., 2010; Reich et al., 2010).

Migration/Colonization

Another kind of origins question relates to the migration of populations within species into new geographic areas. An often-debated migration case study is the peopling of the Americas: From what continent(s) did the populations inhabiting the Americas prior to the arrival of Europeans in the fifteenth century come? How long ago? How many groups of people moved to the Americas, and did they come from different parts of the world? What routes did they travel? While modern DNA analyses have informed many of these debates, ancient DNA analyses have provided key pieces of evidence. Most recently, an ancient DNA study of an individual dating to 10,300 years ago from *On Your Knees* cave in Alaska demonstrated the presence of a novel mitochondrial genetic founder lineage, indicating that the early American colonizers were more genetically diverse than was previously thought (Kemp et al., 2007).

Disease

Disease is an unfortunate but integral part of life. Disease can be inborn (due to a genetic mutation present from birth) or infectious (caused by viruses, bacteria, fungi, protozoa, and parasites). All these disease-causing agents involve DNA and can be targeted in an ancient DNA analysis. Researchers have been looking for the degraded molecular remains of such pathogenic agents as tuberculosis (Donoghue et al., 2004; Wilbur et al., 2009) and leprosy (Haas et al., 2000). For a good recent review of ancient disease studies, see Drancourt and Raoult (2005), and Smith (Chapter 7), this volume.

Genetic Sex

Osteological techniques for estimating the sex of a skeleton are well established for modern populations as well as for those from the contemporary past. However, as Moore (Chapter 4), this volume, points out, application of these techniques to more ancient populations becomes problematic. Additionally, there are no accepted gross morphological methods to estimate sex osteologically in subadults, present or past; genetic techniques of sex estimation could provide an additional line of evidence. Genetic sexing studies use PCR to amplify genomic regions that are specific to the X and Y chromosomes. If only X chromosome regions amplify, then the genetic sex of the skeleton is female, and if both X and Y chromosome regions amplify then the sample is genetically male. However, although this seems straightforward, genetic sexing using degraded samples can be somewhat problematic. Contamination is hard to rule out. Furthermore, it is possible that due to the damaged nature of any particular set of remains, combined with the fact that any individual sample is expected to have more copies of the X than the Y chromosome, a Y chromosomal fragment may fail to amplify and yield a false result (i.e., resulting in a female versus a male sex estimate).

CASE STUDY: THE TRIALS AND TRIBULATIONS OF DNA RESEARCH IN PRACTICE

The Missing Person Case of Leoma Patterson

The story of the missing person case of Leoma Patterson was originally published in 2007 by the Dr. Bill Bass and Jon Jefferson writing duo in their fiction book *Beyond the Body Farm* and offers a good lesson of how degraded DNA studies can go wrong. By way of background, Leoma Patterson went missing in 1978, and five months later, a partial skeleton was found that was tentatively identified as hers. In 2005, members of Leoma Patterson's family had the skeleton exhumed from its grave, and found a forensic genetic testing company in Nevada to test a single bone sample from the exhumed skeleton and compare it to two family samples.

According to the company's one-page report, they examined ten locations on the mtDNA, and detected the presence of two different DNA bases at three of the ten locations. In one paragraph, the report stated that "[p]ossible explanations include that the sample is degraded," and cautioned that, "[i]t is not recommended to use this information for sole identification or comparison purposes." However, in the next paragraph, the report declared that "[i]n comparison to the bone sample, [Leoma Patterson's two maternal descendants] can be excluded as having the same maternal lineage." The family, as well as Bass and Jefferson, took these words at face value and believed that the skeleton was *not* that of Leoma Patterson.

Soon after, Bass and Jefferson contacted the primary author of this chapter for her opinion, which was that not only was the report unclear, worse, it was misleading. Though the statement in the first paragraph was correct, it was not accurate to say that Leoma Patterson's two maternal relatives could be excluded. To explain, the report indicated that the extracted DNA showed more than one DNA base at several (three) DNA locations (a condition that, when naturally occurring, is termed **heteroplasmy**). Although humans occasionally show heteroplasmy, the chances of having three heteroplasmic sites within a few hundred bases of each other (which is what the report showed) is very low. This could only mean that they had more than one individual's sequence on their hands, and that the samples were in fact contaminated.

On the advice of the first author of this chapter, several skeletal samples were sent to Dr. Jason Eshleman, a researcher with extensive experience in degraded DNA. He followed proper decontamination procedures for the samples, attempted to extract DNA, and found no DNA remaining in any of it. It later turned out that this was because the skeleton had been processed in a heavy-duty detergent and soaked in bleach after it had been found, all of which would have significantly deteriorated any possible remaining DNA.

Later, one of the original investigators of the Leoma Patterson case rediscovered a hair mat that had been at the site where the skeleton had been found. That hair mat was sent to Dr. Eshleman, who then took two samples that he and another specialist independently worked on in different laboratories. This time the sample did yield mtDNA. At this point neither specialist had prior knowledge of what the DNA of the maternal relatives looked like, but when they finally made a comparison, the DNA from the hair mat matched those of the surviving maternal relatives. Case solved: the exhumed skeleton was that of Leoma Patterson.

Here you can see that had the sample been sent to an experienced researcher and laboratory from the start, many of the problems would have been avoided, including the misleading information received from the first analysis. The original lab was clearly not used to dealing with skeletal samples and did not grasp the level of ambiguity that potential contamination can introduce.

APPLICATION OF DNA ANALYSIS TO LONG-STANDING ANTHROPOLOGICAL INQUIRIES INTO HUMAN VARIATION, ITS PATTERN, AND ITS EXPLANATION

Without a doubt, genetic studies, whether conducted independently or in concert with morphological studies will influence future anthropological inquiry. Already we have seen their impact on important issues, the single most persistent of which is the biological race concept as it applies to humans. Though anthropologists have rejected the categorical view of biological race, bioanthropologists continue to apply it as a useful heuristic to describe patterns of human biological variation. As we bring more data and analysis to bear on the description and understanding of patterns of human variation, the ways in which the biological race concept is used within bioanthropology are likely to change in response.

Human Genetic Variation: Is it Patterned?

Recent genomic studies argue that it is. A relatively recent set of landmark papers by Rosenberg and colleagues (Rosenberg et al., 2002, 2005) looked at almost 400 STRs in a little over 1000 individuals from 52 globally distributed populations. They argued that despite the fact that over 90% of the STR variation could be found within populations, there was still 3–5% of STR variation that differentiates on a "major" or continental level. This finding is apparently robust (Rosenberg et al., 2005). This means that some human genetic variation can form clusters that correspond with major geographic areas, which in turn broadly correspond to traditionally used racial categories.

What Are the Possible Evolutionary Explanations for the Pattern?

In the last few years there has been intense discussion in the scholarly literature of what evolutionary process(es) produced this continental distribution of human variation. At first, several contemporaneous studies demonstrated that human genetic variation conforms to a clinal pattern. That is, rather than forming tightly bounded clusters, human genetic variation is continuous, and is patterned as a strong association with local geography: populations in close geographic proximity will tend to be more similar to each other in their pattern of genetic variation, and the further apart populations are, the less similar they become. Formally, this is known as a pattern of **isolation by distance**, or IBD. Several scholars have argued that this pattern has resulted from the tendency of people to find mates within close geographic distance from each other, although some will find mates further afield (Konigsberg, 1990; Relethford, 2004; Manica et al., 2005; among others).

At the same time, others were suggesting that instead, the strong correlation between geographic proximity and genetic similarity results from a serial fission process (Ramachandran et al., 2005). Picture a single founder population that grows in size to the point that a daughter population splits from it. The original population persists, while the daughter population grows in size and itself splits. This serial fission process repeats itself, with successive daughter populations spreading out from the original founding population. This will create a *nested* pattern of variation, because each daughter population will consist of only a subset of the variation found in its parent population.

Most recently, Hunley and colleagues (2009) demonstrated that both processes—local mate exchange (leading to IBD) and serial fissions—account for the pattern. Specifically, they demonstrate a nested pattern of population genetic structure that is consistent with a history of serial population fissions, population discontinuities, as well as long-range migrations associated with the peopling of major geographic regions, and gene flow between local populations. This inferred historical process is different from what has been argued previously, and cannot support the thesis that the human species consists of independently evolving biological races.

No doubt, as more and more individuals are sampled, and as more of their genomes are investigated, we will be hearing much more on the topic. Additionally, as our capabilities to glean information from degraded skeletal remains improve, we will be able to obtain more direct information about genetic variation in the past.

FUTURE RESEARCH OPPORTUNITIES

In the Pipeline

Advances in genetics and genomics are happening very quickly so that almost every month a new breakthrough in technology and reduced cost occurs. Though most people refer to the current moment as the "genomic era," some would argue that we are transitioning to a "post-genomic era." The reasoning here is that the genomic era occurred during the development of technologies that have allowed us to sequence entire genomes. That trend started more than ten years ago, so that at this point, we have complete genomic sequences from individual organisms from multiple species, and genomic sequencing efforts are now being focused on increasing within-species sample sizes. For example, the "1000 genomes project" is aiming to sequence in-depth 1000 genomes from geographically dispersed humans (see www.1000genomes.org). Further, the post-genomic era will introduce methods and software to quickly and easily "annotate" genomes (i.e., find and tag locations of interest).

What Does this Mean for Skeletal Biology?

Over the decades, biological anthropologists have used the skeleton for various purposes: assigning racial categories, individual identification, tracking prehistoric population migrations, differentiating different species in the fossil record, and understanding function and adaptation among individuals and populations. Underlying each of these purposes is one or more fundamental assumptions about the relationship between genotype and phenotype in a population, such as the degree of heritability (i.e., susceptibility to natural selection), phenotypic plasticity (i.e., susceptibility to environmental forces), or selective neutrality, to name a few examples.

Importantly for skeletal biology, molecular-based analyses have opened new windows—if not widened existing windows—into biological processes related to morphology and their relationship with environmental factors throughout the course of life. Recent studies have either generated or exploited publicly available genomic-level data on worldwide populations to ask what aspects of the skeleton have evolved neutrally, and which seem to have been under selection. For example, a recent spate of studies are asking whether or not, and what regions, if any, of the human cranium have been evolving neutrally (in which case we can use the cranium, or maybe certain cranial regions, to access population history) or have been under selection (in which case we can look at the history of selection on the cranium or cranial regions) (Roseman, 2004; Sherwood et al., 2008; Smith, 2009). For the future, can we find genes controlling for particular phenotypes? What can we say about the developmental regulation of genes? Thus, some of the more promising future research studies lie in dissecting genotype–phenotype relationships, including accompanying mathematical and computational methods. As we develop a more thorough understanding of the functional interactions among different genomic regions, we stand to gain a more sophisticated and nuanced view of what it means to be human.

CONCLUSION

I Am a Student of Skeletal Biology. If I am Interested in the Possibility of Incorporating Molecular Methods into My Work, What Should I Make Sure to Do and to Learn?

Because of the potential for such exciting developments, students of skeletal biology should strongly consider taking courses in evolutionary biology, genetics, and particularly classes that teach about the relationship between genetics and environment. Because culture is part of our environment, maintaining a strong foundation in the principles of cultural anthropology, as well as an understanding of variation in cultural norms, is also important. Finally, advanced statistics and quantitative and computational methods are a must. If pursuing genetics in anthropology is your calling, volunteer to work in a molecular lab to familiarize yourself with laboratory techniques.

Anthropological genetics is a fascinating as well as fast moving field. The fact that it *is* quick paced should not deter you from becoming involved in the field as a researcher as a solid foundation in general anthropology, biology, genetics, and statistics will allow you to always follow along and make valuable contributions. We hope that this chapter enables you to initiate this process.

ACKNOWLEDGMENTS

The authors are grateful to the editors, Drs. Elizabeth A. DiGangi and Megan K. Moore, for inviting us to contribute to this valuable text. We would also like to thank Drs. Katherine M. Spradley and Bridget F.B. Algee-Hewitt for helpful comments.

REFERENCES

Ausbel, F.M., Brent, R., Kingston, R.E., Moore, D.D., Seidman, J.G., Smith, J.A., Struhl, L. (Eds.), 2002. Short Protocols in Molecular Biology, 4th ed. Wiley and Sons, New York.

Bass, B., Jefferson, J., 2007. Beyond the Body Farm: A Legendary Bone Detective Explores Murders, Mysteries, and the Revolution in Forensic Science. Harper Collins, New York.

Boyd, W.C., 1939. Blood groups. Tabulae Biologicae 17, 113–240.

Boyd, W.C., 1963. Four achievements of the genetical method in physical anthropology. American Anthropologist 65 (2), 243–252.

Cann, R.L., Stoneking, M., Wilson, A.C., 1987. Mitochondrial DNA and human evolution. Nature 325 (6099), 31–36.

Chamberlin, T.C., 1965. The method of multiple working hypotheses. Science 148 (3671), 754–759.

Crawford, M.H., 2007. Foundations of anthropological genetics. In: Crawford, M.H. (Ed.), Anthropological Genetics: Theory, Methods and Applications. Cambridge University Press, Cambridge, pp. 1–16.

Crawford, M.H., Mielke, J.H. (Eds.), 1980. Current Developments in Anthropological Genetics. Vol. II. Ecology and Population Structure. Plenum Press, New York.

Crawford, M.H., Workman, P.L. (Eds.), 1973. Methods and Theories of Anthropological Genetics. University of New Mexico Press, Albuquerque.

DiGangi, E.A., Moore, M.K., 2013. Application of the scientific method to skeletal biology. In: DiGangi, E.A., Moore, M.K. (Eds.), Research Methods in Human Skeletal Biology. Academic Press, San Diego.

DiGangi, E.A., Moore, M.K., 2013. Introduction to skeletal biology. In: DiGangi, E.A., Moore, M.K. (Eds.), Research Methods in Human Skeletal Biology. Academic Press, San Diego.

Donoghue, H.D., Spigelman, M., Greenblatt, C.L., Lev-Maor, G., Kahila Bar-Gal, G., Matheson, C., Vernon, K., Nerlich, A.G., Zink, A.R., 2004. Tuberculosis: from prehistory to Robert Koch, as revealed by ancient DNA. The Lancet Infectious Diseases 4 (9), 584–592.

Drancourt, M., Raoult, D., 2005. Palaeomicrobiology: Current issues and perspectives. Nature Reviews Microbiology 3 (1), 23–35.

Excoffier, L., Heckel, G., 2006. Computer programs for population genetics data analysis: a survival guide. Nature Reviews Genetics 7 (10), 745–758.

Excoffier, L., Lischer, H.E., 2010. Arlequin suite ver 3.5: a new series of programs to perform population genetics analyses under Linux and Windows. Molecular Ecology Resources 10 (3), 564–567.

Fan, H., Chu, J.-Y., 2007. A brief review of short tandem repeat mutation. Genomics, Proteomics and Bioinformatics 5 (1), 7–14.

Futuyma, D., 2009. Evolution, 2nd ed. Sinauer Associates, Massachusetts.

Green, R.E., Krause, J., Briggs, A.W., Maricic, T., Stenzel, U., Kircher, M., Patterson, N., Li, H., Zhai, W., Fritz, M.H.-Y., Hansen, N.F., Durand, E.Y., Malaspinas, A.-S., Jensen, J.D., Marques-Bonet, T., Alkan, C., Prüfer, K., Meyer, M., Burbano, H.A., Good, J.M., Schultz, R., Aximu-Petri, A., Butthof, A., Höber, B., Höffner, B., Siegemund, M., Weihmann, A., Nusbaum, C., Lander, E.S., Russ, C., Novod, N., Affourtit, J., Egholm, M., Verna, C., Rudan, P., Brajkovic, D., Kucan, Z., Gusic, I., Doronichev, V.B., Golovanova, L.V., Lalueza-Fox, C., de la Rasilla, M., Fortea, J., Rosas, A., Schmitz, R.W., Johnson, P.L.F., Eichler, E.E., Falush, D., Birney, E., Mullikin, J.C., Slatkin, M., Nielsen, R., Kelso, J., Lachmann, M., Reich, C., Pääbo, S., 2010. A draft sequence of the Neandertal genome. Science 328, 710–722.

Haas, C.J., Zink, A., Pálfi, G., Szeimies, U., Nerlich, A.G., 2000. Detection of leprosy in ancient human skeletal remains by molecular identification of *Mycobacterium leprae*. American Journal of Clinical Pathology 114 (3), 428–436.

Harpending, H., Jenkins, T., 1973. Genetic distance among Southern African populations. In: Crawford, M.H., Workman, P.L. (Eds.), Methods and Theories of Anthropological Genetics. University of New Mexico Press, Albuquerque, pp. 177–200.

Hartl, D., 2011. Essential Genetics: A Genomics Perspective. 5th ed. Jones and Bartlett, Massachusetts.

Hartl, D., Clark, A.G., 2006. Principles of Population Genetics. Sinauer Associates, Massachusetts.

Hunley, K.L., Healy, M.E., Long, J.C., 2009. The global pattern of gene identity variation reveals a history of long-range migrations, bottlenecks, and local mate exchange: implications for biological race. American Journal of Physical Anthropology 139 (1), 35–46.

Kemp, B.K., Malhi, R.S., McDonough, J., Bolnick, D.A., Eshleman, J.A., Rickards, O., Martinez-Labarga, C., Johnson, J.R., Lorenz, J.G., Dixon, E.J., Fifield, T.E., Heaton, T.H., Worl, R., Smith, D.G., 2007. Genetic analysis of early Holocene skeletal remains from Alaska and its implications for the settlement of the Americas. American Journal of Physical Anthropology 132 (4), 605–621.

Konigsberg, L.W., 1990. Analysis of prehistoric biological variation under a model of isolation by geographic and temporal distance. Human Biology 62, 49–70.

Kruglyak, L., 1999. Prospects for whole-genome linkage disequilibrium mapping of common disease genes. Nature Genetics 22 (4), 139–144.

Manica, A., Prugnolle, F., Balloux, F., 2005. Geography is a better determinant of human genetic differentiation than ethnicity. Human Genetics 118, 366–371.

Mielke, J.H., Crawford, M.H. (Eds.), 1980. Current Developments in Anthropological Genetics. Vol. I. Theory and Methods. Plenum Press, New York.

Moore, M.K., 2012. Sex estimation and assessment. In: DiGangi, E.A., Moore, M.K. (Eds.), Research Methods in Human Skeletal Biology. Academic Press, San Diego.

Ottoni, C., Ricaut, F.-X., Vanderheyden, N., Brucato, N., Waelkens, M., Decorte, R., 2011. Mitochondrial analysis of a Byzantine population reveals the differential impact of multiple historical events in South Anatolia. European Journal of Human Genetics 19 (5), 571–576.

Perry, G.H., Dominy, N.J., Claw, K.G., Lee, A.S., Fiegler, H., Redon, R., Werner, J., Villanea, F.A., Mountain, J.L., Misra, R., Carter, N.P., Lee, C., Stone, A.C., 2007. Diet and the evolution of human amylase gene copy number variation. Nature Genetics 39 (10), 1256–1260.

Ramachandran, S., Deshpande, O., Roseman, C.C., Rosenberg, N.A., Feldman, M.W., Cavalli-Sforza, L.L., 2005. Support from the relationship of genetic and geographic distance in human populations for a serial founder effect originating in Africa. Proceedings of the National Academy of Sciences USA 102 (44), 15942–15947.

Reich, D., Green, R.E., Kircher, M., Krause, J., Patterson, N., Durand, E.Y., Viola, B., Briggs, A.W., Stenzel, U., Johnson, P.L., Maricic, T., Good, J.M., Marques-Bonet, T., Alkan, C., Fu, Q., Mallick, S., Li, H., Meyer, M., Eichler, E.E., Stoneking, M., Richards, M., Talamo, S., Shunkov, M.V., Derevianko, A.P., Hublin, J.J., Kelso, J., Slatkin, M., Pääbo, S., 2010. Genetic history of an archaic hominin group from Denisova Cave in Siberia. Nature 468 (7327), 1053–1060.

Relethford, J.H., 2004. Global patterns of isolation by distance based on genetic and morphological data. Human Biology 76 (4), 499–513.

Ridley, M., 2004. Evolution, 3rd ed. Wiley-Blackwell, Massachusetts.

Roberts, D., 1980. Current developments in anthropological genetics. In: Mielke, J.H., Crawford, M.H. (Eds.), Current Developments in Anthropological Genetics. Vol. I. Theory and Methods. Plenum Press, New York.

Rohland, N., Hofreiter, M., 2007. Ancient DNA extraction from bones and teeth. Nature Protocols 2 (7), 1756–1762.

Roseman, C.C., 2004. Detecting interregionally diversifying natural selection on modern human cranial form by using matched molecular and morphometric data. Proceedings of the National Academy of Sciences, USA 101 (35), 12824–12829.

Rosenberg, N.A., Pritchard, J.K., Weber, J.L., Cann, H.M., Kidd, K.K., Zhivotovsky, L.A., Feldman, M.W., 2002. Genetic structure of human populations. Science 298 (5602), 2381–2385.

Rosenberg, N.A., Mahajan, S., Ramachandran, S., Zhao, C., Pritchard, J.K., Feldman, M.W., 2005. Clines, clusters, and the effect of study design on the inference of human population structure. PLoS Genetics 1, 660–671.

Sherwood, R.J., Duren, D.L., Demerath, E.W., Czerwinski, S.A., Siervogel, R.M., Towne, B., 2008. Quantitative genetics of modern human cranial variation. Journal of Human Evolution 54 (8), 909–914.

III. TECHNOLOGICAL ADVANCES

Smith, H.F., 2009. Which cranial regions reflect molecular distances reliably in humans? Evidence from three-dimensional morphology. American Journal of Human Biology 21 (1), 36–47.

Smith, M.O., 2013. Paleopathology. In: DiGangi, E.A., Moore, M.K. (Eds.), Research Methods in Human Skeletal Biology. Academic Press, San Diego.

Stone, A.C., 1996. Genetic and Mortuary Analyses of a Prehistoric Native American Community. PhD dissertation. University Park, Pennsylvania State University.

Stone, A.C., Stoneking, M., 1993. Ancient DNA from a pre-Columbian Amerindian population. American Journal of Physical Anthropology 92 (4), 463–471.

Stone, A.C., Stoneking, M., 1998. MtDNA analysis of a prehistoric Oneota population: implications for the peopling of the New World. American Journal of Human Genetics 62 (4), 1153–1170.

Wilbur, A.K., Bouwman, A.S., Stone, A.C., Roberts, C.A., Pfister, L.A., Buikstra, J.E., Brown, T.A., 2009. Deficiencies and challenges in the study of ancient tuberculosis DNA. Journal of Archaeological Science 36 (9), 1990–1997.

Williams, G.C., 1996. Adaptation and Natural Selection. Princeton University Press, Princeton, NJ.

PART IV

COMPLETING AND CULTIVATING THE SCIENTIFIC PROCESS

17

Library Research, Presenting, and Publishing

Elizabeth A. DiGangi

INTRODUCTION

As an advanced undergraduate or new graduate student, you probably have quite a bit of experience with doing small-scale literature reviews for term papers in a variety of different subjects. Now that you are preparing to embark on an original research project in skeletal biology, you are starting to discover that the process is a bit more complicated than what you are used to. You may have some unanswered questions about the different stages of the research process beyond data collection and analysis.

This chapter is therefore set up in a "how-to" format and is designed to take away some of the mystery surrounding the other necessary research steps. The chapter begins with library and database research, includes a discussion of how to obtain outside funding, and ends with the final stage of the scientific process: dissemination of information through presentation at conferences and publication. The advice and suggestions presented herein were learned through personal experience (often via trial and error), and I realized that a written guide might be helpful to new students for the navigation of the intricacies of these aspects of the scientific process. This advice is based on my own experience as to what works and what doesn't. Your professors will probably have some additional advice or may have other opinions. Please ensure that you talk to them about their own experiences, especially pertaining to the presenting and publishing process. It will help the quality of your work immensely if you have an expert and mentor walk you through what to do and what to expect. In addition, the information in the chapter's tables is not meant to be exhaustive. Again, your advisor should have further advice and suggestions.

LIBRARY AND DATABASE RESEARCH

Library research has come a long way since just a few years ago, before computers and search engines became entrenched in our vocabulary and culture. It wasn't that long ago that your local college library did not even have a computer, possibly in your lifetime and certainly in your parents' lifetimes. In the past, the intrepid researcher had to take a physical trip to the library to review the literature. Today, however, you can easily search your library's holdings from anywhere in the world, given an Internet connection. You are probably already somewhat familiar with this from having to search for books and articles as an undergraduate. However, there is always more to learn about the search process that will help you with locating the information you seek.

Your first step should be to take a trip to the library. While searching for articles from the comfort of home is certainly a convenience, you need to familiarize yourself with the actual physical building. Online databases and catalogs are fantastic resources, but they do not contain everything ever written. There is a significant amount of work in print that has not been digitized (and may never be digitized), such as theses, dissertations, certain books, etc. You can expect articles and some chapters published after 2000 or so to be online. For anything earlier than that, it will be dependent on the source.

When doing your literature review search and later write-up, keep in mind that it will infrequently be necessary or appropriate to cite sources that are 50 years or older. Circumstances when this would be important include if you are doing a comprehensive historical literature review, if the most recent publication on your question happens to be decades old (unusual), or if you are making a particular point or stating when something historically first appeared in the literature. Situations in which it would not be appropriate to cite decades-old sources would include if you need citations for recent applications of certain methods or theory, or if you need to reference the most updated information for a given topic. For most projects in skeletal biology, relevant literature will be available that is less than 10 or 15 years old. For example, if your topic is "sex estimation from the humerus," you may include the oldest reference on sexing from the skeleton or from the humerus for historical background, but you will focus on the most recent literature that your study uses as its starting point.

Take advantage of having access to librarians, who have bachelor's or master's degrees in library science. They are experts in cataloging and successfully searching for information. University libraries have subject librarians, who specialize in knowing about publications and search engines for specific disciplines. Find out who the subject librarian is for anthropology and go meet that person. Their job is to keep up to date on the latest resources in the field and buy them for the library when applicable. They will be the most knowledgeable person on campus with regard to which databases have articles relevant to skeletal biology. If you are at a school without subject librarians, go talk to one of the general librarians. Part of their job is to help students and faculty with their information search. They can guide you in the right direction with regard to your particular literature review. If searching online databases and catalogs is completely new to you, find out if the library has a free workshop on how to use its resources. It most likely does. Take advantage of it. The library may also offer free workshops on topics such as thesis and dissertation document formatting, and using software such as SPSS® or Photoshop®.

Begin to familiarize yourself with searching the library's catalog. From a computer inside the library, go to "catalog" and take the time to read the "help" file. Even if you are already familiar with how to search the catalog, there may be new features of which you are unaware. Next, enter a broad topic into the search field—such as "biological anthropology" or "human skeletons."[1] Your search will pull up books the library owns that cover these topics. Find out where they are physically located in the stacks. Go to that section of the library and look around. This section will probably have all the books relevant to biological anthropology. (The journals and theses/ dissertations may be located in different sections of the library.) You will see that the books in this section are organized thematically—so the books on human evolution will be grouped together as will the books on skeletal biology. For a variety of reasons, often your computer search of the catalog will not necessarily return all the relevant results. Whenever you go to the stacks to retrieve a book you searched for, take a look at the books adjacent to it. These books will be related to your topic in some way, and might also hold pertinent information that you need.

Sometimes the library does not own a book or journal that you require. In these cases, you will need to use interlibrary loan. This service is usually free for students and faculty. There should be a link somewhere on the library's website to request a loan. Fill out the required information and usually within about a week or so, depending on the physical location and/or rarity of the resource, it will arrive at the library for you (or it may be delivered to you electronically). Interlibrary loan can take some time, which is one reason not to wait until the last minute to do your literature review. The reference you need the most is frequently the reference not available at the very moment you need it. In addition, sometimes the library will own the book you need but someone else has checked it out. In that case, you can request a recall of the book. However, keep in mind that this process can take even longer, as the person who has it may not bring it back right away.

In addition to the catalog, the library will own rights to access a number of different databases and indexes, many of which have full text articles available for download. You can also search these from the library's website—look for the link for "databases." Typically you will be able to search for relevant databases either by the name of the subject (i.e., "anthropology") or by the name or type of the database. Most libraries have also purchased licenses to different journals. This then allows you to click on the name of a journal within the catalog and it will bring you to the link where downloading full text articles can be done.

One database with which you will become the most familiar is Thomson Reuters Web of Knowledge[SM], which contains the database Web of Science[®]. This database holds full text articles in many of the journals with content in skeletal biology. You will come to love this database. Most likely your college or university owns a license to access it. For the social sciences, it has content back to 1956, and for the natural sciences, back to 1900. One of the best features of Web of Science is its "cited reference search." This allows you to find other articles that have cited a particular article. For example, if you are interested in article X, first search for it and then click on "cited reference search." This will bring up every article in the database that has cited article X. You can also go about this backwards, by looking at the references cited by article X as well. This enables you to be a detective, and expedites some of the literature review work.[2]

[1]Note that there are certain conventions to use when searching, known as Boolean operators (e.g., AND; NOT; OR). Each database or library catalog will have a tutorial on these and other conventions. Learning what they are and how to use them will improve your search.

[2]Keep in mind that databases may or may not have information on book chapters and other sources of which you will need to be aware. While the cited reference search feature will show which articles have cited article X, it will not show which book chapters have.

ScienceDirect® and JSTOR® are two other databases that contain back issues of multiple journals in anthropology and some current issues, as well as certain books. One new database that is able to search all search engines and your library catalog simultaneously is called Summon™. Free databases include Google™ Scholar, which also has a citation search feature and can search for free reprints online, and PubMed®, which contains references relevant to biology or medicine. If a study received funding from the National Institutes of Health, PubMed will have the article available as a free download. Scientific WebPlus®, part of Web of Knowledge, is also available freely and searches the general Internet for science topics, which may be useful particularly if you need to know what general information is available for topics such as evolution. Truly comprehensive searches will include dissertations and theses covering the topic of interest. Dissertation Abstracts International, managed by ProQuest®, has thousands of thesis and dissertation abstracts from North America. Depending on how comprehensive your scope is, a simple Google search can also assist as the results may include unpublished sources such as presentations or posters. Table 17.1 lists several databases that will provide a good starting point for your search.

TABLE 17.1   Selected List of Databases

Database/Index Name	Website	Free or Restricted Access	Special Feature
AnthroSource	www.aaanet.org/publications/anthrosource/	Restricted (access through your university) or free if you are AAA member	Sponsored by the American Anthropological Association (AAA); full text anthropology, mostly cultural anthropology
Google™ Scholar	http://scholar.google.com	Free	Cited reference search and free downloads
JSTOR®	www.jstor.org	Restricted (access through your university library)	Backfiles of articles in anthropology, biology (among others)
ProQuest® Dissertation Abstracts International	www.proquest.com	Restricted (access through your university library)	Thousands of thesis and dissertation abstracts from accredited universities in North America; can also search the Dissertation and Theses Full Text Database with worldwide holdings
PubMed®	www.pubmed.org	Free	Free downloads of studies funded by NIH
ScienceDirect®	www.sciencedirect.com	Freely searchable; access to articles restricted	Articles available in physical, life, health, and social sciences
Scientific WebPlus®	http://scientific.thomsonwebplus.com	Free	Searches general Internet for scientific topics; can filter by domain (.edu, .com, etc.)
Web of Science®	http://wokinfo.com/	Restricted (access through your university library)	Searches for references cited by each article; can save references to online bibliographic software (EndNote®Web)

Website addresses are current as of publication.

Bibliographic Software

Before you begin your literature review in earnest, you *must* purchase a copy of bibliographic software, such as EndNote®, ProCite®, or Reference Manager®. These software packages organize all your references, allowing you to directly import search results from many online databases into your computer. The most important feature beyond basic organization is their ability to automatically create your bibliography, using whatever format necessary. For example, if your bibliography must follow *American Journal of Physical Anthropology* formatting, it is as simple as a couple of clicks. Gone are the days of formatting your bibliography manually. In addition, these packages have "cite as you write" features, which allow you to automatically insert references already saved in the program.

Further, a reference organization program will allow you to organize your references in separate files thematically (e.g., "bioarchaeology of Chile" or "Peruvian mummy pathology"), enabling you to quickly find the citations you need based on the topic. Each entry will have an area for freehand notes, so that you can create an annotated bibliography with short paragraphs or bullet points in your own words pertaining to each article's contents. You should consider doing this every time you read a new article for several reasons: (1) when the time arrives to write your literature review, you will not necessarily remember the main points of each article and an annotated bibliography can help prevent you from having to reread everything again; and (2) it will be immensely helpful when it is time to study for your qualification or advanced exams in graduate school for the same reason. Your school's bookstore, computer store, or library website should offer at least one of these packages either free for students or for sale at a discounted student price.

SEARCHING AND OBTAINING OUTSIDE SOURCES OF FUNDING

As a graduate student, the subject of money is in all likelihood at the forefront of your mind most of the time. Large student loans, tuition, books, and living expenses eat up the typical anthropology graduate student's budget, leaving little (if any) left over for necessities such as research-related travel, data collection, and analysis. This underscores the importance of obtaining an outside source of funding.

As you already know, most academic departments offer assistantships to graduate students that cover tuition along with a stipend in exchange for some sort of service (typically teaching). You may be one of the fortunate ones who already have an assistantship. However, if you do not have an assistantship through your department, be aware that other departments/offices on campus will have assistantships available—such as the admissions office, the housing office, the student life office, the office of international education, etc. Further, perhaps one of the professors in your department has received a grant that includes funding for students to help with data collection or analysis. Research these possibilities. Your college or university may also have other funding opportunities for graduate students in the form of fellowships, travel grants, and so on. Talk to your advisor and other professors to learn what exists. The departmental administrative assistant and graduate education office should be aware of these opportunities as well.

In terms of funding that will support your research goals, there are a number of agencies that specifically support thesis and dissertation research. The National Science Foundation offers Doctoral Dissertation Improvement Grants and Graduate Research Fellowships, aimed at funding expenses such as travel away from the home institution, living expenses while conducting data collection, and analysis. The Wenner-Gren Foundation has grants for anthropology students working on their doctoral degree, and includes students at institutions outside the United States. The National Institute of Justice has a variety of different funding opportunities directed towards augmenting and facilitating forensic science (among other things). The Ford Foundation offers fellowships at the predoctoral and dissertation level for students whose goal is to forge careers in academia. For the truly adventurous, the National Geographic Society offers Young Explorer Grants for outstanding field projects. In addition, The Foundation Center lists available scholarships, fellowships, and awards from private and corporate institutions for graduate students. While this site is not freely available for searching for funding opportunities, you can either pay a registration fee or search the site to find out which library (public or university) closest to you has searching privileges. Table 17.2 lists a sampling of the agencies that have funding opportunities and their websites. Your advisor or committee members may be aware of other funding prospects as well.

Ensure that you talk to your advisor about any grant or fellowship for which you plan to apply. They have experience with applying for grants and will be able to give sage advice. When applying for any grant, the first thing you must do is ensure that the grant is a good fit for you and your project. Read the Call for Proposals or solicitations description in its entirety. There may be just one sentence that would disqualify you or your project from a particular grant, and you should not waste your time writing a proposal for a grant for which you are not qualified. In addition, grant writing is a specific skill that takes practice. Ensure that you follow the directions to the letter and ask your advisor or other professors to read over your drafts as you prepare. Your university library or other similar organization may also offer grant-writing workshops that you should take advantage of. See Table 17.3.

TABLE 17.2 Common Agencies with Funding for Anthropology Projects

Agency Name	Website	General Type of Project/Grant
Ford Foundation	www.fordfoundation.org/Grants	Predoctoral and dissertation grants
The Foundation Center	http://foundationcenter.org/	Various scholarships, fellowships, and awards; search the website for "Foundation Grants to Individuals Online"
National Geographic Society	www.nationalgeographic.com/explorers	Young Explorers Grant for fieldwork
National Institute of Justice	http://nij.gov/	Grants for forensic science projects
National Science Foundation	www.nsf.gov	Dissertation Improvement Grants and Graduate Research Fellowships
Wenner-Gren Foundation	www.wennergren.org	Dissertation grants in anthropology

Website addresses are current as of publication.

TABLE 17.3 Golden Rules #1 and #2 for Preparing Abstracts, Presentations, Manuscripts, Grant Proposals

1. **FOLLOW THE DIRECTIONS** laid out in the Call for Papers, Guidelines for Authors, or Call for Proposals.
2. Do not wait until the last minute to start writing/preparing.

GIVING A PRESENTATION

Congratulations—at this point, after completing all the steps discussed throughout this volume, you have arrived at the final stage of the scientific process—disseminating your results to a wider audience. Without this step, your study would essentially be useless, because no one else would be aware of your results. Knowledge in science grows through sharing results in a variety of forums. The two most important forums for communicating scientific results are scientific conferences and publications. Typically studies will be presented in abridged format at conferences to be followed by publication in a peer-reviewed journal. First I will cover conference presentations.

For many, the very thought of public speaking causes anxiety. Some people are more comfortable with speaking in front of groups than others, and some are better at clearly articulating spoken ideas. If you are not one such person, don't despair—with a few key tips and practice, you can certainly learn how to give an excellent presentation. Regardless of your current skill level with public speaking you can only benefit from learning a few more pointers. You should know that your reputation as a scientist will partially be tied to the quality of your presentations at conferences.

Recently I attended a conference and while perusing the books for sale in the exhibition room, I overheard someone point out a book to someone else. This person remarked that the author of that particular book had given "the worst presentation he had ever seen in his life." I am aware of another situation at a conference reception where one attendee, casually speaking within a group of people, remarked that a presentation he saw that day was pointless. Unfortunately, this attendee did not realize that the author of the presentation was standing within the group with which he was speaking. The appropriateness of disparaging colleagues in public where others can overhear should be considered; however, these examples make clear that the ability to articulate your ideas to your colleagues will partially shape your reputation in the field no matter how stellar your publication record. Further, you must be able to communicate clearly in and out of the classroom with your own students.

At Which Conference Should I Present My Study?

The major conference for skeletal biology is of course the annual gathering of the *American Association of Physical Anthropologists* (AAPA). This is held every spring, March or April, in a different city in the United States (or rarely Canada). Three other association meetings are typically held in conjunction with this conference: *Paleopathology Association*, *Human Biology Association*, and *Paleoanthropology Society* every other year (odd years; even years meetings are held in conjunction with the *Society for American*

Archaeology in the spring). If you are interested in forensic anthropology, the major confer-ence would be the *American Academy of Forensic Sciences* (AAFS), held every February. Smaller regional conferences that emphasize forensic anthropology are held every year: *Mountain, Swamp, and Beach Forensic Anthropologists* for the Southeastern United States, the *Northeast Forensic Anthropology Association* for the Northeastern United States, the *Midwest Bioarchaeology and Forensic Anthropology Association* for the Midwestern United States, and the *Mountain Desert and Coastal Forensic Anthropologists* for the Western United States. Regional meetings are more intimate and informal and present a good opportunity for presenting your work without the pressure of a national or international conference. The annual meeting of the *American Anthropological Association* is held every fall, and does have a biological anthropology section. See Table 17.4. You can find information regarding any of these conferences (or others not listed—for example, several other coun-tries have their own biological anthropology association and respective conference) by going online and searching for the respective association's website. You should seriously consider becoming a student member of the AAPA and any other association that covers the topic in which you have the most interest.

You should peruse the abstracts of papers from the past two or so years that have been presented at the conference at which you wish to present (these proceedings will usually be online). This will give you an idea of whether or not your study is thematically appropriate for that particular conference, and on what topics other researchers in the field are currently working. This will narrow down your decision considerably. AAPA occasionally holds a special poster symposium dedicated to studies by undergraduates, and many associations

TABLE 17.4   Associations Holding Conferences with Themes Relevant to Biological Anthropology

Conference Name	Region/Time of Year
• *American Anthropological Association*	United States/fall annually
• *American Academy of Forensic Sciences*	United States/February annually
• *American Association of Anthropological Genetics*	Holds symposia in conjunction with AAPA annually
• *American Association of Physical Anthropologists (AAPA)*	United States or Canada/spring annually
• *American Society of Primatologists*	United States/summer annually
• *British Association for Biological Anthropology and Osteoarchaeology*	Great Britain/fall annually
• *Canadian Association for Physical Anthropology*	Canada/fall annually
• *Human Biology Association*	United States/spring annually
• *Institute of Andean Studies*	California/January annually
• *Latin American Biological Anthropology Association (Asociación Latinoamericana de Antropología Biológica)*	Latin America/fall biannually
• *Latin American Forensic Anthropology Association (Asociación Latinoamericana de Antropología Forense)*	Latin America/fall annually
• *Paleoanthropology Society*	United States/spring annually
• *Paleopathology Association (European meeting)*	Europe/every other year (even)
• *Paleopathology Association (North American meeting)*	United States/spring annually
• *Paleopathology Association (South American meeting)*	South America/every other year (odd)
• *Society for American Archaeology*	United States/spring annually
• *World Congress of Mummy Studies*	Held in conjunction with other conferences; search their website

have student paper prizes. You should look into these opportunities several months in advance.

When Should I Begin Preparing My Study for Presentation?

Most associations in our field that hold annual conferences (such as AAFS and AAPA) require that the study be finished before you submit your abstract—that is, results are presented in the abstract. This can pose a challenge as abstracts are due several months in advance of the conference (August 1 and September 15, respectively).[3] However, no one wants to go to a presentation for which no results are available. I attended a paper once where the presenter repeatedly emphasized the preliminary nature of the results and I could not help but wonder why this person had not waited to present until the results were more defined. Learn the deadlines for abstract submission for the conferences to which you wish to present your results, and conduct the analysis of data and later writing of the abstract accordingly. It will save you time if you work on a presentation and publication simultaneously, as once the presentation has finished you will be well on your way towards sending off your publication for consideration. In addition, you will get a lot of feedback and suggestions from conference attendees that may be worth incorporating before manuscript completion. This feedback will be fresh in your mind when you get home, so it will be beneficial to continue work at that point. Further, never disregard the fact that your presentation and manuscript will involve **a great deal** of work and time on your part.

Abstract Preparation and Submission

Once you have decided for which conference you are going to prepare a presentation, you must submit your abstract. Find out when the deadline is and what the abstract preparation guidelines are. **Adhere to these guidelines strictly**. As with guidelines for grant proposals or journal manuscript preparation, **they exist for a reason**. Not following the directions can be a good reason for rejection. See Table 17.3. The guidelines are *not* suggestions; rather, they are rules. If a particular font and particular layout style are required, use them. There are several people who will be reviewing all the submitted abstracts, and it makes it easier for them if each abstract they read follows the same format and style.

In addition, don't wait until the last minute to write an abstract. You will thank yourself later if you get it submitted in advance. Many conferences now have online submission systems, and before you can upload your abstract, you may have to register with the system, pay your conference registration, etc. You never know when technical problems are going to arise—and they seem to most commonly arise when you are under a time constraint. As most people will wait until the last minute to submit, the online system might become overloaded and move slowly. To avoid any problems that may result in tears and copious sweating on your part, start early.

---

[3]These dates are subject to change. Please verify with each respective association.

Once you have uploaded your abstract, you probably will receive some sort of confirmation of submission depending upon the conference. After several months, you will find out whether or not your abstract has been accepted. Don't despair if it is not accepted—there can be a number of reasons for this. If you did follow all the formatting and style directions, then perhaps there was simply no room for your study or it may not have been topically appropriate. Other possibilities could include a poorly written abstract, noninclusion of results, or evident methodological flaws. If the latter option applies to your study, you need to do a major reassessment of your work in conjunction with your advisor and committee. If your study is not topically appropriate for that particular conference, figure out which conference would be best. If there are issues with the way you wrote your abstract, use this as a learning experience and find someone who can help you with your writing. Refer to the upcoming section on scientific writing for more information.

Abstract Acceptance—What Next?

Once your abstract has been accepted, you will want to begin preparing your presentation. The acceptance letter or e-mail will indicate whether or not you will be doing an oral presentation or a poster. Most likely you will have requested one format or the other during the submission process, but you may not get what you asked for based on the way the program committee has decided to design the program. Major conferences will have guidelines on how to prepare your Microsoft PowerPoint presentation or poster. As with the guidelines for abstract preparation, adhere to these guidelines. See Table 17.3. They exist to help you give the best presentation possible. In addition, it is crucial that you know in advance how much time you will have if giving an oral presentation or what the maximum poster size is so it fits in the space provided. I will not go through every possible guideline here, as these already exist within the Call for Papers for each conference that you can find online; however, I will provide for you some basic tips that will help you become a stronger presenter. See Tables 17.5 and 17.6.

Posters

Posters are great because they allow you to personally interact with other colleagues with regard to your research. In addition, if you are not the best public speaker, doing a poster can be a good alternative because you will only have to speak with one person at a time. If you want to network and meet other people who have the same interests or who are working on similar problems, presenting a poster is a good option. Each conference is slightly different with regard to the poster presentation setup. At AAFS and AAPA, the posters will remain up all day long with a set time for you to stand in front of yours to answer questions. Many presenters will provide their business card as well as a small version of the poster or paper as a handout.

Posters have become fancier and fancier with the advent of software programs and printers that can print out pages three or more feet wide. There are many programs you can use to create your poster, including Microsoft PowerPoint. Whichever program you decide to use, make sure that you set the resolution high enough so that it does not appear grainy or pixelated when it prints. Consider using a border for a more polished appearance.

TABLE 17.5 Dos and Don'ts of Poster Presentations

Do	Don't
• Follow the conference-specific directions for size and formatting	• Include too much text
• Look at posters of others for ideas (examples can be found online)	• Use too small a font
• Set an appropriate resolution and put a border around the poster	• Choose colors or style that are too busy/unclear/hard to read
• Research different printing options and cost	• Forget it on the plane, train, bus, etc.
• Have Plan B ready (e.g., a copy of your poster on your memory drive with you)	
• Bring extra tacks	
• Put your contact information on the tube and take it as a carry-on on the airplane	

TABLE 17.6 Dos, Don'ts, and Nevers of Paper Presentations

Do	Don't	Never
• Become comfortable with public speaking	• Use overly technical language	• Read from a paper that is in publication format
• Follow the conference-specific directions	• Put too much text on each slide	• Read without using slides or other visuals
• Find out how much time you will have	• Use unnecessary animation	• Keep talking after your time is up
• Try to emulate a good public speaker you admire	• Read your paper if you can avoid it	
• Write an abridged version of your study	• Leave a slide up for too long	
• Organize your talk into sections of introduction, methods, etc.	• Use the words "um" or "uh" or other fillers	
• Choose a high-contrast font/background color combination	• Put tables full of numbers on a slide—only put up absolutely necessary numbers	
• Have enough slides so that you can switch about every 30–45 seconds	• Paste figures into a slide without ensuring the font size of the legend or numbers is readable	
• Put it together in advance	• Use the same delivery style that you would with your students	
• Relate the facts about your work		
• Practice, practice, practice		
• Remember that the goal of presentations is to educate the audience about the results		
• Be confident!		

Follow common sense and conference guidelines for size, contents, and colors. For example, yellow-colored font on a white background will not work. Make sure you choose a font size large enough so that it can be read from about three feet away. Many people decide to use some sort of background image that they then superimpose the text over. Do this with caution, as this may make it look too busy. Remember that "presentation is everything" —you can have the best presentation in terms of the science, but if your poster looks messy or unfinished, the presentation will not be perceived well by others. You also do not want to put too much text on your poster. While the idea is for people to read it, most people would prefer for you to explain it so that they do not have to spend 20 minutes reading your poster. Include photos, graphs, and tables of your results when appropriate. Your poster will not include every single aspect of your study—just the highlights.

You can print your poster out at many stores that specialize in photocopying and other office services. Do your homework first with regard to these services. Find out how much printing costs per square foot and if there is an extra cost for color—for example, if the entire background is dark blue with white text, the cost may go up due to how much ink will be used. These services can be expensive, so make sure to check with your college or university, as there may be a lab that has a special printer available for students at a reduced rate, such as in the geography, art, architecture, natural sciences, or engineering departments. There are also many services advertised online that will print out your poster and mail it either to your address or directly to the conference hotel. I personally have never used any of these online services, but they can be convenient and may prevent mishaps such as forgetting the poster in the overhead bin of the airplane (see below). Make sure, however, that you vet any service you are going to use and always have Plan B ready just in case (i.e., bring a copy of your poster on your memory drive with you in case reprinting is necessary).

Buy a cardboard or plastic tube for your poster and bring along extra tacks, as these may not be available at the conference. Make sure that you put your name and contact information on the tube, take it as a carry-on (to prevent the airline from losing it), and **do not forget** your tube on the airplane. It sounds obvious, but it is not an uncommon occurrence. The second editor of this volume went to France for a conference with several others and the person in charge of all the posters forgot them on the plane. The entire group then spent several days before the conference running around trying to figure out how to get the posters reprinted (in a foreign country) given the software they had used to create them. This obviously also cost a small fortune.

Papers

Presenting your work as a paper is an excellent way to reach a large number of people at once, including people who may not necessarily have a particular interest in your area of research. It is important that all of us try to avoid the "tunnel vision" that can be so easy to fall into, where you only focus on your own very specific area of interest (for example, the biomechanics of the foot) and essentially ignore what else is happening in the field. Paper presentations are a great way to combat tunnel vision, as many people will sit through an entire session of papers at one time. In addition, it is important for all of as general skeletal biologists to be aware of what is happening in other subdisciplines in our field. A new method being applied in one area might apply to your own work. Moreover, if you are going to be teaching the discipline (as most likely you will be at some point), you need to be aware of the current trends in areas beyond which you are specifically working.

I have seen many different paper presentations over the years and have come to a few conclusions about what does and does not work. There are a handful of papers that stand out in my mind to this day as the best I have ever seen (due to both the science and the presentation style), and unfortunately a handful that fall into the category of among the worst I have ever seen. However, most presentations fall into the middle, average category. Your goal should be to bring your paper presentation into the realm of "excellent." You might argue that you are terrified of public speaking. In that case, I recommend joining an organization such as Toastmasters—members give speeches every week and you will learn tips on becoming a better speaker. Otherwise, all you need to do is practice in front of others to build your confidence and believe in yourself. Practice in front of the mirror, in front of your dog, in front of anyone who will listen—until it comes just as naturally to you as anything else. Yes, you will get nervous—but you can harness that energy and use it positively during your presentation.

Your first step will be to find out how long you will have for your presentation. For many conferences it is 10 or 15 minutes. Golden Rule #1 of paper presentations is **DO NOT** go over the allotted time. The papers are scheduled in such a way so that different sessions move along simultaneously and attendees can easily move back and forth between sessions to see other papers. If even just one person goes over their time, the entire system is disrupted. In addition, it is very distracting to the audience when someone goes over their time because the session moderator will stand up near the presenter, and the presenter acknowledges this but keeps on going. At that point, everyone stops listening. You can avoid this situation by practicing in advance using a timer. However, if you ever do find yourself in this situation, just stop talking and say you are out of time, or skip ahead to your conclusions when you receive the two-minute warning.

You will need to write an abridged version of your study for your presentation. Alternatively, if you already have a fair amount written (if your presentation is from your thesis or dissertation for example) then will you need to edit what you already have so that it will fit within the time allotted and be appropriate. Remember that the language you use in a written publication, thesis, or dissertation is not necessarily the same type of language you will use in an oral presentation. For example, the phrase, "as discussed above" is appropriate only for a written paper. If you wish to say something similar to this phrase, use instead, "as I just mentioned." In addition, sentences with a complex structure work well when written, but are harder for an audience to understand if read aloud.

Further, language that is too technical, even if you are giving your presentation to an audience that understands the terminology, may not work because you will lose people's focus. I once attended a presentation by a primatologist about baboons. I am not a primatologist and do not know much about baboons beyond the basics, but the presenter had geared his talk towards a general biological anthropology audience. He avoided technical language and spoke in plain English. The result was that his presentation had much more of an impact than if he had spent the time trying to impress the audience with his knowledge of professional jargon. I therefore walked away from that presentation having really learned something—which is the ultimate goal of presentations to begin with.

As you come up with the final pages of what you wish to say during your presentation, make sure that you adhere to the basics of introduction, materials and methods, results, and conclusion. Determine how you will divide these sections up among your slides and what illustrations you will use. Make sure that your presentation has a clear introduction, middle, and conclusion. This organization will help you avoid rambling.

Remember the basic rules of do not put too much text on each slide (four to five lines maximum), do not use unnecessary animations, and do choose a font/background style and color combination that has high contrast so it is easily read from far away. Make sure you have enough slides to be able to switch every 30–45 seconds or so. Avoid leaving one slide up for too long (i.e., several minutes), unless you are continuously talking about it and actively pointing things out on that particular slide. If you have to show a particular slide more than once, insert it into the slide show as many times as necessary to avoid skipping backwards during the presentation. Keep your presentation as simple as possible. You will only have a few minutes and you do not want to overwhelm the audience with information. If they want more information, they can ask you afterwards or they can read your paper once published. See Table 17.6.

You should also give serious consideration to giving a talk, as opposed to reading your paper outright. While giving a talk is more challenging and requires more experience, discipline, and practice, it will be more palatable to the audience. Remember that at a conference you are presenting to your colleagues (who are your peers), rather than to your students, so you should adjust your delivery accordingly. Reading is acceptable, but remember that it will be harder to keep the audience's attention than if you give a talk. If you do decide to read, *under no circumstances* should you stand up and read the paper in the same format it would be for publication (using the same type of language and sentence structure, etc.). Also, *under no circumstances* should you not have any slides or other visuals to go along with your read presentation. See Table 17.6. Watching someone read from their paper without accompanying visuals is academic torture. I attended a presentation in graduate school once where the person literally pulled out their dissertation and started reading. The entire point of giving presentations in the first place is so that the audience will learn something, so reading from your paper without use of visuals is not good pedagogy. You want your presentation to relate the facts about your results, and the best way to do that is by giving a talk (with reading a paper coming in second) with supporting slides.

Put your presentation together several days before the conference and practice, practice, practice. Make sure you test the presentation on a computer other than the one which created it—especially if you use a Mac and the conference will only have PCs, or vice versa. You do not want to discover strange formatting changes at the conference when you put the presentation on a different computer. Don't ignore the practice stage—it will help increase your confidence and help take away stage fright. I have a colleague who on one occasion was still putting her presentation together during the car ride to the conference. Needless to say, this did not leave her much time to practice. Sometimes putting your talk together at the last minute is inevitable; however, it should be the exception rather than the rule. The guideline I try to adhere to is to arrive at the conference with the presentation complete, already rehearsed, and saved on different media (CD, memory drive, e-mail, and the Internet cloud). The last piece of advice necessary with regard to conference presentations is to be confident. No one knows your study better than you do. Speak up and project your presence into the room.

PUBLISHING

Perhaps the most famous mantra in academia is "publish or perish." If your goal is to have a career in skeletal biology and you plan on becoming a professor, then you must become very familiar and comfortable with the process of publishing your original work. While it can be intimidating especially when you have not done so before, it is certainly not impossible. It will require a tremendous amount of work on your part (probably more than you think it will), but it is manageable if you simply complete one step at a time.

Each journal operates a little differently, but typically most will accept manuscripts in the following categories: original research, short reports, case studies, and book reviews. Original research papers are longer than short reports, which are usually just brief reports of ongoing research. Case studies and book reviews are self-explanatory, but keep in mind that book reviews are typically solicited by the editor (i.e., you should not send one in unless specifically asked to do so). As noted, each journal is different in terms of the types of manuscripts they accept for publication. Ensure that the journal you are aiming for publishes the type of study on which you are working. You may send a brief one-paragraph overview to the editor in an e-mail to ask whether they would be interested in considering your study for publication based on the subject matter.

Scientific Writing

Writing well is a critical skill you must acquire if you wish to have a career in anthropology or in research, administration, academia, and beyond. Whether or not you choose to continue with skeletal biology, at some point you will have to write a memo, a report, a proposal, or perhaps even a recommendation letter for someone else. If you cannot write well, anything you write will lose its impact and will reflect poorly on you. All colleges and universities have tutoring centers where you can bring your work for editing. In addition, some colleges have programs where they pair graduate students in English up with students writing scientific papers—the English students get credit for helping you with your writing, and you benefit by learning how to become a better writer. Scientific writing should be straightforward and clear, and even if you are already a good writer, writing in this style takes practice. I strongly recommend that you find someone who is a good writer who can help you in a one-on-one setting if you are writing in a language other than your native one, if you have learning disabilities that impact your writing, or if writing is simply not your strong suit. Your ideas may be brilliant but if you are unable to communicate them in a clear written way, no one will benefit.

Choosing the Right Journal

You are halfway there if you have already presented your study at a conference. You will have written an abridged version of your study for the presentation (discussed earlier) and you can use that as your starting point. If not, then you will need to start from the beginning. You should identify which journal you wish to submit to before you begin major revisions of what you already have or start writing from scratch. Become familiar with the journals in the field (if you are not already) and the themes that each covers.

In order for your work to have the most impact, you should submit your manuscript to a peer-reviewed journal. This means that your manuscript will be read and vetted by other experts in the subject in order to determine if it is suitable for publication. Some journals may use a single-blind process, meaning that the author does not know who the reviewers are, but the reviewers know who the author is. Others may use a double-blind process, meaning that both the reviewers and the author are unaware of each other's identity. In both processes, only the editor will be aware of who all the reviewers are. This peer-review aspect of publication gives legitimacy to the scientific publishing process. Readers of articles in peer-reviewed journals can be reasonably certain that what they are reading is reputable.[4] Be aware that some journals in the field are more prestigious than others and therefore manuscripts submitted to those journals will undergo a more rigorous review process (e.g., journals such as *Science* or *Nature*, which publish the most groundbreaking research from different scientific disciplines).

The premier journal in our specific field is of course the *American Journal of Physical Anthropology* (AJPA) (which incidentally was chosen by the Special Libraries Association Biomedical and Life Sciences Division as being one of the top ten most influential journals of the twentieth century).[5] If your work focuses on paleopathology or bioarchaeology, consider the *International Journal of Osteoarchaeology* or the *International Journal of Paleopathology*. If your interests lie in forensics, take a look at the *Journal of Forensic Sciences* (JFS) or *Forensic Science International*. See Table 17.7 for a listing of relevant English-language journals publishing work in skeletal biology.

Once you have chosen a journal for your manuscript, remember that you can only submit your work to one journal at a time and that some journals may enjoy the first rights to publish your work if you have presented it previously at the affiliated conference. For example, if you present your work at the *American Academy of Forensic Sciences* meeting and you wish to publish it, JFS will enjoy exclusive rights to review your manuscript within six months of the date of the conference. After that time has expired, you are free to submit your manuscript to whichever journal you wish. In addition, once your article is published, you relinquish the copyright to the journal's publisher. This means that you no longer own your article and you cannot publish it in the same form elsewhere.

Authorship Order

You have probably noticed that most articles are authored by several individuals. This then begs the question of how to decide who will be first author, second author, and so on. The answer is simple: the first author is the person who has done/will do the most work on the study and the paper. It then ranks in decreasing order from there. For the natural science disciplines (chemistry, physics, etc.) it is customary to include the lab director's name

---

[4]Keep in mind that the peer-review process is not perfect. The scientists who review papers may miss something. To some extent, they have to take the word of the authors of the paper as to what they did and the results. For this reason, you shouldn't necessarily always believe everything you read. Give higher weight to studies published in more prestigious journals and look at multiple sources to confirm the same information, or validate the study yourself if possible.

[5]http://units.sla.org/division/dbio/publications/resources/topten.html (last accessed March 2012).

TABLE 17.7 Common Journals Publishing Work in Skeletal Biology

Journal	Theme Relevant to Skeletal Biology
• *American Journal of Human Biology*	All human biology, especially as it relates to health and disease
• *American Journal of Physical Anthropology*	All biological anthropology
• *Current Anthropology*	All of anthropology
• *Forensic Science International*	Forensic anthropology
• *HOMO — Journal of Comparative Human Biology*	All biological anthropology and associated fields
• *International Journal of Osteoarchaeology*	Paleopathology; bioarchaeology
• *International Journal of Paleopathology*	Paleopathology; bioarchaeology
• *Journal of Dental Research*	Health and disease as related to dental structures
• *Journal of Archaeological Research*	All of archaeology, including bioarchaeology
• *Journal of Forensic Sciences*	Forensic anthropology
• *Journal of Human Evolution*	Paleoanthropology
• *Yearbook of Physical Anthropology*	All biological anthropology

as last author on the paper if the study was done in a lab. While this custom is not necessarily adhered to in anthropology (with the exception of anthropological genetics), you must make sure that everyone who is involved in the project is in agreement ahead of time as to authorship order. Some will not want their name on a paper with which they had no direct involvement, and others will because their lab's resources were used in the generation of the study. Therefore it is important to get author order cleared up at the beginning. This also will enable the first author to assign tasks to all of the other authors. Sometimes if there are just two authors, the understanding is that both people will do equal amounts of work and the compromise may be that one researcher is first author for study A but will be the second author for study B.

Manuscript Preparation

While each journal is different, your manuscript will essentially follow the basic format of abstract, introduction, materials and methods, results, discussion, and conclusion. You will find requirements for these sections in the Guidelines for Authors, found at each journal's website. In addition to these requirements, choose a title carefully. It should succinctly state the topic of the study. Often for conference presentations, people will choose clever titles to attract attention to their study so that people will attend. An example is a recent poster presented at AAFS: "And Dens There Were Two: The Utility of the Second Cervical Vertebra as an Indicator of Sex and Age-at-Death" (Seet and Bethard, 2010). While creative titles work well for conference presentations, it is better to leave out the creativity and stick to the facts when choosing a title for your manuscript. The same study was published as "Sex Determination from the Second Cervical Vertebra: A Test of Wescott's Method on a Modern American Sample" (Bethard and Seet, 2012). When people are searching for articles, the title is the first thing that will come up and you want the point of your article to be clearly stated to make it easier for them to decide if your article is relevant for their needs. In addition, the abstract should be brief, able to stand on its own (including brief summaries of the introduction, methods, results, and conclusion), and not a pasting of text from the introduction. Many people will read the abstract to determine what your study is about and therefore decide whether or not they need to read the article for more information.

Once you have decided to which journal you are going to submit, you need to download the Guidelines for Authors from that journal's website if you have not already done so. These directions are typically extensive and you must follow them to the letter. They will usually include rules for font type and size, margin size, how to cite references, how to use common abbreviations, which sections the manuscript should contain, and how to format the bibliography. See Tables 17.3 and 17.8. As with abstract guidelines for conferences, the author guidelines for manuscript preparation are <u>not</u> suggestions. **They are requirements**. Not following the requirements will result in your manuscript being sent back to you by the editor possibly even before being sent to reviewers. When in doubt about any of the requirements, use a recent article from that journal as a formatting example.

Pay close attention to the rules for which file formats are acceptable (e.g., which version(s) of Microsoft Word are supported) and the requirements for illustrations. Most journals will not want the tables and figures to be embedded within the document. All will require that the figures be a certain digital resolution and will have a rule about which digital file format photographs should be (i.e., TIFF, JPEG, etc.). It is important to know this early on so you avoid having to retake or reformat photographs later for example. They will also have rules about color illustrations. Printing in color is very expensive, so the editor will want to know if color is absolutely necessary for your article. If so, then the cost of the color printing may have to be assumed by the authors. A reasonable compromise is to ask that the print edition have grayscale illustrations and that the online version have the illustrations in color. Most journals today have online submission and the system will not allow you to finalize your submission if, for example, your photos are too small or large or if you have used an unsupported document creator.

You may be tempted to include a multitude of figures and tables in your manuscript. Unless absolutely necessary, do not give into this temptation. While figures and tables

TABLE 17.8 Typical Formatting/Inclusion Considerations for Manuscript Preparation

- Cover letter to editor
- Cover page with title, author names, contact information, keywords
- Type of manuscript (original research, case study, technical report, etc.)
- Sections of manuscript (abstract, introduction, methods, etc.)
- Type of document creator and file extension (Microsoft Word, etc.)
- Font size and type
- Margin size
- Requirements for figure size and file format
- Requirements for table formatting
- Color illustrations or grayscale?
- Use of special characters (e.g., in formulae or non-English words)
- Type of spelling (American or British)
- Formatting of headings for each section
- Formatting of bibliography
- Formatting of references (endnotes or parenthetical)

are an excellent way to demonstrate your results, you <u>can</u> have too many. You do not want to confuse the reader. In addition, each figure or table will add to your manuscript preparation time considerably—particularly if formatting issues arise (refer to the case study later in this chapter). Keeping this in mind will help you make your decision wisely. Only include those figures necessary to illustrate the main points and where it will help with comprehension of the text. Further, make sure to give yourself enough time when you are ready to upload your manuscript using an online submission system. Depending upon the size of the figures and your connection speed, each one can take several minutes to upload. Plan ahead for this.

In addition to formatting the manuscript in accordance with the journal's requirements, you must ensure that your grammar and spelling are pristine. If you are submitting to a journal published in the United Kingdom, use British spelling for words (e.g., "colour" instead of "color"), and the opposite will apply if submitting to a journal published in the United States. Reviewers and editors will not look favorably on a manuscript whose author(s) did not take the time to use spell check and read the manuscript over carefully before submission. Errors like these will detract from the science in the paper, and this carelessness will cause reviewers to ask themselves if the author(s) had been just as sloppy in the research design of the study. If you have issues with writing well for any reason, it will be to your benefit to find a professional editor or someone who is an excellent writer to help you before submission. You <u>must</u> be able to communicate in a straightforward and clear manner. Refer to the earlier section on scientific writing.

About the Acknowledgments

Every paper should include some acknowledgments. There is always someone to thank: your advisor for their support, the museum/lab where you conducted research, the entity that gave you permission to publish the data (if applicable), the person who gave you the idea for the project, anyone who significantly helped you, and so on. While you can obviously acknowledge who you want, it is proper academic etiquette to acknowledge those individuals and organizations by name without which you could not have done your study. Sometimes authors will acknowledge the anonymous reviewers whose comments helped them improve the manuscript. I personally always choose to acknowledge the individuals who composed the skeletal sample for my project. In addition, you must always disclose any grants or other funding that you received towards support of the project. You may also need to include a disclaimer statement such as, "the results of this project may or may not reflect the views of the granting agency". Read the fine print of any grants you have to find out if the funding agency requires such a statement.

The Submission Process

As mentioned previously, many journals now have an online submission process. This has facilitated submission over the previous process of sending via snail mail multiple hard copies of everything. You will need to create a profile for yourself and the other authors (if applicable) if you are not already registered with the system. You should be prepared to upload several files: (1) your cover letter to the editor (discussed in a moment); (2) cover page (which usually includes the article title; authors' names, order, and contact information; three or so key words which will be used for Internet search engine purposes; and an abbreviated title); (3) the actual manuscript; (4) each figure (graphs, photographs, drawings) separately; (5) tables; and (6) sometimes the bibliography separate from the manuscript. The author guidelines for each particular journal will direct you as to exactly what is required. See Table 17.8.

A cover letter to the editor may not be specifically requested, but you should do one anyway. Essentially, this is your opportunity to "sell" your article to the editor and tell her why your article should be considered for publication in their journal. It should be short, sweet, and to the point. Find out who the editor is and make sure you spell their name correctly and address them appropriately, e.g., Dr. Jane Smith. If you have color figures, this would be a good time to mention it. You also should be ingratiating in the letter. You are asking the editor to consider your manuscript and you need to succinctly explain why your manuscript is worthy of publication in their journal. An example sentence would be similar to, "We appreciate the opportunity to submit our manuscript for consideration to the *Journal of Amazing Things* and look forward to receiving your comments" and so on. Your cover letter should be no longer than one page. You should also mention which author will be the corresponding author at this point, that is, the person who will receive all relevant correspondence from the journal. This may not necessarily be the first author—all authors can decide amongst themselves who wants this designation.

Once your manuscript is ready and you have gone over it for the seemingly thousandth time, set aside some time for the submission process. The system may ask you to suggest reviewers for your article based on the subject matter. This is obviously no guarantee as to which three or four individuals will actually review your manuscript, but it will help give the editor an idea of who may be appropriate given the particular topic. You will receive a confirmation number of your submission and sometimes an automatically generated e-mail. The system will also generate a PDF file that combines all uploaded files. Save this digitally. At this point, you will need to familiarize yourself with three things: (1) patience; (2) receiving constructive criticism; and (3) rejection. It may be several months before you receive the reviewer comments from the editor, so set your manuscript aside and start working on other things!

The Decision Letter

Some time after you have submitted your manuscript and you are just beginning to wonder whatever happened with it, you or the corresponding author will receive an e-mail with the decision letter. This is always an exciting (and sometimes scary) day. The letter will contain the comments of the editor and anonymous reviewers. The editor will inform you if your manuscript was or will be (1) accepted, with minimal revisions; (2) reconsidered for publication if significant revisions are made; (3) not accepted because formatting guidelines were not followed; (4) not accepted because it is not suitable for publication in that particular journal; (5) not accepted because it is not a scientifically sound manuscript—there are major methodological changes that must be made; or (6) some combination of points 3–5.

The Revision Process

Regardless of what the letter says, you will want to read over the comments carefully. If revisions are required, you will probably read the comments over several times. Send the reviews to your coauthors if applicable and come up with a game plan. If revisions are required, the letter will give you a deadline to submit those revisions, typically about two months or so from the date of the letter. Sometimes the revisions are simple and sometimes they are more involved, so get started early. You will make the necessary changes and write a detailed letter to the editor and reviewers explaining how you have responded to each of their comments specifically. Sometimes you may not agree with a change a reviewer is suggesting. In that case, you will address the reason why in the response letter. Once again, you will be ingratiating in the letter and thankful for the insight and helpful comments that have improved the manuscript. Once finished, you will go through the online submission process again with the revised manuscript. This time, however, you will probably not have to wait as long for a new decision letter from the editor.

If your manuscript is not accepted because it is not suitable for publication in this particular journal, you will want to read over reviewer comments (if there are any), make minor changes (if applicable), and resubmit to a journal that is more appropriate. If your manuscript was not accepted because of formatting or writing issues, you need to fix those immediately. Again, get someone to help you with this. If your manuscript was not accepted because it was not a scientifically sound study, then you must read over the comments with an open mind to determine the problems and possible remedies. If there were methodological issues, then you may need to rework your research design. If there were ethical issues, then either abandon the project or rework it so that no ethical issues remain. Hopefully you will never find yourself in any of the above situations (especially after heeding the advice and knowledge in this book)!

After Article Acceptance

Once all the necessary changes have been made and you receive the letter saying your article has been accepted, congratulations! Your hard work has paid off. There is still a little more to do, however. Within a few weeks or months (depending upon the journal's production schedule) you will receive a set of proofs. These are a formatted copy of what your article will look like in print. This is also an exciting day, because here is your article, with your name on it, almost print-ready! This will be your last chance to make any changes to your article. However, these changes will be minor—no adding new paragraphs, figures, or the like. Changes you may need to make might include mentioning someone else in the acknowledgments, adding one new sentence, fixing a number that is incorrect, and things of that nature. You can also request that the copy editor or typesetter move things around or make changes, such as making one figure larger or putting two of the tables side by side.

You must read the proof over very carefully. Do not do this on a computer screen because you will certainly miss things. Print out a copy and read it over in a location with no distractions. You want to make sure that no errors were made when typesetting your manuscript into its current format. Double-check the affiliation information and spelling of each author's name. Send a copy to your coauthors if applicable and ask them to read over the proof as well. Check over the proof as soon as possible and send it back to the copy editor before the given deadline. Within a few weeks, your article will appear online on the journal's website in Early View format and will be fully citable. Soon thereafter, your article will be in print format in the journal. Don't forget to add it to your curriculum vitae, and congratulations, you have successfully published your first article! On to the next one!

CASE STUDY: THE FIRST RIB AND THE PHOTOGRAPHS

A few years ago, several colleagues and I published an article on a new method to estimate age-at-death using the first rib (DiGangi et al., 2009). There were eleven variables on three different morphological aspects of the first rib that we examined and tested to determine which were best correlated with real age. Statistical analysis later discriminated this list to two variables.

We began data collection about three years before manuscript preparation, and while we took photographs at the time, we realized three years later that some of those photographs were not of sufficient quality for publication. It is common for the data collection stage to precede the publication stage by a large amount of time. We learned from our mistake that it is always best to take as many high-quality photographs as possible of each variable you are studying, as you never know what images you will need later for publication. Given that several of our images were low quality or did not illustrate exactly what we needed, we had to do two things: (1) find examples of the variables in a different skeletal collection, as our original study collection was no longer available (this involved going through several hundred boxes), and (2) hire a photographer with a camera that had high-quality zoom to take the necessary photographs. These logistical solutions added a great deal of time (and money) to manuscript preparation.

The final method had two variables (the surface texture of the tubercle facet and geometric shape of the costal face), and therefore we needed to include photos of each different possible scoring phase for each variable (there were nine total possible phases). This meant including 18 photographs in the manuscript, as we included two examples of each scoring phase. Since the print version of the article was to have grayscale images and the online version color images, 18 photographs doubled to 36. This by itself was daunting; however, the reviewer comments asked us to include a supplementary file for online publication on the nine variables and their scoring states that we had studied but had not been discriminated statistically as best correlated with real age. This involved adding *several dozen* more photographs!

As each variable involved different aspects of one of three morphological areas of the first rib (costal face, tubercle facet, or rib head), there were several photographs that illustrated more than one variable (for example, we used the same photo twice to separately show the geometric shape of the tubercle facet and articular margins of the tubercle facet). Having some duplicate photos and some single photos meant that we had to be meticulously organized and very careful with the real age and sex information for the figure legends. The second author and I spent many hours over the phone together checking and rechecking everything. We also had to be prepared for the considerable amount of time it took to upload so many large images.

As you can imagine, the unexpected requirement of the supplementary file not only added several more days of work to the manuscript but additionally contributed to an increase in our collective stress level. While the number of figures we managed was exceptional for a journal article, our experience with organizing the photographs certainly prepared us for future projects that will involve numerous figures. The moral of the story is to be as meticulously organized as possible with photographs and other figures or tables for your project and to be prepared for the unexpected even after you have submitted your manuscript for consideration. This will help in the long run with minimizing errors and stress.

CONCLUSION

Hopefully this chapter has reduced some of the mystery surrounding library searches, presenting, and publishing. Each time you sit down in the library and use its resources, you will become much more comfortable and proficient with finding even the most elusive of sources. Similarly, each presentation you give will build upon previous ones in terms of your knowledge and comfort level with either posters or paper presentations. You may even grow to enjoy the process, as it ultimately involves sharing your results in person with your colleagues. You'll probably even discover that you love being in a room full of people who have the same affinity for anthropology and skeletal biology that you do! Likewise, while the publication process can be wrought with stress, there is no feeling in the world similar to seeing your name in print on a publication and knowing it is the culmination of all of your hard work. The best part of course is the fact that each of your publications contributes to the growth of scientific knowledge—serving to remind you why you wanted to become a scientist in the first place.

ACKNOWLEDGMENTS

The contents of this chapter result not only from personal experience, but from lessons imparted over the years from former professors and current colleagues. Therefore, I thank them for passing on their knowledge. Beth West helped with information for the funding section of this chapter. Dr. Graciela Cabana generously read a draft of this chapter, and I thank her for comments that improved the manuscript.

REFERENCES

Bethard, J., Seet, B., 2012. Sex determination from the second cervical vertebra: a test of Wescott's method on a modern American sample. Journal of Forensic Sciences, in press.
DiGangi, E., Bethard, J., Kimmerle, E., Konigsberg, L., 2009. A new method for estimating age-at-death from the first rib. American Journal of Physical Anthropology 138 (2), 164–176.

Seet, B., Bethard, J., 2010. And dens there were two: the utility of the second cervical vertebra as an indicator of sex and age-at-death. Proceedings of the American Academy of Forensic Sciences 16, 372.

SUGGESTED READING

Bolker, J., 1998. Writing Your Dissertation in Fifteen Minutes a Day: A Guide to Starting, Revising, and Finishing Your Doctoral Thesis. Owl Books, New York.

Day, R., Gastel, B., 2011. How to Write and Publish a Scientific Paper, 7th ed. Greenwood, Santa Barbara, CA.

Luey, B., 2010. Handbook for Academic Authors, 5th ed. Cambridge University Press, New York.

Strunk, W., White, E.B., 1999. The Elements of Style, 4th ed. Longman, New York.

Zerubavel, E., 1999. The Clockwork Muse: A Practical Guide to Writing Theses, Dissertations, or Books. Harvard University Press, Cambridge.

Future Research Considerations in Human Skeletal Biology

Elizabeth A. DiGangi, Megan K. Moore

Surely the astute reader of this volume has noticed the broad diversity of the contributors' experience. Some are senior scholars with the advantage of having successfully completed dozens of research projects, presentations, and publications. Other scholars are recent PhDs or advanced graduate students with the student perspective still fresh on their minds, and yet others fall somewhere in between. Our intent in assembling such an assortment of authors was to bring a variety of viewpoints on the research process to the volume and to illustrate that one need not be a senior scholar to successfully conduct a research project. Even scholars with years of experience were once in your shoes: eager to learn, maybe a little overwhelmed, and perhaps apprehensive of the process ahead. Each chapter in this volume has demonstrated that certain key factors are necessary to begin: (1) knowledge of the scientific method; (2) knowledge of the literature (both historic theoretical foundations and more recent advances); and (3) knowledge of the anthropological questions and methods particular to the area of interest. Other themes are evident as well, which will be discussed herein.

RECOMMENDATIONS FOR DEVELOPING YOUR APTITUDE AS A SCHOLAR

It seems belated to state that you must know your osteology. Each area in skeletal biology will require that the practitioner be an expert in skeletal anatomy, including knowledge of the cellular structure of bone (i.e., histology). Musculoskeletal anatomy is critical as well, as you cannot understand dry bone without understanding the system of muscles, joints, ligaments, and tendons that operated on the once living skeleton. Courses in gross anatomy and physiology will help you gain a deeper understanding of the interconnectedness of the different systems within the human body. An additional understanding of how the skeleton is affected by its environment (physical and cultural) is necessary, making osteology a required subject even for demographers whose main interest is running robust statistical analyses.

If you have not yet taken graduate level courses in skeletal biology, osteology, *and* osteometry, now would be a great time to start. Osteology courses focusing on fragments in particular are suggested. There are increasingly more field schools with either a component or an emphasis on bioarchaeology (typically outside the United States), which are tailored to aspiring skeletal biologists. These offer the student an opportunity to learn how to properly excavate skeletal remains in addition to how to curate and later analyze those remains. For an anthropologist with an interest in skeletal biology, a field school is indispensible in terms of the methodological skill set that you will acquire.

We have learned from experience that the best way to learn a subject is by teaching the subject. Explaining how to identify or analyze bones in addition to explaining anthropological concepts to other people will help to solidify your own knowledge base. Therefore, you should jump at any opportunity to teach anthropology—volunteer as a teaching assistant in the osteology lab or seek out teaching assistantship positions.

In addition to knowing your bones, you *must* be familiar with the literature. As made clear throughout this volume, science builds on what has come before. You are not the first person to do a project in skeletal biology, nor will you be the last. The foundation for your project has been laid by your professors and by their professors before them. As a result, the only way to contextualize your particular project is via thorough knowledge of previous work in order to create a strong foundation for your research design.

Do not ignore literature that is seemingly outside of your specific research focus. There are broad themes of which all biological anthropologists must be aware. These include the evolutionary underpinning of our discipline and the biocultural framework that we apply to the questions and hypotheses we pose. Avoid a tunnel-vision approach, whereby you focus specifically on your own question and ignore developments in theory or method in the other scientific disciplines and in anthropology overall. Theory drives the discipline forward and incorporation of that theory is necessary for work to stay current and relevant, and for scientific advancement.

While few chapters in this volume dove deeply into statistics, it should be apparent that statistical analyses are essential for elucidating patterns, providing estimable error rates, and validating results. Therefore, as authors in the volume have emphasized, fluency with statistical approaches to anthropological questions is necessary. Statistics is not only vital for your own analyses, but also fundamental for critically reviewing the literature. Students of anthropology may be intimidated to enroll in a college-level statistics course, but should nevertheless start now and work their way up to multivariate analyses courses. Developing a strong foundation in statistical theory and practice will make you a better skeletal biologist.

As discussed continually throughout this volume, biological anthropology today takes a population perspective approach to human variation. As skeletal biologists, we investigate the skeleton to answer questions regarding human experience, life history, and population history for both past and present populations. Our unique holistic and biocultural viewpoint has enabled us to move past typology and embrace the population perspective as capable of informing us of the where, when, why, and how for human variation. Ensure that your questions are constructed in such a way that the interaction of culture and the environment is considered in terms of the resulting impact on biology and therefore population history overall.

Try to approach skeletal research as a functional morphologist, investigating the etiology of factors such as trauma, pathology, and cross-sectional shape and the possible implications these had for the life history of the individual. This reflects Washburn's call for a "new physical anthropology" (1951), which while published over six decades ago, still has relevance for the practice of biological anthropology today.

In addition, Blakey (1998) proposed that we be critically self-reflective of our cultural assumptions that creep into the scientific process. Further, he suggested that we realize that science, because human beings practice it, cannot be utterly objective. While we strive for objectivity, subjective interpretations can influence our analyses and conclusions (Blakey, 1998). As a result, it is necessary to take an anthropological viewpoint towards our role as scientists, the research that we do, and the impact it has on society at large. It would be to our advantage if we could acknowledge our limitations as scientists as a result of inherent cultural bias. Consciously taking a critical and self-reflective approach to the questions we choose to pursue, to hypothesis construction, and to the interpretation of results will enable us to more effectively communicate our conclusions. As emphasized in several chapters in this volume, each scientist is a product of their own culture and the associated sociopolitical thought. Therefore, we have a responsibility to society to acknowledge how our own cultural biases affect our questions, methods, results, and conclusions.

TRENDS IN HUMAN SKELETAL BIOLOGY

A critical read of the content in this volume demonstrates that several trends are apparent in contemporary skeletal biology. These include (1) an increased awareness of secular trends; (2) a recognition of the importance of developing population-specific standards for both bioarchaeological and forensic applications of skeletal analysis; (3) an emphasis on validation studies; (4) an increased reliance on robust statistics; (5) advances in technology that permit the posing of anthropological questions in new and creative ways; and (6) the potentiality that biodistance analysis will continue to clarify how evolutionary forces have affected our species' history.

Secular trends, as demonstrated by several chapters in this volume, are important for understanding a variety of processes. The fact that populations change through time due to environmental forces demonstrates the influence that the environment, via evolutionary forces, has on biology. The first author lives in Bogotá, Colombia, where a walk of the streets quickly reveals that males in their fifties and above are a great deal shorter than teenage boys and young males in their twenties. While this observation falls into the first part of the scientific method, the subsequent hypothesis would be that secular change has occurred in the *Bogotano* population over the past few decades, possibly as a result of improved access to medical care, improved nutrition, and improved sanitation for city dwellers (coinciding with sociopolitical change) that has at least affected biological growth. A contrary hypothesis could be that the decreased stature in older males is a result of stature reduction as a result of aging and compression of the soft tissues of the body or collapsing of the vertebrae.

Given that there is a countrywide database on stature kept by the agency that administers identification cards and that there are two modern skeletal collections in Colombia, both hypotheses could be tested. The methodological approach would have to be altered slightly however in order to directly test the latter hypotheses. It is important to note that the age-effects hypothesis for stature reduction is not the null hypothesis of the secular trend hypothesis or vice versa. While secular trends in other populations or in areas other than stature may not be as immediately apparent, it remains clear that they do occur, even on a subtle level, and they contribute to our understanding of population history. Similarly, biological changes throughout the life cycle reflect an individual's life history.

Further, the fact that secular change occurs underscores the importance of developing standards for the biological profile that are population specific in both time *and* space. Standards developed on individuals who died 50 years ago or more are probably not going to be accurate when applied to modern individuals. However, we must test assumptions such as these via comparison of historical samples with modern ones. One way to do this is through the validation of standards. As discussed in several chapters, there are a few methods that we continually rely on to estimate age, sex, ancestry, and stature. These must be tested on different populations and updated for contemporary generations to assure their validity and that they are suitable for application to particular populations. This is because each population has its own specific population history that has affected the resultant variation. As a result, when conceiving your own research project idea, you do not always have to reinvent the wheel: a multitude of possibilities, such as testing and validating existing methods, already exist.

As discussed above, fluency in statistics is an essential component of the skeletal biologist's tool kit. Today we increasingly rely on more robust statistics, as demonstrated by several chapters in this volume. With regard to validation studies in particular, a novel statistical approach (such as Bayesian analyses) can be used to improve upon previous methods or introduce a more sound way to analyze our data. However, it is essential that you fully understand the limitations and assumptions involved with any statistic chosen for data analysis, as some tests will be more appropriate for particular hypotheses and types of data than others.

Statistics are becoming particularly important in forensics, especially in light of the recent critique of the state of the forensic sciences by the National Research Council of the National Academies (2009). Research that uses advanced statistics to determine the probabilities of identification given the presence of particular skeletal features will help fortify forensic anthropological analyses.

Advances in technology even of methods that have existed for decades (e.g., stable isotope analysis and microscopy) are revolutionizing the field. Breakthroughs in DNA have been used not only for identification of human remains in medicolegal contexts, but also for examining the genetic structure of our distant ancestors, for identifying pathogens in human skeletal remains, and for investigating the geographic patterning of human variation. Medical imaging technology has the potential to reveal detailed information about the functional adaptation of the human skeleton and of health and disease in mummified and skeletal remains. All of these advances have the potential to answer numerous questions about the human biocultural past and present that early physical anthropologists never could have imagined.

While some scholars have contended that biodistance analysis is simply typological and harks back to early manifestations of physical anthropology (e.g., Armelagos and Van Gerven, 2003), others have disagreed, stating that biodistance analysis has the potential to clarify how evolutionary forces have affected our species' history, including, among other things, providing insight into ethnogenesis via understanding of how populations interacted with each other in the past (e.g., Stojanowski and Buikstra, 2004). However, fears that analyses such as biodistance are essentially typological should be heeded by scholars undertaking such analyses when constructing hypotheses and during the contextualization of the results and the conclusions.

IMPORTANT CONSIDERATIONS

It should be clear after reading this volume that presenting and publishing your results is a requirement. Imagine if Earnest Hooton had never published *The Indians of Pecos Pueblo*, or Sherwood Washburn decided to not write his manuscript about the direction he thought the discipline should take. What if George Armelagos had not attended the 1965 National Academy of Sciences symposium on the sad state of skeletal analysis hosted by Saul Jarcho or if Jane Buikstra had never formally married archaeology with the study of human skeletons? How might the discipline be different without these seminal contributors or contributions? These pioneers, among others, set the foundation for modern skeletal biology. While your project may not necessarily become a keystone of skeletal biology research, it nevertheless is a contribution that adds to the growth of the discipline.

This volume has further demonstrated that collaboration with scholars in other disciplines is beneficial in terms of the knowledge that can be generated. The biocultural approach essentially calls for interdisciplinary collaboration. As anthropologists, our unique holistic viewpoint requires our vision to take place through a wide lens. A valuable way to answer anthropological questions therefore is through collaboration with colleagues in all areas of science.

VISION TOWARDS THE FUTURE

The field has evolved significantly since Hrdlička, Hooton, and Boas laid its foundation. We have moved from a discipline focused on the analysis and description of human types to one that interprets adaptation and embraces cultural and environmental explanations for human variation. Larsen asserts, "The recent shift in paradigm from emphasis on typology and description of anatomical and pathological variation to that of processual and behavioral interpretation is a breakthrough that is providing the basis for a more meaningful understanding of past adaptation" (1987:410). While this statement was made almost 30 years ago, it remains relevant today. Our goal as skeletal biologists is to explain and interpret the reasons for human variation from a holistic standpoint, acknowledging the complex interaction of culture, environment, and biology.

Students of skeletal biology are therefore encouraged to carry the torch into the next generation, by asking new questions based on developing technologies from different scientific disciplines. What new inventions within engineering, physics, chemistry, geology, and the biomedical sciences can be applied to the study of the human skeleton to automate research protocols, facilitate nondestructive and robust analyses, or provide digital archives of human skeletal remains? What secular changes can be detected in human populations that affect forensic or bioarchaeological analyses? How can current theory in archaeology and other disciplines be applied to emerging questions surrounding gender, agency, and identity in the bioarchaeological record? How can we communicate effectively with the public about the effects of the social race concept while simultaneously improving our ability to identify individuals? The investigation of these questions, among others, will help you shape the future of the discipline.

As a graduate student you will be required to take a qualifying or comprehensive exam most likely at the end of your first year. A question on one of our qualifying exams queried, "Just what can anthropologists learn from those old bones and teeth, anyway?" We hope that this volume has presented tools that will enable you to begin to answer that question for yourself through the development of your own research program in human skeletal biology.

ACKNOWLEDGMENTS

We thank Drs. Maria Smith and Jonathan Bethard for their helpful suggestions during the preparation of this conclusion.

REFERENCES

Armelagos, G.J., Van Gerven, D.P., 2003. A century of skeletal biology and paleopathology: contrasts, contradictions, and conflicts. American Anthropologist 105 (1), 53–74.

Blakey, M.L., 1998. Beyond European enlightenment: toward a critical and humanistic human biology. In: Goodman, A.H., Leatherman, T.L. (Eds.), Building a New Biocultural Synthesis. University of Michigan Press, Ann Arbor, pp. 379–405.

Hooton, E.A., 1930. The Indians of Pecos Pueblo, A Study of Their Skeletal Remains. Vol. 4. In: Papers of the Southwestern Expedition. Yale University Press, New Haven.

Larsen, C.S., 1987. Bioarchaeological interpretations of subsistence economy and behavior from human skeletal remains. Advances in Archaeological Method and Theory 10, 339–445.

National Research Council of the National Academies, 2009. Strengthening Forensic Science in the United States: A Path Forward. The National Academies Press, Washington, D.C.

Stojanowski, C.M., Buikstra, J.E., 2004. Biodistance analysis, a biocultural enterprise: a rejoinder to Armelagos and Van Gerven (2003). American Anthropologist 106 (2), 430–432.

Washburn, S.L., 1951. The new physical anthropology. Transactions of the New York Academy of Sciences. Series II, 13 (7), 298–304.

Glossary[1,2]

3Skull: A three-dimensional data acquisition program, which interfaces a 3-D digitizer with a personal computer to register 3-D coordinates of traditional craniometric landmarks. This program was developed by Stephen Ousley.

Acceleration: The rate of change in velocity over time.

Accentuated line: A hypoplasia, or period of decreased enamel or dentin secretion, that is related to a stressful event in an organism's life during that period of tooth development. See also **linear enamel hypoplasia**.

Accuracy: For accuracy in stature estimation, the actual stature of an individual fits within the standard error of the regression line. Accuracy does not necessarily indicate that an estimate is precise, i.e., it has a narrow range of standard error.

Activation, resorption, formation (ARF): The sequential process of bone remodeling.

Actualism/actualistic research: Experimental **taphonomic** research designed to replicate and observe natural phenomena.

Acute: Disease process of short duration that does not typically disseminate to bone.

Acute injury: An acute injury is one that has a sudden onset and has occurred close to the time frame in question. In forensics, this is often used to denote an injury that has occurred close to or at the time of death.

Adaptive history: This concept of adaptive history is compared with **population history**. Adaptive history is a study of the history of natural selection on one or more traits exhibited by the population sample in question.

Age cohorts: Groupings of individuals lumped together on the basis of chronological age categories (e.g., juvenile, young adult, adult, etc.).

Agency theory: An explanatory alternative within post-processualism to counter the processualist focus on ecological and economic explanation for how archaeological cultures develop and are maintained. Individuals (the agent) in their respective cultural contexts make personal choices that are counter to routine behavior (doxa) and social norms (habitus), all of which have social and physiological consequences. These may be far-reaching (e.g., impetus for cultural change). How these social and physiological consequences are detected (i.e., a methodology) has yet to be articulated.

Allele: An alternative form of a gene that is located at a specific position on a specific chromosome.

Allometry: A change in shape or proportions related to change in size; also the differential growth rates of the different elements within an individual in relation to size and shape. An example of this in human infants and children is demonstrated by the disproportionately large head, which scales down as the rate of growth for the limbs and trunk increases at later stages of growth and development.

Alternative hypothesis: Hypothesis stating that changes in the **independent variable** will lead to changes in the **dependent variable**; opposite of **null hypothesis**.

Alu elements: Transposable elements, also known as jumping genes. These are rare sequences of DNA that can move themselves to new positions within the genome of a single cell.

Ameloblast: Enamel-forming cell.

American School of Anthropology, The: Informal name for the anthropological research being done in the United States during the nineteenth century, especially applying to the craniometric work of Samuel

---

[1]This glossary results from the combined collaboration of all contributors to this volume.

[2]For terms specific to geometric morphometrics, many of the definitions are drawn from a much larger glossary by Slice et al. (2009) on the SUNY Stony Brook Morphometrics website (http://life.bio.sunysb.edu/morph/index.html). This online glossary was an updated version of the glossary provided in the volume *Advances in Morphometrics* edited by Marcus et al. (1996). Expanded definitions and further resources can be found in this larger document. Citations for these references can be found in Chapter 12.

George Morton in Philadelphia (Brace, 2005—reference cited in Chapter 5).

Analytical paleopathology: The problem-oriented methodology for evaluating pathological conditions of human remains. The approach is premised on a sample large enough for (at least) simple statistical analysis.

Anatomical method for stature estimation: A method for living stature estimation that includes the height/length of each of the bones that make up stature (e.g., skull height, height of each vertebra and one sacral segment, pelvic height, femur length, tibia length, and the height of the articulated talus and calcaneus) along with an estimate of soft tissue thickness (e.g. Fully's anatomical method for stature estimation).

Ancient DNA: The **DNA** of long-deceased organisms (generally 100 or more years).

Andresen lines: Long-period lines that are the dentinal (dentin) equivalent of **striae of Retzius,** the periodicity for which is useful for age estimation.

Anisotropic: A material that has different properties in different directions (i.e., transverse direction as compared to the longitudinal direction).

Antemortem: Before death. In the analysis of human skeletal remains, this is usually indicated by signs of vital response (i.e., healing).

Anthropological genetics: A synthetic discipline that applies the methods and theories of genetics to evolutionary questions posed by anthropologists.

Antigen: A substance that stimulates an immune response in the body.

Antimeres: Left/right paired skeletal elements.

Any antemortem stature available (ASTAT): Wilson and colleagues (2010) define ASTAT as any antemortem stature that is available, including cadaver stature, measured stature (as from medical or military records), or forensic stature (as reported on a driver's license or by the family members of the decedent) (citation in Chapter 6).

Area moments of inertia: This cross-sectional property of a bone is a measure of the bone's resistance to bending (i.e., **bending strength**). The area moments of inertia are a measure of the distance of the bone's periosteal surface to the geometric center of the bone (centroid).

ASTAT: See **any antemortem stature available.**

Atlas approach for dental aging: Comparison of the X-rays of a specimen to an illustration drawn from X-rays of individuals with normal development of the dentition for the purposes of age estimation.

Atomic mass: The sum of the number of protons and neutrons of an element.

Atomic number: The number of protons of an element.

Autolysis: More commonly known as self-digestion, refers to the destruction of a cell through the action of its own enzymes.

Axial compression: See **compressive stress**.

Ballistic trauma: Injury to the body from the impact of a high-speed projectile, most commonly from firearms or munitions.

Base: See **nucleobase**.

Basic multicellular units (BMUs): Complex interaction of **osteoclasts** and **osteoblasts** to coordinate apposition and resorption, which is responsible for remodeling.

(William M.) Bass Donated Human Skeletal Collection: A large collection of documented skeletons of modern individuals with known age, sex, height, weight, and other antemortem data (some with photos and medical records, etc.). The individuals typically decompose in the outdoor Anthropological Research Facility at the University of Tennessee in Knoxville and the remains are curated within the Department of Anthropology at the University of Tennessee.

Bayes' theorem: A theorem that incorporates additional ("prior") information into probability estimates. It is fundamental in **Bayesian analysis**.

Bayesian analysis: Methods of statistical inference that incorporate additional ("prior") information into probability estimates, specifically incorporating **Bayes' theorem**. Used for application to age-at-death, sex, stature, and ancestry estimates in anthropology.

Bending energy: Based on the bending energy used in physics to quantify the amount of energy necessary to deform a point on a thin, metal plate in a particular direction. In geometric morphometrics, bending energy is quantified as the amount of energy necessary to displace the coordinates of one landmark from a configuration and exactly map it onto the coordinates for the same landmark on another configuration, thereby depicting the degree of deformation necessary to deform one configuration into another. For more information, be sure to consult Bookstein (1991) and Slice et al. (2009) (citation in Chapter 12, this volume).

Bending strength: The ability of a bone to resist deformation when loaded. The bending strength of a bone is typically measured by a mathematical property of its cross-section (known as **area moments of inertia**).

Bioarchaeology: Field that combines skeletal analysis with archaeology, analyzing human remains in the context of material culture and environment. See **biocultural approach**.

Biocultural approach: The paradigm that emerged in the 1970s, which premises **bioarchaeology**. It is argued that the physical environment, cultural roles, social status, repetitive tasks, nutritional deprivation, diet, and chronic disease all alter the condition of human bone. This alteration, in turn, can be used to interpret the lifestyle, sociopolitical context, health status, and subsistence economy of past cultures.

Biological determinism: The scientifically disregarded belief that biology (i.e., **genotype** and **phenotype**) determines not only physical traits, but sociocultural traits (such as language, intelligence, level of civilization, wealth, etc.) as well. It assumes that categories for different human groups exist and therefore classifies each physical and cultural characteristic accordingly. For example, statements that an individual or a group of individuals is destined for a certain fate (e.g., from poverty to wealth or early death to longevity) dependent upon or due to their physical/cultural traits (country of birth, skin color, head shape and size, language spoken, etc.) are deterministic in nature.

Biological distance (also known as biodistance): How closely related or, alternatively, divergent **populations** are from one another. Biological distance studies are used to explore how evolutionary factors (e.g., **gene flow, genetic drift**) have affected human **population history**.

Biomechanics: The study of the physics, structure, and function of biological organisms.

Biplanar radiography: This technique takes a traditional 2-D X-ray image of an individual (or bone) from two separate directions (e.g., typically from both anteroposterior and mediolateral directions).

Blastic: Characterization of reactive bone change that results in new bone formation. The process is also generically labeled as "osteoblastic".

Blunt trauma: Slow-velocity injury to the body from an impact, an injury from a weapon, or an assault.

Bone histomorphology: The structure of bone tissue at the microscopic level.

Bone matrix: The organic unmineralized portion of the bone, also known as **osteoid**.

Butterfly fracture: A common bone fracture pattern observed resulting from a combination of compressive and tensile forces; results in a fracture that resembles a wedge or butterfly shape.

C_3: Abbreviation for the Calvin photosynthetic pathway, which is one of the three types of photosynthesis. Plants from temperate ecological zones typically fix carbon through this pathway. Their $\delta^{13}C$ values average -26.5%.

C_4: Abbreviation for the Hatch–Slack photosynthetic pathway, which is one of the three types of photosynthesis. Plants from tropical ecological zones typically fix carbon through this pathway. Their $\delta^{13}C$ values average -12.5%.

Calcification: The buildup of calcium during the development of a body tissue. In the case of teeth, this refers to the **hydroxyapatite** mineral that makes up a large portion of the enamel and dentin.

CAM: Acronym for crassulacean acid metabolism. One of the three types of photosynthetic pathway intermediate between C_3 and C_4 pathways. Examples of CAM plants are cacti and other succulents.

Canaliculi: An extensive interconnecting network of tunnels or finger-like extensions that link bone cells (**osteocytes**).

Cancellous: The type of spongy bone located beneath the cortex or surface bone. It is also referred to as diploic bone or the diploë. See also **trabecular bone**.

Canonical scores: The transformed variables from **canonical variates analysis**, the first few of which account for the majority of the variation between the groups being studied.

Canonical variates analysis (CVA): A statistical analysis that computes linear combinations of the original variables to maximally separate groups. For further details, see a statistical text such as Affifi and Clark (1996) or Rencher (1995) (citation in Chapter 12, this volume).

Carabelli's trait: Feature on the mesiolingual surface of the first maxillary molar that ranges from a small groove or pit through to a fully developed additional cusp.

Categorical traits: Skeletal characteristics defined in terms of some quality or categorization, and differentiated from **continuous traits** as qualitative rather than quantitative. These traits include dichotomous traits (presence/absence), ordinal (small, medium, large), and nominal (no logical ordering: square, triangular, round).

Cell cloning: A method of **DNA** amplification, where host cells are manipulated to carry and replicate a foreign DNA sequence.

Cement reversal line: A thin, mineral-deficient layer of the bone matrix that separates a **secondary osteon** from the **lamellar bone**.

Cementum: The calcified tissue covering tooth root surfaces that serves as the attachment point for periodontal ligaments.

Centroid: The geometric center of a three-dimensional object or group of data points. In traditional morphometrics, this is the multivariate mean for a group; in geometric morphometrics, it can refer to the "coordinate-wise average of the landmarks" (Mitteroecker and Gunz, 2009:238) of a configuration (citation in Chapter 12, this volume).

Centroid Size: The square root of the sum of the squared distances from coordinates for a configuration to its **centroid** (Slice et al., 2009). In geometric morphometrics, it is used as a measure of overall size and in Procrustes superimposition, scaling to Centroid Size removes isometric size differences among configurations (citation in Chapter 12, this volume).

Chi-square test: A test (also called Pearson's chi-square or χ^2) that compares multiple sample frequencies (test of independence) or single sample frequencies against an expected result (goodness of fit). It tests the **null hypothesis** that the samples are from the same distribution. The calculated chi-square value (χ^2) is compared to a critical tabular value (χ^2) for acceptance/rejection of the null hypothesis.

Chromosomes: Tightly packed bundles of genetic material containing the DNA blueprint of every organism. In the case of humans, there are 23 pairs of homologous chromosomes.

Chronic: Disease process of long duration which disseminates to bone. See **chronic injury**.

Chronic injury: A persistent or repetitive injury that lasts over a long time frame. In medicine, the term "chronic" is used to denote injury or illness persisting longer than three months.

CI: See **confidence interval**.

Circadian periodicity: In the case of **cross striations** in enamel, assuming a regular, roughly 24-hour cycle.

Clade: A diagram used to illustrate evolutionary relationships between species. It has been used erroneously to demonstrate relationships between human races (as in **polygenism**).

Cladistic thinking: Belief that different human races or ancestral groups have diverged separately from one another and have separate ancestors, which is not the case. See **clade**.

Classical markers: Blood groups and proteins.

Cline: Some trait (i.e., skin color) that exhibits gradual phenotypic or genetic difference over a geographical area that typically results from differences in the environment, although evolutionary factors such as **gene flow** and **genetic drift** may play a role in the observed variation.

Coefficients of correlation: Pearson's *r* measures the strength of the linear relationship between two variables. The Pearson coefficient of correlation is calculated from the covariance of the variables divided by the product of their **standard deviations**.

Compact bone: See **cortical bone**.

Complex traits: See **polygenic traits**.

Compressive stress: A force applied to an object that induces axial shortening.

Computed tomographic imaging (CT): CT performs multiple two-dimensional slices of three-dimensional objects and mathematically reconstructs the cross-sectional image (as a **DICOM** image) from the X-ray measurement of thin slices to create what are essentially three-dimensional radiographs.

Concentric fractures: Circular fractures around the point of impact.

Confidence interval (CI): A range of numbers indicating the precision of a measurement for an estimate. Given a correct statistical model and repeated sampling, a confidence interval will include the true population **parameter** over a proportion of the calculations. Commonly the 95% CI is used, and thus, upon repeated sampling, 95% of the confidence intervals calculated will contain the true population parameter.

Consolidation: This is the early stage in the life of a bone in which the bone increases in density until peak bone mass is reached in the early or mid-thirties.

Continuous traits: Traits measured or identified on a numerical scale. Examples include craniometric data (bizygomatic breadth), postcranial measurements (maximum length of the femur), etc.

Control: Refers to the limiting of **parameters** (e.g., by age, by sex) or a constant (e.g., a point of departure) that is used in order to evaluate the meaning of bioarchaeological parameters.

Cortex: The outer surface of bone. It consists of compact, mature **lamellar** bone. See **cortical bone**.

Cortical bone: The compact bone made up of **osteons** (also known as **Haversian systems**) that predominates the shaft of bones but is also found at the subperiosteal surface of bone.

Covariance: A statistical measure of the mutual interaction of two variables; when normalized this is known as the correlation coefficient.

Co-variates: Variables related to the **dependent variable**. Confounding occurs when uncontrolled co-variates influence both the **dependent variable** and the **independent variable**. Common co-variates with the skeleton include real age and sex.

Craniometrics: Linear distances and angles observed on the cranium and mandible; commonly used for investigating patterns of morphological variation in the craniofacial complex with traditional morphometrics.

Cribra orbitalia: A chronic pathological condition of childhood characterized by discrete areas of perforating pits in the cortical bone of the orbital roof. Smooth-walled pits indicate an active condition. Healing consists of pore-bridging new bone formation that can, by accretion, result in a plaque layer of new bone. The multiple causes of cribra orbitalia include anemia, scurvy, infection, and parasites.

Criteria drift: Despite well-defined categories to classify discontinuous traits or conditions, over the course of data collection, there is an unconscious mental process that slightly redefines scoring criteria. This can result in different classificatory thresholds between initial and final scoring. Drift can be neutralized by rescoring the initial cases.

Cross striations: In dental anthropology, short-period incremental lines in enamel that represent roughly 24 hours' worth of growth (i.e., enamel secretion by **ameloblasts**).

Cross-sectional geometry: The shape of the transverse cross-section of a bone that can be measured to reveal biomechanical properties of bone strength.

Crown module: Average size of the tooth crown given a certain tooth class (e.g., incisors, canines, etc.).

CT: See **computed tomographic imaging**.

Cultural relativism: Evaluating cultures only by their own standards and not by the standards set by your own culture.

Diaphysis: The shaft of a long bone that includes the primary ossification center.

Decalcification: The removal of calcium ions from bone.

Decedent: A deceased individual, typically the unidentified subject of a forensic investigation, for whom identification is sought.

Decomposition: A general term referring to the **post-mortem** breakdown of cells and organs through its two major processes, **putrefaction** (involving bacteria) and **autolysis** (involving enzymes).

Deduction: An approach to scientific inquiry that begins with theory and is followed by **hypotheses** and then finally, **observations**. Contrast with **induction**.

Delamination: A form of material failure common in composite or layered material, such as the compact bone of the skull. Delamination in bone is commonly seen as the separation of the inner and outer cortex, or **compact bone**.

Demarking point: See **sectioning point for sex estimation**.

Demography: A description of a **population**, specifically their ages and sexes.

Dental age approach: Analysis of tooth growth where fractions of completion of individual teeth are considered, which is used for the purpose of age estimation.

Dependent variable: The response variable (variable being measured) in an analysis, in which a change (or lack thereof) is being measured as the result of an **independent variable**. The independent variable will have an effect on the dependent variable, but not typically the reverse. An example of this in research

on human skeletal biology is the effect of age on the presentation of **osteoarthritis**. Age is the independent variable and osteoarthritis is the dependent variable. See **independent variable** and see Chapter 2 for a more complete explanation and exceptions.

Descriptive statistics: A set of statistics used to summarize a sample. Examples include means, frequency distributions, and **coefficients of correlation**.

Determinism: See **biological determinism**.

DEXA: Also DXA. See **dual energy X-ray absorptiometry**.

Diagenesis: The physical and chemical changes that happen to teeth and bones after death *in situ*, such as fossilization, but also includes the chemical and compositional effects of discovery, recovery, handling, and storage.

Diagnostic: Pathological feature that is indicative of, but not necessarily exclusive to, a particular disease process.

DICOM (Digital Imaging and Communications in Medicine) images: Includes the individual transverse 2-D grayscale image slices created during a **CT** scan.

Differential diagnosis: The weighing of the presenting pathological changes against changes characteristic of known disease processes.

Diphyodont: The property of having two sets of teeth (deciduous/primary and permanent).

Diploic (diploë) See **cancellous**.

Discrete traits: Human skeletons exhibit numerous nonmetric attributes or features, which demonstrably vary between populations. They are routinely used in **biological distance** studies. The traits may have a genetic, developmental, or behavioral cause. The attributes may be expressed dichotomously (i.e., presence/absence) or ordinally (i.e., mild to extreme expression).

Discriminant function analysis (DFA): A linear statistical analysis designed to classify unknown specimens based on similarity to a predefined reference sample, providing the probability of classification in the groups included in the analysis. Classification can be based on a linear function that generates a discriminant score based on observed variables from the unknown specimen. For further information, consult a statistical text such as Affifi and Clark (1996) or Rencher (1995) (citation in Chapter 12, this volume). DFA is useful for both sex and ancestry estimation.

DNA: Deoxyribonucleic acid. A nucleic acid contains the genetic instructions used in the development and functioning of all known living organisms (with the exception of **RNA** viruses). The main role of DNA molecules is the long-term storage of information.

Dual energy X-ray absorptiometry (DEXA) (or DXA): A medical imaging technology designed to use X-rays to measure integral bone mass and areal density. It is relatively sensitive to subtle changes in bone density and body composition (the proportion of fat and lean tissue mass).

Elastic deformation: A type of deformation to an object that is reversible. Once acting forces are eliminated or removed from an object, it returns to its original shape. Contrast with **plastic deformation**.

Elliptical Fourier analysis (EFA): Analysis that fits outline data consisting of coordinates through Fourier analysis. For further information see Rholf (1990) (citation in Chapter 12, this volume).

Embedding: The process of fixing small pieces of bone into a plastic resin for histological analysis.

Enamel hypoplasia: See **linear enamel hypoplasia** and **accentuated line**.

Enamel prism: The path of enamel secretion of an **ameloblast**.

Endochondral ossification: The process by which the bones of the skeleton (mostly postcranial) are first ossified from a cartilage template.

Endosteal apposition: The rare mechanism of cortical bone growth (as compared to **endosteal resorption**) in long bones, in which the bone grows inward, decreasing the size of the medullary canal.

Endosteal resorption: The common mechanism of bone growth/aging (as compared to **endosteal apposition**) in which the **osteoclasts** remove bone at the endosteal surface, which increases the diameter of the medullary canal.

Endosteum: Membranous layer covering the internal surface of the medullary cavity.

Entrance wound: The area of impact or defect in which an object enters the body.

Epiphyses: The end of a bone, typically at an articular surface or muscle attachment, that includes the secondary ossification center, which is separated from the rest of bone by a cartilaginous growth plate during growth and is fused and fully ossified in adults.

Epigenetic variants: Nonpathological variations of skeletal tissues that can be better classified as present or absent (or as a point on a morphological gradient, e.g., small to large) rather than quantified by a measurement (this definition is discussed in Chapter 5, this volume).

Equifinality: When the causes are different, but the effect is the same, as in taphonomic effects for example.

Essentialism: Viewing each racial taxonomic category as having certain fundamental features that define it, with the categories being due to separate evolutionary histories. Fits with **polygenist** and **biological**

determinist viewpoints. See Caspari (2003) for more information (citation in Chapter 5, this volume).

Euclidean distance matrix analysis (EDMA): A method for analyzing differences in forms by employing matrices of interlandmark distances calculated from coordinate data. For a detailed explanation of this method, see Lele and Richtsmeier (1991) and Richtsmeier et al. (2002) (citation in Chapter 12, this volume).

Evolution: The changes in **gene** frequencies in a **population** over time.

Evolutionary theory: Theory that provides explanatory mechanisms for evolutionary change, including the forces of **gene flow**, **genetic drift**, **mutation**, and **natural selection**.

Exit wound: The defect occurring when a fired object exits the body.

Experimental research design: A form of **actualistic** methodology that actively seeks to replicate the effect under study by reproducing the hypothetical causal event in a controlled setting.

Extreme extrapolation in stature estimation: If the individual for which stature is being estimated does not fall within the normal population range (e.g., extremely tall or extremely short), the stature estimation is considered to be a case of extrapolation beyond the mean, which requires statistical models that perform well with cases of these extreme **outliers**.

Extrinsic factors: Forces or variables that originate from outside the body. Extrinsic factors in skeletal maturation can include the environmental influence of nutrition or the biomechanical influence of different forces on the skeleton, such as locomotion and gravity.

Feminist archaeology: A perspective borne of criticism for the *a priori* utilization of Western **gender** (usually male-biased) norms (e.g., man the hunter, woman the gatherer) in archaeological explanation. Although there is a fundamental validity to criticism of androgenic (male-focused) archaeological explanation, feminist archaeology as a perspective has been criticized as having a sociopolitical agenda. See **gender archaeology**.

Femur/stature ratio: A mathematical method for stature estimation, the femur/stature ratio is the ratio of the femur length to the total stature and is the most common **long bone/stature ratio** model used to estimate stature in humans and human ancestors.

Fisher's exact test: A test measuring whether a set of sample distributions are the same. This test is for **categorical** data, and is ideal for small sample sizes.

Force: Anything that causes an object to change its shape, direction, or speed. Calculated in terms of mass times **acceleration**.

FORDISC: An interactive computer program, running under Windows, for classifying adults by ancestry and sex using any combination of standard measurements and made-to-order discriminant functions (**discriminant function analysis**). Developed by Richard Jantz and Stephen Ousley. See citation in Chapter 5.

Forensic Databank (FDB): The Forensic Databank was started in 1986 at the University of Tennessee, Knoxville, Department of Anthropology and is a digital archive of cranial and postcranial measurements, nonmetric observations, and demographic information that often includes age, sex, stature, weight, ancestry, occupation, and place of birth of individuals from modern forensic anthropology casework from around the United States. Practicing forensic anthropologists submit data to the databank once their cases have been positively identified. Three-dimensional coordinate data are now also being added to the databank.

Forensic DNA: The **DNA** analysis of recently deceased individuals for medical and legal purposes.

Forensic stature (FSTAT): FSTAT is the stature that is self-reported on a driver's license/identity card or as reported by a family member of a missing or deceased person.

Form: The geometric properties of a configuration that include both size and shape.

Founder effect: Loss of genetic variation that occurs when a very small number of individuals from a larger **population** establish a new population.

Fractional volume: The percentage or ratio of a volume. For example, this can refer to the percentage of primary to secondary bone or vice versa.

Functional adaptation: The ability of bone to respond to extrinsic biomechanical forces by changing its micro- or macrostructural shape properties in order to maintain a balance between being strong enough for support and light enough for locomotion.

Functional morphology: The field of study within osteology based on the notion that the form of a bone reflects its function; i.e., a bone will functionally adapt its shape to the activities needed of it, especially during growth and development.

Gap junction: The space at the surface of each cell. In **osteocytes**, the gap junction helps to dissipate a biomechanical force.

Gender: Gender is a sociocultural construct of maleness or femaleness. Contrast with **sex**: a biological distinction between males and females.

Gender archaeology: An emerging perspective in bioarchaeological enquiry, often substantially premised in social theory and vocabulary, which seeks to identify and assess biological sex-bridging social, economic, and political roles. See also **feminist archaeology**.

Gene: A general term referring to "elements of heredity that are transmitted from parent to offspring in reproduction" (Hartl, 2011: 2) (citation in Chapter 16, this volume).

Gene flow: The movement of **alleles** from one population to another via people mating outside of their own **population**.

Generalized Procrustes analysis (GPA): An iterative process for removing differences due to location, orientation, and scale for multiple coordinate-based configurations. For further details, see Slice (2005) and Rohlf and Slice (1990) (citation in Chapter 12, this volume).

Genetic drift: Changes in the **allele** frequencies in a **population** due to random events, an example of which is a genetic bottleneck.

Genetic marker: Any informative region of the **genome**, either nonprotein coding and therefore selectively neutral, or protein coding and potentially subject to **natural selection**.

Genetics: The study of heredity and the science of variation.

Genome: The entirety of an organism's hereditary information. It is encoded either in **DNA** or, for many types of viruses, in **RNA**.

Genomics: The branch of molecular biology concerned with the structure, function, evolution, and mapping of **genomes**.

Genotype: An individual's genetic makeup or heritable aspects of a **phenotype**.

Geometric mean: This is calculated as the nth root of the product of n variables; can be used to uniformly scale data with size variation.

Gompertz model: See **hazard model**.

Hamann-Todd Human Osteological Collection: This collection of skeletons of 3000 known individuals is from retained cadaver specimens housed at the Cleveland Museum of Natural History. It was developed by T.W. Todd beginning in 1912 with support from the Dean of (Case) Western Reserve University School of Medicine, C. Hamann.

Haversian canal: Canal in the center of an **osteon** that serves as a passage for blood cells, lymph vessels, and nerves.

Haversian system: Also known as an **osteon**, this is the microscopic structure in **cortical (compact) bone** shaped like a long tube in which a central canal (for blood vessels and nerves) is surrounded by concentric layers of mineralized **lamellar bone** and containing many embedded **osteocytes**.

Hazard model: Statistical models of mortality (or time until an event occurs). These provide the "prior" information in **Bayesian analysis**. A commonly used model for anthropology is the Gompertz model.

Hematopoiesis: The process by which immature precursor cells develop into mature blood cells.

Heterodonts: Animals having more than one type of tooth class (i.e., incisors, canines, premolars, molars). Monkeys, apes, and humans are heterodonts.

Heteroplasmy: The presence of a mixture of more than one type of **genome** within a cell or an individual.

Highest posterior density distribution: The probability of an event after *a priori* (prior) information has been taken into account in a **Bayesian analysis**.

Histomorphometrics: Quantification of the variation in the microscopic appearance of bone tissue.

Homeostasis: The body's ability to maintain equilibrium (or balance) in temperature, chemical regulation, etc.

Homologous: Landmarks on the skeleton are considered homologous when they are located in approximately the same location on all specimens.

Howship's lacunae: Enzymatically etched resorptive bays in the bone matrix caused by **osteoclastic** action.

Human variation: The modern perspective with regard to ancestry that has replaced the biological race concept.

Huntington Collection: The Huntington Collection is curated at the Smithsonian Institution in Washington, D.C. and was assembled by Dr. George Huntington (1861–1927) in New York and brought to the Smithsonian by Dr. Aleš Hrdlička. The collection includes 1600 individuals with known age, sex, nationality, and cause of death. Many of the skeletons have been sectioned and dissected, but the preservation quality is high and it is well documented with excellent examples of trauma and pathology.

Hydroxyapatite: An inorganic material that comprises 70% of bone makeup and about 96% of tooth material.

Hyperostosis: The pathological expansion of bone. It can occur in **cancellous bone** (see **porotic hyperostosis**), **cortical bone** (e.g., hyperostosis frontalis interna), or in the ossification of soft tissue such as ligaments (e.g., diffuse idiopathic skeletal hyperostosis or DISH).

Hypothesis: A scientific statement that proposes something about nature. Can be divided into **null** and **alternative hypotheses**.

ImageJ: A free computer software program for image processing and analysis that can calculate area and pixel value statistics, and measure distances and angles, among other calculations.

Independent variable: The independent or experimental variable is the variable that will change throughout the study to demonstrate an effect on the **dependent variable**. An example of this in research on human skeletal biology is the effect of age on the presentation of **osteoarthritis**. Age is the independent variable and osteoarthritis is the dependent variable. See also **dependent variable** and see Chapter 2 for a more complete explanation and exceptions.

Induction: An approach to scientific inquiry following closely the steps of the scientific method: **observation**, **hypothesis** formation, methods, results, conclusion, and later, theory. Contrast with **deduction**.

Inference: Statistical inference is the extrapolation of a sample estimate to a population **parameter** using a statistical test (e.g., **Fisher's exact test**) to account for sample variation.

Interobserver error: (also **Observer error**) Criteria for the classification of **continuous** or discontinuous traits or conditions that are differentially perceived between individuals (visually or metrically). This results in different scores or thresholds reported between observers, which are a source of data error.

Intramembranous ossification: The process of ossification that begins within membranes (*in utero*) of some of the cranial and flat bones as opposed to **endochondral ossification** of long bones from a cartilage model.

Intraobserver error: Source of data error that results from variations in measurements or observations by a single observer (researcher) of **continuous** or discontinuous traits. Repetition of measurements is an important method to overcome intraobserver error.

Intrinsic factors: Forces or variables that originate within the body. During growth and development, bone is greatly affected by intrinsic or systemic factors within the body, such as genetic constraints and hormone levels.

Inverse calibration: A Bayesian approach widely used in biological anthropology. It is at odds with **allometry** and thus the "inverse" in which stature (y) is regressed on long bone length (x), and stature is considered the **dependent variable** and long bone length the **independent variable** (see Hens et al., 2000) (citation in Chapter 6, this volume).

Involution: The stage in the life of a bone following peak bone mass (the consolidation phase) when bone loss exceeds bone formation, starting at around age 30.

Ischiopubic index: This index is calculated by the length of the pubis multiplied by 100 and then divided by the length of the ischium. Both measurements are subject to high **inter-** and **intraobserver error** as it is difficult to locate the intersection point for both lengths within the acetabulum after the bones have fused.

Isolation by distance (IBD): A population **genetic** model describing the tendency of individuals to find mates from nearby **populations** rather than distant populations.

Isometric scaling: In contrast to **allometry** and differential growth of body parts, isometric scaling occurs when changes in body size do not correlate with changes in body proportion.

Isotopes: Variations of chemical elements that differ in the number of neutrons but have the same number of protons.

Isotope fractionation: A change in **isotope** ratios due to chemical processes.

Isotope ratio mass spectrometers (IRMS): Instruments utilized for analyzing precise isotopic ratios of various elements. See also **mass spectrometry**.

Isotropic: Material properties are the same in all directions.

Kendall's shape space: The theoretical geometric space underlying analysis of multidimensional configurations described by Kendall (1984). It is a curved, multidimensional space where configurations of two or more dimensions can be plotted as a single point. For further details, see Kendall (1984) and Slice (2001) (citation in Chapter 12, this volume).

Kyphosis: Postural slumping that results from excessive outward curvature in the mid-thoracic region and can be the result of collapsed vertebral bodies as a result of **osteoporosis** fracture (also known as the dowager's hump) or simply from poor posture.

Lacunae: Small spaces within the bone matrix where **osteocytes** reside.

Lamellar bone: Also known as **compact bone**, it is mature, compact (i.e., dense), organized in layers, and mechanically strong. Also called lamellae.

Least squares regression: In a simple linear **regression**, the fitting of a straight line through a set of points (e.g., femur length compared to stature) in which the sum of the squared residuals (the vertical distance squared of each point in relation to the line) is as small as possible.

Life history: Can refer to one of two things: in the case of modern humans, most often the course of an individual's life including stress and growth events that manifest skeletally. In the case of species, life history refers to the pace of life events including the timing of major life events (e.g., menstruation) and duration of growth and reproductive events (e.g., age at first reproduction, number of offspring).

Likelihood ratio: The probability of observing data under one **hypothesis** divided by the probability of observing the same data under an alternative hypothesis.

Linear enamel hypoplasia: In normal tooth crown development, enamel is smoothly and uniformly horizontally deposited. When the process is disturbed by a developmental stressor (e.g., disease or malnutrition), enamel is erratically or insufficiently deposited resulting in grooves or pits on the tooth crown.

Load: Any force or acceleration applied to an object or a structure.

Locus (plural loci): A fixed position on a **genome**.

Log (logarithmic) transformation: A transformation of a variable using a logarithm (typically base 10). Generally used in statistical regression, when the **independent** and **dependent variables** demonstrate a nonlinear relationship, specifically an exponential relationship.

Long bone/stature ratio model: The ratio of bone length to stature to estimate an unknown stature from a single bone length. This is calculated from the population average length of the bone compared to the population average of stature. The bone makes up an average percentage of the overall stature. This percentage can be multiplied by the length of bone to yield a stature estimate. The **femur/stature ratio** is an example of the long bone/stature ratio model.

Lordosis: Postural slumping that results from excessive inward curvature in the lower curve of the spine at the lumbar vertebrae, also known as "sway back."

Lytic: Description of a hole, hollow defect, or lesion in bone caused by the destruction or removal (lysis) of bone.

Macrostructure (of bone): Bone macrostructure is a combination of external and internal geometric properties, as well as the orientation of **trabecular bone** (Ruff, 1981) (citation in Chapter 14, this volume).

Magnetic resonance imaging (MRI): A type of **tomography** in which radiofrequency waves pass through the body as a large superconducting magnet spins around the subject to create multiple two-dimensional image slices of three-dimensional objects.

Mahalanobis distance (D^2): A distance measure introduced by P. C. Mahalanobis in 1936 to gauge similarity of an unknown set of measurements to a known reference sample. Also, the generalized distance between group **centroids**.

Major axis (MA): Major axis or principal axis is a common Model II type regression. In stature estimation neither **dependent** nor **independent variables** are assigned and error is associated with both (Konigsberg et al., 1998) (citation in Chapter 6, this volume).

Masculinization of skull: Masculinization of the skull occurs with older age in females after a decrease in systemic estrogen levels with the onset of menopause, rendering **sex** assessment from cranial traits more difficult (Krogman and İşcan, 1986; Buikstra and Ubelaker, 1994) (citation in Chapter 4, this volume).

Mass spectrometry: A technology that is able to measure the elemental composition of a material (such as bone) by ionizing the material with an electron beam and then measuring the mass of the ions. See also **isotope ratio mass spectrometers**.

Material properties: Material properties include chemical composition (percentage of collagen and **hydroxyapatite**) and bone density (Ruff, 1981) (citation in Chapter 14, this volume).

Mathematical method for stature estimation: A mathematical method to estimate stature that applies a mathematical equation to the length of one or two skeletal elements to estimate the unknown stature of an individual. The **long bone/stature ratio model** (or **femur/stature ratio**) and **least squares regression** are two examples of mathematical models to estimate stature.

Maximum likelihood: A statistical method for estimating the **parameters** of a model by selecting values that produce a distribution with the highest probability.

Measured stature (MSTAT): The stature reported on medical or military records that include the standardized measurement of living stature.

Mechanosensory cells: The ability of **osteocytes** to act as strain receptors in the process of **mechanotransduction** (Pearson and Lieberman, 2004) (citation in Chapter 14, this volume).

Mechanotransduction: The process in which cells sense mechanical stimuli. The process of mechanotransduction is possible because the bone cells have a connected cellular network (CCN) of **canaliculi** and this network functions like its own nervous system (Pearson and Lieberman, 2004) (citation in Chapter 14, this volume).

Mesenchymal cells: Stem cells that can differentiate into multiple types of cells.

Meta-analysis: A comparison across multiple studies related to a common **hypothesis**.

Micro-CT: A variation of **CT** that scans at an extremely high resolution (as small as 1 μm) to view some histological structures (but not at the cellular level). The level of radiation at this resolution is lethal to living subjects. A reduced resolution of 50 μm is used for living subjects.

Microenvironment: The environment immediately surrounding a decomposing body that influences or is influenced by it, including temperature, moisture, pH, and associated organisms. The body and its microenvironment change through time due to processes of **decomposition**, consumption by scavengers, dispersal, and assimilation involving plants, animals, and microorganisms that become associated with the decomposing body.

Microstructure (of bone): Microstructure of bone is characterized by the **modeling** and **remodeling** of **Haversian systems** and **trabeculae**.

Microwear: Microscopic etchings on the tooth surface; often examined for evidence of diet.

Modeling: Bone modeling involves the sculpting of bone during growth and development and initial bone mineralization in the embryonic stage.

Modern synthesis: The converging of Darwin's theory of **natural selection** with **population genetics** theory to compose modern **evolutionary** theory.

(Molecular) marker: A "marker" is any informative region of the **genome** that is either nonprotein coding and therefore selectively neutral, or is protein coding and therefore potentially subject to **natural selection**.

Monogenic traits: Traits whose inheritance are presumed to be due to the action of single or very few **genes**.

Monogenism: Belief that all the races originated from the Biblical Adam and Eve and that following this, the other races originated as a result of changes in the environment and population movements (Brace, 2005) (citation in Chapter 5, this volume). Contrast with **polygenism**.

Morphoscopic traits: The cranial nonmetric traits used in forensic anthropological research that are quasi-continuous variables of the cranium that can be reflected as soft-tissue differences in the living.

Mortuary treatment: The way a body is prepared after death, which will affect preservation and impact subsequent **taphonomic** forces.

MSY: Male-Specific Y; the part of the Y **chromosome** inherited from the biological father. Also known as **NRY** (Nonrecombining Y).

mtDNA: Mitochondrial **DNA**. Contained in the mitochondria (powerhouses) of every cell. Present in a higher copy number than nuclear DNA.

Multivariate analyses: Statistical analysis that includes multiple variables (e.g., multiple **regression**, multivariate **discriminant function analysis**).

Multivariate analysis of covariance (MANCOVA): Statistical analysis that tests for differences between multivariate group means while allowing for effects of **co-variates**. For further information, consult a statistical text such as Affifi and Clark (1996) or Rencher (1995) (citation in Chapter 12, this volume).

Multivariate analysis of variance (MANOVA): Statistical analysis that tests for differences between multivariate group means. For further information, consult a statistical text such as Affifi and Clark (1996) or Rencher (1995) (citation in Chapter 12, this volume).

Mutation: A change in the **DNA** sequence of an organism.

Multifactorial methods: Age-at-death estimation methods that combine estimates from multiple skeletal indicators.

Natural experiment: Experiment involving **observation** of changes produced by real events in nature. In relation to human skeletal remains, this form of research involves observation of changes to osseous, dental, and soft tissues.

Natural selection: The process by which **alleles** become more or less common in a **population** due to factors impinging on the survival and reproduction of their bearers.

nDNA: Nuclear DNA. See **DNA**.

Neutral axis: The axis along the bone shaft in which there are no longitudinal stresses. The neutral axis typically goes through the center of the medullary canal. If an object is symmetric, the neutral axis and the centroid are one and the same.

Neutron number: The number of neutrons in an **isotope**.

New Physical Anthropology: Proposed by Sherwood Washburn in 1951 as a movement of the discipline away from **typology** and towards research focusing on **human variation** and **populations** (citation in Chapters 1, 5, and 14, this volume).

Nonparametric methods: Statistical methods that do not rely on assumptions that the data are drawn from a given probability distribution.

Nonspecific infection (or nonspecific indicators of stress): Nondiagnostic reactive changes to bone, which cannot unequivocally be ascribed to a particular pathological cause. Although labeled as infection, the reactive changes also include inflammation caused by mechanical injury. Contrast with **specific infection**.

NRY: Over 95% of the Y chromosome is inherited relatively intact from the biological father and is referred to as the NRY, or NonRecombining Y (also MSY, or Male-Specific Y).

Nucleic acid: Biological molecules essential for life, including **DNA** and **RNA**.

Nucleobase: Or simply, "base." A group of nitrogen-based molecules that form nucleotides (along with sugar and phosphate). The primary nucleobases are cytosine, guanine, adenine (**DNA** and **RNA**), thymine (DNA), and uracil (RNA), abbreviated as C, G, A, T, and U, respectively.

Nucleotide: The combination of a sugar, phosphate, and a single **nucleobase**.

Null hypothesis: **Hypothesis** stating that changes in the **independent variable** will not lead to changes in the **dependent variable**. Stated in negative or conservative terms; also known as the hypothesis of "no difference."

Observation: To perceive something or note an occurrence or fact. Can be used as a synonym for "data collection" as the data are essentially being observed.

Observer error: See **interobserver error** and **intraobserver error**, also **criteria drift**.

Odontometrics: Linear measurements of tooth crowns.

Osteoarthritis: Noninflammatory reactive damage to cartilaginous joint surfaces that has multiple causes (e.g., trauma, excessive physical stress, obesity, or idiopathic). It is identified by porotic pitting and a surface polish (eburnation) caused by bone-on-bone contact. Osteoarthritis is often accompanied by reactive changes (osteophytes) at the joint margins.

Osteobiography: A term used to specifically describe the assessment of a single case or of several individuals within their cultural context. Coined by Frank Saul. See Chapter 1, this volume.

Osteoblasts: Cells that deposit **osteoid** to build bone.

Osteoclasts: Cells that resorb bone.

Osteocytes: Bone maintenance cells that are former **osteoblasts** that have become trapped in their own secreted matrix.

Osteogenic: Bone forming.

Osteoid: Immature **bone matrix** laid down by **osteoblasts** that will harden to become bone.

Osteological paradox: The recognition that an absence of skeletal evidence of chronic health is not necessarily indicative of good community health. Individuals without evidence of chronic stress may have died at an early or acute phase of the disease and may actually have been more frail. In contrast, individuals who exhibit skeletal markers of chronic physiological stress reflect long-term survival with a chronic condition (Wood et al., 1992) (citation in Chapters 1, 2, 3, and 7, this volume).

Osteometrics: Linear measurements and angles that capture dimensions of the human skeleton.

Osteomyelitis: A direct infection of the bone or a blood-disseminated infection of bone. The reactive changes can resemble advanced **periostitis**. It is osteologically recognized by a cavity that penetrates the bone cortex (cloaca), the presence of detached necrotic (i.e., dead) bone (known as "sequestrum"), and an enveloping shell of new bone (known as "involucrum").

Osteon: See **Haversian system**.

Osteopenia: A subclinical loss of bone mineral density. This decrease in density is the precursor to **osteoporosis**.

Osteoporosis: A disease characterized by the loss of bone mineral density that is 2.5 standard deviations below average peak bone mass and associated with an increase in the risk of fracture.

Osteoprogenitor: Osteoprogenitor cells are those derived from mesenchymal tissue during embryonic development, which have the ability to differentiate into a number of different bone cell types.

Osteoware: A computer software program available at no cost from the Smithsonian Institution used for documenting human skeletal remains that has incorporated the guidelines in Buikstra and Ubelaker (1994), *Standards for Data Collection from Human Skeletal Remains* (cited in Chapter 2), via a relational database. http://osteoware.si.edu/

Outliers: Observations that appear to deviate markedly from other observations of the **sample** in which they occur.

Paleodemography: A description of **populations** from the past. See **demography**.

Paleopathology: Generically, the study of ancient diseases. Methodologically, it refers to the diagnosis of any and all pathological conditions, the determination of **pathognomonic** and **diagnostic** criteria, and the determination of the antiquity, sociocultural circumstances, and geographical distribution of pathology.

Paradigm: A shared theoretical framework from which explanations, methodology, and ideas for **hypothesis** testing are generated.

Parameter: An underlying population quantity, usually what we are trying to estimate using sample statistics.

Parsimony, Law of: States that the simplest (most logical and least complicated) explanation for an **observation** is the likeliest explanation, as the likelihood of complicated explanations being correct is going to be very low. See Chapter 2, this volume, for an example.

Pathognomonic: Pathological changes that are exclusive to particular diseases.

PCR: Polymerase chain reaction; a technique enabling geneticists to make multiple copies of **DNA** to increase the **sample** for analysis.

Percutaneous bone lengths: Anthropometric measurements of bone lengths in living individuals that are taken from palpable landmarks on the surface of the skin.

Perikymata: Lines that appear on the surface of teeth corresponding to long-period **striae of Retzius** lines in enamel.

Perimortem: At or around the time of death. In the analysis of skeletal remains, this term is generally used to describe trauma or treatment of the body that occurred immediately before or after death while bones are still fresh enough to respond similarly to living tissue, i.e., their collagen content is still to the level where the bone is "wet". Bones can remain in this state for some time after death, depending upon the deposition environment.

Periosteum: A double-layered fibrous protective covering on the outer bone surface.

Periostitis: Reactive change on bone stimulated by inflammation of the surrounding tissue (**periosteum**) caused by disease or injury. The change can take the form of bone deposition or removal (**lysis**).

Peripheral quantitative computed tomography (pQCT): A type of computed **tomography** that allows for scanning of smaller peripheral parts of the body (e.g., arms, hands, and feet) and is often used to take bone mineral density readings. pQCT has lower radiation than **CT**.

Periradicular bands: Surface manifestations of **Andresen lines** that are the dentin equivalent of **perikymata**.

Phenice method: A visual **sex** assessment method that examines the traits of the subpubic concavity, the medial ischiopubic ramus, and the ventral arc (Phenice, 1969) (citation in Chapter 4).

Phenotype: The expressed characteristics of an organism, combining both environmental and **genetic** factors, such as those that help a hare outrun a hungry cheetah or those involved in adult human stature.

Phylogeny: The study of the **evolutionary** relatedness of organisms.

Physiological stressors: The generic term or label for extremes of malnutrition, mechanical load, and/or chronic disease that can interrupt the normal growth and maintenance of the human body.

Plastic deformation: A type of deformation that is not reversible once a force is relieved from an object. The object will not return back to its original shape. Contrast with **elastic deformation**.

Plasticity: The capacity of the human body to adjust growth and development in the face of malnutrition, mechanical load, and/or chronic disease stress. See **physiological stressors**.

Plexiform bone: Rectangular, brick-like shaped bone. It stems from mineral buds that grow first perpendicular and then parallel to the outer edge of bone surface. This type of bone is common in nonhuman animals that grow large quickly but is rarely seen in humans.

Poisson's ratio: Ratio used to compare the deformation of an object in the longitudinal axial direction as compared to the perpendicular axis.

Polar moments of area: The cross-sectional property of a bone to predict its resistance to twisting or torsion (i.e., **torsional strength**). The symbol "J" is typically used to represent the polar moments of area.

Polygenic traits: Traits whose inheritance are presumed to be due to the action of multiple **genes**; also, **complex traits**.

Polygenism: Belief dating back to Renaissance Europe that each race (Caucasoid, Mongoloid, etc.) had its own unique origin, with the Caucasoid race being the oldest and therefore most evolved and the Negroid race being the youngest and the least evolved (Brace, 2005) (citation in Chapter 5, this volume). Contrast with **monogenism**.

Population: A group of human individuals who are contemporaneous, live in relatively the same geographic area, have a shared culture (language, traditions, belief systems, etc.), and who tend to find mates from within the same group. Biological anthropology has as its focus the study of human populations.

Population genetics: A field of biology that studies the composition of biological **populations**, and the changes in biological composition as a result of the four main evolutionary processes (**mutation, genetic drift, gene flow**, and **natural selection**).

Population history: The study of similarities or differences in population structure between two or more **populations** due to a shared ancestry or mate exchange. When embarking on an investigation of population history, you are essentially attempting to understand what factors have shaped **genetic** variation in your sample, except for **natural selection**. This concept is compared with **adaptive history**.

Population-specific standards: Methodological standards and equations for estimating aspects of the biological profile (e.g., age, sex, stature formulae) that have been developed on the same **population** of the targeted individual, thus increasing the accuracy of estimations.

Population structure: The study of how **populations** are subdivided, if at all, into local or subpopulations.

Porotic hyperostosis: The pathological condition of porotic pitting of the outer cortex of the skull accompanied by the thickening of the diploë (**cancellous** bone).

Postcranial metrics: Linear measurements, angles, and circumferences observed on elements from the postcranial skeleton.

Posterior probability: The probability that an unknown case belongs to a certain group under the assumption that the unknown belongs to one of the groups in the function, based on relative distances to each group, the sum of which equals one. In a **Bayesian analysis**, this is the probability of an event or outcome given previously collected evidence. It is proportional to the product of the **likelihood** and the probability of the event or outcome prior to the evidence.

Postmortem: Literally means after death. In the analysis of skeletal remains, any process or modification of remains that occurred after death when bones are no longer fresh enough to respond as a living tissue. It represents **taphonomic** change.

Post-processualism: Originating in the United Kingdom in the late 1970s as primarily a criticism of processualist archaeology (see **processual archaeology**), it is now a controversial conglomeration of various viewpoints derived from cultural anthropology, postmodernism, and feminism. A positive result of post-processualism is a broader range of interpretations but it has been criticized as not generating a methodology.

Phenotype: The expressed characteristics of an organism, combining both environmental and genetic factors, such as those that help a hare outrun a hungry cheetah or those involved in adult human stature.

Precision in stature estimation: Precision will have a low standard error, or a smaller spread of points, but accuracy may be low in which this interval does not include the actual stature.

Prediction interval: An estimate of an interval (often in **regression analysis**) within which a future data point will likely fall.

Pretoria Bone Collection: This skeletal collection from retained cadavers of known individuals includes 290 complete skeletons, 704 dissociated skulls, and 504 complete postcranial remains. The collection began in 1942 and is housed at the Department of Anatomy and the Medical School at the University of Pretoria in South Africa.

Primary lamellar bone: The original concentric bone layers of young bone.

Primer: A strand of nucleic acid that serves as a starting point for **DNA** synthesis.

Principal component analysis (PCA): A linear analysis that transforms correlated variables from ungrouped data into uncorrelated variables known as principal components (PC). Each PC is a linear combination of the original variables that maximizes the **variance**. For further information, consult a statistical text such as Affifi and Clark (1996) or Rencher (1995) (citation in Chapter 12, this volume).

Principal components analysis: A multivariate statistical procedure that combines several variables into a single variable for analysis.

Probability density function: A probability distribution for a **continuous** variable.

Problem: Refers to the larger overall picture for a given scientific conundrum as compared to **the question**, which is more specific towards addressing a particular aspect of the problem. See Chapter 2 for an example.

Processual archaeology: The directed problem-solving primary paradigm of archaeological inquiry also referred to as the "New Archaeology." It is premised in the view that human culture (i.e., aspects such as social organization, subsistence strategy, and production) is reflected in and can be retrieved from the material remains using quantitative (i.e., scientific) methods. It has been criticized as being too environmentally deterministic (i.e., citing environmental causes for culture change), androgenic (male-biased), and ignoring the role(s) of individuals as agents of cultural change. See **post-processualism**.

Procrustes shape coordinates: The coordinates for configurations that have been fitted via a **Procrustes superimposition**.

Procrustes superimposition: A method for removing differences in location, orientation, and size from multiple configurations defined by coordinate data. For further details, see Slice (2005) and Rohlf and Slice (1990) (citation in Chapter 12, this volume).

Pseudopathology: Changes to skeletal tissues (or other tissues) that mimic or are confused with pathological conditions. May be **taphonomic**.

Pseudotrauma: Changes to skeletal tissues that mimic or are confused with the effects of trauma. May be **taphonomic**.

Putrefaction: Decomposition involving the breakdown of cells and organs due to bacteria and fermentation.

p-value: Under the **null hypothesis**, the probability of observing a test statistic as extreme or more extreme than the one calculated. In statistical inference, if we calculate a p-value smaller than a cutoff (usually 0.05), we reject the **null hypothesis** (see **statistical significance**).

Quantitative bone histology: Measures the amount of variation in the microscopic appearance of bone tissue.

Question: Refers to answering a specific scientific conundrum that is part of a larger overall scientific **problem**. See Chapter 2 for an example.

Racial typology: Prior to the adoption of the biocultural approach, skeletal analysis was primarily metric, particularly craniometric. The purpose of metric analysis was to determine the racial composition of skeletal samples, as populations were perceived as

more or less hybrids of arguably primary discrete races. The concept of the pure race was discredited with the **modern synthesis** of the early twentieth century. See also **typology** and **biological determinism**.

Radiating fractures: Fractures that travel away from the area of impact in a linear fashion.

Radiography: Medical imaging technology that uses X-rays to examine the internal structure of the body or of a bone. Multiple different modalities use radiography, including **CT**, **DEXA**, and **traditional x-rays**.

(Ranked) ordinal scores: Categorical data that have an underlying increasing or decreasing distribution.

Reduced major axis (RMA): A **regression analysis** appropriate for describing relationships between two traits or biological variables with measurement error. The slope of an RMA regression is calculated by the slope of an ordinary **least squares regression** divided by the **coefficient of correlation**. RMA regression is also referred to as a standardized major axis (SMA) regression and is considered a Model II type equation[1] (Konigsberg et al., 1998) (citation in Chapter 6, this volume).

Reference sample: A sample with known age and sex information that we apply to the **target sample** for estimating **demographic parameters**. Ideally, the characteristics of the reference sample make it appropriate for application to the target sample (i.e., they have similar **population histories**).

Regression analysis: A statistical analysis that describes the relationship between **independent** and **dependent variables**. For further information, consult a statistical text such as Affifi and Clark (1996) or Rencher (1995) (citation in Chapter 12, this volume).

Remodeling: Bone remodeling involves the removal and replacement of old bone with new bone.

RNA: Ribonucleic acid, a nucleic acid with a similar chemical structure to **DNA**. Unlike DNA, it performs multiple essential organismal functions, such as catalyzing biological reactions, controlling gene expression, and cell signaling.

Robustness index: Tooth index reflecting crown area.

Sacral corporobasal index: An index that was developed to discriminate sex and is measured as the corpus width of S1 × 100 and divided by the base width.

Sample: A subset of a whole intended to represent the whole (i.e., *Homo sapiens*, bones, teeth, DNA, etc.), that is available for study and used to derive conclusions about the whole. Ideal samples are both

---

[1]See http://prometheuswiki.publish.csiro.au/tiki-index.php?page=RMA+regression

smaller than the overall whole and representative of the whole.

Scientific racism: The use of science to justify discrimination against different groups of people on the basis of physical and sociocultural characteristics.

Sclerosis: The process of the hardening of a tissue. The reactive process in bone results in particularly dense and thick (sclerotic) bone with an ivory-like surface texture.

Secondary osteon: Formed by the replacement/ **remodeling** of existing bone. See **osteon**.

Sectioning point for sex estimation: The sectioning point is calculated by taking the mean for a measurement for males and the mean for the females and then taking the average of those male and female mean values. Typically, any values above the sectioning point represent a sex estimation of male and any values below the sectioning point indicate a sex estimate for female (but see discussion in Chapter 11, this volume). See also **demarking point**.

Secular change/trends: How time brings about changes in biology via **evolutionary** forces due to changing variables in the environment (i.e., nutrition, exposure to pathogens, access to medical care, sanitation, etc.). Often used to refer to greater height and weight (among other trends, such as earlier onset of first menstruation) of recently born individuals compared to those born several decades or centuries ago.

Segmentation: The process of selecting regions or surfaces from three-dimensional images and then separating the objects into three-dimensional surface models based on grayscale threshold values.

Semilandmarks (sliding landmarks): Coordinates from points along curves or arcs that are fitted by allowing the coordinates to slide along a vector tangent to the curve or arc until an algorithmic criterion is met. Once the semilandmarks are fitted, they can be used as homologous landmark coordinates for subsequent analyses. For further information, see Bookstein et al. (1999) and Gunz et al. (2005) (citations in Chapter 12, this volume).

Sequence polymorphism: Differences in tooth emergence sequences, designated by brackets. Reported for species or **populations** when the unique sequence occurs in greater than 15% of the population.

Seriation: Seriation of a bone involves the selection of a trait of interest (e.g., **sex** estimation from the mastoid process) and then ordering the bones from a large **sample** of individuals based on the absence or the least expression of the trait to the greatest

expression of the trait. One end of the spectrum would be male and the other end female.

Sex: Sex is a biological distinction between males (who have both X and Y **chromosomes** and have testes) and females (who have no Y chromosome and have ovaries), whereas **gender** is a sociocultural construct of maleness or femaleness, or a combination thereof.

Sex assessment: Visual **sex** assessment is the relatively simple, gross observation and assessment of sex from the skull and/or pelvis. While these traits are difficult to quantify metrically, the visual observations are immediate and require no equipment, only knowledge and experience. Contrast with **sex estimation**, below (Spradley and Jantz, 2011) (citation in Chapter 4, this volume).

Sex estimation: Sex estimation involves the metric analysis of skeletal features (e.g., diameter of femoral head or scapular width) and has only recently become the standard in both forensic anthropology and bioarchaeology because it involves less subjectivity and lower inter- and intraobserver error than **sex assessment** (Spradley and Jantz, 2011) (citation in Chapter 4, this volume).

Sexual dimorphism: The difference between males and females of a species in terms of body size, body shape, and/or difference in the timing of development.

Shape: The geometric properties of a configuration that are invariant to size.

Shape index: The ratio of maximum (I_{max}) to minimum (I_{min}) **bending strength** in the femoral midshaft. Dividing the maximum moment of inertia by the minimum (I_{max}/I_{min}) gives a unitless "shape" variable. It has been suggested that a high I_{max}/I_{min} ratio (or shape index) correlates strongly with greater levels of activity.

Sharp trauma: Trauma inflicted with an edged weapon.

Sharpey's fibers: Bundles of fibers that connect the membranous **periosteum** to the underlying **cortical bone**.

Shear stress: A stress that is applied perpendicular to the axis, or coplanar to the material cross-section in opposite directions causing the material to deform internally, like sliding one flat hand against another in opposite directions.

Sigma: In bone histology, the total amount of time required to move through the six phases of bone **remodeling**.

Significance: See **statistical significance**.

SNP: Single nucleotide polymorphism. A difference in a single base in a particular location on the **genome**.

Specific infection/diseases: The antithesis of **nonspecific infection**. Certain pathological bone changes or bone predilections can diagnostically discriminate between a disease or inflammatory processes.

Stadiometer: A calibrated device to measure the stature of a living individual with a vertical, metric ruler and a horizontal paddle that rests atop the head.

Standard deviation: The square root of the **variance**; it measures the dispersion of a distribution, i.e., how much spread there is around the mean.

Standard error: The estimate of the **standard deviation** of a sample statistic (e.g., sample mean, **sample proportion**).

Standard error of estimate: Used in **regression analysis** to examine how well a least squares line equation fits a dataset.

Statistic: A quantity that is calculated from a **sample** that is used to estimate a **parameter**.

Statistical regression: A statistical analysis relating a **dependent variable** to one or multiple **independent variables**. See also **regression analysis** and **least squares regression**.

Statistical significance: An expression that designates that a research result from a statistical analysis is unlikely to be the result of chance, usually determined from a **p-value**.

STR: Short tandem repeat. A **genetic** variant consisting of a linear repetition of a characteristic sequence motif. For example, AGTC may be repeated four times in one individual's **genome**, but be repeated five times in another person's genome.

Strain: A geometrical measurement of the amount of displacement in a given material.

Stress: The measure of forces acting on an object.

Stress markers: Generic term or label for the quantifiable bone changes consequential to malnutrition, mechanical load, and/or chronic disease.

Striae of Retzius: Incremental pattern of light and dark bands in the cross-section of enamel that is the result of the development of the tooth enamel; this pattern can provide estimates of age.

Subperiosteal expansion: In normal long bone growth and aging, **osteoblasts** build new bone on the subperiosteal surface, which increases the diameter of the bone's cross-section.

Summary tooth size: A dental index that calculates the overall size of the dentition.

Survivorship function: Proportion of a birth cohort that is alive at any given age. For example, at age 0 (i.e., birth), survivorship is 1.0, while if everyone in that cohort is dead by 85 years, survivorship is 0.0.

Synergistic: The compounding or mediating effects of multiple factors (pathological conditions, **taphonomic** effects, etc.) on each other in a single individual.

Taphonomy/taphonomic: Of or relating to taphonomy; The study of what happens to remains after death.

Target sample: The skeletal **sample** with unknown ages and/or sexes for which we wish to estimate a **population** level and individual **demographic** parameters (ages and sexes).

Tensile stress: Stress acting to lengthen or stretch an object.

(Robert J.) Terry (Anatomical Skeletal) Collection: Anatomy Professor Dr. Robert Terry (1871–1966) collected the remains of 1729 individuals for a skeletal collection of known age, sex, ancestry, cause of death, and pathology. Files contain the autopsy records, anthropometric measurements, skeletal inventories, and dental charts. There are photographs, death masks (face imprints), and hair samples associated with each case. The collection is now housed at the Smithsonian Institution in Washington, D.C. Age-at-death ranges from 16 to 102 years, with dates of birth from 1822 to 1943.

Thin-plate spline (TPS): A geometric morphometric method for evaluating shape differences in terms of grid deformations of one coordinate-based configuration when exactly mapped onto the coordinates for another configuration.

Thin section: A section of bone sliced at a desired thickness prepared for light microscopy histology.

Tomography: The process of performing multiple two-dimensional image slices of three-dimensional objects.

Torsion: The biomechanical force of rotation or twisting.

Torsional strength: The cross-sectional property of a beam to predict a bone's resistance to twisting or **torsion**, measured by the **polar moments of area**.

Trabecular bone/trabeculae: Also known as spongy bone or **cancellous bone**, this is one of the two types of bone responsible for giving bone its strength, which is composed of a honeycomb-like structure. Also see **cortical bone**, its complement, and the definition for **cancellous bone**.

Traditional X-ray: Radiographs or traditional X-rays are generated by a cathode-ray tube and have a specific wavelength that allow them to pass through the body (or bone). The difference in the amounts of absorption of the X-rays by the different tissues of the body causes differential shadowing on photographic paper.

Trajectorial theory of cancellous bone: The functional adaptation of bone as described in **Wolff's law** in which the **trabeculae** will align themselves along the trajectory of principal strain.

Transition analysis: A technique for modeling the age at which a skeletal indicator transitions from one phase to the next.

Transverse isotropy: Material properties that are the same in all transverse planes.

T-score: A standard score in statistics to designate how many **standard deviations** an individual is from the mean. In bone density scans, the T-score compares the subject to the optimal bone density of a young healthy individual. The **Z-score** compares the subject's density to sex, age, height, weight, and ancestry-matched individuals. Both T- and Z-scores are used to quickly diagnose **osteoporosis**.

Typicality probabilities: A statistic that measures the likelihood that an unknown case belongs to a group based on the absolute distance (**Mahalanobis distance**) of the individual from each group in an analysis. If the typicality probability for a case equals 0.45, then 45% of the sample making up that particular group is as far or farther from the group's **centroid** (center of the distribution, i.e., three-dimensional mean). If this is less than 0.05, this could indicate an error.

Typological approach: See **typology** and **racial typology**.

Typology: Creating categories just for the sake of creating categories without basis in science or using the characteristics of one or a few individuals as being definitive of an entire group (especially with **biological determinism**). See also **racial typology**.

Ultrasonography (also ultrasounds): In medical ultrasonography, short pulses of sound waves travel through the body and reflect (i.e., echo) off different tissues. When the echo is received, the delay in time for the reflection is mathematically translated into different tissue types and interpreted as a grayscale image.

Uniformitarianism, Principle of: Natural mechanisms by which processes occurred in the past are the same mechanisms by which processes occur today (i.e., wind erosion, mutation rates of **genes**, **natural selection**, etc.). Using this principle, we are able to come to conclusions about things we cannot see or measure directly today.

Variance: Variance is a measure of statistical dispersion from the mean and is the square of the **standard deviation**. It is calculated as the average of each measurement "x" minus the population mean squared.

Viscoelastic: Material properties that change depending on the rate of the **force** applied.

Volkmann's canals: Canals that traverse the bone matrix and connect **Haversian canals** to help maintain bone cell nourishment.

Voxel: In three-dimensional medical imaging such as **CT**, the data are recorded as voxels, which are essentially three-dimensional pixels.

Wedl: A type of microbial attack characterized by tunneling in bone; it can be seen histologically.

Wolff's law: Often interpreted as the general theory of the **functional adaptation** of bone, that healthy bone will reinforce itself along the lines of principal strain in the **trabeculae** (see **trajectorial theory of cancellous bone**) and then resorb bone that is no longer biomechanically necessary.

Woven bone: Newly deposited temporary, immature bone that has an irregular matrix (randomly oriented collagen fibers) and is not integrated into the cortex. It can have a fibrous, pitted or honeycomb appearance.

Y5 pattern: Feature on mandibular molars where the fissure pattern presents as a "Y" that opens to the distobuccal cusp. This is a shared trait among hominoid primates.

Young's modulus: The measure of the stiffness of a material.

Z-score: A method for transforming data into a standard normal distribution with mean 0 and **standard deviation** 1; calculated as the original variable minus the mean divided by the standard deviation. In bone density scans, the Z-score compares the subject's density to sex, age, height, weight, and ancestry-matched individuals to quickly diagnose **osteoporosis**. See also **T-score**.

Index

Page numbers followed by "f" indicates figures and "t" indicates tables.

Printed and bound by CPI Group (UK) Ltd, Croydon, CR0 4YY

03/10/2024

01040301-0002